The Changing School Scene. Challenge to Psychology
by Leah Gold Fein

Troubled Children: Their Families, Schools, and Treatments
by Leonore R. Love and Jaques W. Kaswan

Research Strategies in Psychotherapy
by Edward S. Bordin

The Volunteer Subject
by Robert Rosenthall and Ralph L. Rosnow

Innovations in Client-Centered Therapy
by David A. Wexler and Laura North Rice

The Rorschach: A Comprehensive System, in two volumes
by John E. Exner

Theory and Practice in Behavior Therapy
by Aubrey J. Yates

Principles of Psychotherapy
by Irving B. Weiner

Psychoactive Drugs and Social Judgment: Theory and Research
edited by Kenneth Hammond and C. R. B. Joyce

Clinical Methods in Psychology
edited by Irving B. Weiner

Human Resources for Troubled Children
by Werner I. Halpern and Stanley Kissel

Hyperactivity
by Dorothea M. Ross and Sheila A. Ross

Heroin Addiction: Theory, Research, and Treatment
by Jerome J. Platt and Christina Labate

Children's Rights and the Mental Health Profession
edited by Gerald P. Koocher

The Role of the Father in Child Development
edited by Michael E. Lamb

Handbook of Behavioral Assessment
edited by Anthony R. Ciminero, Karen S. Calhoun, and Henry E. Adams

Counseling and Psychotherapy: A Behavioral Approach
by E. Lakin Phillips

Dimensions of Personality
edited by Harvey London and John E. Exner, Jr.

The Mental Health Industry: A Cultural Phenomenon
by Peter A. Magaro, Robert Gripp, David McDowell, and Ivan W. Miller III

Nonverbal Communication: The State of the Art
by Robert G. Harper, Arthur N. Wiens, and Joseph D. Matarazzo

Alcoholism and Treatment
by David J. Armor, J. Michael Polich, and Harriet B. Stambul

A Biodevelopmental Approach to Clinical Child Psychology: Cognitive Controls and Cognitive Control Theory
by Sebastiano Santostefano

Handbook of Infant Development
edited by Joy D. Osofsky

Understanding the Rape Victim: A Synthesis of Research Findings
by Sedelle Katz and Mary Ann Mazur

Childhood Pathology and Later Adjustment: The Question of Prediction
by Loretta K. Cass and Carolyn B. Thomas

Handbook of Minimal Brain Dysfunctions
edited by Herbert E. Rie and Ellen D. Rie

Intelligent Testing with the WISC-R
by Alan S. Kaufman

HANDBOOK OF
MINIMAL BRAIN DYSFUNCTIONS
A Critical View

HANDBOOK OF MINIMAL BRAIN DYSFUNCTIONS

A Critical View

Edited by

HERBERT E. RIE
Case Western Reserve University

ELLEN D. RIE
Case Western Reserve University

A WILEY-INTERSCIENCE PUBLICATION

JOHN WILEY & SONS, New York • Chichester • Brisbane • Toronto

Library of Congress Cataloging in Publication Data

Main entry under title:

Handbook of minimal brain dysfunctions: a critical view

  (Wiley series on personality processes)
  "A Wiley-Interscience publication."
  Includes index.
  1. Minimal brain dysfunction in children.
I. Rie, Herbert E., 1931–   II. Rie, Ellen D.
[DNLM: 1. Minimal brain dysfunction—In infancy and
childhood—Handbooks. WS340.3 H236]
RJ496.B7H36   618.9′28′58   78-25656
ISBN 0-471-02959-9

Printed in the United States of America

10 9 8 7 6 5 4 3 2 1

Contributors

IRA BELMONT, Ph.D., Professor of Psychology, Yeshiva University.

LILLIAN BELMONT, Ph.D., Research Scientist V, Epidemiology of Brain Disorders Research Unit, New York State Psychiatric Institute; Senior Research Associate, Division of Epidemiology, School of Public Health, Columbia, University.

KENNETH BERRY, Ph.D., Associate Professor of Medical Psychology, Nebraska Psychiatric Institute, The University of Nebraska, College of Medicine.

JAMES H. BRYAN, Ph.D., Professor, Department of Psychology, Northwestern University.

TANIS BRYAN, Ph.D., Associate Professor, College of Education, University of Illinois at Chicago Circle; Director, Chicago Institute for Learning Disabilities.

ADEN BURKA, Ph.D., Instructor, Pediatric Psychology, University of Maryland, School of Medicine.

DENNIS P. CANTWELL, M.D., Associate Professor, Department of Child Psychiatry, School of Medicine, University of California at Los Angeles.

VALERIE J. COOK, Ph.D., Associate Professor, George Peabody College for Teachers, Nashville, Tennessee.

S. THOMAS CUMMINGS, Ph.D., Director of Psychology, York Woods Center, Ypsilanti, Michigan; Adjunct Professor, Department of Psychology, University of Michigan.

D. CRAIG FINGER, Ph.D., Director, Adolescent Day Treatment Program, York Woods Center, Ypsilanti, Michigan.

JACK M. FLETCHER, Ph.D., Developmental Services and Child Development Research Units, Texas Research Institute of Mental Sciences.

MALCOLM M. HELPER, Ph.D., Professor, Department of Pediatrics and Department of Psychology, The Ohio State University.

RONALD S. ILLINGWORTH, M.D., Children's Hospital, Department of Child Health, Sheffield, England.

THOMAS J. KENNY, Ph.D., Associate Professor and Director of Pediatric Psychology, University of Maryland Hospital.

JANE W. KESSLER, Ph.D., Professor, Department of Psychology, Case Western Reserve University; Director, Mental Development Center.

HERBERT C. LANSDELL, Ph.D., Fundamental Neurosciences Program, National Institute of Neurological and Communicative Disorders and Stroke.

v

ALEXANDER R. LUCAS, M.D., Head, Section of Child and Adolescent Psychiatry, Mayo Clinic; Professor of Psychiatry, Mayo Medical School.

HAROLD MARTIN, M.D., Associate Professor of Pediatrics and Psychiatry, John F. Kennedy Child Development Center, University of Colorado Medical Center.

GARY B. MESIBOV, Ph.D., Assistant Professor of Psychology, Division for Disorders of Development and Learning, University of North Carolina.

ELLEN D. RIE, Ph.D., Adjunct Assistant Professor, Department of Psychology, Case Western Reserve University; Principal Investigator and Project Director, Research on Learning Disabilities.

HERBERT E. RIE, Ph.D., Professor and Chairman, Department of Psychology, Case Western Reserve University.

DONALD K. ROUTH, Ph.D., Professor, Department of Psychology, University of Iowa.

SELMA G. SAPIR, Senior Faculty, Member of Graduate Programs in Learning Disabilities and Director of the Learning Laboratory, Bank Street College of Education.

PAUL SATZ, Ph.D., Professor, Department of Clinical Psychology, Neuropsychology Research Laboratory, University of Florida.

RICHARD J. SCHAIN, M.D., Professor and Head, Division of Pediatric Neurology, UCLA School of Medicine.

MARK A. STEWART, M.D., The Ida P. Haller Professor of Child Psychiatry, University of Iowa.

ABRAHAM TOWBIN, M.D., Medical Director, Mental Retardation Research Institute, Newton, Massachusetts.

PAUL S. WEINER, Ph.D., Department of Pediatrics, University of Chicago.

GABRIELLE WEISS, M.D., Director, Department of Psychiatry, The Montreal Children's Hospital.

EMMY E. WERNER, Ph.D., Professor of Human Development, University of California at Davis.

THEODORE H. WOHL, Ph.D., Director of Psychology, Cincinnati Center for Developmental Disorders.

Series Preface

This series of books is addressed to behavioral scientists interested in the nature of human personality. Its scope should prove pertinent to personality theorists and researchers as well as to clinicians concerned with applying an understanding of personality processes to the amelioration of emotional difficulties in living. To this end, the series provides a scholarly integration of theoretical formulations, empirical data, and practical recommendations.

Six major aspects of studying and learning about human personality can be designated: personality theory, personality structure and dynamics, personality development, personality assessment, personality change, and personality adjustment. In exploring these aspects of personality, the books in the series discuss a number of distinct but related subject areas: the nature and implications of various theories of personality; personality characteristics that account for consistencies and variations in human behavior; the emergence of personality processes in children and adolescents; the use of interviewing and testing procedures to evaluate individual differences in personality; efforts to modify personality styles through psychotherapy, counseling, behavior therapy, and other methods of influence; and patterns of abnormal personality functioning that impair individual competence.

IRVING B. WEINER

Case Western Reserve University
Cleveland, Ohio

circumspect, and often painstaking review of an extensive and multifaceted literature. Every chapter was prepared expressly for this volume. The outline of the book, found in the table of contents, includes nine major sections, of one to five chapters each. These span topics ranging from the concept and history of minimal brain dysfunctions, to most of the principal concerns of both researcher and practitioner.

As a reference work, this volume offers the available foundations for the formulation of a reader's own perspective of a variety of conceptually, if not empirically, related childhood disorders. It does not collectively offer a definitive reformulation of the relevant concepts. Indeed, the repeated concerns about the adequacy of current knowledge suggest that the effort would be premature.

The editors thank their author-colleagues, recognizing that the nature of the field does not lend itself to effortless characterization. The editors also thank those who assisted with the editorial process.

Finally, if this volume serves no other purpose, it will have been a worthwhile undertaking if it generates greater compassion, circumspection, and respect toward the children to whom the designation "minimal brain dysfunction" is applied.

HERBERT E. RIE
ELLEN D. RIE

Cleveland, Ohio
January 1979

Contents

11. Perceptual Organization and Minimal Brain Dysfunctions   **253**

Ira Belmont

12. Effects of MBD on Learning, Intellective Functions, and Achievement   **272**

Ellen D. Rie

HANDBOOK OF
MINIMAL BRAIN DYSFUNCTIONS
A Critical View

PART ONE

The Concept of Minimal Brain Dysfunctions

CHAPTER 1

Definitional Problems[1]

Herbert E. Rie

Absence of verifiable fact about a group of vexing problems seems inevitably to result in the adoption of strongly held views that tend to be indefensible. For a time the amount of controversy, of contradiction, of conceptual confusion, of questionable interpretation of observations and tangentially relevant references in the literature on minimal brain dysfunction (MBD) suggested that verifiable facts were scarce indeed. It remains to be seen whether we continue to suffer from absence of fact or from a failure to incorporate accruing data into current conceptualization. In time, through the comfort of familiarity, initially plausible hypotheses tend to be transformed imperceptibly into "fact" and to resist displacement.

Debate has been stimulated not only about the several elements of the designation, MBD, but also about the very existence of such a "disorder," about practice affecting children so designated, and about the professions that ought properly to be involved. If one writer questions whether the disorder may reasonably be regarded as "minimal," another inquires whether "minimal" refers to a problem in the brain or to its educational or behavioral effects. If one author marshalls evidence for a dysfunction referable to the brain, another cites the absence of demonstrable lesions, characteristic neurological findings, and laboratory evidence of neurophysiological anomalies.

It is remarkable in this context not only that substantial numbers of school children are diagnosed as having minimal brain dysfunction, but also that a generally accepted definition has been in existence for some dozen years. Though the tolerant limits of the definition may have served rather diverse interests equally well, its value is being increasingly questioned. The definition of minimal brain dysfunction and/or the concept itself has variously been regarded as a "sophisticated statement of ignorance" (Grinspoon and Singer, 1973), a "simulacrum of symptomatology" (Twitchell, 1971), a "myth" based on invalid diagnostic criteria (Schmitt, 1975), a misnomer due to naiveté about brain-behavior relations (Benton, 1973), and the unwitting confusion of a psychologic construct with a biomedical fact (Birch, 1964).

A POPULAR DEFINITION

The events culminating in the establishment of a national task force that formulated the most prevalent definition of MBD in 1966 are discussed in Chapter 2.

[1]Much of the research of the author and his colleagues that is related to the principal themes of this volume was supported by the Office of Program Evaluation and Research, Division of Mental Health, Ohio Department of Mental Health and Mental Retardation.

They include the familiar threads of identification earlier in this century of post-encephalitic dysfunctions, the observation and description of so-called organic driveness by Kahn and Cohen (1934), the psychological findings in individuals with known brain damage by such investigators as Werner and Strauss (1939) and Strauss and Lehtinen (1947), the studies of later adaptation of individuals known to have been at high risk perinatally, the speculations about dyslexia and other learning problems, the proliferation of designations for one or more elements of presumed syndromes, and finally the recognition that greater order and coherence were required.

The widely adopted definition was formulated by the first of three task forces which had terminology and identification as its primary focus (Clements, 1966). The initial portion of the definition stated:

The term 'minimal brain dysfunction syndrome' refers in this paper to children of near average, average or above average general intelligence with certain learning or behavioral disabilities ranging from mild to severe, which are associated with deviations of function of the central nervous system. These deviations may manifest themselves by various combinations of impairment in perception, conceptualization, language, memory, and control of attention, impulse, or motor function. [P. 9]

It was elaborated to note that similar symptoms "may or may not" occur in cases of cerebral palsy, epilepsy, mental retardation, blindness, or deafness.

The section headed "definition" further included the observations that "these aberrations" could be the consequence of genetic variations; of biochemical irregularities; of perinatal "brain insults," illness, or injury occurring during the period of maturation of the central nervous system; "or from unknown causes." Finally allowance was made for possible permanent, "central nervous system alterations" as a result of early, severe sensory deprivation.

With respect to etiology, the definition was necessarily imprecise but, despite occasional rather circumspect wording, there was no doubt left that the "certain learning or behavioral disabilities" were the consequence of aberrations *in the central nervous system.* Indeed, in formulating a definition, it was the intention not only to eliminate the seeming terminological confusion that obtained but also to emphasize the role of "organicity" in certain (albeit ill-defined) problems of childhood. This was explicitly a response to two conditions: (1) the recognition that brain disorder "can manifest itself as learning and behavioral irregularities" (p. 6) and (2) the belief that organicity ". . . is frequently ignored in the final diagnosis of the child."

Since the effects of brain *damage* or *injury* (at least of certain kinds) were familiar enough, it also became necessary to contrast the problems subsumed under the designation "minimal brain dysfunction" from these more obvious manifestations. The task force observed that "the vital implication is that educational programing and rehabilitation for these children must be different than for the brain-damaged mentally subnormal groups." It was also noted that the term "brain damaged" had been applied to most children having "organic" problems regardless of etiology and that the term had taken on an "all-embracing 'wastebasket'" character. This is of course the same complaint that subsequently met the concept of "minimal brain dysfunction." Apparently the professional world will not be deprived of its wastebaskets.

Finally the task force was equally intent on differentiating between "minimal brain dysfunction" (with symptomatology in one or more "of the specific areas of brain function, but in mild, borderline, or subclinical form'') and mental retardation. Hence it is repeatedly stressed that overall intellectual functioning is not reduced to the ''subnormal ranges.'' The group of children so designated are by definition of near average, average, or above average general intelligence.

Summary

At the risk of redundancy, but with a view to the several problems generated by the definition which we shall now consider, the seemingly critical elements of the definition are summarized. Ignoring for the moment the additional problems of symptom definition, the concept and definition of MBD emphasize:

1. The link between certain abnormal motor, sensory, and intellective functions and ''dysfunction'' in the brain.

2. The minimal nature of the noted behavioral and/or educational problems and/or of the brain dysfunction, apparently in the sense that demonstrable central nervous system (CNS) impairment does not exist and/or that the effects of the brain dysfunction are subtle, or perhaps more subtle than the effects of demonstrable CNS impairment.

3. The belief that the noted behavioral and/or intellectual problems are of ''specific kinds,'' which are presumably different from behavioral and/or intellectual problems that are the consequence of non-CNS dysfunctions.

4. The occurrence of intellectual problems ''*without* evident lowering of general intellectual capacity,'' although the somewhat contradictory modification of this assertion also appears: that overall intellectual functioning is not reduced to subnormal ranges.

5. The wide variety of causes of the CNS dysfunction, ranging from genetic to environmental, for example early sensory deprivation.

MBD Symptoms and Brain Dysfunction

The first of these definitional emphases, the link between certain abnormal behavior and dysfunction in the brain, has generated considerable heated debate. The issue is the focus of at least two chapters in this book and will be considered here only in a general sense as it bears on definitional clarity.

The concept of minimal brain dysfunction is often traced to the work of Strauss and Werner who had studied so-called exogenous and endogenous groups of mentally defective children. The exogenous group contained a large proportion of children who were characterized by symptoms ostensibly seen in the (present) syndrome of minimal brain dysfunction. These included hyperactivity, emotional lability, disordered perception, impulsivity, distractibility, abnormal rigidity and perseveration. While the last two of these have not typically been stressed in descriptions of MBD, it apparently seemed logical to assume that if these symptoms of brain damage manifested themselves in lesser degree, they could be attributed to less severe CNS impairment.

Birch (1964) has observed that little evidence exists that the children in question actually have brain damage and that many children with known and independently verified brain damage do not exhibit the MBD patterns of behavior. He further rejected the notion of Strauss and Lehtinen (1947) that ''all brain lesions, wherever localized, are followed by a similar kind of disordered behavior.'' It seems likely that this early belief encouraged the adoption of a definition of an identifiable *syndrome* of MBD.

Schmitt (1975) argues that electroencephalographic findings have been of limited use in evaluating MBD. Clemmens and Kenny (1972) found that the classical neurological examination contributed little to the diagnosis of learning disabilities, minimal brain dysfunction, and hyperactivity. Like many others Becker (1975) notes the absence in children diagnosed as having MBD of ''diagnostically, radiographically, or clinically'' demonstrable evidence of gross structural, morphological, or architectural lesions.

In short children who are being diagnosed as having MBD (and perhaps learning disabilities and hyperactivity) by whatever criteria, do not have neurological problems of the kinds that have previously been identifiable by means of classical neurological examination or typical electroencephalography. In light of the definition of MBD, it would be surprising indeed if this were not the case. It is simply a reflection on the selection of the children, the majority of whom have no gross, demonstrable neurological impairment. Together with other problems, the difficulty in establishing a link between brain and behavior where typical criteria are disallowed has caused some disenchantment with the concept of MBD and led to the suggestion that it should be discarded (Schmitt, 1975; Twitchell, 1971).

If the usual criteria of neurological impairment cannot be utilized, then the presumed link must obviously be demonstrated by other means. Accordingly there has been a shift of emphasis from hard neurological signs to soft neurological signs (suggestive minor abnormalities in functions presumably referrable to the central nervous system), including the inability to perform adequately on tasks requiring coordination, balance, appreciation of laterality, and the ability to comprehend and reproduce motorically instructions given verbally.

Schmitt (1975) argues that soft signs are an invalid criterion for establishing the diagnosis of MBD on the grounds that they are transient phenomena and disappear with age, ''At best they are evidence for neurological immaturity.''

Kinsbourne (1975) similarly stresses the need to view soft signs from a developmental perspective noting that ''soft signs differ from hard signs in that the child's age is the factor that determines whether the sign represents an abnormality.'' He has observed elsewhere (Kinsbourne, 1973) that reliance on a variety of soft signs ''blurs essential distinctions. . . . If we bracket lack of dexterity and hyperactivity together as signs of MBD, we will soon be treating clumsiness with stimulant drugs.''

While the perspective of soft neurological signs as essentially developmental rather than pathognomonic phenomena seems to be based, in the above instances, on clinical experience, some more definitive data are appearing in partial support of this inference. Rie, et al., (1978) found that half of the soft neurological signs evaluated in their studies factored with age in a factor analysis of their data, but the other half did not. Some soft signs clearly factored with variables serving as independent indexes of neurocognitive dysfunction. Work in this area has obviously suffered from the absence of a standard battery of soft signs evaluated by standardized procedures in children selected by the same criteria. Problems of this kind have been endemic to work with MBD.

In the absence of definitive findings through traditional electroencephalography, a number of investigators have explored visually or auditorily evoked responses or potentials (Conners, 1972; Satterfield, 1971; Satterfield, 1973; Prichep, Sutton, and Hakerem, 1976; Shields, 1973). While some investigators have interpreted the findings to mean that children with so-called MBD are cortically underaroused, the findings are far from consistent as yet. Since the focus of a number of these studies has been hyperactive children, it is uncertain to what extent they bear implications for other children with MBD. It is too early to conclude that the link between atypical CNS functioning and atypical behavior in MBD will be established by this approach.

Though it goes beyond the scope of a discussion on definition, it should be noted that other more characteristically biomedical phenomena are also being explored, including autonomic reactions under various conditions (Cohen, Douglas, and Morgenstern, 1971; Zahn et al., 1975) and speculation is increasing about neurophysiological abnormalities (Wender, 1973). Becker (1975) believes that recent developments "have brought about a more refined set of specific concepts which suggest that neurometabolic, genetic, and enzymatic abnormalities may be at the very foundation of the MBD syndrome."

If the major definitional emphasis on brain dysfunction as the basis for the noted MBD behaviors is still without precise, empirical verification, it may be that the right kinds of data have not consistently been studied in consistently and adequately defined subgroups. Clinical experience and logic certainly argue for the existence of behavioral and/or intellectual problems that are the consequence of various as yet undetectable neurological problems. Rutter (1977), on reviewing the evidence for "brain damage" in what he terms "psychiatric disorder" in children concludes that it is "highly likely that in addition to those children with cerebral palsy and obvious neurological conditions, there are many others with some degree of damage or dysfunction of the brain." Whether they happen to manifest this damage or dysfunction in the multiple ways said to constitute the syndrome of minimal brain dysfunction is of course another matter.

Still the definition appears to rely on the *conviction* that certain kinds of behavioral and/or intellectual problems are "organically" determined, but the long symtom list of MBD, which is yet to be considered, cannot and does not imply general criteria for distinguishing organic from nonorganic behaviors.

Minimal Dysfunction

Like most elements of the definition of MBD, the term "minimal" has stirred controversy. It seems to refer both to presumed minimal neurological impairment and to minimal behavioral and/or intellectual effects. As previously noted the term was adopted at least partly because of the belief in an organic etiology of certain childhood problems in the absence of demonstrable organic abnormalities. But it was adopted as well to distinguish the problems from those of demonstrably and more profoundly affected individuals, including those in the "subnormal ranges" of intellectual functioning.

Birch (1964) contended " . . . that attaching the adjective 'minimal' to the term . . . does not increase the descriptive accuracy of the term or add to either its scientific validity or its usefulness." Benton (1973) has referred to differential consequences of demonstrable brain damage in young and older primates and cats to criticize the concept of minimal dysfunction in the brains of MBD children, especially if it is postulated that their dysfunction(s) originated perinatally or in early development. Given the lower probability of sequelae of early insults in animals and the absence of gross behavioral and intellectual problems even in some cases of hemispherectomy, he contends that any brain problem that results in the behavior of the MBD syndrome cannot reasonably be regarded as minimal. And it may well be that the dysfunctions are simply too subtle for detection on neurological examination rather than minimal in nature, particularly if they should prove more often to result from neurophysiological rather than anatomical or morphological problems.

It is obvious as well that some of the children designated by the term MBD have very substantial and enduring problems (see Chapter 4), surely as relatively incapacitating as those of some individuals with demonstrable damage. They are therefore minimally affected only in contrast to a given reference group and then necessarily with respect to given functions.

At present the term "minimal" seems more nearly to serve a connotative than a denotative function.

Specificity of Dysfunction

Among the most troublesome aspects of the definition of minimal brain dysfunction (Clements, 1966) is the relative vagueness with which the question of specificity of dysfunction is dealt. Reference is made to problems in "any of the areas of brain function," to "abnormal manifestations of motor, sensory, or intellectual function," to "specific kinds of learning, thinking, and behavioral sequelae," and to the conviction that "these children are *different* in certain learning and behavioral patterns. . . ." But it is not precisely clear in which ways they are different and, indeed, given the multiple determinants especially of late-developing complex intellective functions, it was surely impossible to distinguish precisely the consequences of subtle neurologic impairment from the consequences of environmental impact on an othersise intact organism. It is evident, as Birch (1964) observed, that "the behavioral disturbances of children who come to our notice are developmental products and not merely manifestations of a damaged portion of the brain."

Nevertheless the idea of unique, identifiable patterns of functioning that are the consequence of neurologic dysfunction continues to be attractive. Thus Wender 971) asserted that "the behavioral pattern associated with minimal brain dysunction is rather distinct and easily identified." Similarly Bakwin and Bakwin (1966) claimed that "the behavioral manifestations of cerebral damage, whatever the etiology, are fairly uniform and characteristic." Though these assertions may be more appropriate to instances of "damage" than of "dysfunction," and though they may reflect a popular conviction, unique and easily identified patterns of minimal dysfunction continue to be elusive and subject to debate.

In support of the contention of symptom specificity, a substantial list of symptoms of MBD was culled from the literature (Clements, 1966). While a number of the 15 symptom categories are referable to demonstrable neurologic impairment, the list *in toto* represents most categories of maladaptation. In short even the definitional elaboration represented by the illustrative listing of symptoms of MBD fails to convey convincingly the qualitative differences between maladaptation attributable to subtle impairment of the central nervous system and maladaptation attributable to other causes. This is not to suggest either that differences do not exist or that more recent research has not helped to clarify this issue. Rather the generally accepted definition does not, and perhaps at the time could not, offer the criteria by which symptoms or constellations of symptoms could be reliably identified as primarily organic or primarily not organic. It is evident in several of the categories of symptoms that the more obviously "organic" symptoms appear at one end of the list (that is those which are more typically the consequences of demonstrable brain damage) and the less obviously organic symptoms appear at the other. Unfortunately it is often the latter symptoms that are regarded as part of MBD and which MBD shares with nonorganic disorders. For example in the category of "Disorders of Motor Function," one finds first on the list "frequent athetoid, choreiform, tremulous, or rigid movements of hands," which would rarely be attributed by anyone to psychogenic or sociogenic disorders. Hence these symptoms would appear to be quite distinctly organic. Unfortunately they are not the hallmarks of MBD either and would therefore be helpful in identifying only a minority of MBD children. At the other end of the list one finds "hyperactivity" which—although regarded as a hallmark of MBD by many—is often situation-specific, and is recognized to occur for a sufficient variety of reasons to lead some investigators to distinguish between organic and nonorganic hyperactivities (Cantwell, 1975; Bower and Mercer, 1975; Conners, 1967). Nearly all of the seven symptoms listed under "physical characteristics" are not unique or even common among children with MBD. They range from "excessive drooling in the young child" to enuresis and encopresis and are often the consequence of unfortunate socialization practices. The same absence of potential for differentiation characterizes the first category headed "Test Performance Indicators," which is particularly important by virtue of the frequency with which such data are utilized. The items in this category range from "spotty or patchy intellectual deficits," to "poor showing on group tests," to "characteristic subtest patterns on the Wechsler Intelligence Scale for Children." While scatter and Verbal-Performance disparities exist among children diagnosed as having MBD, they and poor group test performances occur as well among children with disorders not attributable to subtle neurological impairment. In our own data (Rie and Rie, 1978) WISC subtest scatter proved to be as great in subjects deemed to be free of neurocognitive dysfunction as in subjects who would generally have been classified as MBD (see Chapter 12).

In fact many of the categories of symptoms and many of the symptoms within categories occur as well on a psychogenic as on a sociogenic basis. It is this large number of symptoms that has made it virtually impossible to identify the MBD child on the basis of this definition with any assurance. Though diagnostic problems are the concern of Chapter 15, it is evident from the definition and its illustrative elaboration in the symptom list, that a great variety of problems can be "diagnosed" as minimal brain dysfunction which differ etiologically, symptomatically, and prognostically. It is the apparent occurrence of such uncertain diagnoses that has led to the concern that MBD has become the same "wastebasket" diagnosis as its predecessor "brain damage" was said to be. The reader may wish to consult other relevant chapters in this volume for consideration of the extent to which clinical and research data have provided a basis for a more precise and more readily applicable definition.

MBD without Effect on Intellectual Functioning

It has already been noted that the definition of MBD (Clements, 1966) clearly excludes children who are deemed to be mentally retarded. The exclusion was intentional having as a partial purpose the mobilization of resources on behalf of children who were not as readily identifiable as children with "subnormal" intellectual functioning and who were ostensibly being confused with children having psychogenic problems.

See Chapter 12 for a detailed discussion of the relationship among minimal brain dysfunctions, intellectual functioning, and achievement. For the present it is of interest that three somewhat different perspectives of the intellectual functioning of children with MBD are offered on the same page of the task force monograph (Clements, 1966, p. 9). First it is specified that the children in question are subtly affected in their "learning and behavior, *without* evident lowering of general intellectual capacity." Next one of two basic premises states that the symptomatology appears in "mild, borderline, or subclinical form, without reducing overall intellectual functioning to the subnormal ranges." Finally in the definition itself the children are described as of "near average, average, or above average general intelligence." The last of these avoids the issue of the effect of the brain dysfunction on intellectual functioning, simply delimiting the range of intellectual functioning that will be viewed as properly fitting the concept of MBD. The second of the above specifications clearly allows for the possibility of reduced intellectual functioning as a result of the brain dysfunction and excludes children with "subnormal" functioning. The first of the above contentions on the other hand suggests that there is *no* evident effect of the brain dysfunction on intellectual functioning.

This contention, which appears to be popular among advocates of MBD children, has some curious implications. If children with MBD have learning disabilities, as many are said to have, then the implication would appear to be that *different* underlying mental processes affect performance on measures of scholastic achievement and on measures of intellectual functioning. That is, a deficit (learning disability) would become evident on the former, but no deficit would become evident on the latter. The implication is questionable at best on logical grounds, on the grounds of characteristically high correlations between measures of intellectual functioning and scholastic achievement, and on the basis of accruing data. Adding still further contradiction, the monograph section on symptomatology lists "characteristic subtest patterns on the Wechsler Intelligence Scale for Children, including 'scatter' within both Verbal and Performance Scales; high Verbal-low Performance; low Verbal-high Performance." While scatter may actually be no more characteristic of children with MBD than of children with psychogenic problems, the Verbal-Performance disparities seem to be generally acknowledged and are confirmed by our own data (Rie, et al., 1978; Rie and Rie, 1978). Is it reasonable however to describe such disparities while contending that overall intellectual level is unaffected? That is, if one or the other of the two major subscales of the WISC is reduced by virtue of MBD, then the (composite) Full Scale IQ is necessarily reduced as well. The pattern of Verbal-Performance disparities is presumably described as characteristic of children with MBD because it distinguishes them from children without MBD. Hence normal children must be assumed not to have such disparities—at least to the same degree—and therefore would be expected, as a group, to have higher mean IQs. This is necessarily the case unless one also assumes that the group of children with MBD had greater than normal potential initially. This claim is not typically made and would, in any case, be unverifiable.

These contradictory contentions concerning the intellectual functioning of children with MBD suggest that several rather different goals needed to be served in the formulation of a definition, and these were apparently difficult to reconcile. In some sense the definition may have had more hortative value than empirical justification.

Variety of Determinants

The ostensible syndrome of MBD is attributed by definition to virtually any factor that can affect neurologic functioning adversely. These include "genetic variations, biochemical irregularities, perinatal insults or other illnesses or injuries sustained during the years which are critical for the development and maturation of the central nervous system, or from unknown causes." Further the definition allowed for "the possibility that early severe sensory deprivation could result in central nervous system alterations which may be permanent."

These determinants are recognizable as those which had previously been held accountable for brain *damage* and with the inclusion of unknown causes and early deprivation, they seem to exhaust the logical possibilities. This definitional emphasis may therefore be more useful for directing research interests than for clinical purposes. For example, one still cannot conclude that a child is free of MBD even if all of the presumed (known) determinants have been ruled out. However research has been directed at the relations between symptoms and several of these categories of determinants that may prove helpful in clarifying the nature of the ostensible syndrome. Thus Towbin (see Chapter 8) has stressed perinatal hypoxia as a determinant, Wender (1973) has hypothesized about biochemical determinants to which research has recently been directed, Martin (see Chapter 7) has reviewed the effects of childhood injuries, and Werner (see Chapter 9) has shown the significance of interaction between perinatal factors and environment for ultimate adaptation.

Whatever the determinant, the emphasis in this definition is the effect upon brain functioning that ultimately manifests itself in behavioral and/or educational problems, rather than upon the child's adaptation directly. In the absence of definitive data on the central nervous system consequences of severe, early sensory deprivation, one is left to speculate about such possibilities from research with animals. Doubt necessarily remains about the degree of severity of deprivation that can be withstood without permanent "central nervous system alterations" (not to mention the problem of gauging "severity"); about the choice of intervention if there is, or is not, permanent CNS alteration; and about the potential irreversibility of severe early deprivation. The difficulty in identifying a causal agent, a problem that is not unique to MBD, is confounded by the absence of a clearly specifiable, invariant core of symptoms by which the existence of the disorder can be confirmed. The definitional reference to a syndrome is of course based on the assumption that a common set of symptoms exists, for a syndrome is "a group of signs and symptoms that occur together and characterize a particular abnormality'' (Webster's, 1975). The validity of that assumption is considered next.

MINIMAL BRAIN DYSFUNCTION AS SYNDROME

The designation of various, presumed minimal brain dysfunctions as a syndrome is unfortunate and seems quite unnecessary, if only on the grounds that the definition itself specifies that ''the child with minimal brain dysfunction may exhibit these minor symptoms in varying degree and *in varying combinations.*'' [Emphasis added] The definition of a syndrome is thereby violated, and one might generously conclude that ''syndrome'' was simply a poor choice of term. However the consequences of that usage have been substantial and cannot be ignored. They necessitate consideration of the empirical justification for continued reliance on the concept of a syndrome and its implications.

Apart from the confusion and controversy that have been stirred, the effect has been felt both in research and in clinical practice. In practice, if one assumes that a syndrome exists, it seems reasonable to deal more or less similarly with all instances of its occurrence regardless of the presenting complaint, that is regardless of the particular aspect of the symptom complex that has occasioned referral. It has long been evident that ''minimal brain dysfunction,'' ''hyperkinesis,'' ''learning disabilities,'' and a number of other less popular designations have been used virtually synonymously (Rie, 1975). Yet a learning problem, with or without accompanying symptoms, is likely to require psychoeducational intervention while severe, persistent hyperactivity may require temporary treatment with a stimulant drug. However it is quite clear that stimulant drugs will not effect any general improvement in scholastic achievement (Barkley and Cunningham, 1977; Rie, et al., 1976a, 1976b) nor are psychoeducational interventions likely to alter severe, persistent hyperactivity. The rather vague references to ''treatment of minimal brain dysfunction'' with stimulant drugs (Erenberg, 1972; Friedman, Dale, and Wagner, 1973; Garfinkel, Webster, and Sloman, 1975; Levitis, 1974; Levy, 1976; Millichap, 1973) and to unspecified ''benefits'' or ''improvement'' (Report of Conference, 1971; Barcai, 1971) amply attest to this lack of discrimination among potentially different problems requiring different approaches.

In research the problem is obvious. It is impossible to know whether samples are comparable from study to study if the general designations are used without detailed characterizations of the samples. It is often difficult to know to which population one may generalize from a given study, it is impossible to establish prevalence rates, it is extremely difficult to speak conclusively about intervention effects, and replication is almost a hopeless task. Many of the following chapters recount and illustrate these problems.

Most of the data challenging the concept of a syndrome were unavailable when the definition of MBD was proposed. Unfortunately the definition with its unsubstantiated assumption has enjoyed wide currency while the findings refuting the assumption have not.

Schulman, Kaspar and Throne (1965) undertook a cluster analysis of data obtained on ''brain damaged'' individuals and concluded that no syndrome of brain damage exists. Werry (1968) factor analyzed 67 variables with data obtained on 103 children selected because of hyperactivity and ''increased frequency of minor neurological abnormalities, slow diffuse dysrhythmias on the EEG, and a variety of perceptual, perceptual-motor, and attentional defects." He found a very low degree of interrelatedness among "neurological, cognitive, behavioral, medical-historical, and EEG dysfunctions . . .," and concluded that the "measures reflect about ten basically unrelated dysfunctions." Routh and Roberts (1972), obtained 16 measures and ratings on 89 children, including most of the 10 variables reported to occur most frequently as part of the "syndrome" (Clements, 1966). Though the study lacked some elements that would have made it more definitive, it offered no support "to the idea of such a syndrome." Crinella (1973) administered a battery of neuropsychological tests to 90 children, of whom 53 had either verified brain lesions or suspected minimal brain dysfunction. The battery was factor analyzed. Profiles for the 53 impaired subjects were intercorrelated and the correlational matrix was cluster analyzed, "resulting in the identification of eight clusters or 'syndromes'." Crinella concluded that "a unitary MBD syndrome was contraindicated." Loney, Langhorne, and Paternite (1978), responding to findings both from the literature and from a series of their own studies, undertook a "multistage multivariate investigation [of] the hyperkinesis/minimal brain dysfunction syndrome" in 135 boys. The analysis resulted in "two relatively independent symptom dimensions: *Aggression,* accounting for 44.6% of the factor variance, and *Hyperactivity,* accounting for 23.4%." They argue for consideration of these symptom dimensions in clinical research as a basis for forming and studying more homogeneous subgroups. Rie, et al., (1978) factor analyzed a variety of data, including soft neurological signs, obtained on children selected because of underachievement. Among the several factors that emerged, three different patterns of "neurocognitive dysfunction" were identifiable. Several of the other major symptom groups of the ostensible syndrome of MBD also emerged, more or less independent of each other. It is noteworthy that 11 of 22 soft neurological signs factored with age, suggesting that those signs are more indicative of developmental level than of lasting brain dysfunction.

The data, of which this review offers but a small sampling, lend no credence to the concept of a syndrome of minimal brain dysfunction. Rather they indicate a considerable variety of symptom complexes that may, at the extremes, overlap minimally or perhaps not at all. To the extent that the usage in the definition of "minimal brain dysfunction" has tended to obscure these facts, the definition once again requires modification.

CONCLUSION

The definition of the "minimal brain dysfunction syndrome" (Clements, 1966) that was widely adopted is more speculative than definitive, was tentative in the absence of data that have subsequently accrued, and was apparently intended to serve a variety of purposes that seem, in retrospect, not to be entirely compatible. In the intervening years it seems to have been forgotten, as Clements and Peters (1973) reminded their colleagues, that "the original concept of MBD presented ten years ago was not intended as a final statement on the subject." Whether a final statement will ever be possible remains to be seen, but it is clearly time to revise the original.

The next approximation to a definition of disorders that are the consequence of presumed CNS impairment must rest on a more solid empirical base. To the extent that it is partly the purpose of the following chapters to examine that base and its relation to theory and practice, a definition cannot reasonably precede them. However the problems addressed in this chapter point to certain areas that need reconceptualization in striving for a more precise definition:

1. If symptoms occur concomitantly some of the time but not consistently enough to be characterized as a syndrome, it seems logical to hypothesize that some are secondary to the manifestations of CNS impairment rather than manifestations of the impairment itself. If the presumed impairments can be more precisely identified, then perhaps one might wish to explore whether the manifestations of a given CNS impairment tend to interact with the environment so as to increase the probability that particular patterns of maladaptation will occur.

2. The pathognomonic significance for CNS impairment of given symptoms or categories of symptoms requires greater empirical support or an explicit theoretical rationale that is consistent with knowledge in the neurosciences. For definitions of "minimal brain dysfunctions" to be convincing and to have relevance for practice and research, the consequences of such dysfunctions must be distinguishable from the consequences of other determinants of adaptation.

3. The broad designations of behavioral and educational problems, for example hyperactivity or learning disabilities, are clearly inadequate and should be discarded in favor of terms that have more precise referents. The multiple meanings of current designations and the possibility of two or more etiologies for any of them robs such designations of much of their utility. It is probably time, for example, to substitute designations referring to particular, underlying mental processes that have a verifiable relation to the CNS for the vague designation "learning disabilities."

4. It may be preferable to formulate new definitions of the various problems currently termed "minimal brain dysfunction" without reference even to this most general term. In the absence of a syndrome, it is illogical to continue to use a designation that represents one. But more importantly the various kinds of problems that have been subsumed under this heading may differ significantly and ought to bear names that are more descriptive of their unique characteristics. For example brain dysfunctions that eventuate in scholastic deficiencies of certain kinds ought not to bear the same name as brain dysfunctions that eventuate in problems of motor control.

5. The relation between CNS impairment and variations in rate of development requires clarification. The distinction between developmental lags and brain dysfunction should have prognostic significance, should preclude misdirected efforts and false hope, and should alert one to the potential problems of early screening.

The flaws in the current definition(s) of MBD would probably encourage one to stipulate still more conditions for new definitions. However no flaw in the popular definition of MBD obviates the fact that neurologic impairments can and do affect human adaptation adversely in a variety of ways and in different degrees. Similarly no amount of repetition of the elements of that definition can any longer establish a given syndrome and justify the synonymous use of terms that are descriptive of grossly different kinds of behavioral or educational problems. Indeed it is no longer reasonable to speak of "minimal brain dysfunction" in the singular. It is partly the inadequacy of the definition and its implications that occasioned this volume in which the concept of minimal brain dysfunctions is critically reviewed.

REFERENCES

Bakwin, H., and R. M. Bakwin. *Clinical Management of Behavior Disorders in Children.* Philadelphia: Saunders, 1966.

Barcai, A. "Predicting the response of children with learning disabilities and behavior problems to dextroamphetamine sulfate." *Pediatrics*, 47, 73–79, (1971).

Barkley, R. A., and C. E. Cunningham. "Stimulant drugs and academic performance in hyperkinetic children: A review," In *Symposium on Hyperactivity in Children,* Annual Convention of the American Psychological Association, San Francisco, August, 1977.

Becker, R. D. "Minimal cerebral dysfunction." *Journal of Learning Disabilities*, 8 (7), 30–32, (1975).

Benton, A. L. "Minimal brain dysfunction from a neuropsychological point of view," in F. F. de la Cruz, B. H. Fox, and R. H. Roberts, eds., *Minimal Brain Dysfunction,* pp. 29–37, New York: New York Academy of Sciences, 1973.

Birch, H. G. "The problem of 'brain damage' in Children," in H. G. Birch, ed., *Brain Damage in Children: The Biological and Social Aspects,* pp. 3–12, Baltimore: Williams & Wilkins, 1964.

Bower, K. B. and C. D. Mercer. "Hyperactivity: Etiology and intervention techniques. *Journal of School Health*, 45, 195–201, (1975).

Cantwell, D. P. "Clinical picture, epidemiology and classifications of the hyperactive child syndrome," in D. P. Cantwell, ed., *The Hyperactive Child: Diagnosis, Management, Current Research,* New York: Spectrum, 1975.

Clements, S. D. *Minimal Brain Dysfunction in Children—Terminology and Identification.* U.S. Public Health Service Publication No. 1415. Washington, D.C.: 1966.

Clements, S. D., and J. E. Peters. "Psychoeducational programming for children with minimal brain dysfunctions," in F. F. de la Cruz, B. H. Fox, and R. H. Roberts, eds., *Minimal Brain Dysfunction,* pp. 46–51, New York: New York Academy of Sciences, 1973.

Clemmens, R. L., and T. J. Kenny. "Clinical correlates of learning disabilities, minimal brain dysfunction and hyperactivity." *Clinical Pediatrics*, 11, 311–313, (1972).

Cohen, N. J., V. I. Douglas, and G. Morgenstern. "The effect of methylphenidate on attentive behavior and autonomic activity in hyperactive children." *Psychopharmacologia*, 22, 282–294, (1971).

Conners, C. K. "The syndrome of minimal brain dysfunction: psychological aspects." *Pediatric Clinics of North America*, 14, 749–767, (1967).

———— "Psychological effects of stimulant drugs in children with minimal brain dysfunction." *Pediatrics*, 49, 702–708, (1972).

Crinella, F. "Identification of brain dysfunction syndromes in children through profile analysis: Patterns associated with so-called 'minimal brain dysfunction'." *Journal of Abnormal Psychology*, 82, 33–45, (1973).

Erenberg, G. "Drug therapy in minimal brain dysfunction: A commentary." *Pediatric Pharmacology and Therapeutics*, 81, 359–365, (1972).

Friedman, R., E. P. Dale, and J. H. Wagner. "A long-term comparison of two treatment regimens for minimal brain dysfunction: drug therapy versus combined therapy." *Clinical Pediatrics*, 12, 666–671, (1973).

Garfinkel, B. S., C. D. Webster, and L. Sloman. "Methylphenidate and caffeine in the treatment of children with minimal brain dysfunction." *American Journal of Psychiatry*, 132, 723–728, (1975).

Grinspoon, L., and S. B. Singer. "Amphetamines in the treatment of hyperkinetic children." *Harvard Educational Review*, 43(4), 515–555, (1973).

Kahn, E., and L. H. Cohen. "Organic drivenness: A brain stem syndrome and an experience." *New England Journal of Medicine*, 210, 748–756, (1934).

Kinsbourne, M. "School problems, diagnosis and treatment." *Pediatrics*, 52, 697–710, (1973).

———— "Editorials: MBD—a fuzzy concept misdirects therapeutic efforts." *Postgraduate Medicine*, 58 (3), 211–212, (1975).

Levitis, K. A. "Need for medication in minimal brain dysfunction." *Pediatrics*, 54, 388, (1974). [Letter]

Levy, H. B. "Minimal brain dysfunction/specific learning disability: A clinical approach for the primary physician." *Southern Medical Journal*, 69, 642–653, (1976).

Loney, J., J. E. Langhourne, and C. E. Paternite. "An empirical basis for subgrouping the hyperkinetic/MBD symdrome." *Journal of Abnormal Psychology*, 87(4), 431–441, (1978).

Millichap, J. G. "Drugs in the management of minimal brain dysfunction," in F. F. de la Cruz, B. H. Fox, and R. H. Roberts, eds., *Minimal Brain Dysfunction*, pp. 321–334, New York: New York Academy of Sciences, 1973.

Prichep, L. S., S. Sutton, and G. Hakerem. "Evoked potentials in hyperkinetic and normal children under certainty and uncertainty: A placebo and methylphenidate study." *Psychophysiology*, 31, 291, (1971).

Report of Conference on the Use of Stimulant Drugs in the Treatment of Behaviorally Disturbed Young School Children. *Journal of Learning Disabilities*, 4, 523–530, (1971).

Rie, E. D., and H. E. Rie. "Reading deficits, intellectual patterns and hemispheric functions." (1978) forthcoming.

Rie, E. D., H. E. Rie, S. Stewart, and S. R. Rettemnier. "An analysis of neurological soft signs in children with learning problems," in *Brain and Language*, 6, 32–46, (1978).

Rie, H. E. "Hyperactivity in children." *American Journal of Diseases of Children*, 129, 783–789, (1975).

Rie, H. E., E. D. Rie, S. Stewart, and J. P. Ambuel. "Effects of methylphenidate on underachieving children." *Journal of Consulting and Clinical Psychology*, 44(2), 250–260, (1976a).

———— "Effects of Ritalin on underachieving children: A replication." *American Journal of Orthopsychiatry*, 46(2), 313–322, (1976b).

Routh, D. K., and R. D. Roberts. "Minimal brain dysfunction in children: Failure to find evidence of a behavioral syndrome." *Psychological Reports*, 31, 307–314, (1972).

Rutter, M. "Brain damage syndromes in childhood: Concepts and findings." *Journal of Child Psychology and Psychiatry*, 18, 1–21, (1977).

Satterfield, J. H. "Auditory evoked responses in hyperkinetic children." *Electroencephalography and Clinical Neurophysiology*, 31, 291, (1971).

———— "EEG Issues in children with minimal brain dysfunction." *Seminars in Psychiatry*, 5, 35–46, (1973).

Schmitt, B. D. "The minimal brain dysfunction myth." *American Journal of Diseases of Children*, 129, 1313–1318, (1975).

Schulman, J. L., J. C. Kaspar and F. M. Throne. *Brain Damage and Behavior: A Clinical-Experimental Study.* Springfield, Ill.: Thomas, 1965.

Shields, D. T. "Brain responses to stimuli in disorders of information processing." *Journal of Learning Disabilities,* 6, 501–505, (1973).

Strauss, A. A., and L. E. Lehtinen. *Psychopathology and Education of the Brain-Injured Child,* 2 vols. New York: Grune & Stratton, 1947.

Twitchell, T. E. "A behavioral syndrome," review of *Minimal Brain Dysfunction in Children* by P. H. Wender. *Science,* 174, 135–136, (1971).

Webster's New Collegiate Dictionary, 1975 ed., s.v. "syndrome."

Wender, P. H. *Minimal Brain Dysfunction in Children.* New York: Wiley, 1971.

———— "Some speculations concerning a possible biochemical basis of minimal brain dysfunction," in F. F. de la Cruz, B. H. Fox, and R. H. Roberts, eds., *Minimal Brain Dysfunction,* pp. 18–28, New York: New York Academy of Sciences, 1973.

Werner, H., and A. A. Strauss. "Types of visuo-motor activity in their relation to low and high performance ages." *Proceedings of the American Association of Mental Deficiency,* 44, 163–168, (1939).

Werry, J. S. "Studies of the hyperactive child IV: An empirical analysis of the minimal brain dysfunction syndrome." *Archives of General Psychiatry,* 19, 9–16, (1968).

Zahn, T. P., F. Abate, B. C. Little, and P. H. Wender. "Minimal brain dysfunction, stimulant drugs, and autonomic nervous system activity." *Archives of General Psychiatry,* 32, 318–387, (1975).

CHAPTER 2

History of Minimal Brain Dysfunctions

Jane W. Kessler

THE PERIOD PRIOR TO 1941—THE MEDICAL ERA

The historical antecedent of the term "minimal brain dysfunction" is "brain damage" or "brain injury," terms which belonged to the domain of medicine, specifically neurology and psychiatry. With one or two notable exceptions the literature describing the behavioral results of brain damage in children appeared in medical journals and physicians were clearly deemed responsible for the diagnosis. Psychologists played a secondary role and educators were only slightly interested because the deficits resulting from brain damage were not considered remediable. It was assumed that nothing could be done if the problem behavior was the result of damage to the brain.

The early work followed two major lines of investigation. The first was observation of the psychological after-effects, or sequelae, of known organic events such as head trauma, encephalitis, premature birth, birth injury, and so on. The second approach was the reconstruction of etiology from presenting symptoms leading to hypotheses regarding hyperactivity; specific learning difficulties in language, reading, and writing; and major developmental disorders such as childhood schizophrenia. During this early period clinicians operated on the assumption of a dichotomy between *functional* and *organic* disorders. Because of the discouraging implications of an organic diagnosis, such diagnoses were made conservatively, contingent on documented history and hard neurological signs. In the following review of the classics of this period, one can identify the predecessors of contemporary concepts, but the frame of reference has shifted from a static disease model to a more dynamic model of brain functioning.

Postencephalitis

The World War I epidemic of encephalitis lethargica affected a large number of children and there were countless reports of the behavior which followed (Paterson and Spence, 1921; Burt, 1922; Hohman, 1922; Ebaugh, 1923; Kennedy, 1924; Stryker, 1925; Strecker, 1929). Stryker listed 27 characteristic encephalitic sequelae in children including sleep reversals, emotional instability, irritability, obstinacy, lying, thieving, impaired memory and attention, personal untidiness, tics, depression, poor motor control, and general hyperactivity—altogether a dismal picture with side remarks of "adjustment to environment impossible." Treatment outside the home was considered imperative. One such treatment program at the University of Pennsylvania Hospital School was described by Bond and

Appel (1931). Of 48 children, all but two improved and 26 were discharged home. The treatment was comparatively simple, namely to keep the child busy under constant supervision. Instructions for those in charge emphasized praise for things well done; disregard of minor faults, eccentricities, enuresis, and so on; a strict prohibition of physical punishment; and the use of withdrawal of privileges as punishment. The specific means used to influence the children's behavior included explanation, praise, rewards, occasional suggestion, substitution of more desirable activity, dramatization and humor, neglect, deprivation, isolation, and at all times the authority of the persons in charge. In modern parlance this would be considered a medley of milieu, cognitive, and behavior therapies. It is interesting that this account of treatment success did little to alleviate the general pessimism.

One of the pioneers in child psychiatry, Lauretta Bender, took charge of the children's service at Bellevue Psychiatric Hospital in New York City in 1934. In her words (Bender, 1975):

It was assumed in the 1930's that most of the children in residence were disturbed because of some form of brain damage, such as encephalitis, and that they had a rather poor prognosis. Indeed the ward had been opened in 1920 to accept children who were thought to have a post-encephalitis syndrome following encephalitis lethargica and to send them to Kings Park State Hospital, which had also just opened a ward for the chronic care of such children. [P. 427]

In point of fact they proved relatively few in number. In 1942, Bender recounted her experiences with 55 such children who constituted only 1.4% of the admissions to Bellevue in the period between 1934 and 1940.

At that time Bender (1942) described the post-encephalitis syndrome as follows:

The behavior disorder as such, or personality pattern, is characterized by the psychopathic personality type of reaction with a hyperkinesis that is not modifiable by psychotherapy of the insight or reassurance type or environmental control, except over long periods. It is best understood as an organic driveness of brain stem origin. ... This hyperkinesis leads the child to contact the environment continually, by touching, taking and destroying. It also leads to continuous contact with persons with over-affection and abusiveness, clinging and nagging. As the personality becomes integrated, there is a tendency for asocial behavior in every field, sexual gratification, stealing and destroying property, resisting routine and truanting, running away, etc. Although the child has some awareness that he cannot control his behavior, he is not concerned with guilt or anxiety but with fear of results and apprehension. The behavior can be partially controlled under supervision but not by trying to treat or train the ego drives. [P. 361–362]

Reflecting on these clinical observations at a later date, Bender (1975) placed more emphasis on the perceptual problems:

Hyperkinesis, in my opinion was secondary to the perceptual problems of these children and to their inability to get gratification from perceptions, from contact with the world of reality, or from their drive to experience reality in perceptual experiences of the world, their own bodies, their body images, and their self-images. Hyperkinesis, therefore, was due to their poorly patterned motorperceptual experiences and impulses. [P. 429]

It was in this context that she developed her famous test (1938). In her thinking, she was very much influenced by Gestalt psychologists who elaborated the universal principles of perceptual organization and followed Gesell in emphasizing the innate maturational principles of central nervous system development.

Before leaving this subject to history, it is interesting to give some more recent reports. Gibbs, et al., (1964) followed 250 children who had suffered from encephalitis of various kinds and found a 10% overall frequency of behavior disorders which does not exceed the usual reported prevalence rate. Sabatino and Cramblett (1968) studied the behavioral sequelae of 14 children who had suffered well-authenticated attacks of California viral encephalitis and concluded that a significant proportion exhibited symptoms of the hyperkinetic syndrome although personality disorder (neurotic) symptoms were equally increased. Werry (1972) points out that such results are often cited as evidence of post-encephalitic behavior disorder without regard for what would be found in a control group.

A group of studies from Boston Children's Hospital reported later learning difficulties in children who had recovered from lead encephalitis (Byers and Lord, 1943) as well as measles encephalitis (Meyer and Byers, 1952). Although some of these children were clearly retarded as the result of gross cerebral damage, others appeared normal but showed selective impairment with sensorimotor defects, attentional problems, and reasoning deficits.

Head Injury

Some scant attention was given to behavior disorders which followed cerebral trauma. Strecker and Ebaugh (1924) described 30 children with histories of head injury and concluded that the disorders were similar to the post-encephalitic disorders. They reported only 6 of the children as improving over time. Blau (1936) described 22 children who showed mental changes following head trauma and suggested that the disorder might be the result of a localized lesion of the prefrontal association areas. At a later date (1954) Blau reconsidered this suggestion and proposed that the behavioral disturbance resulted more from the reaction of the parents and child to the injury than to the organic injury per se. Subsequent studies continued to minimize the role of head injuries in the production of behavior disorders (Dencker, 1958; Harrington and Letemendia, 1958).

Birth Trauma

Injury during birth was studied, usually in retrospect, as a causative factor in mental retardation and cerebral palsy. Doll, Phelps, and Melcher, (1932) estimated that from 6 to 10% of their mentally deficient subjects (institutionalized at Vineland Training School) were found to be birth-injured. One of the major contributors to this field, Schilder (1931) commented that birth is often a trauma in which lesions of the brain substance occur. In this context he was discussing hyperkinesis and "how many organic motor factors may determine what is usually called naughtiness, aggressiveness, and sadism" (1931; 1964, p. 191). He continued with a discussion of the "two-way principle" meaning that an organic function may be changed by psychic causes as well as by somatic ones, a fact that is often ignored in our either-or diagnostic thinking. He added that every organic disease and deficiency is also a psychological problem of enormous importance.

One of the few reports by a psychologist in this early period is that of Shirley (1939). She followed some prematurely born children (defined as birth weight under 5 pounds and gestation periods under 8.5 months) for varying periods of time up to 5 years of age. On the basis of incidental observations, she defined a behavior syndrome as characteristic of prematurely born children. Symptoms included auditory and visual hypersensitivity; lingual-motor, fine motor, and loco-motor difficulties; hyperactivity or sluggishness; short attention span; high susceptibility to distraction; irascibility; and stubbornness. This reads very much like the current description of minimal cerebral dysfunction, so we see that these children have been with us for some time! Shirley raised the question as to whether the behavior syndrome was the direct result of the prematurity (that is brain damage) or other factors associated with the care of the premature. Later studies tended to focus more narrowly on IQ results which were generally somewhat lower than sibling controls. The investigators noted that socioeconomic status played a confounding role, both because of the higher incidence of prematurity in poverty groups and also because of the continuing deprivational aspects of the poverty environment (Knobloch, et al., 1956; Douglas, 1956; Drillien, 1958; Dann, Levine, and New, 1964). Very recently Klaus and Kennell (1970) have stressed the role of secondary factors, namely the interference with mother-infant bonding because of the long period of separation after a premature birth.

The implication of birth injury as the cause of childhood behavior disorders led to a number of studies using neonatal difficulties as the independent variable. Although the results were published well after 1941, the major conclusions will be reported at this point because they belong to the "medical model" approach. In a very careful psychological study Graham, et al., (1962; 1963) investigated the effects of clearly established anoxia or other severe pre- or peri-natal complications on later personality and cognitive development in 350 preschool-age children. They used seven measures first standardized on normal preschool children and found that the performance of brain-injured children was significantly inferior to that of the control subjects on all measures except the Peripheral-Distraction Test. It is interesting to note that the anoxic children, presumably injured during or before birth, suffered significant impairment of vocabulary but not of perceptual-motor ability, which is the direct opposite of the adult pattern following brain injury. Graham, et al., reported questionable differences in the frequency of behavior problems as judged by mothers and examiners. These results were similar to those reported on a total of 250 children by Schacter and Apgar (1959) and Fraser and Wilks (1959), but dissimilar to the results reported by Prechtl (1960). Of 400 children, re-examined between two and four years of age, Prechtl identified the so-called brain damage syndrome in 70% of those who had a history of complications as well as an abnormal neurological status in the newborn period; and in only 12% of those who were normal in both these respects. In ascribing the differences solely to organic causes there are the same problems of socioeconomic differences, and possible differences, in parent-child relationships previously mentioned in connection with prematurity.

After-Effects of Brain Injuries in War

This is the title of a landmark publication by Goldstein (1942) which, although dealing with adult patients, had a tremendous impact on people working with children. These words set the stage for his diagnostic approach:

There is a widespread opinion that it is possible to distinguish psychogenic symptoms from those organically produced. However, this is most difficult and requires very careful examination. Experiences with brain-injured soldiers in particular have taught us that many a symptom considered psychogenic may be due to an organic cause. . . . The whole dichotomy itself is probably at fault, for, as has been said before, the organic patient will react to his condition with functional symptoms also which may be no less disturbing to the patient. . . . The decision as to whether disturbing symptoms are functional or organic should not be based simply on the evidence of existing physical phenomena. Absence of organic signs does not rule out the possibility of an organic character of some symptoms. On the other hand, objective findings—for instance, pneumoencephalographic deviations —should be no reason for considering every symptom which the patient presents as organic in nature. [P. 65]

Goldstein discussed a number of secondary symptoms. He described the *catastrophic reaction* to failure or frustration as revealing the struggle of the brain-injured adult to deal with reality. Another group of secondary symptoms were described as *substitute performances,* or defensive maneuvers. These included isolation, avoidance of change, excessive orderliness, and denial. In discussing the symptoms which are direct sequelae of the brain injury, Goldstein talked about general effects rather than specific impairments related to localized injuries. He felt that there was a systematic disintegration which prolonged excitation (perseveration, for example), distractibility, and blurring of the boundaries between "figure and ground." He particularly emphasized the problems related to an impairment in abstract thinking. Goldstein and Scheerer (1941) delineated eight behavioral difficulties resulting from impairment in abstract thinking, which were "positively ascertained as sequelae to cerebral pathology" (p. 4). Overall these problems relate to difficulties in flexibility, selfobservation, performing acts on verbal direction, categorization, and planning ahead. A number of tests were devised to assess abstract thinking involving sorting tasks and reproduction of designs with blocks or sticks.

Many of these concepts and techniques provided the hypotheses for the experimental work of Werner which will be discussed when we consider the Werner-Strauss syndrome. In reviewing this early work, one is struck by the wealth of clinical material and the effort to fit it all into a unified theory of cortical functioning. One of the few specific references to childhood problems is contained in a postscript to a case report of an idiot savant (Scheerer, Rothman, and Goldstein, 1945). They interpreted the special skills of the autistic child, like those of the idiot savant, to be the result of extraordinary exercise of specific concrete activities compensating for the limitations in abstract thinking. Thus they anticipated an organic explanation for autism with particular reference to the symbolic-cognitive problems, that is very similar to Rutter's contemporary explanation of autism (1974).

The second approach to the study of organic factors in childhood problems in this predominantly medical era was reconstruction of etiology—in the absence of known history.

Hyperactivity

In 1934 Kahn and Cohen described some cases in which hyperkinesis was the predominating feature. They termed this "organic driveness" and considered it referable to the brain stem. This classic paper was followed by a discussion which questioned the evidence for implicating the brain stem, the possibilities of cortical damage touching off release phenomena, and the role of personality in adapting to the driveness. In 1937 Bradley wrote the first article written on the use of amphetamines in children's behavioral problems. Bradley and Bowen (1941) later reported on a series of some 100 children representing a mix of schizoid and withdrawn children on one hand, and aggressive, attacking children on the other. Both groups responded by coming closer together to a desirable midpoint. This observation touched off a series of papers defining the hyperkinetic impulse disorder (Laufer, Denhoff, and Solomons, 1957) and attempts to understand the neurological mechanisms involved. Laufer describes his "nagging concern" over the fact that so many children who presented this picture had no clear diagnostic evidence of involvement of the central nervous system and nothing in their history that would provide an acceptable etiological statement (Laufer, 1975). He noted that they tended to be firstborn males and hypothesized some injury at birth. After some complex laboratory studies, Laufer localized the major site of difficulty in the diencephalon (thalamic region). The frequent association of poor school work with hyperkinesis was explained partly as reflecting the interference with attention and partly as a result of visual-motor difficulties. As a personal note it is interesting how much of this early work was contributed by the staff of the Emma Pendleton Bradley Home which was established in 1931 at Providence, Rhode Island, as a memorial to a post-encephalitic child. Bradley was the pediatrician director, Laufer was chief psychiatrist, and Denhoff was the neurologist. Psychologists included Jasper and Lindsley, both famous in electroencephalography.

Specific Learning Difficulties

Coming from another direction, but equally interested in the problem of localization in the central nervous system, a number of physicians undertook the task of explaining specific learning problems in speech, reading, and basic academic subjects. They took their lead from adults who lost a similar function following brain damage. One of the earliest such cases was Monsieur C. who lost his ability to read after a stroke. He was still able to express himself fluently, understand everything said to him, remember minute details, write without difficulty, but unable to name letters or even read what he himself had written. For the first time an autopsy was possible and the underlying pathology could be identified. It was suggested that he could not transmit information from the undamaged part of his visual center in the right hemisphere of his brain to the areas in the left hemisphere where the concepts and names of lexical items are processed. Even before this discovery of Dejerine in 1892, Broca (1861) had demonstrated a connection between injury to the left hemisphere of the human brain and an impairment of language ability. Many case reports about particular disorders (alexia, agraphia, aphasia, agnosia, apraxia) followed Broca's discovery with accompanying anatomic localizations for each—some contradicting others.

In 1917 a Scottish ophthalmologist, Hinshelwood, described a number of children who were "congenitally word blind." They had no trouble seeing lines and forms, recognizing numbers, and were fluent talkers. Hinshelwood compared them to Monsieur C. after his stroke and suggested that they lacked the necessary connections between the visual and speech centers of their brains.

The conditions of developmental aphasia and developmental dyslexia have been the subject of continuing debate and controversy. Criteria for diagnosis were difficult to agree upon because it is rare to find a child who shows an isolated deficit like that experienced by Monsieur C. The approach of relating specific cognitive defects to discrete brain lesions fell into disrepute. Much more attention was given to the semantic issues involved in definition than to the therapeutic issues. One of the significant contributors with a fresh approach was Orton, a psychiatrist at the University of Iowa. He related children's difficulties in acquiring language skills to developmental disturbances in cortical dominance (Orton, 1937). He noted that these children tended to reverse letters, numbers, syllables, or whole words. He coined the term "strephosymbolia" (twisted symbols). Orton felt that the current term of "congenital language defects" overstressed the inherent difficulties and underemphasized important environmental factors, such as methods of teaching and emotional and social factors. He preferred the use of the term "developmental disorder." He ascribed the reversals to a failure to erase the memory images from the nondominant side. This idea was attractive, partly because of his optimism regarding educability of such children. This concept enjoyed a renaissance with the work of Doman, Delacato and their co-workers (1960) at the Norwood Rehabilitation Center in Philadelphia, later reorganized as the Institutes for the Achievement of Human Potential.

Currently Orton's conceptualizations regarding cerebral dominance have little credibility. There has never been any substantiation for the notion that mirror images are projected onto the brain, and many theorists regard this conjecture as illogical. For instance Corballis (1974) noted that one might as well expect the right and left sides of a camera lens to project mirrored versions of a single image. Educators noted that reversals are the most common errors made by beginning readers (Moyer and Newcomer, 1977) and many investigators reported on the relationship of mixed cerebral dominance and reading skill. After her review Vernon (1958) suggested that there might be a "congenital disposition" toward the occurrence of certain related defects: reading disability, speech defects, motor incoordination, and mixed laterality. She saw these difficulties as a kind of syndrome, a cluster of symptoms resulting from a lack of cortical maturation. This idea leads us back to Lauretta Bender. The shift in her thinking from post-encephalitic behavior disorders to maturational lag in childhood schizophrenia illustrates well the progression in the medical model from the concrete to the abstract.

Maturational Lag

Bender stayed on the organic path in child psychiatry, influenced as she reports by her work with neurologist Herrick, her husband, Schilder, and Orton. Bender (1975) stated that maturational lag indicates a

lack of differentiation of patterning (as envisaged by the embryologists) in the development or maturation of perceptual-, mental-, and reflex-motor patterning, so that the child functions less maturely in some or all areas. The chief characteristic is a less mature level of patterning in perceptual, mental, motor, and also visceral and autonomic behavior. There is no structural defect, no function is lost or defective, and maturation will continue, if slowly, and may even tend to accelerate after puberty. Maturational lags occur most specifically in minimally brain-damaged children, children with learning disabilities, and schizophrenic children. [P. 435]

Obviously this was a very encompassing concept which linked a wide variety of childhood disorders. For instance, on aphasia she commented (1962) that:

The developmental lag in those children who have language disorders is a total developmental lag which will also be seen in motor areas and in personality organization, in space and time perception, and in cortical unilateral dominance. [P. 25]

If you want to see the greatest variety of aphasic disorders in children, and to see them change from one into another; or to see a child speak normally and then become aphasic and go through all kinds of aphasic anomalies and then learn to speak more normally again; if you want a chance to observe the greatest number of aphasic anomalies in early childhood, you should look for the schizophrenic children. [P. 27]

One might add parenthetically that most of the participants in this conference disagreed with this notion of combining aphasic and schizophrenic symptoms.

Bender (1961) stated that:

Schizophrenia in childhood is a biological disorder in central integration and in maturation processes involving behavior with a lag characterized by embryonic features, especially plasticity. [P. 536]

[She defined plasticity (Bender, et al., 1963) as a] primitive level of organization of physiological (homeostasis), neurological (motility), and psychic and behavioral functioning (including self concept, body image, and language skills) in children who have problems in maturation. [P. 305]

Cautiously Bender and others suggested that plasticity might be a symptom of diffuse brain injury, but basically it was used in a descriptive sense. The primary cause of the child's problems was in the "congenitally determined" immaturity of his nervous system functioning.

In an overview of this medical era, we see a relatively small number of medically trained workers persistently investigating the organic factors in childhood psychopathology. They worked in relative isolation, with little to offer in the way of treatment. Beginning in the 1940s, they were increasingly apart from the mainstream in child guidance and child psychiatry which were dominated by psychodynamic theory derived from psychoanalysis. As Laufer (1975) remarked rather wistfully in his personal reminiscences:

This was a very uncomfortable situation in which to be. Even to hint to fellow candidates (in psychoanalysis) that there might be an organic component of significance in some of the children under discussion was an invitation to be dealt with in a manner remarkably close to ostracism. [P. 110]

In truth the dichotomy between the organic and the psychogenic disorders of childhood was initiated by those interested in the latter. Riding high on their discoveries about the long-lasting effects of early maternal care and infantile trauma, child psychotherapists were blind to contributory organic factors. Besides, what could you do if the brain were really damaged? It was only with the advent of specific therapeutic suggestions in the area of special education and the beginning disillusionment with psychotherapy results that organic explanations came back in style.

CONTRIBUTIONS FROM PSYCHOLOGISTS AND EDUCATORS: 1941–1960

As the reader has doubtlessly noted, our calendar demarcations are not precise. Many of the physicians who began their work in the 1930s continued after 1941, refining, modifying, and extending their earlier concepts. Beginning in the 1940s something new was added by experiments, theories, applied programs reported by psychologists, educators and professionals from the allied fields.

Werner-Strauss Syndrome

Hallahan and Cruickshank (1973) have provided a personal history of the originators of this new movement. A. A. Strauss, a psychiatrist and the only physician in the new wave, emigrated from Heidelberg to Spain in 1933 when Hitler came to power. After three years in Barcelona, he accepted an appointment as research psychiatrist at the Wayne County Training School in Northville, Michigan. At the same time Heinz Werner, as associate professor of psychology at the University of Hamburg, emigrated first to The Netherlands and then to the research department at the Training School. Werner and Strauss collaborated in efforts to learn whether the psychological manifestations of brain injury found in adults by Goldstein would also be observable in children. This mutual interest stimulated some 13 experiments comparing groups of mentally retarded children in residence at the Training School. The groups were relatively small, around 20 children in each, with IQs ranging from 60 to 80. The "exogenous" mentally retarded group consisted of children who had no history of retardation in the family and whose history indicated a prenatal, natal, or postnatal disease or injury to the brain. In some studies the two groups were selected on the basis of differences in performance on intelligence tests rather than neurologic criteria. In the exogenous group the mental ages scored on performance tests were one year or more below the Stanford-Binet mental age; in the endogenous group, the mental ages scored on performance tests were three or more years above the Stanford-Binet mental age. It is difficult to ascertain if the same children were used in repeated studies.

The experimental methods were ingenious and explored many facets of behavior. Perception was studied most thoroughly and many differences between the exogenous and the endogenous retarded of the same mental age were described. Werner and Thuma reported differences in ability to see apparent motion (1942b) and in the critical flicker fusion frequency (1942a). The brain-injured child had more difficulty recognizing figures imbedded in a homogenous background on tachistoscopic exposure because he was more distracted by the ground (Werner and Strauss, 1941). The Marble Board test (Werner and Strauss, 1939) involved a visual-motor task, the reproduction of a model figure on another marble board. The pattern of the exogenous group was incoherent and characterized by unrelated, discontinuous lines and moves. Werner and Bowers (1941) investigated the reproduction of auditory perceptual patterns by having the child sing a musical pattern played for him on the piano. As was found on the visual-motor tasks, the auditory-motor experiment revealed that the vocalization of the exogenous children lacked melodic-harmonic synthesis and satisfactory endings, whereas the responses of the endogenous subjects resembled normal children's more global responses. This was taken as evidence that the impairment in the exogenous children was of a general perceptual nature rather than specific to the visual modality.

A number of studies of concept formation were made. Strauss and Werner, using a sorting test procedure, demonstrated that the exogenously retarded child is especially apt to group objects in uncommon, far-fetched, and peculiar ways. He often selected objects for grouping on the basis of some unusual or apparently insignificant detail (1942). Werner and Carrison (1944) found more animistic thinking in brain-injured mentally retarded children; these children identified with objects and events in nature as much as with people. The theoretical explanation that the authors offered for this follows the line of reasoning which relates everything about the child's behavior to the organic defect.

1. In an organism which is driven hither and yon by outside stimulation, the essential difference between oneself as a person, who masters the external world by planful action, as opposed to objects without this ability is less obvious.

2. The pathological condition of fixation, perseveration, rigidity could also obstruct the child's understanding of purposeful activity as a characteristic of a person in contradistinction to a thing.

3. The behavior characteristics of lack of emotional control and motor disinhibition (organic driveness) also reduces the self-directed behavior of the individual and reduces his awareness of the difference between spontaneous, personal activity and external occurrences in the world of things. [P. 60]

Two other studies illustrate the interests of these researchers. Werner studied the tendency toward perseveration as a particular aspect of rigidity defined as "lack of variability and adaptability" of response (1946). By means of a behavior rating scale, Strauss and Kephart (1940) had institutional teachers and cottage parents rate a group of retarded children "blind," that is without knowing the psychological diagnosis. The exogenous group was reliably differentiated from the others in such ways as being "erratic, uncoordinated, uncontrolled, uninhibited, and socially unaccepted."

In his first major publication (Strauss and Lehtinen, 1947), Strauss proposed four criteria for the diagnosis of brain injury:

1. A history of trauma or inflammatory processes before, during, or shortly after birth.
2. Slight neurological signs.
3. The existence of immediate family with normal intelligence.
4. The presence of psychological disturbancces in perception and conceptual thinking of the order described in the research.

According to Strauss it would be legitimate to base the neurological diagnosis on the fourth criterion alone. The main reason that Strauss' work attracted so much attention however was that he offered extensive educational recommendations. In a survey of the first 500 admissions to the Wayne County Training School, Strauss and Kephart (1939) had found that exogenous children as a group declined 2.5 IQ points during residence in the institution over four to five years. The endogenous children on the other hand had increased 4.0 points during institutionalization. In a further investigation of this difference, Kephart and Strauss (1940) looked at those subjects whose intelligence test scores could be traced from a period of time prior to admission at the school to a period of time afterward. Whereas the exogenous children showed a steady decline in IQ over the years, the endogenous children experienced decline only until the time of institutionalization. Apparently the exogenous children were not benefiting from an educational program designed for both groups. It was hypothesized by the Wayne County group that the reason for this discrepancy was the inability of the exogenous children to profit from a highly stimulating environment and curriculum—perhaps an unusual way to characterize an institutional environment! Werner and Strauss (1940) suggested that unessential distractions should be minimized and essential elements stressed. This strategy was elaborated first by Strauss (1943) and then by Strauss and Lehtinen (1947). This educational philosophy was basically as follows

"Since the organic lesion is medically untreatable, our efforts may extend in two directions: in manipulating and controlling the external, overstimulating environment and in educating the child in the exercise of voluntary control." [P. 131]

Werner did not participate directly in the authorship of this book and the diagnosis and treatment of the brain-injured child was identified with Strauss.

The early work, as already indicated, dealt with mentally retarded children, but it was not long before similar investigations were undertaken with children of normal intelligence. One of the first was the doctoral dissertation of Jane Dolphin, written under the supervision of Cruickshank who had been in close contact with Werner and Strauss. Dolphin and Cruickshank worked with a population of cerebral palsied children of near average, average, and above average IQ. These children, when compared to their nonhandicapped peers, demonstrated deficiencies in the discrimination of figure from background (Dolphin and Cruickshank, 1951*a*), in concept formation ability (Dolphin and Cruickshank, 1951*b*), in visual motor performance (Dolphin and Cruickshank, 1951*c*), and in tactual-motor performance (Dolphin and Cruickshank, 1952). These studies continued for some time and were consistent in supporting the hypothesis that cerebral palsied children displayed the same psychological characteristics found by Werner and Strauss in their exogenous, mentally retarded subjects. Cruickshank and Dolphin (1951) recommended adoption of the educational recommendations of Strauss and Lehtinen. Thus the work of Cruickshank and his students extended the ideas of Werner and Strauss, but still in relationship to children with independent evidence of brain injury, that is cerebral palsy.

In a second volume of the 1947 classic, Strauss and Kephart (1955) devoted much attention to the brain-injured child of normal intelligence. The difference between this child and a "normal" child was very much emphasized:

Everything which we do as normal individuals we do in terms of patterns. These patterns become so instilled in us, and patterned behavior becomes so ingrained, that we cannot get it out. For this reason we cannot appreciate the problem of the brain-injured fully because we cannot truly experience it. We cannot reproduce in ourselves unpatterned behavior and therefore we cannot empathize with the individual who has few patterns. Because our patterns group and regroup themselves constantly and are always in a state of flux, meeting new demands of new situations, we find it impossible to imagine the plight of the individual in whom it is not so. We cannot see what he sees, we cannot feel what he feels, and we cannot follow the processes which bring him to a certain end result. To us his performance seems only bizarre. [P. 214]

Further Developments in Perceptual-Motor Theories

Although Lehtinen wrote little after her coauthorship with Strauss in 1947, Kephart, an educator, forged ahead. Kephart emphasized the importance of motor development which he believed preceded perceptual development. In 1960 Kephart pointed out that:

> Early studies in the area of posture have investigated the postural adjustment of the child while he was not moving. Present studies investigate his posture during the process of movement. The emphasis has swung from highly specific motor skills (which can be learned as splinter skills and have limited relationship to the activities of the total organism) to investigations of general movement patterns and the ranges involved in these general patterns. [P. 41]

In Kephart's view the body is the zero point, or point of origin, for all movements and perceptual understanding of outside objects will be disturbed if the body image is disturbed. Laterality, the ability to distinguish the left from the right side of the body and to control these individually or simultaneously, was considered prerequisite to the differentiation of left and right in space. This would result in the failure to discriminate between a "b" and a "d," not because of mirror images as hypothesized by Orton, but because of the absence of a proper kinesthetic, body reference point.

Kephart collaborated with still another leading investigator in this field, namely Getman, an optometrist. They worked together on a program for the perceptual development of retarded children (Getman and Kephart, 1956) and operated a camp for brain-injured children and their parents in 1957 and 1958. As would be expected from his optometric background, Getman stressed ocular motor systems, but he proposed a comprehensive program for the development of perceptual motor skills which included practice in general coordination, balance (walking beam), eye-hand coordination, eye movements, form recognition (templates), and visual memory (Getman, et al., 1964). In 1960 Getman operated the camp for brain injured with Barsch, who in turn developed another program, known as "movigenics," built around 12 components of motor movement and spatial awareness (Barsch, 1967). Superficially this seems to have a lot in common with sensory integration therapy developed by Ayres, (1963), an occupational therapist. Following a somewhat different line independent of these investigators, Frostig, founder and director of the Marianne Frostig Center of Educational Therapy in Los Angeles, developed a visual-motor test and specific educational materials (Frostig, Lefever, and Whittlesey, 1961) which had a clear relationship to beginning reading instruction.

Cruickshank points out that Kephart, Getman, Barsch, and, to a certain extent, Frostig all shared the Werner and Strauss orientation. In addition to the specific educational activities advocated, they shared a concern for control of the stimulus environment. Cruickshank particularly urged the use of cubicles to reduce external distractions, although he noted difficulties with lighting and the management of auditory distractions. However all shared a developmental approach wherein one indirectly deals with the learning problems by first building up prerequisite perceptual-motor skills.

In a historical review of this period and these trends, one cannot omit the highly controversial Doman-Delacato method. Doman, a physical therapist, and Delacato, an educational psychologist, worked together on a theory of "neurological organization" with a central therapeutic concept of patterning (Doman, et al., 1960). This was done by:

1. Placing the child on the floor for training activities to remediate damaged areas of the brain.
2. Externally manipulating the child into body patterns characteristic of the level of the damaged brain.
3. Imposing dominance and unilaterality by restraining one or the other hand.
4. Administering carbon dioxide therapy to increase blood circulation to the brain.
5. Stimulating the senses to improve body awareness.

This set off a torrent of debate and criticism in the professional literature culminating in official cautionary statements and critical position papers published by several prestigious organizations such as the American Academy of Neurology and the American Academy of Pediatrics. Doman and Delacato were criticized for making undocumented claims of cure and for the extreme demands put on parents. Also their neurological theories were questioned and great doubt was expressed regarding the possibilities for direct "brain training" (Robbins and Glass, 1969). Hallahan and Cruickshank (1973) point out that a major difference in the training regimen of the neurological-organization theory proponents and the programs of other perceptual-motor theorists is in the emphasis on passive versus active involvement. Following a strict one-to-one correspondence between training and the alteration of brain structure, Doman and Delacato recommended procedures which require external manipulation of the child's limbs, whereas Kephart, Getman, Barsch, Cruickshank, and Frostig all emphasized the active involvement of the child in the training process.

Language Theorists

Although less visible than the perceptual-motor theorists in the 1950s, some workers were concentrating on language disorders. In 1941 Katrina de Hirsch, a speech pathologist trained abroad, started the first language disorder clinic in this country, the Pediatric Language Disorder Clinic, which was functionally part of Pediatric Psychiatry at Columbia-Presbyterian Medical Center. In her first published paper regarding dyslexia (1952), she described many associated disturbances of a nonlanguage nature such as visual-motor problems, figure-ground disturbance, and distractibility. She became very much interested in the problem of predicting reading problems and noted that many of the predictors, such as the human figure drawing and the Bender Gestalt, bore no obvious relevance to reading. She suggested a generalized defect in the ability to experience and respond in terms of Gestalten led to a weakness in integrative competence (1968). Following Bender she considered these phenomena to be manifestations of central nervous system dysfunction. Katrina de Hirsch (1965, 1973) invoked the idea of plasticity as a central sign of maturational lag:

Plasticity might be observed along a continuum. There are at one end children in whom plasticity is pervasive, ego organization is diffuse, ego boundaries are fluid, and there is trouble with reality testing. At the other end there are those youngsters who are in no way bizarre or deviating, who are able to form meaningful relationships and whose plasticity shows mainly in inability to stabilize perceptual experiences and to maintain a 'linguistic Gestalt'. [P. 477]

In treatment recommendations, she concurred with the perceptual-motor theorists in recommending that reading instruction be postponed until success is achieved with "perceptual-motor" and oral language education (1968).

Another early investigator who followed an independent course was Samuel Kirk who had been at the Wayne Training School even before Strauss and Werner. After some 15 years of clinical experience, much graduate work by students, and a great deal of field testing, Kirk and his colleagues produced the Illinois Test of Psycholinguistic Abilities (Kirk, McCarthy, and Kirk, 1961). This is a battery of 12 subtests utilizing the Osgood model of communication to assess reception and expression, automatic versus representational levels of meaning, in both auditory-vocal and visual-motor channels. Although the test is directed toward assessment of psycholinguistic abilities, five of the items involve visual-motor functioning. In their introduction, the test authors declared that the test would be useful for children labeled "learning disabled," "minimally brain injured," or "perceptually handicapped" in order to get an individual profile to use as the basis for educational remediation.

Educational Impact

Throughout this period there was an increasing emphasis on delineating specific educational techniques for the so-called brain-injured child and there was a corresponding proliferation of educational programs. Many of these started as residential schools, for instance the Cove Schools in Wisconsin directed by Strauss and the Pathway School in Pennsylvania directed by Rappaport. However there were obvious economic and emotional disadvantages to residential treatment and there was a nationwide drive to establish special classes in the community. Cruickshank, et al., (1961) provided a detailed description of special classes for brain-injured and hyperactive children that became a prototype for many such classes. The classroom researched by Cruickshank had specially equipped rooms designed to reduce environmental distractions, and the teaching techniques were highly structured and exacting. At the end of a year, after comparing the experimental group receiving the structured program to the control group receiving the traditional special-class curriculum, they found that the former showed significant improvement on the Bender-Gestalt and the Syracuse Visual Figure Background Test, but it was not possible to evaluate academic achievement since so many could not get base scores on a pre-test. In 1959, a year after the demonstration program ended, follow-up study showed that the experimental group had lost their gains. Other similar programs were evaluated in the public schools. For instance in 1958 the Columbus Board of Education and the Ohio State Division of Special Education started a three year program for brain-damaged children. Class enrollment was restricted to eight pupils, all functioning within the normal range of intelligence. All children were required to have a thorough neurological examination including an electroencephalographic study. The reception of this experimental program was so overwhelming in terms of numbers identified as "needing special education'' and the success of those enrolled that it led to the establishment of standards for ''neurologically handicapped children'' for units throughout the state (Holt, 1962). In the period of 1950 to 1960, many parent groups were formed to press for special education services. Among the first such groups were the Fund for Perceptually Handicapped Children (Evanston, Illinois) and the New York State Association for Brain-Injured Children, both organized in 1957. The California Association for Neurologically Handicapped Children was organized in 1960. The growth of such local organizations was rapid and they were extremely effective in calling attention to these special children.

It is worth noting that there was at this time relatively little interest in drug therapy or special diets; the focus was on education and the target was public school officials. Werner and Strauss provided the theoretical base, neurologists legitimatized the diagnosis, and Cruickshank provided much of the technology. Behavior therapy was yet to be developed as a technique in special education. A former student of Cruickshank, Norris Haring (1965) introduced behavior modification as a means of providing a structured environment. Finding that attention could be maintained by establishing contingency reinforcement procedures, this approach began to take precedence over the special, and somewhat artificial, physical environment originally proposed by Strauss and Lehtinen and developed by Cruickshank.

Critique

This discussion will be limited to the Werner and Strauss studies and their application in practice. One major criticism was the logical fallacy involved in the circular reasoning regarding diagnosis. As Sarason pointed out in 1949, children were included in the exogenous retarded group who exhibited certain behavior characteristics and psychological test results even without positive neurological evidence. So it was not surprising that they showed similar characteristics on psychological measures which overlapped with the original selection criteria. Parenthetically it should be pointed out that the early work of Strauss and Werner demonstrated for all time that retarded children have important individual differences which are independent of the degree of retardation.

The assertions of Strauss, Werner, and colleagues stimulated a great deal of research of a replication nature. Keller (1962) did not obtain the same differences in critical flicker fusion frequency or perception of apparent movement in another study at Wayne County Training School. Also with retarded children, Cruse (1962) did not find that the performance of brain-injured children was more detrimentally affected by increased distraction and Weatherwax and Benoit (1962) found no differences in capacity for abstract thinking between groups. Rubin (1969) found no evidence to support the assertion that mentally retarded, brain-injured children manifest figure-ground pathology. On the other hand the several studies coauthored by Cruickshank and one by Vegas and Frye (1963) did confirm the Werner and Strauss hypothesis. Some theorists suggested that these differences might represent a ''maturational lag'' rather than a basic difference in neurological functioning, citing the work of Kagan. In an experiment involving a task of visual analysis, Kagan (1966) found that with children 6 through 10 years, there was a marked increase with age in correct labeling of the figural component accompanied by poorer recognition of the background component.

There were also numerous studies attempting to evaluate the effectiveness of special education programs emerging from the Strauss work. One of the earliest critiques was that of Gallagher (1957) who worked with matched groups of brain-injured and familial mentally retarded children. He raised serious questions as to whether the differences between the groups were sufficiently great or consistent to warrant using drastically modified educational and training programs for the brain injured. He also described the individual differences within the group of brain injured and the role of personality disturbances in preventing them from reaching their full efficiency. In 1973 Hallahan and Cruickshank did a masterful analysis of some 42 articles appearing between 1965 and 1970 evaluating the effectiveness of one or another form of perceptual-motor training. In their opinion only seven studies were methodologically sound and deserving of close attention. Two of these involved investigation of Delacato's procedures for neurological organization training (O'Donnell and Eisenson, 1969; Robbins, 1966) and were essentially negative. The other studies reported equivocal findings which led the review authors, Hallahan and Cruickshank (1973), to state, "It is obvious that from these few studies little may be concluded concerning the effectiveness of perceptual-motor training, in general, let alone particular programs" (p. 212). After some trial and error, educators found that no one method fit all the problem cases and one began to read more and more about the importance of individual assessment and prescriptive teaching. The one feature which did survive as crucial was the low pupil-teacher ratio, 8:1.

Paralleling the educators' observations that even those children designated as brain injured needed different programs was the mounting evidence against the "unitary concept" of brain damage. In 1947 Strauss and Lehtinen stated that "all brain lesions, wherever localized, are followed by a similar kind of disordered behavior" (p. 20). Some of the psychological refutation of this will be presented in the next section. It became increasingly clear that many of the early statements were over-simplifications of the diagnostic and treatment problems presented by hyperactive or learning disabled children.

During the 1940s and the 1950s, the separation continued between those concerned with organic factors and those concerned with psychological factors. By and large child psychiatrists and clinical child psychologists relegated the "organic" cases to the neurologists and special educators and neglected them much as they ignored the mentally retarded. "Functional" learning problems were studied and treated under the rubric of "underachievement" with emphasis on motivational blocks, family models, disguised aggression, inhibition as a defense against "knowing" or "succeeding," or as the neurotic expression of conflicts displaced from pre-genital functions, such as "taking in" (oral phase), "producing" (anal phase), "exhibiting" (phallic phase), and so on, (Kessler, 1966). In the early 1960s, some few efforts at bridging the gap appeared. Rappaport wrote an article for the *Psychoanalytic Study of the Child* (1961) consisting of a case study of a youngster with major and multiple neurologic symptoms, probably related to kernicterus at birth. The boy had a hearing loss, athetosis, aphasia, and was generally slow with a Cattell IQ of 54 at age 18 months and an Arthur Performance IQ of 60 at age 8 years. Rappaport describes the twice weekly psychotherapy with the boy, the concomitant parent guidance, and the McGinnis method of speech therapy. In his discussion (1961) he states that the behavior disturbance in brain-injured children is

(1) not due solely to damaged brain tissue per se and therefore is not untreatable; (2) is due to a considerable degree to the disturbance which that damage causes in the epigenesis of the ego; (3) the deviant ego maturation fostering a disturbed parent-child relationship that in turn inhibits proper ego development; and (4) disturbances both in ego development and in the parent-child relationship can be alleviated by psychotherapy and adjunctive therapies. [P. 425]

It is interesting that this case is a mentally retarded child because more and more mentally retarded children were excluded from the special designation of "brain injured."

Another early treatment report was provided by Doris and Solnit (1963), describing four nonretarded children with brain damage and a wide variety of associated problems:

In psychotherapeutic work with these children, the principles of verbalization, clarification, and interpretation are the same as in the treatment of the neurotic child without brain damage. However children with a central nervous system deficit often are unable to use thought, memory, and language with as much cathexis and discharge as neurotic children without organic deficits. . . . It becomes necessary to utilize the therapy hour for purposes beyond those of the development of insight and the resolution of internalized conflicts. [P. 631]

They describe the ego handicaps of the brain-damaged child as:

Perceptual impairment; relative inability to postpone discharge or accept substitute gratifications; poor motility control; disturbed body image; defective speech development and control; differentiated or diffuse difficulty in the use of the symbolic process (e.g., a visual-motor handicap or speech deviation); relative inability to transform impulses, i.e., to sublimate and to have available the psychic energies necessary for the trial-action functions of speech, thought or memory; and inability to cope simultaneously with outer stimulation and inner needs. [P. 633]

In both these papers there was no doubt as to the primary diagnosis of brain damage in the children treated. The authors were attempting to elucidate the effect of the brain damage on parent-child relationship and on the normal developmental tasks of childhood.

1960–1968—THE WIDENING WORLD: FROM "BRAIN DAMAGE" TO "MINIMAL CEREBRAL DYSFUNCTION"

The Problem with "Brain Damage"

In 1964 Birch pointed out that the *fact* of brain damage in children and the *concept*, "the brain-damaged child," are two different things.

As a fact, brain damage refers to any anatomic or physiologic alteration of a pathologic kind present in the nerve tissues of the brain. Obviously the functional consequences of such anatomic or physiologic change are most diverse and may range from an entire lack of discernible functional alteration to complete paralysis, amentia, and death. Thus children with cerebral palsy, hemiplegia, mental deficiency deriving from hydrocephalus, epilepsy as a result of cortical scarring, and those who are normally functioning but who have porencephalic cysts all in fact have brain damage. The concept 'the brain-damaged child' does not necessarily apply to all of these children but is, rather, a term that has been used to designate a certain pattern or set of patterns of behavioral disturbance. [Pp. 3–4]

He added that many children with known and independently verified brain damage do not exhibit the patterns of behavior presumably characteristic of "brain damage."

Two extensive review articles dealing with brain damage in children appeared in 1964. Rapin, writing primarily for pediatricians, reiterated the "two-way principle" enunciated by Schilder in 1931:

"The point which the author wishes to make is that hyperactivity, distractibility, and forced responsiveness are not pathognomonic of brain damage, but that they may be seen just as well in functional derangements of the subcortical mechanisms which influence the activity of the reticular formation. In other words, cortical damage with decreased cortico-fugal control of sensory inputs is only one possible explanation for the observed behavior. Increased activity in the reticular formation secondary to anxiety is another. [P. 23]

After lengthy discussion of laboratory research, she reviewed the research on the use of psychologic tests in the assessment of brain-damaged children. This includes scatter or unevenness in intelligence test items; visual-motor tests such as the Bender-Gestalt, Marble Board Tests, Block Design, and Rorschach; and the Halstead-Reitan battery. In general she agreed with the generally pessimistic conclusions of other reviewers regarding the diagnostic specificity of such tests for differentiating between organically and emotionally caused deficits. Herbert's review (1964) was equally critical. Many of the studies reviewed reported significant mean differences between groups but with such an overlap of scores between groups that individual diagnosis would be hazardous. In the discussion Herbert states:

Undoubtedly the major weakness of tests of brain damage is the absence of an adequate theory of brain function upon which they can be based. It is common practice to use the diagnostic tests to make a dichotomous classification of 'brain-damaged' versus 'non-brain-damaged' children. [P. 210]

He quotes Wortis' statement (1957) that:

There is, in short, no 'brain-injured child,' but only a variety of brain-injured children whose problems are quite varied and whose conditions call for more refined analyses than some of the current generalizations on the brain-injured child provide. [P. 206]

Herbert concludes by suggesting that:

Psychologists could make a more valuable contribution by the development and application of tests which describe the various psychological deficits resulting from brain-injuries and which have implications for the academic and social training of the child, rather than by evolving diagnostic tests of dubious clinical value. [P. 212]

One particularly elaborate research study of this question was done by Schulman, Kaspar, and Throne (1965) with a population of 35 mildly retarded adolescent boys attending the Kennedy School for Exceptional Children in Illinois. They correlated eight "indicators" of brain injury: WISC IQ; WISC Scatter; WISC IQ differences (performance versus verbal); Binet Scatter; Bender Gestalt; Draw-a-Person; EEG; and Neurological examination. Nineteen of the 28 correlations were nonsignificant; specifically the neurological examination did not relate significantly to any of the other measures, including the EEG. Those relationships which were found were related to intellectual level rather than amount of damage. They describe the lack of covariance as "disquieting," but acknowledge the restricted range of functioning represented by their retarded population. In their conclusions they state that the only variable which approached unequivocal support as a correlate of brain damage, regardless of extent or location of damage, was distractibility; on the other hand no evidence was adduced to support the hypothesis that hyperactivity is a correlate of brain damage. This led to a second study of 36 school-age children with neurological evidence of brain damage and a control group, both within the normal range of intelligence. Briefly, they found that in three of four distractibility tasks, more brain-injured subjects than control subjects were distractible (but with the inevitable individual exceptions). The activity measures indicated more hyperactivity in the structured situation, but not in the free situation. This lead Kaspar, et al., (1971) to conclude that

> These results support the hypothesis put forth earlier that the effect of brain damage is not to increase the amount of activity a child generates in a free situation, . . . but to make it more difficult for the child to reduce his activity level in situations in which such a reduction is expected or required. [P. 333]

This investigation highlights the problem of reliability in behavioral assessment, for instance with regard to hyperactivity. It also foreshadows a shift of emphasis to the area of attention. In 1971 Dykman, et al., wrote that for learning disability children, "There is a more basic defect than misperception, and this is faulty attention" (p. 57). For explanation they return to the Bender idea of a maturational lag.

> Neurological immaturity could well explain the attentional deficits of learning disability children. . . . One of the most outstanding characteristics of the neurologically immature child is his poor coordination, both gross and fine actions. Motor incoordination can be related to and correlated with faulty attention, we believe, in at least two ways. [P. 89]

In the above quotation, one can see that the search for a unifying common denominator persists. Despite the change in terms and focus, a unitary, neurological explanation is considered. This persistence is all the more remarkable in view of the many discussions regarding the possible variations of brain damage with respect to etiology, extent, type of lesion, locus, duration of damage, time of life, and developmental stage at time of injury. The resultant disorders are equally varied (Birch, 1964). Many professional workers were nonplussed by the continued use of the diagnosis of "brain damaged" as if it were a single phenomenon in the face of so much contrary evidence. Neurologists were loath to call a child brain damaged on the basis of behavior problems or learning difficulties in the absence of corroborating history or independent neurologic evidence. In addition parents were shocked by the diagnosis and concerned about explaining it to the child. All in all despite the excellent educational programs established for the brain-damaged or neurologically handicapped child (nonretarded), many were reluctant to use this presumptive diagnosis simply to gain access to the special education.

Minimal Brain Damage

One solution to the dilemma was to soften the diagnostic impact by attaching the adjective "minimal" to the term "brain damage." Among the first to use this term was the pediatrician-psychiatrist team of Knobloch and Pasamanick (also wife and husband). After examining 500 premature and 492 full-term infants at age 40 weeks, they described a continuum of cerebral damage (1959), ranging from severe abnormalities such as cerebral palsy and mental deficiency, to minimal damage. Minimal cerebral damage was identified in 100 infants (almost 10%) by:

Minor but clearly defined deviations from the normal neurological and behavioral developmental patterns, usually with more or less complete compensation by 15 to 18 months as determined by the standard neurological examination. These developmental abnormal neurological signs persist well into the preschool period but require special techniques and a knowledge of maturity to elicit and interpret them. [P. 1384]

They remarked that perhaps behavior problems in children which have been explained on the basis of tension in their mothers are more the cause than the result of such observed parental tension.

The above study started with differences in neurological status in infancy and projected the behavioral consequences, but Pasamanick and his colleagues investigated the same issue in retrospect as well. They studied the early medical records of about 500 children who had been referred because of behavior problems to the special services division of the Baltimore Department of Education. The frequency of pre- and peri-natal complications in this group was compared with a normal control group of 350 children from the same classrooms matched for race, sex, and birthplace. They found that the behaviorally deviant group as a whole exhibited a statistically significant excess of early complications and that the behavioral syndrome most significantly associated with these complications was hyperactivity. This led them to hypothesize a continuum of reproductive casualty with severe to minimal sequelae (Rogers, Lilienfeld and Pasamanick, 1955; Pasamanick and Knobloch, 1960). In a later critique Werry (1972) pointed out that the quantitative differences were small with considerable overlap between groups. Thus many normal children had early complications and many behaviorally disturbed had none. Nevertheless these studies established the idea of a continuum with regard to both cause and after-effects.

In a discussion of this work, Harrison and McDermott (1972) commented that:

We have found in our clinical experience that the most difficult diagnostic issue involves the question of 'normal organicity.' It is the area in which clinicians often hotly disagree and become polarized in their clinical approaches. While it is crucial that large scale epidemiologic and longitudinal studies such as Pasamanick's continue, it is vital to balance these with individual in-depth studies of children with disorders ascribed to minimal brain damage. [P. 825]

Even a cursory review of the literature will document their statement about the controversy. One specific question bandied back and forth is the value of soft signs in neurologic diagnosis. In 1960, Kennard defined soft signs as those associated with more complex motor behavior and described equivocal signs as those which are slight or inconsistently present, but most workers combine the two categories. Kinsbourne (1973) stated that:

A soft sign is a finding that is normal in a young child but that, in the normal course of maturation, should go away. If it persists unduly long, then it qualifies as an abnormality. It represents a developmental delay or lag in the differentiation of a sensory or motor system. Soft signs have two aspects. On the one hand, a soft sign represents a persistence of a primitive form of response. On the other hand, it represents a failure in a certain performance. [P. 701]

In the absence of uniform criteria for judging soft signs, it is not surprising that reported results have been contradictory. Kennard (1960) reported so many equivocal signs, also in the majority of the control children, that the diagnostic significance is somewhat obscure. Hertzig, Bortner, and Birch (1969) compared the neurologic findings of 90 children attending a special educational facility for the brain injured with 15 controls. In the special group, 29% were reported to have "classical" neurologic syndromes and an additional 65% showed soft signs of central nervous system dysfunction—compared with 6% of the controls. The most frequently occurring soft signs involved disturbances of balance, coordination, and speech. Since a requirement for placement in this program was an independent medical confirmation of the presence of brain injury, the findings are hardly surprising. In a recent study Adams, Kocsis, and Estes (1974) examined 368 fourth graders who were divided into "normal learners," "borderline," and "learning disabled" according to IQ achievement test discrepancies. They found no relationship for most of the soft neurological signs. Graphesthesia and diadochokinesia were significantly depressed in the learning disabled group but the authors concluded that the magnitude of difference was not great enough for clinical usefulness. Again the results are not surprising when one considers the selection of subjects. The learning disabled children in this study were identified on the basis of a statistical definition which rather arbitrarily included almost 40% of all fourth graders! These two studies, which at first seem so divergent in their conclusions, betray the investigators' biases in the differences in methodology. Hertzig, Bortner and Birch (1969) firmly assert that:

> Children labeled 'brain damaged' do in fact have clear evidence of central nervous system abnormality, though of great neurologic heterogeneity. The usefulness of the label, therefore, may be to prevent us from attributing undue weight to the etiologic role of social environment or parental care. [P. 437]

Fifteen years later Adams, Kocsis, and Estes (1974) argue that:

> It is apparent that 9 and 10 year old learning disabled children cannot be reliably distinguished from normally achieving children on the basis of the soft neurological signs outlined in this study. [P. 618]

It is obvious that these latter-day learning disabled children were not the same children as those identified as "brain damaged" in the early days of the "movement."

Minimal Brain Dysfunction

Many agreed with Birch (1964) in his statement that:

> Regardless of any adjectives, we have the overriding obligation to demonstrate, in terms of replicable, valid and clearly defined criteria, that the multiplicity of aberrant behaviors we now attribute to 'minimal brain damage' are, in fact, the result of damage to the brain. [P. 5]

Since this turned out to be an impossible task, a subtle shift in terminology from "minimal brain damage" was proposed by Clements and Peters (1962). In this paper, which forecast an important monograph of the same title published by the National Institute of Neurological Diseases and Blindness in 1966, Clements and Peters decried the tendency, to weave a complete causative fabric out of the fragile threads of stereotypes such as sibling rivalry, rejecting parents, repressed hostility, oedipal conflict, repressed sexuality, etc., much of which may well be secondary and epiphenomenal rather than primary. [P. 185]

They asserted that child guidance workers were prone to assume psychogenicity when no easily recognizable organic deviation could be found and argued for indirect support of organicity on the basis of the following points:

(1) The similarities between the perceptual defects and symptoms of children and adults with known brain damage and children in which a brain-damage history cannot be firmly established, yet who have similar symptoms;

(2) the fact that the symptoms cluster together to make recognizable entities. This is, of course, especially true of the hyperactivity syndrome and specific reading disability, but is also true of the subtler variations that do not fit precisely into these categories;

(3) the statistical studies which show a positive correlation between complications of pregnancy and the incidence of later appearing learning and behavioral symptoms;

(4) the studies of Hallgren (1950) and Hermann (1959) showing that there is a heredity basis for some cases of dyslexia;

(5) organicity as a basis for the clinical entities being discussed is lent support by the fact of the high ratio of males to females for hyperactivity, dyslexia, impulsive acts, etc.;

(6) the good response of most of these children to drugs and remedial instruction without benefit of psychotherapy, if they are detected early enough;

(7) the ever present and oft disparaged fact that innumerable siblings reared under sufficiently equivalent conditions do not show these particular learning and behavior symptoms and that countless children reared under psychopathogenic conditions from the mildest to the most severe do not develop learning and behavior symptoms. [P. 195]

To some extent these points have already been reviewed, but to recapitulate briefly, this line of argument ignores "the two-way principle" that similar difficulties may be caused by a variety of reasons; that certain symptoms would naturally coexist (for example hyperactivity and learning problems) regardless of underlying cause; and that many children with known brain damage or history of perinatal insult do not exhibit the classical syndrome—just as many children appear to be immune to psychopathogenic environmental conditions.

Inevitably articles appeared describing children with the label "minimal brain dysfunction." For example Stevens, et al., (1967) compared 26 children "assigned to the MBD category by a clinical evaluation" with 26 normal controls of the same age, sex, and socioeconomic class. Despite the efforts at control, it is worth noting that 8 of the MBD children and none of the control children were reported as "taken from natural parents before age 5 years" for reasons not stated. On a battery of tests the MBD children were slower to respond, less able to follow verbal instructions, and poorer in tone discrimination and tapping. The difference in Verbal IQ on the WISC was significant in favor of the control children (mean IQ of 114 compared with 103 for the MBD); also the difference in total WISC IQ was statistically significant (113 compared with 102). However the difference in Performance IQ scores was not significant nor was the Verbal-Performance discrepancy different in the two groups. Stevens, et al., (1967) conclude that, "the deficits in performance suggest subtle deviant function of the central nervous system, whether of an acquired or genetic origin" (p. 285).

This study illustrates the dilemma of interpreting IQ differences when comparing a deviant group with a control group. Even when subjects are restricted to those scoring in the broad range of "normal," it is common to find significant overall IQ differences. In fact when IQs are precisely matched, other test differences tend to disappear. There are two possible explanations for the frequently reported mean IQ differences: (1) the effect of the minimal cerebral dysfunction may cause the lower IQ or (2) the other deficits observed in the MBD child may be "normal" for the lower IQ. It is important to note in this connection that when the term "minimal" was affixed to "brain damage" or "brain dysfunction," children with *definite* indications of brain damage were excluded. This led to the paradoxical situation in which children who scored below 80 IQ (for whatever reason) were again considered as a homogeneous, mentally retarded group, taking us back thirty years to the point when Strauss and Werner began their original work!

Although much remained the same with the new term, there was an important conceptual difference in "minimal cerebral dysfunction" with regard to presumed etiology. As suggested in 1962 and amplified in Clements (1966), the possible causes were broadened to include:

Genetic variations, biochemical irregularities, perinatal brain insults, or the results of illnesses and injuries sustained during the years critical for the normal development and maturation of the central nervous system. The definition also allows for the possibility that early severe sensory deprivation could result in central nervous system alterations which may be permanent. [P. 10]

It would have been semantically awkward to speak of genetic variations as a possible cause of brain *damage* (which implies that something has happened to a normal brain), but genetic variations in brain *functioning* are not only possible but probable. Cantwell (1975) gave considerable support to this hypothesis in a careful study of parents of hyperkinetic children. Parents of 50 hyperkinetic and 50 normal comparison children were interviewed at some length. The data indicated that most of the interviewed parents in the control group were free of any psychiatric illness whereas nearly half of the parents of the hyperkinetic children had some psychiatric diagnosis, particularly alcoholism, sociopathy, and hysteria. This study was followed by a similar one evaluating the adoptive parents of 39 hyperkinetic children. The relative absence of psychopathology in these parents compared with the biological parents was cited to support the case for the genetic transmission of the hyperkinetic syndrome. The idea of genetic variations introduces the related concepts of inborn temperament (Thomas, Chess, and Birch, 1968), innate perceptual sensitivities (Escalona, 1968), congenital differences in physiological reactivity (Grossman and Greenberg, 1957), and so on. In discussing the possible antecedents of differences in reflective versus impulsive cognitive styles, Kagan (1966) mentioned "constitutional predispositions."

Since the extremely impulsive boys in our studies were also excessively restless and distractible, it is possible that these children suffered subtle cerebral damage early in life. It is possible, of course, that biological variables, unrelated to central nervous system deficit, predispose some infants and preschool children to hyperactivity and impulsive reactions. [P. 519]

The widening of the etiological lens brings into view many individual differences which, although innate, would justifiably be considered examples of "normal organicity."

Clements (1966) included early deprivation as another possible cause of "minimal cerebral dysfunction" which blurs the distinction between "organic" versus "environmental" etiology. It implies, probably correctly, that fixation in development can occur from organic factors affecting central nervous system maturation, or lack of stimulation in critical periods for learning. Perhaps the mode of interference is not so important as the timing. There are several strands of evidence to support this view. For instance Provence and Lipton (1962) observed behavior in children who had been institutionalized in infancy which closely resembled behavior ascribed to "brain-damaged" children. Goldfarb (1955) examined adolescents who had been institutionalized for their early years and described serious learning difficulties and behavior problems such as hyperactivity, inability to concentrate, and impulsivity which are also reminiscent of the "Strauss syndrome." Cawley (1966) found Head Start children to be severely lagging on tests of eye motor coordination, form constancy, position in space, spatial relations, motor speed, auditory attention, visual attention, language output, and stimulus organization and sequencing—disabilities which he attributed to "developmental lag." In their review of the bioneural results of deprivation, Hallahan and Cruickshank (1973) reported studies which indicated a higher proportion of brain damage in the lower socioeconomic classes although this does not agree with the distribution in public school class enrollment in learning disabilities classes (Franks, 1971). It is probable that a poverty child of minority status with minimal cerebral dysfunction characteristics will test below the cutoff point of 80 IQ and fall into the category of mental retardation. In summarizing this material Hallahan and Cruickshank (1973) point out the many ways that the poor suffer disadvantages and remind us that,

Since all learning is neurologically based, any dysfunction of the neurological system, whether diagnosed, specified, and isolated or not, is of vital importance to the understanding and planning by psychologists and educators who must implement community-based programs for children. [P. 57]

However it is a fact that the diagnosis of "minimal cerebral dysfunction" served to absolve the parents of blame. Both in the original article in 1962 and the 1966 monograph edited by Clements, the alternative to the organic hypothesis is seen as parental mishandling and the parents are therefore to blame. This is a most unfortunate misreading of the psychodynamic point of view. Of course there are some parents who have in fact done a conspicuously poor job of rearing their children (even though some still thrive to an astonishing degree). However child development is a complicated process and there are many failures in which the parents have had only a secondary role. Temperamental differences make one child vulnerable and unable to assimilate an event which is inconsequential for another child. A parent may respond more readily to one child than to another, for many reasons. Fortuitous events such as physical illnesses, family crises, disasters experienced vicariously by the child, experiences initiated by people outside the family, are also important in shaping behavior. Add to all of this the distorted perceptions and misunderstandings created by the primitive thinking and unspoken fantasies of the young child and the inevitability of inner conflict between contradictory drives or wishes. With all that we know about the multiple causation of behavior (normal or abnormal), it is astonishing that we still deal in credit and blame. If one really had only two choices, that is organicity or blame-the-parents, many would lean toward the former even in the absence of real proof (Aronson and Kessler, 1968).

Landmark Conferences

Few topics elicited so much discussion around the conference table as the subject of minimal cerebral dysfunction. Strother (1972) reviewed three conferences concerned with the specific topic of dyslexia but with a wide variety of sponsors. The first was held in 1961 under the auspices of the Association for the Aid of Crippled Children; the second was convened in 1966 by the American Committee on Optics and Visual Physiology and the Neurological and Sensory Disease Program of the United States Public Health Service; the third was held in 1967 under the auspices of the United States Office of Education. This conference recommended the appointment of a national commission which eventually concluded that, "there was no prospect of arriving at a definition of 'dyslexia' which could be accorded general acceptance" (Templeton, 1969). In 1962 the Oxford International Study Group on Child Neurology held a conference addressed primarily to problems of definition and diagnosis. The term "minimal cerebral dysfunction" was recommended in place of "minimal brain damage" primarily on the basis of a consensus at this conference that brain damage should not be inferred from behavioral signs alone.

There were a number of conferences which led to significant publications. For instance Birch's book on brain damage in children (1964) was an outgrowth of a meeting held in 1962 sponsored by the Association for the Aid of Crippled Children. In January 1963 the Easter Seal Research Foundation sponsored a conference at the University of Illinois on children with minimal brain impairment which led to a larger conference in Washington, D. C., with the added sponsorship of the United States Public Health Service Division of Chronic Diseases. A direct outcome of this conference was the establishment of three task forces to prepare papers on different aspects of the problem. The report of Task Force I, published as a monograph of the National Institute of Neurological Diseases and Blindness and edited by Clements (1966), reviewed the problem of identification and terminology. The monograph mentions 38 terms used to describe or distinguish the conditions grouped as minimal brain dysfunction in the absence of findings severe enough to warrant inclusion in an established category, for example cerebral palsies, mental subnormalities, sensory defects. Others could be added to this list, such as "the Dysynchronous child" or "central nervous system deficit." It is interesting that the Task Force III report, edited by Chalfant and Scheffelin (1969), reviewed the research under the title of "Central Processing Dysfunction in Children." The original monograph listed a total of 99 signs and symptoms exhibited by children with minimal cerebral dysfunction, although it recommended that an effort be made to identify more homogeneous subcategories.

Another historically important conference was a seminar on brain-injured children assembled by Cruickshank in October 1965, with 27 experts from a variety of disciplines. While a multitude of concerns was examined, much time was devoted to the most pressing problem encountered during the entire seminar—definition. This topic, more than any other, revealed differences of opinion and provoked heated controversy. Gallagher (1966) urged that these children be identified in educational terms and many complained about the medical bias of "minimal cerebral dysfunction." In a recent review of this seminar, Hallahan and Cruickshank (1973) state:

All told, the results of this discussion on terminology and definition were both promising and discouraging. While the general consensus, especially among educators, pointed to the need for an educationally relevant definition, no such definition was adopted. Nor has any consistent terminology been agreed upon to date. A child in Michigan would be called perceptually handicapped; in New York, brain injured; in California, neurologically impaired or educationally handicapped. In Florida or Maryland, he would be said to have special learning disabilities. [P. 71]

Hallahan and Cruickshank also point out that the conferees' general disposition toward an exclusively behavioral definition (in 1965) reflected the decreasing concern with etiology apparent in their survey of the literature published between 1960 and 1965. Nevertheless the debate continued. As late as 1972 in a conference sponsored by the New York Academy of Sciences and the National Institute of Child Health and Human Development, physicians and educators argued about the very existence of minimal brain dysfunction. The medical group concerned itself particularly with comprehensive diagnosis following a medical model, with the assessment of biological concomitants and antecedents of the condition, and with the role of medical management (for example drug therapy). The educators were concerned primarily with assessment of learning problems and techniques of special education.

Political Resolution: Emergence of Learning Disability

On April 6, 1963, in Evanston, Illinois, Kirk spoke at a conference sponsored by the Fund of Perceptually Handicapped Children, Inc. Among other things, Kirk stated that he had not found medical labels then in current usage to describe children with educational deficits particularly helpful and went on to say:

Recently, I have used the term 'learning disabilities' to describe a group of children who have disorders in development in language, speech, reading, and associated communication skills needed for social interaction. In this group I do not include children who have sensory handicaps such as blindness or deafness, because we have methods of managing and training the deaf and the blind. I also exclude from this group children who have generalized mental retardation.

At that meeting the group voted to organize itself as the Association for Children with Learning Disabilities (ACLD) and a new special education category was born. In 1968 the first annual report of the National Advisory Committee on the Handicapped was published. It provided a definition of learning disability which was an elaboration of Kirk's description in 1963, provided an incidence estimate of 1 to 2 million, and acted as a spur to legislation. The succession of legislative events at the federal level started in 1969 with Senator Yarborough's *Children with Learning Disabilities Act,* and Representative Pucinski's introduction of a similar bill in the House. This act amended *Title VI* of the *Elementary and Secondary Education Act,* known as the *Education of the Handicapped Act of 1967,* by specifically providing authority to the U. S. Office of Education to establish programs for learning disability pupils. The definition adopted by the 91st Congress states that:

> Children with special learning disabilities exhibit a disorder in one or more of the basic psychological processes involved in understanding or in using spoken or written language. These may be manifested in disorders of listening, thinking, talking, reading, writing, spelling, or arithmetic. They include conditions which have been referred to as perceptual handicaps, brain injury, minimal brain dysfunction, dyslexia, developmental aphasia, etc. They do not include learning problems which are due primarily to visual, hearing, or motor handicaps, to mental retardation, emotional disturbance, or to environmental disadvantage.

At about the same time another new term was born, "developmental disabilities," in order to include disabilities which originate before the age of 18 years, are permanent, constitute a substantial handicap, and which are attributable to mental retardation, cerebral palsy, epilepsy, autism, or dyslexia. The crucial difference between "developmental disabilities" and "learning disabilities" is one of degree rather than origin. The recent law, *Education for All Handicapped Children* (P.L. 94–142), established the right of every child, regardless of handicap, to receive free and appropriate education from age 5 through 21 years, in the least restrictive environment with a written individual educational plan. It also spelled out a due process for parents who have questions regarding the placement or educational plan. The individual plan is an effort to get away from the tyranny of categorical labels and homogeneous curricula for heterogeneous groups, but funding still flows according to the channels of diagnostic categories.

For economic reasons, if no other, the arguments about definition go on. In November 1977, a 47-member national task force submitted to Congress and HEW a proposal to sharpen the definition of developmental disabilities by emphasizing the severity and chronicity of handicap rather than the medical label, so that mild mental retardation and epilepsy, for example, would be excluded. In 1977 Hallahan and Cohen discussed the definitional problems of learning disabilities on several scores. They commented on the problem in measuring "psychological processes," assumed to be the core of learning disabilities, and the difficulty with the "exclusion clauses."

> The fact of the matter is that little research has been generated to justify the inclusion of the exclusion clauses. In particular, there is no research to support the claim that the mildly retarded and disturbed and the environmentally disadvantaged differ much from the learning disabled in the behaviors they do and do not exhibit. In light of this, it is not surprising that teaching methods for the mildly retarded and disturbed and the environmentally disadvantaged do not differ widely from those for the learning disabled. [P. 133]

They conclude with a proposal that, "Learning disabilities would now refer to any child with a discrepancy between his performance and potential ability" which is essentially the concept of underachievement in vogue in the 1950s.

This excursion into the present completes a cycle. The theoretically pure idea of learning/behavioral problems related to brain damage was increasingly contaminated by the practical efforts to help more and more children. The concept of minimal brain dysfunction opened the doors wide to bring in children with varied symptoms from equally varied causes. Generic similarities no longer obtained and the urgency of individual planning became obvious. As the educators took over the treatment, with a combination of special teaching methods, low pupil-teacher ratio, and behavior modification techniques, etiologic considerations faded and the child with his individual characteristics emerged.

REFERENCES

Adams, R. M., J. J. Kocsis, and R. E. Estes. "Soft neurological signs in learning-disabled children and controls." *American Journal of Diseases of Children,* 128, 614–618, (1974).

Aronson, L. J., and J. W. Kessler. "Point: Counter point on minimal brain dysfunction." *Clinical Psychologist,* 21(3), 125–128, (1968).

Ayres, A. J. "The development of perceptual-motor abilities: A theoretical basis for treatment of dysfunction." *American Journal of Occupational Therapy,* 17, 221–225, (1963).

Barsch, R. H. *Achieving Perceptual-Motor Efficiency.* Seattle, Wash.: Special Child Publications, 1967.

Bender, L. *A Visual Motor Gestalt Test and Its Clinical Use.* Research Monograph No. 3. New York: American Orthopsychiatric Association, 1938.

——— "Postencephalitic behavior disorders in children," in J. B. Neal, ed., *Encephalitis: A Clinical Study,* pp. 361–385, New York: Grune & Stratton, 1942.

——— "The brain and child behavior." *Archives of General Psychiatry,* 4, 531–548, (1961).

——— "The semantics of childhood aphasia," in *Childhood Aphasia. Proceedings of the Institute on Childhood Aphasia,* pp. 16–32, San Francisco: California Society for Crippled Children and Adults, 1962.

Bender, L. "The concept of plasticity from a neurological and psychiatric point of view." *American Journal of Orthopsychiatry,* 33, 305–307, (1963). [Digest]

——— "A career of clinical research in child psychiatry," in E. J. Anthony, ed., *Explorations in Child Psychiatry,* New York: Plenum, 1975.

Birch, H. G., ed., *Brain Damage in Children: The Biological and Social Aspects.* Baltimore: Williams & Wilkins, 1964.

Blau, A. "Mental changes following head trauma in children." *Archives of Neurological Psychiatry,* 35, 722–769, (1936).

——— "The psychiatric approach to posttraumatic and postencephalitic syndromes." in R. McIntosh, ed., *Neurology and Psychiatry in Childhood. Proceedings of the Association for Research in Nervous and Mental Diseases,* v. 34, pp. 404–424, Baltimore: Williams & Wilkins, 1954.

Bond, E. D., and K. E. Appel. *The Treatment of Behavior Disorders Following Encephalitis.* New York: Commonwealth Fund, 1931.

Bradley, C. "The behavior of children receiving benzedrine." *American Journal of Psychiatry,* 94, 577–585, (1937).

Bradley, C., and M. Bowen, "Anphetamine (benzedrine) therapy of children's behavior disorders." *American Journal of Orthopsychiatry,* 11, 92–103, (1941).

Broca, P. "Remarques sur le siege de la faculte du langage articule, suives d'une observations d'aphemie." *Bulletin de le Societe Anatomique de Paris,* 330–357, (1961).

Burt, C. "Note on the mental after-effects of sleeping sickness in school children." *British Journal of Psychology Medical Section,* 2, 237–238, (1922).

Byers, R. K., and E. E. Lord. "Late effects of lead poisoning on mental development." *American Journal of Diseases of Children,* 66, 471–494, (1943).

Cantwell, D. P. "A model for the investigation of psychiatric disorders of childhood: Its application in genetic studies of the hyperkinetic syndrome," in E. J. Anthony, ed., *Explorations in Child Psychiatry*, pp. 57–81, New York: Plenum, 1975.

Cawley, J. F. *An Assessment of Intelligence, Psycholinguistic Abilities, and Learning Aptitudes among Preschool Children*. Washington, D. C.: Project Head Start, ED–014 –323, 1966.

Chalfant, J. C., and M. A. Scheffelin. *Central Processing Dysfunctions in Children: A review of Research*. NINDS Monograph No. 9. Bethesda, Md.: U.S. Department of HEW, 1969.

Clements, S. D. *Minimal Brain Dysfunction in Children—Terminology and Identification*. NINDB Monograph No. 3. Washington, D.C.: U.S. Public Health Service, 1966.

Clements, S. D., and J. E. Peters. "Minimal brain dysfunctions in the school-age child." *Archives of General Psychiatry*, 6, 185–197, (1962).

Corballis, M. C. "The left-right problem in psychology." *Canadian Psychologist*, 15, 16–33, (1974).

Cruickshank, W. M., and J. E. Dolphin. "The educational implications of psychological studies of cerebral palsied children." *Exceptional Children*, 18, 3–11, (1951).

Cruickshank, W. M., F. A. Bentzen, F. H. Ratzberg, and M. T. Tannhausser. *A Teaching Method for Brain-Injured and Hyperactive Children*. Syracuse, N.Y.: Syracuse University Press, 1961.

Cruse, D. B. "The effects of distraction upon the performance of brain-injured and familial retarded children," in E. P. Trapp and P. Himelstein, eds., *Readings on the Exceptional Child*, pp. 492–500, New York: Appleton-Century-Crofts, 1962.

Dann, M., S. Z. Levine, and E. V. New. "A long-term follow-up study of small premature infants." *Pediatrics*, 33(6), 945–956, (1964).

Dejerine, J. "Contribution a l'etude anatomo-pathologique et clinique des differentes varietes de cecite verbale." *Memoire de la Societe de Biologie*, 4, 61, (1892).

Dencker, S. J. "A follow-up study of 128 closed head injuries in twins using co-twins as controls." *Acta Psychiatrica et Neurologica Scandinavica*, 33, (Supplement 123), pp. 125, (1958).

Doll, E. A., W. M. Phelps, and R. T. Melcher. *Mental Deficiency due to Birth Injury*. New York: Macmillan, 1932.

Dolphin, J. E., and W. M. Cruickshank. "The figure-background relationship in children with cerebral palsy." *Journal of Clinical Psychology*, 7, 228–231, (1951a).

——— "Pathology of concept formation in children with cerebral palsy." *American Journal of Mental Deficiency*, 56, 386–392, (1951b).

——— "Visuo-motor perception of children with cerebral palsy." *Quarterly Journal of Child Behavior*, 3, 198–209, (1951c).

——— "Tactual motor perception of children with cerebral palsy." *Journal of Personality*, 20, 466–471, (1952).

Doman, R. J., E. B. Spitz, E. Zucman, C. H. Delacato, and G. Doman. "Children with severe brain injuries: Neurological organization in terms of mobility." *Journal of the American Medical Association*, 174, 257–262, (1960).

Doris, J., and A. J. Solnit. "Treatment of children with brain damage and associated school problems." *Journal of the American Academy of Child Psychiatry*, 2(4), 618–635, (1963).

Douglas, J. W. B. "Mental ability and school achievement of premature children at 8 years of age." *British Medical Journal*, 1, 1210, (1956).

Drillien, C. M. "Growth and development in a group of children of very low birth weight." *Archives of Diseases of Children*, 33, 10, (1958).

Dykman, R. A., P. T. Ackerman, S. D. Clements, and J. E. Peters. "Specific learning disabilities: An attentional deficit syndrome," in H. R. Myklebust, ed., *Progress in Learning Disabilities*, Vol. 2, pp. 56–94, New York: Grune & Stratton, 1971.

Ebaugh, F. "Neuropsychiatric sequelae of acute epidemic encephalitis in children." *American Journal of Diseases of Children*, 25, 89–97, (1923).

Escalona, S. K. *The Roots of Individuality*. Chicago, Ill.: Aldine, 1968.

Franks, D. J. "Ethnic and social status characteristics of children in EMR and LD classes." *Exceptional Children*, 37(7), 537–538, (1971).

Fraser, M., and J. Wilks. "The residual effects of neonatal asphyxia." *Journal of Obstetrics and Gynaecology of the British Empire*, 66, 748–752, (1959).

Frostig, M., D. W. Lefever, and J. R. B. Whittlesey. "A developmental test of visual perception for evaluating normal and neurologically handicapped children." *Perceptual and Motor Skills*, 12, 383–394, (1961).

Gallagher, J. J. "A comparison of brain-injured and nonbrain-injured mentally retarded children on several psychological variables." *Monographs of the Society for Research in Child Development*, 22 (2), (1957).

————— "Children with developmental imbalances: A psychoeducational definition," in W. Cruickshank, ed., *The Teacher of Brain-Injured Children*, pp. 21–34, Syracuse, N.Y.: Syracuse University Press, 1966.

Getman, G. N., and N. C. Kephart. "The perceptual development of retarded children," Luverne, Minnesota. [Mimeographed]; Lafayette, Indiana: Purdue University, 1956.

Getman, G. N., E. R. Kane, M. R. Halgren, and G. W. McKee. *The physiology of readiness, an action program for the development of perception for children*. Minneapolis: Programs to Accelerate School Success, 1964.

Gibbs, F., E. Gibbs, H. Spies, and P. Carpenter. "Common types of childhood encephalitis." *Archives of Neurology*, 10, 1–11, (1964).

Goldfarb, W. "Emotional and intellectual consequences of psychologic deprivation in infancy: A re-evaluation," in P. Hoch and J. Zubin, eds., *Psychopathology of Childhood*, pp. 105–120, New York: Grune & Stratton, 1955.

Goldstein, K. *After-Effects of Brain Injuries in War*. New York: Grune & Stratton, 1942.

Goldstein, K., and M. Scheerer. "Abstract and concrete behavior: An experimental study with special tests." *Psychological Monographs*, 53(2), Whole No. 239, (1941).

Graham, F. K., C. B. Ernhart, D. Thurston, and M. Craft. "Development three years after perinatal anoxia and other potentially damaging newborn experiences." *Psychological Monographs*. 76(3), Whole No. 522 (1962).

Graham, F. K., C. B. Ernhart, D. Thurston, and M. Craft. "Brain injury in the preschool child: Some developmental considerations." *Psychological Monographs*, 77(10, 11), Whole No. 573 and 574, (1963).

Grossman, H. J., and N. H. Greenberg. "Psychosomatic differentiation in infancy." *Psychosomatic Medicine*, 19, 293–306, (1957).

Hallahan, D. P., and S. B. Cohen. "Learning disabilities: Problems in definition. Behavioral Disorders." *Journal of the Council for Children with Behavioral Disorders*, 2(3), 132–140, (1977).

Hallahan, D. P., and W. M. Cruickshank. *Psychoeducational Foundations of Learning Disabilities*. Englewood Cliffs, N.J.: Prentice Hall, 1973.

Hallgren, B. "Specific dyslexia: A clinical and genetic study." *Acta Psychiatric et Neurologica Scandinavica*, (Supplement 65), pp. 287, (1950).

Haring, N. G., and R. J. Whelan. "Experimental methods in education and management of emotionally disturbed children," in W. C. Morse, ed., *Conflict in the Classroom: The*

Education of Emotionally Disturbed Children, pp. 389–405, Belmont, Cal.: Wadsworth, 1965.

Harrington, J., and F. Letemendia. "Persistent psychiatric disorder after head injury in children." *Journal of Mental Science*, 104, 1205–1218, (1958).

Harrison, S. I., and J. F. McDermott. *Childhood Psychopathology: An Anthology of Basic Readings.* New York: International Universities Press, 1972.

Herbert, M. "The concept and testing of brain damage in children: A review." *Journal of Child Psychology and Psychiatry*, 5(3,4), 197–217, (1964).

Hermann, K. *Reading Disability.* Springfield, Ill.: Thomas, 1959.

Hertzig, M. E., M. Bortner, and H. G. Birch. "Neurologic findings in children educationally designated as 'brain-damaged'." *American Journal of Orthopsychiatry*, 39(3), 437–447, (1969).

Hinshelwood, J. *Congenital Word Blindness.* London: H. K. Lewis, 1917.

Hirsch, K. de, "Specific dyslexia or strephosymbolia." *Folia Phioniatrica*, 4, 231–248, (1952).

———— "Clinical spectrum of reading disabilities: Diagnosis and treatment." *Bulletin of the New York Academy of Medicine*, 44, 470–477, (1968).

———— "The concept of plasticity and language disabilities." *Speech Pathology and Therapy*, 8, 1, (1965). Reprinted in S. G. Sapir and A. C. Nitzburg, eds., *Children with Learning Problems*, pp. 477–485, New York: Brunner/Mazel, 1973.

Hirsch, K. de, and J. J. Jansky. "Early prediction of reading disability," in A. H. Keeney and V. T. Keeney, eds., *Dyslexia*, pp. 21–32, St. Louis, Mo.: Mosby, 1968.

Hohman, L. B. "Post-encephalitic behavior disorders in children." *Johns Hopkins Hospital Bulletin*, 33, 372–375, (1922).

Holt, E. E. *A Demonstration Project for Brain Damaged Children in Ohio.* Columbus: Ohio Department of Education, 1962.

Kagan, J. "Developmental studies in reflection and analysis," in A. H. Kidd and J. L. Rivoire, eds., *Perceptual Development of Children*, pp. 487–522, New York: International Universities Press, 1966.

Kahn, E., and L. H. Cohen. "Organic driveness: A brain stem syndrome and an experience." *New England Journal of Medicine*, 210, 748–756, (1934).

Kaspar, J. C., J. G. Milichap, R. Backus, D. Child, and J. L. Schulman. "A study of the relationship between neurological evidence of brain damage in children and activity and distractibility." *Consulting and Clinical Psychology*, 36(3), 329–337, (1971).

Keller, J. E. "The use of certain perceptual measures of brain injury with mentally retarded children," in E. P. Trapp and P. Himelstein, eds., *Readings on the Exceptional Child*, pp. 485–492, New York: Appleton-Century-Crofts, 1962.

Kennard, M. A. "Value of equivocal signs in neurologic diagnosis." *Neurology*, 16(6), 753–764, (1960).

Kennedy, R. "Prognosis of sequelae of epidemic encephalitis in children." *American Journal of Diseases of Children*, 28, 158–172, (1924).

Kephart, N.C. *The Slow Learner in the Classroom.* Columbus, Ohio: Merrill, 1960.

Kephart, N. C., and A. A. Strauss. "A clinical factor influencing variations in IQ." *American Journal of Orthopsychiatry*, 10, 343–350, (1940).

Kessler, J. W. *Psychopathology of Childhood.* Englewood Cliffs, N.J.: Prentice-Hall, 1966.

Kinsbourne, M. "School problems." *Pediatrics*, 52, 697–710, (1973).

Kirk, S. A. "Behavioral diagnoses and remediation of learning disabilities." *Proceedings of the Annual Meeting Conference on Exploration into the Problems of the Perceptually Handicapped Child.* Evanston, Ill.: vol. 1, pp. 1–7, 1963.

Kirk, S. A., J. J. McCarthy, and W. D. Kirk. *Illinois Test of Psycho-linguistic Abilities, Experimental Edition.* Urbana: University of Illinois Press, 1961.

Klaus, M. H. and J. Kennell. "Mothers separated from their newborn infants." *Pediatric Clinics of North America,* 17(4), 1015–1037, (1970).

Knobloch, H., R. Rider, P. Harper, and B. Pasamanick. "The neuropsychiatric sequelae of prematurity: A longitudinal study." *Journal of the American Medical Association,* 161, 581–585, (1956).

Laufer, M. W. "In Osler's day it was syphilis," in E. J. Anthony, ed., *Explorations in Child Psychiatry.* New York: Plenum, 1975.

Laufer, M. W., E. Denhoff, and G. Solomons. "Hyperkinetic impulse disorder in children's behavior problems." *Psychosomatic Medicine,* 19, 39–49, (1957).

Meyer, E., and R. K. Byers. "Measles encephalitis: A follow-up study of sixteen patients." *American Journal of Diseases of Children,* 84, 543–579, (1952).

Moyer, S. B., and P. L. Newcomer. "Reversals in reading: Diagnosis and remediation." *Exceptional Children,* 43(7), 424–432, (1977).

O'Donnell, P. A., and J. Eisenson. "Delacato training for reading achievement and visual-motor integration." *Journal of Learning Disabilities,* 2, 441–446, (1969).

Orton, S. T. *Reading, Writing, and Speech Problems in Children.* New York: Norton, 1937.

Pasamanick, B., and H. Knobloch. "Syndrome of minimal cerebral damage in infancy." *Journal of the American Medical Association,* 170, 1384–1387, (1959).

——— "Brain damage and reproductive casualty." *American Journal of Orthopsychiatry,* 30, 298–305, (1960).

Paterson, D., and J. C. Spence. "The after-effects of epidemic encephalitis in children." *Lancet,* 2, 491–493, (1921).

Prechtl, H. F. R. The long-term value of the neurological examination of the newborn infant. *Developmental Medicine and Child Neurology,* 2, 69–74, (1960).

Provence, S., and R. C. Lipton. *Infants in Institutions.* New York: International Universities Press, 1962.

Rapin, I. "Brain damage in children," in J. Brennemann, ed., *Practice of Pediatrics,* Vol. 4. Hagerstown, Md.: Prior Publications, 1964.

Rappaport, S. R. "Behavior disorder and ego development in a brain-injured child," in A. Freud, ed., *Psychoanalytic Study of the Child,* Vol. 16, pp. 423–450, New York: International Universities Press, 1961.

Robbins, M. A. "A study of the validity of Delacato's theory of neurological organization." *Exceptional Children,* 32, 517–523, (1966).

Robbins, M. P., and G. V. Glass. "The Doman-Delacato rationale: A critical analysis," in J. Hellmuth, ed., *Educational Therapy,* Vol. II, pp. 321–379, Seattle, Wash.: Special Child Publications, 1969.

Rogers, J., A. Lilienfeld, and B. Pasamanick. "Pre- and para-natal factors in the development of childhood behavior disorders." *Acta Psychiatrica et Neurologica Scandinavica,* (Supplement 102), pp. 157, (1955).

Rubin, S. S. "A reevaluation of figure-ground pathology in brain-damaged children." *American Journal of Mental Deficiency,* 74, 111–115, (1969).

Rutter, M. "The development of infantile autism." *Psychological Medicine,* 4, 147–163, (1974).

Sabatino, D., and H. Cramblett. "Behavioral sequelae of California encephalitis virus infection in children." *Developmental Medicine and Child Neurology,* 10, 331–337, (1968).

Sarason, S. B. *Psychological Problems in Mental Deficiency.* New York: Harper, 1949.

Schachter, F., and V. Apgar. "Perinatal asphyxia and psychological signs of brain damage in childhood." *Pediatrics*, 24, 1016–1025, (1959).

Scheerer, M., E. Rothman, and K. Goldstein. "A case of idiot savant: An experimental study of personality organization." *Psychological Monographs*, 58 (4), Whole No. (1945).

Schilder, P. "Organic problems in child guidance." *Mental Hygiene*, 15, 480–486, (1931). Also in L. Bender, ed., *Contributions to Developmental Neuropsychiatry*, pp. 188–193, New York: International Universities Press, 1964.

Schulman, J. L., J. C. Kaspar, and F. M. Throne. *Brain Damage and Behavior: A Clinical-Experimental Study*. Springfield, Ill.: Thomas, 1965.

Shirley, M. "A behavior syndrome characterizing prematurely born children." *Child Development*, 10(2), 115–128, (1939).

Stevens, D. A., J. A. Boydstun, R. A. Dykman, J. E. Peterson and D. W. Sinton. "Presumed minimal brain dysfunction in children." *Archives of General Psychiatry*, 16(3), 281–286, (1967).

Strauss, A. A. "Diagnosis and education of the cripple-brained, deficient child." *Journal of Exceptional Children*, 9, 163–168, (1943).

Strauss, A. A., and N. C. Kephart. "Rate of mental growth in a constant environment among higher grade moron and borderline children." *Proceedings of the American Association on Mental Deficiency*, 44, 137–142, (1939).

——— "Behavior differences in mentally retarded children as measured by a new behavior rating scale." *American Journal of Psychiatry*, 96, 1117–1123, (1940).

——— *Psychopathology and Education of the Brain-Injured Child*, vol. II, Progress in Theory and Clinic. New York: Grune & Stratton, 1955.

Strauss, A. A., and L. E. Lehtinen. *Psychopathology and Education of the Brain-Injured Child*, 2 vols. New York: Grune & Stratton, 1947.

Strauss, A. A., and H. Werner. "Disorders of conceptual thinking in the brain-injured child." *Journal of Nervous and Mental Diseases*, 96, 153–172, (1942).

Strecker, E. "Behavior problems in encephalitis." *Archives of Neurology and Psychiatry*, 21, 137–144, (1929).

Strecker, E., and F. Ebaugh. "Neuropsychiatric sequelae of cerebral trauma in children." *Archives of Neurology and Psychiatry*, 12, 443–453, (1924).

Strother, C. R. "Minimal cerebral dysfunction: An historical overview." From *Proceedings of the Conference on Minimal Brain Dysfunction*, (March 20–22, 1972). New York Academy of Sciences, in S. G. Sapir and A. E. Nitzburg, eds., *Children with Learning Problems*, New York: Brunner/Mazel, 1973.

Stryker, S. "Encephalitis lethargica — the behavior residuals." *Training School Bulletin*, 22, 152–157, (1925).

Templeton, A. B. *Reading Disorders in the U.S.: Report of the Secretary's (HEW) National Advisory Committee of Dyslexia and Related Reading Disorders*. Washington, D.C.: U.S. Department of HEW, 1969.

Thomas, A., S. Chess, and H. G. Birch. *Temperament and Behavior Disorders in Children*. New York: New York University Press, 1968.

Vegas, O. V., and R. L. Frye. "Effects of brain damage on perceptual motor performance." *Perceptual and Motor Skills*, 17, 662, (1963).

Vernon, M. D. *Backwardness in reading: A study of its nature and origin*. Cambridge, Mass.: Cambridge University Press, 1958.

Weatherwax, J., and E. P. Benoit. "Concrete and abstract thinking in organic and nonorganic mentally retarded children," in E. P. Trapp and P. Himelstein, eds., *Readings on the Exceptional Child*, New York: Appleton-Century-Crofts, 1962.

Werner, H. "Abnormal and subnormal rigidity." *Journal of Abnormal and Social Psychology*, 41, 15–24, (1946).

Werner, H., and M. Bowers. "Auditory-motor organization in two clinical types of mentally deficient children." *Journal of Genetic Psychology*, 59, 85–99, (1941).

Werner, H., and D. Carrison. "Animistic thinking in brain-injured, mentally retarded children." *Journal of Abnormal and Social Psychology*, 39, 43–62, (1944).

Werner, H., and A. A. Strauss. "Types of visuo-motor activity in their relation to low and high performance ages." *Proceedings of the American Association on Mental Deficiency*, 44, 163–168, (1939).

——— "Causal factors in low performance." *American Journal of Mental Deficiency*, 45, 213–218, (1940).

——— "Pathology of figure-background relation in the child." *Journal of Abnormal and Social Psychology*, 36, 236–248, (1941).

Werner, H., and B. D. Thuma. "Critical flicker frequency in children with Brain Injury." *American Journal of Psychology*, 55, 394–399, (1942a).

——— "A deficiency in the perception of apparent motion in children with brain injury." *American Journal of Psychology*, 55, 58–67, (1942b).

Werry, J. S. "Organic factors in childhood psychopathology," in H. C. Quay and J. S. Werry, eds., *Psychopathological Disorders in Childhood*, New York: Wiley, 1972.

Wortis, J. "A note on the concept of the 'brain-injured' child." *American Journal of Mental Deficiency*, 61, 204–206, (1957).

PART TWO

Demography of Minimal Brain Dysfunctions

CHAPTER 3

Epidemiology

Lillian Belmont

This chapter is concerned with a review of studies which have reported the prevalence of conditions which can be subsumed under the general rubric, "minimal brain dysfunction." Our focus is solely on population studies and does not deal with the very extensive research found in the clinical literature on minimal brain dysfunction. We shall begin by dealing with two issues: a definition of epidemiology and a definition of minimal brain dysfunction.

DEFINITIONS

Epidemiology

The definition of epidemiology has been modified over time; current definitions (MacMahon and Pugh, 1970; Susser, 1973) are the ones which guide this presentation. MacMahon and Pugh (1970) define epidemiology as "the study of the distribution and determinants of disease frequency in man." Susser's (1973) definition of epidemiology is somewhat broader: "the study of the distributions and determinants of states of health in human populations." Common to all definitions is the focus on populations, because within the population one should be able to enumerate all instances of the condition under study, not, for example just the instances of those who seek medical assistance.

In brief the epidemiologic approach attempts both to determine the relative frequency (rate) of a condition by relating the number of cases to an appropriate total population, and also to study how rates vary according to such variables as age, sex, social class, ethnicity, and geography. Epidemiologic study should answer two questions: (1) How prevalent is the condition under study? and (2) Is the relative frequency of the condition the same or different between the young and the old, between males and females, between those in the country and those in the city, among (or between) social classes? This phase of epidemiologic study is called descriptive epidemiology. Its intent is to describe the prevalence of a condition in the population and to determine how the rate varies according to certain standard independent variables.

The second phase of epidemiologic study is called analytic. Knowing the distributions of rates according to the kinds of variables enumerated above (age, sex, social class, and so on), hypothesized determinants (causes) may be studied in order to test whether particular variables are causally associated with a given condition. Such hypothesized causal relationships are briefly mentioned in our discussion.

55

We define a rate (relative frequency) as the number of cases (numerator) divided by the number in the population (denominator). "Cases" refer to individuals with the condition under study. A "case" is a quick way of specifying the child who has the diagnosis "minimal brain dysfunction" or a cognate term.

Classic epidemiologic studies dealt with well-defined conditions, in that the diagnosis was clear or indisputable, for example mortality. Morbidity, illness or disability, poses a difficulty for all endeavors: What should be considered evidence of morbidity (caseness)? In addition to the critical issue, case definition, epidemiologists, as well as other workers, try to be alert to biases which may have been introduced into the findings because of such factors as low response rate and self-selection of individuals. Such considerations guide the review of the studies that are presented.

This chapter is concerned with the descriptive epidemiology of minimal brain dysfunction. Epidemiology is concerned with disordered states of health, broadly conceived. For our purposes we should be able to assume that minimal brain dysfunction represents such a disordered state of health.

Minimal Brain Dysfunction

It is beyond our scope to trace the evolution of the term, "minimal brain dysfunction." Instead we start with the report (Clements, 1966) issued as a result of the meeting of a task force of experts[1] who discussed and attempted to come to some agreement on the definition of the term. Views were polarized as to underlying etiology and what emerged was the following definition:

> The term 'minimal brain dysfunction syndrome' refers . . . to children of near average, average, or above average intelligence with certain learning or behavioral disabilities ranging from mild to severe which are associated with deviations of function of the central nervous system. [The disabilities may be shown by] various combinations of impairment in perception, conceptualization, language, memory and control of attention, impulse, or motor function. [Further, during the school years,] a variety of learning disabilities is the most prominent manifestation of the condition which can be designated by this term." [Pp. 9–10]

Symptoms and signs of minimal brain dysfunction culled from the literature were listed under 15 different categories. The 10 most frequent characteristics were: hyperactivity, perceptual-motor impairments, emotional lability, general coordination deficits, disorders of attention, impulsivity, disorders of memory and thinking, specific learning disabilities, disorders of speech and hearing and equivocal neurological signs, and EEG irregularities. Clements (1966) pointed to the "protean" nature of the disability and urged the specification of subcategories within minimal brain dysfunction, such as reading retardation and hyperkinetic syndrome.

The unspecific nature of the definition of MBD was further compounded by later elaboration offered by other workers. Wender (1971, 1975) stressed behavioral problems, including hyperactivity, impulsivity, difficulties in interpersonal relations; and/or perceptual-cognitive problems, learning disorder or impaired learning in school. In fact Wender (1971) indicated that "a substantial fraction of

---

[1] A similar polling of the opinions of British experts is contained in a volume which appeared in 1963 (MacKeith and Bax).

MBD children (of the order of magnitude of one-half to two-thirds) manifest learning difficulties in school" (Wender, 1971). In contrast Clements and Peters (1973) argued that the educational term for minimal brain dysfunction is specific learning disability (SLD); and learning disability is also said to have behavioral manifestations (Dykman, Peters and Ackerman, 1973). Most recently, Cantwell (1977) described the hyperkinetic syndrome as a set of behaviors "with no implications of etiology," that is not necessarily associated with CNS deviations. In addition to the cardinal symptoms of hyperactivity—distractibility, impulsivity, and excitability—other symptoms which are often present include cognitive and learning difficulties. According to Cantwell, "learning difficulties are of major importance in the hyperkinetic syndrome" (p. 527). The terms MBD, SLD, and hyperkinesis appear to be at least overlapping conditions, or at worst different descriptions of the same group of children.

Not surprisingly no simple, valid, reliable, and uniformly accepted tool is currently available which could be put to use in a study of the prevalence of this overinclusive condition. According to Wender (1975) "there is no critical test for MBD." Senf (1973) after reviewing various definitions of learning disability concluded that *none* of the many definitions are "sufficiently detailed to enable reliable diagnosis." Eisenberg (1972) pointed out that the diagnosis of hyperkinesis, or minimal brain dysfunction, "depends upon clinical acumen; there are no pathognomonic findings."

It is apparent then that the investigator who studies the condition has unclear guidelines as to the kind of child who should be included in a count.

To study the extent of the condition and its variations, it is left to the investigator to define an appropriate population and decide on some operational definition of the condition under study. Therefore difficulties were also involved in our selection for review of studies that fit the conditions somehow related to minimal brain dysfunction.

SELECTION OF STUDIES FOR REVIEW

We did not locate a single study of the prevalence of minimal brain dysfunction as such. One recent report (Nichols, et al., 1976) was concerned with presumed symptoms of MBD. Two studies (Prechtl and Stemmer, 1962; Wolff and Hurwitz, 1966) of a neurologic sign, choreiform movements, were included here because such data have been used as evidence of MBD (Wender, 1971). Because of the blurred boundaries between MBD and learning disability on the one hand and between MBD and hyperactivity on the other, it seemed reasonable to review studies of both learning disability and of hyperactivity. A total of 12 studies were included.

The general features of the studies are presented in three tables, which summarize:

1. Case definitions and populations studied (Table 3–1).
2. The demographic characteristics of the cases (Table 3–2).
3. Other relevant findings (Table 3–3).

PREVALENCE OF MINIMAL BRAIN DYSFUNCTION

The prevalence of minimal brain dysfunction has been estimated to be 5 to 10% (Wender, 1971). The higher figure derives in part from the inclusion of the choreiform syndrome (Prechtl and Stemmer, 1962) as evidence of minimal brain dysfunction (see Table 3–1). The study was considered by us to contain insufficient information to serve as an estimate of prevalence.

In the course of a report on 50 children seen for neurologic evaluation, Prechtl and Stemmer (1962) devoted one paragraph to the presence of the choreiform syndrome or movement, muscle twitches present when subject stood still with eyes closed, in "children at ordinary schools." The paragraph begins with the undocumented statement, "In another study . . . additional evidence is accumulating" which suggested that those with the choreiform syndrome are "poor readers at school and show a highly significant lower performance in school compared to a control group" (p. 122). Other problems (for prevalence estimates)

Table 3–1.   Case Definitions and Characteristics of Populations Studied for Prevalence Rates

Study and Location	Diagnosis and Case Definition	Population (N)				Prevalence
		Total	Boys	Girls	Age/Grade	
Prechtl and Stemmer (1962) Netherlands	Choreiform movement and described as "poor readers"	?	876	671	no information	Boys: 5% severe 15% slight. Girls: 1% severe, 4% slight
Wolff and Hurwits (1966) Newtown, Mass.	Choreiform movement	872	463	409	10–12 years Grades 4–6	11.4%
Nichols, Chen, and Pomeroy (1976) Collaborative perinatal project	MBD syndrome: "abnormal" on neurologic, achievement, and hyperactivity factor scores	29593 approx. =			Grades 1 and 2	0.2% (N=54)
Silverman and Metz (1973) U.S. schools	Specific learning disability: number of pupils (a) receiving and (b) requiring special services as reported by principals	2% sample of U.S. elementary and secondary schools				(a) 1.4% (b) 2.6%
Rutter, Tizard, and Whitmore (1970) Isle of Wight, U.K.	Specific reading retardation: reading 28 months or more below level of predicted reading age	2334 approx. =			9–11 years	3.7%

Study and Location	Diagnosis and Case Definition	Population (N)				Prevalence
		Total	Boys	Girls	Age/Grade	
Myklebust, Killen, and Bannochie (1971) Illinois; 4 participating school systems	Learning disability: learning quotients 84 or below. Borderline: learning quotients 85–89	2767 approx. =			Grades 3 and 4	Total 8.2% (Learning disability = 4%) (Borderline = 4.2%)
Meier (1971) 8 Rocky Mountain states; "representative stratified sample;" 20 locations	"Individual" learning disability: those teacher thought "were having unusual difficulty in learning"	2400	not given		7–11 years Grade 2	15% (?) 11.8% (?) 4.2% (?)
Werner, et al., (1968) Kauai, Hawaii	Hyperkinetic symptoms: "unable to sit still, marked inability to concentrate, distractible, extremely irritable"	750	369	381	10 years	5.9%
Miller, Palkes, and Stewart (1973) Suburb near St. Louis, Mo. 4 schools	Hyperactivity: those called hyperactive and distractible by teacher; plus at least 5 other symptoms	849	440	409	Grades 3–6	5.5%
Krager and Safer (1974) Baltimore Co., Md., elementary schools	Hyperactivity: child receiving psychotropic medication for hyperactivity in 1971 and in 1973	70,554 (1971) 65,897 (1973)	not given		elementary grades	1.07% (1971) 1.73% (1973)
Lambert, et al., (1978) 2-county area, San Francisco metropolitan area	Hyperactivity: as defined by home, by school, and by physician	5212	2793	2519	Grades K-5	1.19% (3 sources) 3.30% (school only)
Bosco and Robin (1978) Grand Rapids, Mich. 1/2 of school system; grades K–9	Hyperkinesis: Physician diagnosed reported by (a) parent and (b) teacher	7250 approx. =			Grades K–9	2.92% (parent) 3.18% (teachers)

include: no age or grade information; the proportion of those with the neurologic sign is read from a bar graph; a selection bias may exist—876 boys and 671 girls are in the elementary school, whereas the number of boys and girls are approximately equal in most school populations; and the degree of association between the presence of the neurologic sign and associated learning difficulties cannot be evaluated.

Following Prechtl and Stemmer (1962), Wolff and Hurwitz (1966) reported that the prevalence of choreiform movements among "normal" 10-to 12-year-old children in the fourth through sixth grade was 11.4% (99 cases). The rate among boys was 17.2% and among girls 5%, a sex ratio of 3.4 to 1.

Wolff and Hurwitz (1973) later reported on the "functional implications" of the presence of unequivocal choreiform movements for minimal brain damage in a group of 95 boys and 25 girls who were 10 and 11 years old, presumably identified in the course of their prevalence study of choreiform movements (Wolff and Hurwitz, 1966). It is not clear how there could be more cases (N=120) than had been identified in the prevalence study (99). The investigators concluded that the cases did not differ from a sex, age, and social class matched control group on measures of IQ or achievement. Critical to note is that the presence of the neurologic sign was not associated with objective measures of intelligence or achievement. Some differences between the cases and controls were culled from teachers' comments (school records); there were significantly fewer "favorable reports" for cases and certain behaviors were more often noted in the records of the cases. However since teacher reports might not note "significant" behaviors if they did not interfere with classroom activities, these findings of more subtle behavioral differences are only suggestive.

Nichols, Chen, and Pomeroy (1976) focused on the frequency of the association among three symptoms which served as indicators of minimal brain dysfunction. They used data from the 7-year examination of over 29,000 children followed as part of the Collaborative Perinatal Project.[2]

The children were given a psychological examination, including WISC, Wide Range Achievement, Bender Gestalt. A behavioral record form consisting of 15 behavioral items was filled out by the psychologist who had administered the psychological tests. At about the same time (that is age seven) children were given a neurological examination.

Nichols, Chen, and Pomeroy (1976) used these relatively independent ratings— test scores, results of neurological examination, and psychologists' behavior ratings—to study the association among often-cited indicators of minimal brain dysfunction. After rescoring and recalculating achievement scores controlling for grade level and IQ, the data from the various sources were factor analyzed.

Four factors were defined. The first, called low achievement, contained loadings from the psychometric measures. The second, called hyperactivity, contained items from the behavioral observations as did the third, called immaturity.

[2] The Collaborative Perinatal Project is a large scale investigation described as a "prospective investigation of relationships between adverse conditions surrounding birth and neurological and cognitive deficits in infancy and early childhood" (Broman, Nichols, and Kennedy, 1975). Women enrolled in 12 hospitals during their pregnancies were studied and the children of these pregnancies were evaluated during the first year of life, at ages three, four, and seven. Chapter 2 of Broman, Nichols, and Kennedy contains a detailed description of the study.

Table 3–2.   Rates by Sex, Age/Grade, Social Class, and Other Variables

Study	Sex: Male/Female	Age/Grade	Social Class (Income, Occupation)	Other Variables
Prechtl and Stemmer (1962)	4:1	——	——	——
Wolff and Hurwitz (1966)	3.4:1	No difference	——	——
Nichols, Chen, and Pomeroy (1976)	3.5:1	——	Generally similar findings across race and sex groups	——
Silverman and Metz (1973)	——	Rate higher in elementary school	Rates higher in schools in low income areas, especially at secondary level (3.3% vs. 1.2%)	——
Rutter, Tizard, and Whitmore (1970); Rutter and Yule (1975)	3.3:1	Rate higher at 14 years than at 9–11 years	Overrepresented among social class III, manual	6 to 8% in London 10 year olds
Myklebust, Killen, and Bannochie (1971)	4.1:1 (learning disability) 1.9:1 (borderline)	——	——	——
Werner, et at., (1968)	2.7:1	——	No difference by social class	Rate associated with "educational stimulation" at home
Miller, Palkes, and Stewart (1973)	6.8:1	No consistent pattern by grade	——	——
Krager and Safer, (1974)	——	——	Rates higher in above median income schools	Rates higher for schools with special classes
Lambert, et al., (1978)	6.8:1 (3 sources) 8.0:1 (school)	Highest rate: grade 4 Highest rate: grade 3	Higher proportion of cases from "low" occupational level	Higher rate for school-identified blacks, grades 3–5
Bosco and Robin (1978)	3.7:1	5–11 years = 1.29% (Total = 2.92%)	No difference by social class (Duncan scale)	——

The fourth factor contained items from the neurologic examination. Similar findings were reported by Werry (1968) for clinic cases of hyperactive children.

The population consisted of 29,593 children—the proportions of blacks and whites and of boys and girls were approximately equal—all of whom were in either first or second grade at the time of testing. In defining the "MBD cohort" all children with IQs below 80, those with cerebral palsy or other major neurological abnormality were excluded, presumably to fit the definition of MBD (Clements, 1966). A cutoff point of 8% at the left of the distribution was used to identify separately those who were "abnormal" for low achievement, hyperactivity, and neurologic signs.

Of 29,593 children who had complete information (test scores, behavioral observations, and neurologic examination) about 1% were "abnormal" for any combination of two factors: 0.7% abnormal on low achievement and neurologic signs, 0.9% abnormal on hyperactivity and neurologic signs, 1% abnormal on hyperactivity and low achievement. Only *54 children* (42 boys, 12 girls) or 0.2% of the children were "abnormal" on all three factors. The association among symptoms of this MBD syndrome occurs with very low frequency.

These findings were in the first report of an ongoing analysis. MBD symptoms have also been related (Nichols, 1977*a*, 1977*b*) to antecedent events, perinatal complications and aspects of the children's test behavior during the eight months of psychological evaluation (see Table 3–3). The strength of the study is that a very large nonclinic population was studied using independent ratings. A possible problem is that prevalence is predetermined by the particular cutoff point used.

PREVALENCE OF LEARNING DISABILITY

The prevalence of learning disability in the United States population has been variously estimated from 1 to 30%; for legislative purposes it "was recommended that 1 to 3% of the school population be considered as the prevalence estimates, at least until research provides objective criteria for identifying these children more clearly" (Lerner, 1976).

Estimates of SLD, from a U.S. Office of Education 1970 survey, were based on the responses of 85% of the principals of 2000 sampled schools (Silverman and Metz, 1973); the principals were asked to "estimate the number of learning disabled pupils" in their schools and to include conditions, such as perceptual handicaps, brain injury, minimal brain dysfunction, and so on, but to exclude, among others, mental retardation and "environmental disadvantages." A complication is that principals are likely to have their own different interpretations of what SLD includes, which will affect their estimates (Senf and Grossman, 1975). A lower estimate, 1.9% elementary school and 1% secondary school, was based on the number of learning disabled students receiving some sort of special instruction. A higher estimate, 3.1% for elementary school, also included those children who were learning disabled but were not receiving any special instruction. Rates were

Table 3–3.   Other Findings

Study	IQ and/or Achievement Test Scores	Behavioral Rating	Medical and/or Neurologic Findings
Wolff and Hurwitz (1966, 1973)	Boys: No difference from controls in IQ or achievement test scores. Girls: Significant difference from controls (-11.5 points) in IQ *favoring cases:* no difference in achievement test scores	Cases had fewer "favorable" reports and somewhat more "unfavorable" reports	——

Table 3–3. Other Findings—*continued*

Study	IQ and/or Achievement Test Scores	Behavioral Rating	Medical and/or Neurologic Findings
Nichols (1977 *a*, 1977 *b*)	Statistical association between low Bayley scores and abnormal MBD factor scores; those with high Bayley motor scores at decreased risk of abnormal MBD factor scores; low predictive power	Statistical associatiors between speed, intensity, duration of response, etc., and abnormal MBD factor scores; low predictive power	Statistical association of some "perinatal factors" with abnormal MBD factor scores: low predictive power
Rutter, Tizard, and Whitmore, (1970); Rutter and Yule (1975)	Mean IQ 102.5, approximately 109 in general population; N.S.	Boys: (teacher questionnaire) Poor concentration: 84% Overactive: 40% Fidgetiness: 40% 1/3 exhibited anti social behavior. Higher than general population	Possible neurologic abnormality (18.6% vs. 13% for controls; N.S.). Poor complexity of language (15.1% vs. 6.2%, p (.01)
Myklebust, Killen, and Bannochie (1971); Myklebust (1973)	Mean IQ:LD = 104, borderline = 106; control group, mean IQ not given; cases lower on all IQ and achievement measures than controls	Those with emotional disturbance excluded; cases "less independent" than controls	EEG: 25% abnormal (cases) vs. 27% (controls). Neurologic: over all classification of "abnormal" — 50% cases vs. 37% control; N.S.
Meier (1971)	284 LD cases, lower on all quotients than controls; significance levels not reported. Among subset of 101 children: PPVT 93 for cases vs. 104 for controls	Short attention span, distractibility, reads slowly, substitutes words: items checked for at least 2/3 of 284 children. Among 101 children: 20% hyperactive, 40% general behavior problems, 65% "high strung"	Some comparisons between 101 cases and 19 controls — Soft neurologic signs: 90% vs. 75%; Organic brain syndrome: 95% vs. 55%; Lags in development: 25% vs. 5%; Prematurity: 20% vs. 5%. No significance level reported
Werner, et al., (1968)	——	——	Severity of perinatal stress was not associated with hyperkinetic symptoms
Miller, Palkes, and Stewart (1973)	Mean IQ of cases (N=22) 12 points lower than control boys. Only 3 of 6 girls had IQ scores	——	——

63

higher for schools in low income areas than for schools in other areas, especially pronounced among secondary schools, 3.3% versus 1.2%.

The Isle of Wight[3] prevalence survey (Rutter, Tizard, and Whitmore, 1970) was concerned with a number of handicapping conditions including "specific reading retardation." Those identified by screening tests were given individual examinations including a short WISC (four subtests) similarities, vocabulary, block design, object assembly; and the Neale Analysis of Reading Ability, an oral reading test which has quantitative scores on rate, accuracy, and comprehension.

Rutter, Tizard, and, Whitmore, (1970) distinguished two kinds of poor reading: (1) *reading backwardness* was defined as a reading age score for accuracy or comprehension which was at least 28 months below the child's chronological age; (2) *specific reading retardation* was defined as a reading age score which was at least 28 months "below the level predicted on the basis of the child's age and short WISC IQ." The prediction of expected reading age was achieved by the use of regression equations. The distinction comes from the generally accepted notion that more intelligent children should do better in school than less intelligent children.

The equations used to predict expected reading age were developed using the short WISC and the reading scores of 147 randomly selected control children. Since the multiple regression analysis was based on only 147 children, on statistical grounds the prediction of expected achievement may not have been reliable (Thorndike and Hagen, 1969).

The specificity with which the concept of specific reading retardation was elaborated may be useful in clarifying who are learning disabled. There were 155 backward readers (prevalence = 6.64%) and 86 children with specific reading retardation (prevalence = 3.68%). The 155 backward readers were composed of: 79 mainly low IQ children who were reading 28 months or more below their CA; and 76 essentially normal children who were reading 28 months or more below their CA *and* were also reading at least 28 months below predicted reading age, based on IQ. Thus the 76 children also formed a large part of the specific reading retardation group.

The specific reading retardation group of 86 children, 66 boys and 20 girls, was made up of 70 children who had IQs just about average, 10 high IQ children identified solely on the basis of discrepancy of 28 months from predicted reading age and 6 low IQ (borderline) children.

The mean IQ of the 86 children was 102.5 (Rutter and Yule, 1975). Thus the specific reading retardation group was mainly composed of those with *severe*, at least 28 months, reading retardation who were of average intelligence, and thus would be expected to be functioning better at school. These children were also poor in spelling and arithmetic. Note that on the Isle of Wight few children with very high IQs were found to have specific reading retardation.

---

[3] The Isle of Wight study (Rutter, Tizard, and Whitmore, 1970) was a comprehensive epidemiologic survey. A two-stage process was used to estimate the prevalence of handicapping conditions—intellectual, educational, psychiatric, and neuropsychiatric—among the total population of 9- 11-year-old children. Group tests of intelligence and achievement were used to screen for intellectual and educational retardation. Parents' and teachers' questionnaires were used to screen for behavioral symptoms. Children who were identified by screening procedures were individually examined by the study team as were a subset of children not identified by the screening procedures. This summary of procedure necessarily short-circuits the many solved and unsolved issues considered in the conduct of the survey.

Rutter and his colleagues (1970) presented data on behavioral characteristics of the specific reading retardation group, from teachers' and parents' questionnaires, as well as the rate of psychiatric disorder among them (Table 3–3).

More recently using a similar regression equation, but not as detailed an individual examination of the children, the Isle of Wight study of specific reading retardation was replicated in an area of London (Berger, Yule, and Rutter, 1975; Rutter and Yule, 1975); the rate was higher than among Isle of Wight children. Some of these data are presented in Tables 3–2 and 3–3.

The remaining two studies of learning disability (Myklebust, Killen, and Bannochie, 1971; Meier, 1971) used the learning quotient developed by Myklebust (1968), a measure of underachievement, or ratio of actual achievement to expected achievement. The learning quotient lacks specificity in that there is no indication of the actual degree of achievement inadequacy, making it difficult to interpret the meaning of any given prevalence estimate. Of two children who have the same low learning quotient for example, one with a high IQ will be more able in reading than another with an average IQ who may be severely reading retarded. Unlike the Isle of Wight model, there is no built-in standard of what constitutes severe retardation.

Myklebust (1973) screened a total population of 2767 third- and fourth-grade children in four Illinois school systems; these school systems were said to represent "average to high-average opportunity for learning." On the basis of the screening tests he reported that 15% of the school population were underachievers, that is had learning quotients below 90 (Mylkebust, 1973). He then excluded children with "sensory impairments, mental retardation, emotional disturbances or obvious motor disorders." Myklebust stated that the remaining children (N=228; prevalence = 8.2%) had either a WISC Verbal or Performance IQ of 90 or above. The children were divided into two groups: (1) borderline group of 116 children (76 boys and 40 girls) and (2) learning disability group of 112 children (90 boys and 22 girls). Separate control groups were used, one for each of the above groups. The controls were of the same sex, same classrooms, and "were equivalent socioeconomically."

The borderline group had learning quotients (LQs) between 85 and 89, whereas the LQs of the learning disability group were 84 or lower. The LQs of 85 or less or of 85–89 had to be present on *one* or more of 21 selected tests. The control children "had to attain an LQ of 90 or above on all of the 21 test criteria." The 21 tests used in selection are not reported. Thus the method assured that the control groups would be homogeneous with respect to achievement, whereas the learning disabled groups would be quite heterogeneous with respect to achievement, deficient on only one or more of 21 different tests.

The mean WISC IQs of the borderline and learning disability cases were said to be 106 and 104 respectively; the IQs of controls were not reported, although the control groups' mean performance on *all* measures, IQ subtests and achievement scores, were clearly superior to those of the cases. It was not possible to determine on achievement measures, for example reading comprehension age score, whether the differences between the learning disabled and control groups represented any significant degree of retardation. The difference between the groups was occasionally large, 2.7 years difference between the learning disability group and the control group. Since reading level and IQ were confounded however, it was not possible to determine the contribution of either reading or IQ to the final difference.

The children, cases and controls, were also given EEGs, neurologic and opthalmologic examinations (see Table 3–3).

A potentially informative, frequently cited study of the prevalence of learning disability among second-graders (Meier, 1971) is uninterpretable. There were a number of unexplained features concerning the nature of the learning disabled group: ages ranged from 7 to 11 years among second graders, there was no information on the number of boys and girls or on social class. Moreover the differential diagnosis is suspect: the learning disabled group achieved a mean learning quotient of 94.8 which is above the standard of 85–89 for borderline and of 84 or below for learning disabled children (Myklebust, 1968).

The most serious problem is that a variety of prevalence figures can be inferred from the report, with Meier's summary indicating a rate of 15%. Teachers identified 478 children as having "unusual difficulty in learning" from "approximately" 2400 second-graders. However 117 were excluded for what would appear to be low IQ and/or cultural disadvantage. The remaining 361 children (15%) were considered by the author as cases who were to be followed up with individual psychological examination for differential diagnosis: 77 of these children were lost to followup. The remaining 284 children (11.8%) were called "bona fide" learning disability cases. Yet a smaller group of 101 children (4%) could be defined as the learning disabled group, learning quotients essentially below 90.

Puzzling was Meier's (1971) report that

There was a larger percentage of subclinical ('soft') neurological signs manifest among the experimental group (about 90%) as compared to the controls (about 75%) or 'normal' children in general . . . [and] . . . about 95% of the ILD children were classified in the organic brain syndrome category, compared to about 55% of the controls." [P. 15]

While the differences between groups are in the expected direction, the high rate among the normal controls raises questions of interpretation.

PREVALENCE OF HYPERACTIVITY

Prevalence figures of hyperactivity (for example Cantwell, 1977) and of minimal brain dysfunction have come from the same studies. Five studies are reviewed in this section; two of them (Werner, et al., 1968; Krager and Safer, 1974) were not directly concerned with the prevalence of the condition but were included nonetheless because rates can be inferred from them.

The informative study by Werner, et al., (1968) was included here because others have cited it in the context of prevalence estimates of hyperactivity. The report refers to a prospective follow-up study of 750 Hawaiian children, all 10 years old (born in 1955). Their status was assessed in a comprehensive fashion using data collected from a variety of sources including schools and parents.

Information from comprehensive screening and subsequent examinations was used to make decisions on the presence of a number of different problems, such as school achievement, intellectual and emotional problems including hyperkinetic symptoms. Hyperkinetic symptoms were identified through behavior checklists, presumably from parents and teachers and from personality tests. The prevalence of hyperkinetic symptoms in this population was 5.9%. Hyperkinetic symptoms occurred more frequently among boys (8.7%) than among girls (3.2%), a sex ratio of 2.72 to 1. Since the focus of this review is on the prevalence of hyperactivity, the many other important findings of this study are not reported.

A similar rate (5.5%) was reported by Miller, Palkes, and Stewart (1973) who studied the prevalence of hyperactivity in four elementary schools of a suburban school system near St. Louis. Third- through sixth-grade teachers were first asked to identify those of their pupils who showed fidgetiness, restlessness, inattentiveness, and so on. Later the senior author interviewed the teachers individually using a standard questionnaire. A child was classified as hyperactive if the teacher considered him to be both overactive and distractible and had 5 or more symptoms from a 28-item list, which included 3 items on school achievement. A total of 47 children (41 boys and 6 girls) of 849 were classified as hyperactive. Hyperactivity was approximately seven times more common among boys than among girls. The rates for boys varied between 5.8% and 12.6% across the grades, but not in any systematic fashion. The mean IQ of the hyperactive boys was in the normal range but significantly lower than that of a control group (see Table 3–3).

Additional information which was inherent in the data but was not reported includes: the number of hyperactive children who were also doing poorly scholastically, (learning disabled); the number of initially selected fidgety, and so on, children who after formal questioning were not regarded as hyperactive by the teacher—which would have given some indication of possible teacher overestimation of the condition; differences in the contribution of individual teachers to prevalence (rater bias?).

Krager and Safer's (1974) report "on the use of medication for hyperactivity" by elementary school children was included as an indication of a minimum prevalence estimate of hyperactivity, that is only the proportion of treated cases.[4] School nurses submitted lists of names of children at given elementary schools known to be receiving medication for hyperactivity.

The major finding was that in 1971 1.07% of the public elementary school population was on medication for hyperactivity, whereas in 1973 the rate had risen to 1.73%. The rise was also noted in the parochial schools (0.35% versus 0.62%). Rates were higher in schools located in above median income areas than in those located in below median income areas.

Those schools which had special education classes had an above average proportion of children on medication at the two time periods (1.5% in 1971; 2.3% in 1973). This finding is meant to suggest that the proportion of hyperkinetic children is larger in special classes than in regular elementary school classes. The kinds of special classes included are not given.

It has been argued (for example Huessy, 1976; Lambert, et al., 1978; Bosco and Robin, 1978) that not all children remain hyperactive over time. Thus for our purposes it would have been useful to know the proportion of new cases, on medication in 1973, and the proportion of old cases, on medication at both times, represented in the 1973 rate.

Lambert, Sandoval, and Sassone in California and Bosco and Robin in Michigan are conducting extensive surveys of hyperactivity; initial data are available from both of these studies.[5]

---

[4] This chapter is not directly concerned with medication for hyperactivity. Recent reviews of this issue include Lambert, et al., 1978; Sprague and Gadow, 1976.

[5] I should like to thank both groups of workers for making their manuscripts available for inclusion in this chapter.

Lambert, Sandoval, and Sassone, (1978) prepared a detailed report of how prevalence varied according to who made the designation of hyperactivity: parents, school personnel, and/or physicians. The study refers to hyperactivity among a representative population of over 5000 children, in kindergarten through fifth grade (191 classes) during the 1973-1974 school year, who were attending public, private, and parochial schools in two California counties.

Three sources—parents, schools, and physicians—were systematically canvassed in order to identify all children who were considered to be hyperactive. Such a designation required: (a) from the parent a response to a letter and an affirmative response to an interview question regarding the presence of hyperactivity; (b) from the physician a diagnosis of hyperactivity, hyperkinesis, or minimal brain dysfunction with hyperactivity, or a prescription for stimulant medication, and (c) from school personnel their opinion that the child was hyperactive.

Parents had to agree to participate in the study. Thus to some unknown extent those enumerated were self-selected by the parents' willingness to participate in the study. If a parent refused to be interviewed after being contacted by the school or by the physician, such a child was considered to be hyperactive by one or two sources, school and/or physician, but not by home.

Rates are reported for each source separately and for combinations of sources. The most inclusive designation of hyperactivity was the one in which all three sources—parent, school, physician—considered the child to be hyperactive. The overall rate was 1.19% (62 children); rates ranged from 0.59% (5 children) in the third grade to 1.49% (13 children) in the fourth grade.

An additional 3.3% of the children were considered hyperactive by the school only. Lambert, et al., (1978) suggest that peaks in prevalence are related to critical periods in the child's life at school: first entry, stress on achievement from third grade on.[6] All other rates (for example parent only, physician-school, parent-physician, and so on) taken together account for less than 0.5%.

Rates of hyperactivity varied by sex, grade in school, occupational and ethnic status (see Table 3–2).

Bosco and Robin (1978) recently studied the prevalence of physician-diagnosed hyperkinesis as reported by parents and teachers of kindergarden through ninth-grade children in Grand Rapids, Michigan. Questionnaires were sent to parents requesting varied information, including whether their child had ever received a medical diagnosis of some variant of minimal brain dysfunction or hyperactivity or learning disability, or if medication or some other treatment had been prescribed. Information on family structure and parent occupation was also obtained. Teachers were sent questionnaires and asked to report anonymously the number of children who had been medically diagnosed as hyperkinetic using the same set of terms as were given to parents.

Questionnaires were returned by 7250 parents, a 67% response rate. From these returns a prevalence rate for hyperkinesis of 2.92% (167 boys and 45 girls) was reported. This was the rate for "ever-diagnosed" children and the authors estimated that the current rate, including children treated in the last five years, was probably about 2%. It should be noted that, while the parent response rate may be

---

[6] Lambert, et al. indicated that teacher estimates of hyperactivity require more careful attention since in a separate behavior-temperament survey the teachers identified many more children than previously identified as hyperactive (7.75%) while omitting approximately one-half of those so designated previously.

considered relatively high, one-third of the target population did not respond. This may introduce bias of an unknown extent.

Bosco and Robin (1978) report that the rate for children between the ages of 5 and 11 years, 1.29%, is similar to that found by Lambert, et al., (1978).

Teachers (75% response rate) reported that 3.18% of the children had been physician-diagnosed as hyperkinetic. Children were not identified and the authors were unable to verify the diagnosis. The authors believe however that parents and teachers were referring to the same children.

When teachers were themselves asked to identify children with symptoms of hyperkinesis, an additional 3.6% were enumerated. Similarly in response to the Conners Parent-Teacher Questionnaire, parents rated an additional 5% of children as hyperkinetic, that is two or more standard deviations (SD) from mean. However it would be important to know whether these children were considered to be "problems" by their parents. Rates did not vary by social class in this study (Table 3-2).

Frequently in the studies of hyperactivity a physician's diagnosis without elaboration served as the only case definition. Whether the criteria used for identifying a child as hyperactive are the same or different depending on the source (physician, parent, teacher) has not been reported but may become available from the two ongoing studies (Lambert, et al., 1978; Bosco and Robin, 1978).

An unknown number of parents with hyperactive children may not have responded to requests for information for perfectly understandable reasons. However those who do not respond may differ in significant ways from those who do (Cox, et al., 1977). In previous times it was possible to estimate the bias such underreporting might introduce. Recognition of the ethical responsibility of investigators to assure protection of privacy of subjects makes it exceedingly difficult to make such estimates now (Gordis, Gold, and Seltser, 1977).

SUMMARY

General Findings

Basically two findings were consistent across studies: (1) There was a preponderence of males with minimal brain dysfunction, learning disability, or hyperactivity. Such sex ratios have been observed for many conditions, including learning and behavior disorders (Bentzen, 1963). The meaning of the considerably higher rates for boys than for girls is poorly understood (Rutter, Tizard, and Whitmore, 1970); (2) Rates of MBD (one study) and of hyperactivity were frequently lower than rates of learning disability. Except for the sex ratio, no firm generalizations emerged across studies for other demographic characteristics (see Table 3-2), two of which are next discussed.

Demographic Variables

Age and/or grade data, where present (two studies of learning disability), indicated that the rate of learning disability tended to be higher among older children. In contrast across studies of hyperactivity no consistent pattern by grade was found. However in two of three studies of hyperactivity there is the possibility that rates were higher among older children, but different age ranges were examined across studies.

Not all studies reported variations in rates by social class. What indications are available from learning disability studies suggest that rates are higher in low income areas and among working class groups. Studies of hyperactivity presented conflicting information partly due to different methods used to assess social class.

UNRESOLVED ISSUES

Table 3–3 presents whatever additional findings were available from a few of the prevalence studies. We have used these data to speculate concerning both underlying etiology ("cause") and the definition of syndromes (overlap).

"Cause"

In this section we examine the available evidence that relates to "cause" either through concurrent associations with a given condition or through associations with events antecedent to the condition.

In three of the learning disability studies neurologic and/or medical data were reported. The learning disabled groups in all cases had a higher proportion of children with some kind of neurologic abnormality than was found in control groups; none of these differences were reported to be statistically significant however. Thus the evidence suggests that neurologic involvement is not a necessary concomitant of learning disability (see Wolff and Hurwitz, 1973).

Two studies reported on the associations between antecedent events and current symptoms. Nichols (1977a) found statistically significant associations between some perinatal factors and "abnormal" MBD factor scores at age seven years. However these associations had low predictive power. Thus on the one hand "most of the children with low birth-weight were not affected" (did not have abnormal MBD factor scores), and on the other hand, "most of the affected children did not have low birthweights." Similar conclusions emerged concerning associations between MBD factor scores and Bayley test scores (and behavior ratings) obtained when the children were eight months old. These were findings based on univariate analyses; multivariate analyses are now in progress.

Werner, et al., (1968), using a much smaller sample, found no association between the severity of perinatal stress and hyperkinetic symptoms at age 10 years.

Thus from prevalence studies, the issue of the associations between neurologic "risk factors" and behavioral/learning problems is an unresolved one.

Same or Different Condition?

When minimal brain dysfunction, learning disability, and hyperactivity were reviewed, the blurred definitions suggested either overlapping conditions or different descriptions of the same children. Throughout the review of individual studies we looked for evidence of overlap.

Children with Learning Disability

All three studies (Rutter, Tizard and Whitmore, 1970; Myklebust, 1968; Meier, 1971) found learning disabled children at some, frequently minor, disadvantage in terms of IQ. However we found both the Myklebust and Meier studies unsatisfactory in sorting out the IQ characteristics of learning disabled children.

Children with specific reading retardation (Rutter, Tizard and Whitmore, 1970) were rated as overactive, fidgety, and as showing concentration problems significantly more frequently than the general population, over 2000 girls and boys were rated; this finding emerged from both teacher and parent questionnaires and for both boys and girls. Meier (1971) noted that short attention span and distractibility were rated as present for over two-thirds of 284 "bona fide" (teacher identified) learning disability cases; no comparative data on controls were provided. Mylkebust (1973) considered the learning disabled "less independent" (immature?) than controls.

Thus a safe speculation is that children with specific reading retardation, or those called learning disabled, or underachievers share characteristics of those defined as hyperactive.

Children with Hyperactivity

The data here tend to be more circumstantial; the connection between hyperactivity and learning problems tended to be mentioned indirectly. Across studies there was a tendency in one way or another to suggest a link between hyperactivity and learning problems. Thus, for example poor achievement was included among possible rated symptoms used to define hyperactivity (Miller, Palkes, and Stewart, 1973) and rates of medication use were higher in schools with special education classes (Krager and Safer, 1974). We speculated that the finding that the largest proportion of children with hyperkinetic symptoms was found in homes with low educational stimulation (Werner, et al., 1968), might suggest a link between school achievement problems and hyperkinetic symptoms. Lambert, et al., (1978) did not specifically mention learning problems in the diagnostic terms listed in the prevalence study. But we inferred that such problems might have been included because a survey of medical practitioners conducted in the same area as the prevalence study showed that the diagnosis most frequently used for hyperactive children was "hyperactive—learning—behavior disorder, etiology unknown" (Sandoval, Lambert, and Yandell, 1976).

Thus we speculated that there may be a substantial, though partial, overlap in children designated as learning disabled or hyperactive. Perhaps the ongoing California and Michigan studies will be able to estimate the extent of the overlap.

Rates

Another way of looking at possible overlap among conditions is to consider overall prevalence. Rates for MBD and for physician-diagnosed hyperactivity were found to be lower than rates for learning disability. However when the rate of hyperactivity included teacher judgment, it was similar to that reported for learning disability. This trend is particularly clear in the California study (Lambert, et al., 1978) in which the rate (1.19%) becomes considerably higher once the independent designation of hyperactivity by schools is included (1.19% + 3.30%). From this perspective questions may be raised concerning definition, which may be related to the different professional concerns of education and of medicine. Teachers for example may designate as hyperactive those children whose predominant difficulty is learning. This may be done because "hyperactive" has the connotation of learning problems for them or because such a designation may represent a more direct referral for medical intervention. Alternatively teachers see all the children while physicians see only those selected cases referred to them. In any case the rates for the "two" conditions are similar.

POSTSCRIPT

We located only one prevalence study of MBD. Studies which specifically included "minimal brain dysfunction" among diagnostic terms purport to be studies of hyperactivity, and in one case a study of learning disability. This suggests that investigators have been avoiding an undefinable condition (MBD) and have been attempting to replace it with a condition (hyperactivity) which descriptively appears to have specific behavioral referents. It is unclear how specific "hyperactive" is when used in prevalence studies. Researchers, if not clinicians, appear to have discarded the term minimal brain dysfunction. Thus one cannot legitimately write of the "epidemiology of minimal brain dysfunction," nor can its prevalence be determined. Certainly for research, minimal brain dysfunction has not been a useful concept.

REFERENCES

Bentzen, F. "Sex ratios in learning and behavior disorders." *American Journal of Orthopsychiatry*, 33, 92–98, (1963).

Berger, M., W. Yule, and M. Rutter. "Attainment and adjustment in two geographic areas. II. The prevalence of specific reading retardation." *British Journal of Psychiatry*, 126, 510–519, (1975).

Bosco, J. J., and S. Robin. "Hyperkinesis: How common is it and how is it treated?," in C. K. Whalen and B. Henker, eds., *Hyperactive Children: The Social Ecology of Identification and Treatment.* New York: Academic Press, [1978] in press.

Broman, S., P. L. Nichols, and W. A. Kennedy. *Preschool IQ: Prenatal and Early Developmental Correlates.* Hillsdale, N.J.: Erlbaum, 1975.

Cantwell, D. P. "Hyperkinetic syndrome," in M. Rutter and L. Hersov, eds., *Child Psychiatry—Modern Approaches*, p. 524–555. Oxford: Blackwell, 1977.

Clements, S. D. *Minimal Brain Dysfunction in Children—Terminology and Identification.* NINDB Monograph No. 3. Washington, D.C.: 1966.

Clements, S. D. and J. E. Peters. "Psychoeducational programming for children with minimal brain dysfunctions," in F. F. de la Cruz, B. H. Fox and R. H. Roberts, eds., *Minimal Brain Dysfunction*, pp. 46–51. New York: New York Academy of Sciences, 1973.

Cox, A., M. Rutter, B. Yule, and D. Quintan. "Bias resulting from missing information:

Some epidemiological findings." *British Journal of Preventive and Social Medicine*, 31, 131–136, (1977).

Dykman, R. A., J. E. Peters, and P. T. Ackerman. "Experimental approaches to the study of minimal brain dysfunction: A follow-up study," in F. F. de le Cruz, B. H. Fox, and R. H. Roberts, eds., *Minimal Brain Dysfunction*, pp. 93–108. New York: New York Academy of Sciences, 1973.

Eisenberg, L. "The clinical use of stimulant drugs in children." *Pediatrics*, 49, 709–715, (1972).

Gordis, L., E. Gold, and R. Seltser. "Privacy protection in epidemiologic and medical research: A challenge and a responsibility." *American Journal of Epidemiology*, 105, 163–168, (1977).

Huessy, H. R., and A. H. Cohen. "Hyperkinetic behaviors and learning disabilities followed over seven years." *Pediatrics*, 57(1), 4–10, (1976).

Krager, J. M., and D. J. Safer. "Type and prevalence of medication used in the treatment of hyperactive children." *New England Journal of Medicine*, 291, 1118–1120, (1974).

Lambert, N. M., J. Sandoval, and D. Sassone. "Prevalence of hyperactivity in elementary school children as a function of social system definers." *American Journal of Orthopsychiatry*, 48, 446–463, (1978).

Lambert, N. M., M. Windmiller, J. Sandoval, and B. Moore. "Hyperactive children and the efficacy of psychoactive drugs as a treatment intervention." *American Journal of Orthopsychiatry*, 46, 335–352, (1976).

Lerner, J. W. *Children with Learning Disorders*, 2nd ed. Boston: Houghton Mifflin, 1976.

MacKeith, R., and M. Bax, eds., *Minimal Cerebral Dysfunction—Papers from the International Study Group Held at Oxford, September 1962*. Little Club Clinics in Developmental Medicine No. 10, 1963.

MacMahon, B., and T. F. Pugh. *Epidemiology: Principles and Methods*. Boston: Little, Brown, 1970.

Meier, J. H. "Prevalence and characteristics of learning disabilities in second grade children." *Journal of Learning Disabilities*, 4, 1–16, (1971).

Miller, R. G., Jr., H. S. Palkes, and M. A. Stewart. "Hyperactive children in suburban elementary schools." *Child Psychiatry and Human Development*, 4, 121–127, (1973).

Myklebust, H. R. "Learning disabilities: Definition and overview," in H. R. Myklebust, ed., *Progress in Learning Disabilities*, Vol. I, pp. 1–15. New York: Grune & Stratton, 1968.

——— "Identification and diagnosis of children with learning disabilities: An interdisciplinary study of criteria," in S. Walzer and P. H. Wolff, eds., *Minimal Cerebral Dysfunction*, pp. 55–77. New York: Grune & Stratton, 1973.

Myklebust, H. R., J. Killen, and M. Bannochie. "Learning disabilities and cognitive processes," in H. R. Myklebust, ed., *Progress in Learning Disabilities*, Vol. II, pp. 213–251. New York: Grune & Stratton, 1971.

Nichols, P. L. "Minimal brain dysfunction: Associations with perinatal complications." (Paper presented at the Biannual Meeting of the Society for Research in Child Development, New Orleans, March 1977*a*.)

——— "Minimal brain dysfunction: Associations with behavior in infancy." (Paper presented at the 85th Annual Convention of the American Psychological Association, San Francisco, August 1977*b*.)

Nichols, P. L., T. C. Chen, and J. D. Pomeroy. "Minimal brain dysfunction: The association among symptoms." (Paper presented at the 84th Annual Convention of the American Psychological Association, Washington, D.C., September, 1976.)

Prechtl, H. F. R., and C. J. Stemmer. "The choreiform syndrome in children." *Developmental Medicine and Child Neurology*, 4, 119–127, (1962).

Rutter, M. and W. Yule. "The concept of specific reading retardation." *Journal of Child Psychology and Psychiatry*, 16, 181–197, (1975).

Rutter, M., J. Tizard, and K. Whitmore. *Education, Health and Behavior*. London: Longman, 1970.

Sandoval, J., N. M. Lambert, and W. Yandell. "Current medical practice and hyperactive children." *American Journal of Orthopsychiatry*, 46, 323–334, (1976).

Senf, G. M. "Learning disabilities." *Pediatric Clinics of North America*, 20, 607–640, (1973).

Senf, G. M., and R. P. Grossman. "State initiative in learning disabilities: Illinois Project SCREEN, Report III: Local and state opinion regarding the concept of learning disabilities." *Journal of Learning Disabilities*, 8, 587–596, (1975).

Silverman, L. J., and A. S. Metz. "Numbers of pupils with specific learning disabilities in local public schools in the United States: Spring 1970," in F. F. de la Cruz, B. H. Fox, and R. H. Roberts, eds., *Minimal Brain Dysfunction*, pp. 146–157. New York: New York Academy of Sciences, 1973.

Sprague, R. L. and K. D. Gadow. "The role of the teacher in drug treatment." *School Review*, 109–140, (November 1976).

Susser, M. W. *Causal Thinking in the Health Sciences: Concepts and Strategies in Epidemiology*. New York: Oxford, 1973.

Thorndike, R. L., and E. Hagen. *Measurement and Evaluation in Psychology and Education*, 3rd ed. New York: Wiley, 1969.

Wender, P. H. *Minimal Brain Dysfunction in Children*. New York: Wiley, 1971.

—— "The minimal brain dysfunction syndrome." *Annual Review of Medicine*, 26, 45–62, (1975).

Werner, E. E., J. M. Bierman, F. E. French, K. Simonian, A. Conner, R. S. Smith, and M. Campbell. "Reproductive and environmental casualties: A report on the 10-year follow-up of the children of the Kauai pregnancy study." *Pediatrics*, 42, 112–127, (1968).

Werry, J. S. "Studies on the hyperactive child: IV. An empirical analysis of the minimal brain dysfunction syndrome." *Archives of General Psychiatry*, 19, 9–16, (1968).

Wolff, P. H., and I. Hurwitz. "The choreiform syndrome." *Developmental Medicine and Child Neurology*, 8, 160–165, (1966).

—— "Functional implications of the minimal brain damage syndrome," in S. Walzer and P. H. Wolff, eds., *Minimal Cerebral Dysfunction in Children*, pp. 105–115. New York: Grune & Stratton, 1973.

CHAPTER 4

Follow-up of Children with Minimal Brain Dysfunctions: Outcomes and Predictors[1]

Malcolm M. Helper

When told that their child has MBD, parents frequently ask, "Will he (or she) grow out of it?" To give a useful answer the professional needs to know both the outcome of the condition generally and the factors to consider in making a prediction for the individual child. Even more importantly he needs to know what treatments, if any, can be expected to make a difference in longer term course of the child's problems. Finally the professional needs to have a theoretical model from which to work in answering these practical questions and in designing further research on longer term outcome.

This chapter summarizes available studies regarding the course and later status of children diagnosed as having MBD or one of its subtypes. In so doing it also examines rather carefully and critically the research methods used in this very difficult area. Finally it offers interpretation of the meaning of the findings for practice and for further research.

SELECTION AND PRESENTATION OF STUDIES

In attempting to select follow-up studies related to MBD, one is immediately faced with problems posed by the diffuseness of the concept and by the great variety of terms referring to the condition and its symptoms, problems well documented elsewhere in the volume. For this chapter it was necessary to decide which follow-up studies had a sample which could reasonably be called MBD. It was decided at the outset that studies of children labelled either hyperactive or learning disabled would be included in the review, even if they had only the behavioral or only the cognitive-perceptual symptoms, and even if the authors did not use the generic diagnostic category MBD. Studies of the following kinds of subjects were eliminated from detailed review:

1. Perinatal risk only. Follow-up studies of children identified as at-risk for brain dysfunction only by a history of perinatal problems were not included. Whatever its merits in simplicity and objectivity, the use of a single historical fact as a basis for diagnosis of MBD has not characterized

[1]The author gratefully acknowledges the assistance of Steven Feldgaier in locating publications for this chapter.

the field. In any event Sameroff and Chandler (1975) have recently presented an excellent review of the consequences of perinatal insult.

2. Underachievement only. The line between learning disability and underachieving is often blurred in studies of clients of reading clinics. Children in these clinics may not be well evaluated for neurological and perceptual problems, and the samples may therefore intermix children having information processing deficits with children failing to read for other reasons. Where there was doubt the study was included in this review.

3. Major brain insult. Most of the studies that were included clearly stipulated that children with major brain damage had been excluded from the group followed up; a few clearly included some such subjects along with more traditionally defined cases of MBD. Such studies were included.

4. Mental retardation. The studies reviewed varied in the IQ adopted as a lower limit. Eighty was the most frequently used low-end cutoff point, though some studies used 70, and at least one (Koppitz, 1971) evidently included children scoring in the 60s. Preston and Yarington (1967) included at least one child scoring in the 50s. Other studies did not assess IQ at all. Studies which involved a small minority of retarded children, or children of unknown intelligence, were not excluded from this review, provided the subjects had been otherwise diagnosed as MBD, hyperactive, or learning disabled.

Appropriateness of sample aside, the following characteristics eliminated a study from further consideration:

5. Follow-up interval less than two years. Short term studies of the effects of drug, educational methods, counselling, and so on, were excluded. The study by Sleator, von Neumann, and Sprague (1974) was not tabulated because of the short duration of the follow-up interval at the time of that report. With the passage of time information on the longer term development of children taking stimulant medication is likely to come out of this prospective study.

6. Lack of systematic assessment of MBD. Studies which relied solely on history obtained at follow-up to make retrospective diagnosis of MBD (for example Hammar, 1967; Shelley and Riester, 1972) were excluded. Also excluded were studies in which subjects' old records were not approached with preset criteria of MBD (Robins, 1977; Mellsop, 1972) valuable as these studies are for providing insight into the fate of other diagnostic groups. Anecdotal reports were also excluded.

7. Sample size smaller than 10. Reports of individual cases or of small series of cases were not included.

8. Side effects of medication. Studies concerning the longer term effects of stimulant drugs on physical growth are not considered in detail. Growth retardation was considered an outcome of medication, not of hyperactivity.

In practice determining which studies fell within the above guidelines did not prove difficult, as the authors of work fitting them almost always made clear their interest in some concept of MBD.

Tabulation of Data

The literature search described above yielded 33 studies. Salient facts about subjects and methods used in each of the studies are listed in Table 4–1.

For Table 4–1 entries were necessarily abstracted from a much larger quantity of information, necessitating the exercise of some judgment by the author. Further exercise of judgment was called for by the fact that the different studies reported widely varying types of information, especially in regard to initial diagnosis and interim events.

Studies are grouped first by age of subject at time of follow-up. Studies in which most subjects were 12 and under at follow-up are presented first, those in which they are mostly between 12 and 18 come next, and those in which the majority are 19 and over are presented last. As will be seen the largest number of studies concern adolescents; only five had a majority of subjects 12 and under at follow-up and only five concerned subjects 19 and over. Within each of these age groupings, studies are arranged according to most prominent symptom picture or subtype of MBD at time of diagnosis. Studies in which the children were initially selected for learning difficulties are listed first, followed by those concerning children whose behavioral problems predominated at diagnosis.

METHODOLOGICAL ASPECTS OF FOLLOW-UP STUDIES

In addition to summarizing the methodological features of the various studies, this section will add interpretative comments.

Subject Characteristics

Sex Ratios

Samples are uniformly male dominated and generally lopsidedly so. In studies which are not limited by design to boys, ratios range from 64 male, 4 female (Weiss, et al., 1971) to 34 male, 13 female (Eaves and Crichton, 1974–1975). Only one study (Trites and Fiederowicz, 1976) considered a group of girls (N=10) separately. Few of the other studies indicate whether their small contingents of girls exemplify the same pattern of outcome as the boys, who by sheer weight of numbers must mainly determine it.

Age

Studies listed vary somewhat in regard to the age of children at diagnosis. In general studies done in a clinical setting selected children averaging about eight years of age, for example Minde, Weiss, and Mendelson, (1972); Weiss, *et al.*, (1971); Gottesman, Belmont, and Kaminer (1975); Riddle and Rapaport (1976); Silver and Hagin (1964); and so on. Studies done in schools on regular class pupils tended to have a very narrow age range as investigators tended to select single classes or grade levels. Huessy and Cohen (1976) thus started with a cohort of all of second graders in a set of schools in Vermont. The youngest cohort of subjects at diagnosis was a group of four-year old nursery school children followed up by

Table 4–1. Subjects and Measures Used in Follow-up Studies of Children with Learning Disability and/ or Hyperactivity

	Subjects				Follow-up		
Reference	Cases	Controls	Age	IQ	Interval	Method	Treatment
A. Subjects mostly 12 years and under at follow-up:							
1. Subjects selected mainly for reading disability:							
Rourke and Orr (1977)	19M 1st and 2nd graders below 21st centile on MAT Reading test	23M in same grades above 49th centile on same test	M=92 months range= 87–100 months for both groups	M=101 for cases 108 for controls	4 years	Tests	None reported
Hinton and Knights (1971)	57M, 10F referred to pediatric neuro-logist for school learning problems	None	M=9.8, range = 6–14 years	M=96, range = 80–125	M=36, months; range = 24–44 months post diag-nosis	Inter-view, school records	28 got educational help, 25 drugs, 10 psycho-therapy
Eaves and Crichton (1974–1975)	34M, 13F patients referred to medical clinic; 39 diagnosed as MBD	None	5–8 years	——	4–6 years post diag-nosis at average age 12.2 years, range 9.1–13.9	Inter-view, ques-tion-naire	Special educational help for 79%
Yule (1973)	73 Ss reading 2.4+ years be-low level ex-pected for age; ("backward"); 71 backward readers whose reading level is also 2.4+ years below that ex-pected for IQ and age combined ("retarded")	184 non problem readers from same classes selected at follow-up. Sex not reported for any group	9–11 years	At follow-up only; M=86 for backward, 98 for back-ward-retarded group	4 to 5 years	Tests. ——	None reported
2. Subjects selected mainly for hyperactivity:							
Minde, et al., (1971)	34M, 3F from hospital clinic diagnosed as "severe, sus-tained hyper-activity"	34M, 3F classmates selected at follow-up	M about 7 years	Cases M=101; controls 112 at follow-up. All 85 or above at outset	4–6 years post diag-nosis, at about 12 years of age	School records, teacher ratings	Some tutoring, some drugs
Riddle and Rapaport (1976)	72M from Pediat.O.P. Clinic diag-nosed as hyperactive; SES was middle class	57M from schools retested at follow-up	M=about 8 for cases; 10.6 at follow-up for controls	Not given	2 years, when cases average 10.6 years	Tests; ratings; inter-views	Stimulant drugs for all; special education, psycho-therapy for majority
Campbell, Endman, and Bernfeld (1977)	12M, 3F from nur-sery school (M of SES is 33 for cases, 27 for controls (Hollingshead)	14M, 2F from same nursery school	M=47 months for cases and 48 months for controls	M=104 for cases, 111 for controls	M=46 months for both cases and controls	Class obser-vation, ratings, self-esteem test	No drugs 2/15 hyper-active, 1/16 controls in special class

Reference	Cases	Controls	Age	IQ	Interval	Method	Treatment
			Subjects			**Follow-up**	

B. Subjects mostly 12–18 years at follow-up:
1. Subjects selected mainly for learning disorders:

Reference	Cases	Controls	Age	IQ	Interval	Method	Treatment
Balow (1965)	131 (20%F) in 3 school summer reading classes for learning disorder children	One untutored learning disorder group	Group mean range 10.5–12	Group mean range 100–110	2–4 years after diagnosis	Tests	Remedial education for two groups
Buerger (1968)	72 Ss in grades 3–7 who had received 50 + hours instruction in school reading clinic	72 poor readers with comparable ability and achievement scores	Not given	Not given	Maximum of 5.6 years	Tests, school marks, school records	112 hours remediation over 16 months
Koppitz (1971)	152M, 25F referred to learning disorder classes	None	M=8 yr. 11 mo.; range = 6–12 years	M=92; range from under 80 (n=31) to over 119 (n=7)	5 year maximum	Tests, school records	Learning disorder classes
Muehl and Forell (1973 –1974)	36M, 7F reading clinic clients about 3 grades retarded in reading. M = 8th percentile on Iowa Test of Basic Skills	None	M=11.5	M=101	About 5 years after diagnosis at about 10th grade	Test	Some remediation
Gottesman, Belmont, and Kaminer (1975)	49M, 9F referred by schools to medical clinic for evaluation of reading disability	None	M=10.1 range 7–15 years	M=88 all 70 or above	3–5 years after diagnosis	Tests	Remedial education (various programs)
Trites and Fiedorowicz (1976)	27M (group I), 10F (group III) with specific learning disorders; 10M (group II) with organic learning disorders, all from neuro psychology laboratory	None	Means: Group I 11.6, Group II 11.5, Group III 8.9	Means: Group I 106, Group II 92, Group III 103	Means: Group I 2.5 years, Group II 2.8 years, Group II 2.6 years	Test WRAT	All Ss have remedial education
Dykman, Peters, and Ackerman (1973)	31M diagnosed as learning disorder ante rospectively in child guidance clinic	22M from school also selected at outset	9.5–12	M=105 for cases; M=110 for controls	Follow-up at age 14 for all Ss	Neurologic evaluation; tests; laboratory; interview	All have some remedial education

Table 4–1. **Subjects and Measures Used in Follow-up Studies of Children with Learning Disability and/or Hyperactivity**—*continued*

Reference	Cases	Controls	Age	IQ	Interval	Method	Treatment
		Subjects				Follow-up	
Ackerman, Dykman, and Peters (1977 *a*, 1977 *b*)	62M with learning disability	31M selected at outset	8–11 years	90 or above on WISC verbal *or* performance scale	3–6 years all Ss re-evaluated at age 14	Tests	29/62 receive drugs; 53/62 have remedial education
2. Subjects selected mainly for hyperactivity:							
Weiss, et al., (1971)	60M, 4F diagnosed in hospital clinic as "severe, sustained" hyperactivity	19 to 32 normals tested at follow-up only	M=8.8 years, range 6–13 years	M=104; 84 or above	M=4.4 years post diagnosis for cases. M age = 13.3 years	Ratings, Tests	All had chlorpromazine, some had other drugs; most had counseling, 15% had remedial education
Cohen, Weiss, and Minde (1972)	20 M diagnosed as hyperactive 5 years earlier	20M classmates	About 10 at diagnosis	M=108 for cases and controls	5 years at M age of about 15	Tests: MFF, EFT, Stroop color-word	Drugs, some remedial education
Minde, Weiss, and Mendelson (1972)	81M, 10F diagnosed as above. Modal SES = 3 on 5 point scale	20 normal matched on age, sex, and SES	About 8 1/2	84 or above	M=4.5 years at M age of 13.4	4–6 hours 'clinical evaluation ratings	Drugs, counseling, and/or tutoring
Hoy, reported in Weiss and Minde (1974)	20 hyperactives from above sample	20 from above sample	As above	As above	As above	Self-concept test	As above
Weiss, et at., (1974)	72 hyperactives from hospital clinic in 3 sub groups by drug given	N=22 no-drug Ss	M about 8	Not reported	5 years	Interview, ratings, tests, school records	Chlorpromazine (N=24), methylphenidate (N=26), and drug (N=22) groups all had crisis counseling
Mendelson, Johnson, and Stewart (1971)	75M, 8F from private psychiatric practice. All hyperactive or distractible and 75 had 4 or more other symptoms from list of 35. SES M=38 on 1 (low) to 5 scale	None	M=9.9 SD=2.4	M=96 range= 60–120	M=3.5 post diagnosis; range = 2–5 years, pt. M age= 13.4, SD=1.2 years	Parent interview and ratings	92% drugs, most had counseling
Stewart, Mendelson, and Johnson (1973)	81 from Mendelson, et al., (1971) above	None	As above	As above	As above	Interview of child and mother	As above

| Reference | Subjects | | | | | Follow-up | |
	Cases	Controls	Age	IQ	Interval	Method	Treatment
Huessy and Cohen (1976)	95-118 (73% M) pupils scoring in worst 20% on teacher ratings in 2nd, 4th, or 5th grades. Initial cohort was 501 2nd graders	41 (67% M) under 70th percentile on same instrument	2nd grade at 1st rating	M=95 for hyper-actives, 107 for controls	7 years after first rating	School and public records, teacher ratings	Remedial education for some

C. Subjects mostly 19 years or older at follow-up:
   1. Subjects selected mainly for learning disability:

Reference	Cases	Controls	Age	IQ	Interval	Method	Treatment
Robinson, and Smith (1962)	44 Ss from University of Chicago Reading Clinic in 1948 (sex not given)	None	7–18 years, Median=14	85–147 Median=120	10 years	Inter-view, ques-tion-naire	33/44 tutored in clinic
Silver and Hagin (1964)	21M, 3F with learning dis-orders from O.P. mental hygiene clinic: subdivided into "organic" and "develop-mental categories	11 with be-havior prob-lems only from same clinic	Median about 8 in both groups	Child values not reported: as adults cases have Median of 105, controls 112	10–12 years post diagnosis at Ss age 19 to 20	Tests, neuro-logical eval-uation	Not re-ported
Rawson (1968)	20M dyslexics in private school	36 M non-dyslexics in same school	6–14 years	M=131 (cases and con-trols com-bined)	17–35 years at M age 33 years	Inter-view	Gillingham-Orton tutoring
Preston and Yarington (1967)	50 (44M, 6 F) from University of Pennsylvania Reading Clinic with Mdn reading retar-dation of two or more grades	None (population norms used for compar-isons)	6–17years, M=12	53–123, M=98	8 years	Inter-view	46/50 had remedial reading in clinic
Laufer (1971)	66 private patients	None	3–13 M=8	"Normal distri-bution"	Patient age 15–26 years, M=20	Ques-tion-naire	All had stimulant drugs, 31 for 6 months or more

   2. Subjects selected mainly for hyperactivity:

Reference	Cases	Controls	Age	IQ	Interval	Method	Treatment
Menkes, Rowe, and Menkes (1967)	11M, 3F diag-nosed retro-spectively as MBD from psy-chiatric clinic records. All had hyperactivity and learning disability plus motor-visual or speech deficits	None	2.6–15.5 years	70 or above	14–24 years M=24	Clinical eval-uation, EEG	No drugs, supportive manage-ment for 11 patients

Table 4–1.   Subjects and Measures Used in Follow-up Studies of Children with Learning Disability and/ or Hyperactivity—*continued*

	Subjects				Follow-up		
Reference	*Cases*	*Controls*	*Age*	*IQ*	*Interval*	*Method*	*Treatment*
Huessy and Townsend (1973); Huessy, Metoyer, and Townsend (1974)	46M, 12F, 26 sex-unspecified Ss from private and clinic consultations with 3 or more of 8 symptoms of hyperactivity or learning disability	None	3–16 years	Not given	5–11 years past diagnosis, at pt. age 9–24 years	Questionnaire, interview, records	All had drugs
Borland, and Heckman (1976)	20M guidance clinic patients diagnosed retrospectively as hyperactive	20M (18 were brothers of cases)	Range 4–11; M=7.4 for cases; about 5.4 for controls	80 or above; patient average 102; control 105 on school tests	About 23 years at patient age 30	Interview, school and public records	Some had counseling

Campbell, Endman, and Bernfeld (1977). Studies done in school settings but involving special class pupils had a wider age spectrum, but this does not necessarily mean that the older children had not been previously diagnosed. In some instances (Muehl and Forell, 1973–1974; Balow, 1965) age of subjects was dictated by the level of the special reading program in which they were enrolled; the subjects were not necessarily new to such programs. Some of the subjects in Rawson's (1968) private school group had been enrolled in the school precisely because of a previous diagnosis of learning disability, a diagnosis which might have been known years earlier.

The widest range of ages is to be found among subjects in studies in which diagnostic criteria for MBD were applied retrospectively to clinic records of patients who had originally been diagnosed before the concept of MBD was current. Menkes, Rowe, and Menkes (1967) used subjects ranging from 3 to 15 at first diagnosis, while Borland and Heckman's (1976) subjects ranged from 4 to 11 years. Studies based on patients seen in private practice also tended to include subjects of a wide range of ages. Laufer's (1971) patients ranged from 3 to 13 at onset of treatment; Huessy and Townsend (1973), Huessy, Metoyer, and Townsend (1974) had cases ranging from 3 to 16; and Mendelson, Johnson, and Stewart (1971) studied a sample in which the ages of the subjects had a standard deviation of 2.4 years, implying a range of something over 6 years. Cases seen in private practice may have been diagnosed elsewhere earlier. The presence of older children does not imply that their condition went unnoticed earlier.

Even though the older children labelled MBD may well have the same subvariety of the condition as the younger ones, there is no guarantee that this is so. Satz, Radin, and Ross (1971) present evidence that older learning-disabled (LD) children show a different constellation of deficits than younger LD children. As will be noted, a few studies reviewed here found age at diagnosis to correlate with some outcome variables. Trites and Fiederowicz (1976) found that the girls diagnosed in their neuropsychology laboratory averaged two years younger than the boys. Thus there is a good basis for advocating that subjects of different ages be kept separate in future follow-up studies.

Intelligence

Mean IQs, with the notable exception of those in Rawson's (1968) sample, are typically below 100 despite the usual exclusion of subjects scoring below 80 or some other arbitrary point. This pattern suggests some excess of cases scoring below 100 since no study excluded subjects with high IQs. Even Rawson noted that her "dyslexic" cases did not achieve IQs above 135, while the mean for all 56 subjects (dyslexic and nondyslexic combined) was 131.

Follow-up Interval

The mean interval between diagnosis and follow-up varied between about two years (Riddle and Rapaport, 1976) and about 24 years (Rawson, 1968; Menkes, Rowe, and Menkes 1967). Rawson had the greatest range of follow-up intervals within any one study, with intervals for individual subjects as short as 17 years and as long as 35 years.

Combined with variations in age of subjects at diagnosis, these differences in follow-up intervals lead to very large differences in age of subjects at follow-up. This meant that very different amounts and segments of the life span were being compared within a given study. This makes it difficult to evaluate the data on arrest, mental hospitalization, divorce, or any other outcome for which risk accumulates as a function of age. This problem is partially solved by the practice of evaluating subjects in prospective studies as they reach a given age (14 in Ackerman, Dykman, and Peters 1977a; 1977b). School-based studies, such as that of Huessy and Cohen (1976) can rather readily standardize age both at initial diagnosis and at follow-up.

Design

Only a minority of studies employed control groups, and only a few of these control groups were actually subjected to the same initial diagnostic procedures as the MBD group. Ackerman, Dykman, and Peters (1977a; 1977b) used this design; Silver and Hagin (1964) had a control group which was further matched with the MBD group in that its members had been referred to the same clinic. The controls differed only in that they had received a different diagnosis.

Studies of school cohorts by Rawson (1968) and Huessy and Cohen (1976) use pupils scoring above the cutoff point on a diagnostic measure as controls. Clearly subjects (Ss) above and below this point may differ on many factors other than the score on the assessment instrument. Since in Huessy and Cohen's study at least, these other factors—socioeconomic status (SES), sex ratio, intelligence—are not controlled either statistically or through matched subgroups, these variables remain as possible explanations for the differences found. For instance in this study IQ averaged 95 in the hyperactive group, but 107 in the controls. This lack of rigor does not impair the predictive value of the diagnosis; it simply leaves unclear the real basis for successful prediction.

Some studies selected control only at follow-up (Weiss, 1971; Riddle and Rapaport, 1976). This means that the controls will match the cases as they are at follow-up, not necessarily as they were at diagnosis. If IQ of the subjects do in fact decrease over time for instance, controls drawn at follow-up and matched on IQ may well produce a group of Ss who have always had lower intelligence, not a group which has a similar history of IQ decline. If the controls drawn at follow-up are matched to the cases as regards current IQ, these controls of course could not show that a history of MBD was associated with lower (or higher) current IQ. However these IQ-matched controls drawn at follow-up can serve the very useful purpose of ruling out low current IQ as the cause of deficits in other functions (for example reading) at follow-up. Minde, et al., (1971) were able to look at their data both ways. Considering all of the cases and controls and without matching for IQ, they noted a significant 10 point superiority of the controls over the cases. By then selecting subsamples of controls and cases matched on IQ, they were able to show that IQ difference could not account for differences in certain outcome variables, as the cases remained inferior even after the matching equated the subsamples on IQ.

A more basic drawback of control groups which are selected and evaluated only at follow-up is that they do not permit conclusions about the developmental course of neuropsychological or information processing functions which are deficient in younger MBD subjects, but which progress to normal levels as the MBD child grows older. For example Dykman, Peters, and Ackerman (1973) demonstrated slower simple reaction times in MBDs than in controls at time of diagnosis. This difference disappeared when the subjects were retested at age 14. These authors had tested reaction time (RT) in both LDs and controls at both ages. If they had tested the controls only at follow-up, they could have concluded only that learning disabled children were not deficient in simple reaction time. They could not have concluded that simple reaction time was a variable on which MBD subjects do "grow out" of an early deficit. This analysis of specific functions over time is particularly important in understanding a developmental disorder such as hyperactivity or learning disorder.

Likewise it is conceivable that MBD children "grow into" some deficits, that is MBD and control children may not differ on some functions (for example arithmetic skills, knowledge of letter sounds, compliance with complex rules) at an early age, but may differ at a later age. Only a complete design, involving the testing of controls and cases both at diagnosis and follow-up, can demonstrate such patterns.

Finally the fact of being evaluated, the possible attachment of a label, and the persisting special concern of parents and others are all missing in controls selected at follow-up only. Ideally one control group would be selected from children evaluated in the same setting as the MBD children but found to have some other identifiable problem. Silver and Hagin (1964) appear to be the only investigators who have followed this procedure.

Borland and Heckman's (1976) control group is worthy of special mention. They compared 20 boys diagnosed as MBD with their own brothers, except for two cases where the brothers could not be recruited; brothers-in-law were substituted. This design provided excellent control of familial and social factors and resulted in no IQ difference between cases and controls. The brothers however were on the average two years younger than the cases, suggesting that the variable of birth order may have had some significance in the diagnosis of MBD. Brothers, as might be expected, had not been evaluated systematically at the time of diagnosis of the MBD index child. For the most part only follow-up information is available for the controls. Nonetheless the authors were able to show interesting differences on SES changes and work habits between MBD and non-MBD boys from the same families.

Treatment

Several studies report rather extensive periods of medications for some or all of their subjects; in fact some of the studies started as investigations of the longer term effects of drugs on hyperactivity or MBD. For example Minde, Weiss, and Mendelson (1972) used chlorpromazine with 66 subjects and dextroamphetamine with 38 in a pharmacotherapeutic study, but only 12 were still taking the drug at follow-up four to six years later. Fourteen children were taken off medication after three years or less because of "sufficient improvement," 46 were taken off (most after six months or less of treatment) because of lack of desired effects or occurrence of untoward side effects. Laufer (1971) reports that 24 of 55 patients treated with stimulant drugs took the medication for six months or less, while the other 31 took it for six months to five years. Thus the natural history of medication, a seemingly simple and straightforward form of intervention, is in fact characterized by much variability.

Where counseling or psychotherapy was provided, it was typically offered according to perceived need or in response to parent request. No study was found which attempted controlled or randomized evaluation of psychotherapeutic methods with MBD children or their parents over a period of two years or more.

MBD children, especially those diagnosed specifically as having a learning disorder, often received one or more kinds of special educational handling. Some of this management was evidently related only loosely to the child's particular needs. Perhaps the most frequent educational intervention for the LD child is repetition of a grade. Hinton and Knights (1971) found that 34 of 67 children referred to a pediatric neurologist because of school problems repeated one or more grades. Thirty-one of the 34 had failed before the referral was made. In these cases repetition of the grade could not have been part of a comprehensive plan for the child based on the clinical evaluation. Minde, *et al.*, (1971) found that 57% of these cases repeated one or more grades in a four to six year period following diagnosis.

No study was found in which a program combining medical, psychotherapeutic and educational management was carried out over a period of years.

Measures

Only a few studies have used the same measures at follow-up as on evaluation, and only two (Ackerman, Dykman, and Peters 1977*a*, 1977*b*; Silver and Hagin, 1964) presented before and after data on controls as well. These studies offer the most definitive information about the persistence of the symptoms defining MBD and point the way for future work on this question. The primary need is for these kinds of data covering a longer time interval.

Since learning problems are one major manifestation of MBD, and since reading skill can be readily assessed, one would expect a wealth of data on changes in reading and reading related skills in MBD children. Such data are available, but only over shorter follow-up intervals. Studies of subjects who are adults at follow-up have uniformly failed to assess reading skills in any standardized, quantitative way. Rawson (1968) did not secure any quantitative measures of reading ability from her subjects at follow-up, although she reported extremely high academic and professional achievement by her ex-dyslexics, and simultaneously reported that they still found reading and spelling somewhat difficult. Actual scores on reading tests would have been very useful in determining whether the superlative career achievements occurred in spite of real reading deficits or not. Menkes, Rowe, and Menkes (1967) did not secure reading scores on their subjects, though they had been selected initially as having learning problems as well as behavior problems. Borland and Heckman (1976), whose subjects were also adults when reassessed, also failed to make any quantitative study of reading skills. Studies of children and adolescents previously diagnosed as hyperactive, typically did give some consideration to their educational progress.

Several studies use centile scores in reporting reading levels and calculate reading gains and losses in various groups in terms of difference in these centile scales. It must be recognized that the centile scale does not have equal-interval properties. Thus a change of 5 centile points from the 50th to the 45th centile represents a much smaller change in the presumed underlying dimension than a 5 centile change from the 6th to the 1st centile. Nonetheless outcome data are presented here in centiles where the original authors used them; no attempt was made to translate them into Z-scores or standard scores.

Ratings of "improvement," usually from parents, have been obtained rather frequently, undoubtedly because of the ease with which they can be obtained and their practical clinical utility. However they obviously are colored by the raters' changing expectations as well as by any real changes in the subject. Also ratings of improvement are difficult to make on a nondiagnosed control group, the subjects of which presumably did not have any condition which needed improvement.

Several investigators have included measures of mood, self-esteem, and insight. Ratings by the patient himself and by others have been the major source of data, though one study (Riddle and Rapaport, 1976) used the TAT, with surprisingly consistent results. Rather remarkably no one has evidently collected MMPI profiles of adults diagnosed as MBD in childhood. Perhaps the reading level of many of these individuals remains too low to permit this approach.

Assessment of the status of the grown-up MBD—of his or her situation in life—has relied heavily on use of public and semipublic records. These have included information from schools, from courts, mental hospitals, and mental health clinics, among other sources. Such sources may or may not provide base rates for the population as a whole. Such base rates when available can serve as a rough approximation to information available from a control group when such a group is lacking. However base rates (for example of court referral for juvenile delinquency) almost never are given for subpopulations comparable to the MBD group on social class, intelligence, school achievement, and so on. Therefore it is not clear whether the elevated rates of unfavorable outcomes in the MBD group are really attributable to MBD or instead are a reflection of other, incidental characteristics of the sample. Robins (1977) points out that official records are becoming increasingly unavailable to researchers who wish to select controls or evaluate outcomes. This makes the researcher's ideal of controlled samples and objective outcome measures very difficult to attain.

OUTCOME

Functioning versus Status

For purposes of this review, two aspects of outcome will be distinguished: the functioning of the child and his adjustment or status. The former is seen as internal to the child, whether determined by maturation (or lack of it) or by past experience; the latter is determined by the reactions of others to whatever his functioning may be (or may be perceived to be). We shall thus be concerned with the functional characteristics and traits that originally defined the child as MBD—his activity level, explosiveness, neurological soft signs, specific disabilities, attention span, and so on. Along with the later extent of the original signs and symptoms of MBD, we shall also look at other traits which may not have been studied initially, but which are nonetheless interpretable as part of the child's functioning—his typical mood, self-esteem, goal persistence, conscientiousness, and so on. For the second, or externally determined aspect, of the individual's adjustment (his status), we shall consider such matters as his economic self-sufficiency, his marital status, level of education achieved, his involvement with the criminal justice system, and his experience in custodial institutions. Psychiatric diagnosis however shall be considered to reflect functioning, not social condition.

It is recognized that any such distinction between function and status is to some extent artificial, and may ride roughshod over theories which hold that nothing about an individual can be described without reference to a particular situation. However this categorization does seem to have practical and heuristic value for the orderly review of outcome measures, if for no other purpose.

For example the same measure of functioning can be meaningfully administered at different stages in the life span. In contrast criteria of status change rather drastically between the school years and adulthood. Thus data on alcoholism, divorce, and unemployment are very difficult to identify with those on grade repetition, special school placement, school dropout, popularity, and so on, whereas tests of intelligence, neuropsychological functions, and basic academic skills can be compared directly. Scores on behavioral variables such as activity level, impulsiveness, and aggressiveness occupy an intermediate ground, since they are typically obtained from rating scales and the frame of reference of the rater undoubtedly shifts from one age level to the next. While scores on such instruments thus nominally represent functional characteristics of the individual, they in fact reflect his status to some extent.

Functioning and Status in Later Childhood

Only one study was found of the later childhood functioning of young children selected for learning disorder. Rourke and Orr (1977) in a four-year study of first and second grade boys who were retarded (N=19) or average (N=23) readers found that the retarded readers tended to show increases ranging from 12 to 14 centile points on various reading tests but remained well below the 50th centile for the tests and very greatly below the control group. While the authors emphasized the small size of the gains, these subjects at follow-up were on average reading at less than one standard deviation below the test norms, putting them within the average range as broadly defined. It should be noted that these subjects were not extremely retarded in reading to start with, as they scored on average between the 10th and 30th centiles on the various reading tests in the first or second grade. As compared with results for more grossly retarded readers (see the discussion on adolescents), these results are rather favorable. These investigators did not report however on the school marks or grade failures of their subjects, nor did they comment in any way on their behavioral adjustment.

Hinton and Knights (1971) found a high frequency of school problems in their follow-up of preadolescent children three years after original referral for diagnosis of some combination of learning and behavior problems at school. Only 26 of the 67 children were in the appropriate grade for age, the others failed one or more grades or had been placed in special class. However two facts affect the interpretation of these findings: actual or imminent grade failure was evidently one frequent reason for referral, and school progress was highly correlated with measures of general verbal ability. Thus the findings would not necessarily apply to a randomly selected sample of children suffering from specific information processing disabilities only, not general lack of verbal ability.

Eaves and Crichton (1974) report on the school status of preadolescents who had earlier been diagnosed retrospectively as having minimal brain dysfunction. Unlike Rourke and Orr (1977), these authors did not directly assess the child's functioning but rather collected information about the child's placement and grade in school. Like Hinton and Knights (1971), these workers found the cases to have a high rate of grade repetition, poor academic marks, and frequent referrals for special classes or special programs, but failed to rule our general intelligence as a possible factor in these academic failures. Only 3 of the 39 cases diagnosed as MBD were found to be free of both learning and behavior problems at follow-up at an average age of about 12, indicating a strong tendency for problems to persist regardless of the child's ability.

Minde, *et al.*, (1971), however, did study the possibility that IQ, not hyperactivity, accounted for grade failure. They found that a subgroup of their hyperactive sample matched with normal classmates on IQ did not exceed these controls significantly in number of grades repeated, but did have significantly poorer marks and less favorable behavior ratings by teachers.

Minde, *et al.*, also found that their subjects, selected for hyperactivity at about age eight, were rated as less hyperactive two to five years later, but were still rated as significantly above normal levels on this and associated variables.

Riddle and Rapaport (1976) present perhaps the most comprehensive follow-up study of tested and rated functions of hyperactive preadolescent children. Their subjects, boys selected primarily for hyperactivity at about age 8, were rated both at the outset and at a two year follow-up by teacher and parents. The teachers rated them as significantly less hyperactive and as having significantly less conduct disorder at follow-up than on the initial evaluation. Parent re-ratings at age 10 on the Conners Parent Symptom Questionnaire also showed a significant decline in the hyperactivity factor but failed to show a significant reduction on the conduct disorder factor. Reading and arithmetic as assessed by the Wide Range

Achievement test were significantly poorer at follow-up in the hyperactive sample than in a nonhyperactive control group, but only the mathematics scores for the hyperactive group appeared to be below the national average for this test. The average standard score for reading in the hyperactive group was 98 (for controls it was 107). Furthermore the hyperactive boys showed no decrease in standard score in reading on this test over the two year interval, though they did show a slight but significant decrease in mathematics (from a standard score of 91 to one of 89). Thus achievement does not seem to have suffered drastically in this sample of hyperactive boys from middle class families.

Riddle and Rapaport (1976) report evidence of depressive tendencies at age 10 in their cases. The hyperactive boys produced TAT stories rated as more indicative of depression than those produced by controls. On the other hand self-rated self-esteem on the Simmons-Rosenberg scales was not different in the cases and controls, but was lower in older than in younger subjects in both groups. As will be seen depressive and self-critical reactions are noted even more prominently in follow-up of older MBD subjects.

Despite the decrease in hyperactivity and the evident maintenance of adequate progress in reading, the perceived adjustment of hyperactive boys in this study remained poor. Only 2 of 72 parents were free of serious concern about their sons, with two-thirds expressing most concern about impulsive or immature behavior. No data were gathered on the extent and nature of parental concerns in the control group. Teachers and parents both rated the hyperactive children as less well accepted by peers than controls, though parents' diaries of their children's actual hours of peer contacts did not show even a trend toward a difference between cases and controls.

All studies reviewed in this section indicate that the school performance (as opposed to learning) of the MBD child is very poor in the years immediately following diagnosis. Even when IQ is controlled and reading scores approximate grade norms (Riddle and Rapaport, 1976) marks are much below average. When reading problems predominate at diagnosis, only a minority of children are found in the age-appropriate grade at follow-up. However many questions remain as to why the short term school outcomes are so poor. The two studies (Hinton and Knights, 1971; Eaves and Crichton, 1974) which most carefully assess class placement and teachers' marks failed to include tests of actual skills related to reading and mathematics, and the studies which did assess reading skills (Riddle and Rapaport, 1976; Rourke and Orr, 1977) did not report on class placement. Strange as it may seem it is thus very much an open question as to just what factors in the child and in the school setting lead to such rampant grade repetition by children diagnosed as learning disabled.

Parents' perception of their child's problem, like school placement, appears to have complex determinants. Only 2 of 72 parents in the Riddle and Rapaport (1976) study were free of major concerns about their children at follow-up, even though hyperactivity had decreased and academic achievement appeared only slightly below average. On the other hand 75% of the parents in Hinton and Knights' (1971) study judged their child to be improved in school, despite the fact that only 39% of the children were actually in the age-appropriate regular grade. Parents' ratings of their child's peer acceptance did not correlate significantly with that of teachers in Riddle and Rapaport's study.

The two studies which selected subjects primarily for hyperactivity (Minde, *et al.*, 1971; Riddle and Rapaport, 1976) agree in reporting that hyperactivity and associated symptoms decrease over the two to five year period but remain very noticeably and disturbingly above normal levels. Unfortunately the studies which did not select children for hyperactivity per se report little information on behavioral functioning of their subjects at follow-up. It seems fairly clear that hyperactivity has ominous implications for academic performance and behavioral adjustment in older preadolescents, but it is not known what the implications of learning disability alone are for behavioral adjustment in this period.

Data on the later functioning of children identified as hyperactive in the preschool years are just becoming available. Campbell, Endman, and Bernfeld (1977) reported on the behaviors in first and second grade of children first described by only their mothers as hyperactive ("situational hyperactives") or by both mothers and nursery school teachers as hyperactive ("true hyperactives)." Detailed classroom observations showed that both previously defined hyperactive groups elicited more "negative" (that is critical), feedback from teachers than did controls, while only the true hyperactives were observed to be out of seat more often than classmate controls. Teacher ratings on the Conners Scale depicted both true and situational hyperactives as more active than controls, but only the true hyperactives as less attentive than controls. In general results suggested that true and situational hyperactive children differed primarily in the degree to which they possessed symptoms of the syndrome in question, rather than in kind of symptoms.

This carefully designed study also found evidence that the presence of a hyperactive child in a classroom affected interactions between the teacher and other children in that class. Teachers criticized the classroom control child in the classes containing a hyperactive child more frequently than the classroom control child in the classes of the nonhyperactive children being followed longitudinally in the study.

While these data indicate that hyperactive preschoolers remain discriminably different as a group during their early school years, tallies of their overt behavior in the classroom were not overwhelmingly different from those of controls. The very large differences in teacher ratings and the evidence that teacher interactions with other children in the class are adversely influenced by a hyperactive child strongly suggest that even detailed behavior ratings do not fully capture the qualities of behavior of the hyperactive child that are particularly upsetting to teachers. Learning difficulties were not assessed in the Campbell, Endman, and Bernfeld (1977) study, but the average WISC IQ of these hyperactive children at age 6.5 was 116 (as compared with a mean IQ on the Stanford-Binet at age 4.5 of 104). Thus these children could not have been disappointing to teachers because of low or declining general ability.

Functioning and Status in Adolescence

As was true in follow-up studies of subjects in late childhood, studies of adolescents who had only learning disabilities as children usually do not refer to any behavioral problems the children may have had or may have developed, while adolescent follow-ups of hyperactive children usually attend to later learning problems of their subjects as well as to their behavior problems. We shall first consider adolescent outcome of children with learning disabilities when only the academic achievement of the subjects is considered. We shall then move to those few studies which selected subjects initially for learning disabilities, but which consider behavioral outcome in adolescence as well as academic achievement. Finally we will consider adolescent outcomes of children selected mainly for hyperactivity.

In an early study, Balow (1965) reported that 10 to 12 year old children reading at a middle to later third grade level gained about .75 month grade equivalent per month of instruction over periods of up to four years after participating in an intensive summer reading program. He contrasted this with a rate of about .55 month gain per month prior to the program and the much higher rates of 4.8 and 6.6 months gain per month for two different classes during the intensive program itself. He attributed the evident increase in rate of gain during the follow-up period to continuation of some remedial assistance and blamed the failure to maintain the very rapid rate of gain attained during the brief summer program to the mildness of these follow-up remedial efforts.

Koppitz (1971) in a much larger and somewhat longer study of learning disabled children in special LD classes, found yearly average gains ranging from 1.1 grade equivalent per year for those who stayed in a special class only one year down to .34 year per calendar year for those who stayed a full five years in the program. Because return to regular class was based on rate of progress, the data do not necessarily indicate that staying in the special classes retarded educational progress; they only indicate that there are a number of children (71 out of 177 in this study) whose rate of reading progress remains very slow over the longer term despite special educational efforts. The 21 adolescents who left the program at ages 14 and 15 after five years of instruction were reading at an average grade level of 4.7, while the six leaving at 16 and 17 averaged only a 2.8 grade level. The 50 leaving at age 11 through 13, also after 5 years, averaged a reading grade level of about 3.4. All of these subjects could justifiably be called reading disabled. Koppitz reported very little on any behavioral manifestation of MBD in this large sample (177 cases) as the 26 children with serious behavior problems were referred for residential treatment at the outset. She did note that these referred children tended to be viewed as explosive, anxious, aggressive, and/or delinquent.

Trites and Fiederowicz (1976) presented a study of children followed up about 2.5 years after being diagnosed as having a reading disability. Two groups of boys totaling 37, averaged 11.5 years of age, early fifth grade placement, and early third grade reading level (on the Wide Range Achievement Test) at diagnosis. After remedial help for all cases, 2.5 years later the group designated as having "specific reading disability" had an average reading grade of 4.6 while the group diagnosed as "organic" averaged a 4.0 reading grade on the WRAT. Centile standings for the two groups did not change appreciably over the interval, moving only from an average of 13 to 14 in the "specific" group and from 9 to 8 in the "organic" group. A separate group of 10 girls was about 2.5 years younger at diagnosis than the boys and was reading at a 2.3 level on the WRAT. This group gained an average of 1.3 grades in the 2.5-year interval, achieving a 3.6 grade level when they were 11.5 years of age and in the late fifth grade. Their average centile standing was higher initially (26) and dropped to 15 at follow-up. Results for spelling generally paralleled those for reading, but arithmetic scores were less impaired both at diagnosis and follow-up, though interim progress was no better than for spelling and reading. This study, like that of Koppitz (1971), points to the refractory nature of many severe learning disorders. Average rates of gain in this study would range from less than three months to about five months per year for boys and to not over seven months per year for the girls (in spelling only). In every group the discrepancy between age-expected and actual achievement widened for all subtests of the WRAT over the interval between diagnosis and follow-up. These authors made no report of behavior problems in their subjects, nor did they comment on their emotional adjustment.

Muehl and Forell (1973) reported on the somewhat more encouraging progress of 43 children seen initially at the age of 11.5 in the University of Iowa reading clinic. Averaging 101 in IQ, the initial sample of 63 had a rate of EEG abnormalities of 63%. In reading the 43 subjects followed up had an average score at the 8th centile on the Iowa Test of Basic Skills at outset, about three grades below age expectation. At follow-up, when the average grade placement was about the tenth, the subjects achieved an average score at the 18th centile on the reading subtests of the Iowa Tests of Educational Development. Final reading scores were higher in those who had been younger at diagnosis and those with higher verbal IQ scores. The sample was generally of middle or upper middle SES, and those at the highest SES tended to read better at follow-up, though this was not necessarily independent of verbal IQ and age at diagnosis. EEG findings and amount of remedial training were not predictive of reading scores at follow-up.

In a study that parallels that of Muehl and Forell (1973) in some interesting ways, Gottesman, Belmont, and Karniner (1975) found less gain in reading than these earlier authors. They examined 58 reading-disabled children in a medical clinic at an average age of about 10 years and retested reading ability 3 to 5 years later, after 38 of the 58 had had special educational handling at school and 25 had been tutored in the clinic. As a group the subjects declined about 3 centile points on the WRAT over the follow-up interval, dropping from a mean of 9th centile to a mean of 6.3. Younger children who had had higher centile scores initially—and thus had more to lose—did in fact lose more. This sample as a whole had roughly equivalent reading scores to those in Muehl and Forell's sample (9th versus 8th centile in Muehl and Forell, albeit on different tests), but lower IQs at diagnosis than those studied by Muehl and Forell (88 versus 101), and the sample came primarily from working or lower class families, rather than the middle class or higher families of Muehl and Forell's children. The subjects in the Gottesman, Belmont, and Kaminer study tended to lose ground as measured by centile scores, whereas Muehl and Forell's tended to gain. Both studies found signs of organicity and provision of special reading instructions to be unrelated to outcome. Gottesman, Belmont, and Kaminer (1975) found that one-third of all the children in their study, and one-half of those 15 or older at the time of follow-up, could read and comprehend at a fourth grade level or better on the ABLE test, a result they found mildly encouraging. These authors report an average gain of 3.8 months grade equivalent (on the WRAT) per year, a slow pace but one that if it continued long enough eventually resulted in functional reading. Like Muehl and Forell, Gottesman, Belmont, and Kaminer provide no information about behavioral status at follow-up, despite the fact that 38% of the children were considered to be psychiatrically abnormal at time of first evaluation.

Yule (1973) presented four- and five-year follow-up achievement test data on children in the Isle of Wight studies. Children with reading deficits were designated as either "backward" or "retarded" readers on the basis of achievement and intelligence test scores at age 9, 10, or 11. Backward readers were those whose reading achievement at that time was simply 2.4 years or more below chronological age expectation; "retarded" readers were those whose reading achievement scores were 2.4 years or more below the expectation obtained when age and IQ were both represented in the regression equation. Most retarded readers by the age—IQ criteria were also backward by the age—only criterion. Only 10 children in a population of 2300 were found to be retarded readers, but not backward readers by these definitions; they were excluded from follow-up study.

The total group of 144 backward readers (which included the 73 backward-retarded readers) continued to show very slow progress in reading, achieving at age 14.5 years only the reading level obtained by the average 9 to 10 year olds on the tests used. When the subgroup of 71 backward-only readers was compared with the 73 backward-retarded group at follow-up, the backward-retarded had significantly lower achievement levels than the backward-only group. This was true despite the fact that the backward-retarded group had higher IQ scores both at selection and at follow-up. At follow-up the IQ difference amounted to 13 points in favor of the backward-retarded group. As the author points out, the statistical criterion for the backward-retarded group, with its inclusion of IQ, "pulls" for subjects with higher IQ scores. When initial differences in IQ and achievement were controlled statistically, the backward-retarded group remained inferior in reading achievement at follow-up, but was significantly superior in mathematics as compared to the backward-only group. This study suggests that the presence of severe reading disability at age 9 to 11 has ominous implications for future reading progress and that presence of high IQ cannot be considered to offer much hope for reading progress, though it may offer some for progress in mathematics. No attention was given to behavioral or emotional reactions in this study.

Complete results of the first reevaluation of the boys participating in a large, truly prospective study of learning disability have recently been published (Ackerman, Dykman, and Peters, 1977a, 1977b), following an earlier report based on incomplete data (Dykman, Peters, and Ackerman, 1973). In this study, which was planned from the outset as a longitudinal investigation, 8 to 11 year old boys identified as learning disabled were further cross classified according to 3 levels of activity (hyper-, normo-, and hypo-active) and 3 degrees of neurological dysfunction (positive, equivocal, and negative). Control subjects—boys without evidence of learning disability—were also included. A wide range of measures was obtained at both initial evaluation and follow-up: intellectual and achievement tests; laboratory measures of reaction time; classical and "soft" neurological signs. Behavior ratings by teachers and parents were added at follow-up, as was a tabulation of instances of clearcut antisocial behavior. Follow-up measures were obtained for each boy as he reached his 14th birthday.

Academic achievement remained deficient in these learning disabled boys. Initially about 2 years retarded in reading according to the norms of the Gray Oral Reading test, the deficiency widened at follow-up to 2.5 years. Compared to the control subjects, the average deficit in the learning disabled group was 4 years. The average centile score of the LD subjects on initial evaluation on the Gray test was 20; it was also 20 on follow-up. Two thirds of the learning-disabled boys had repeated one or more grades, while only 2 of 31 controls had done so.

However learning outcomes were not completely bleak. Average reading level on the Gray for the learning disabled subjects was 6.0 grade at age 14. While this compares very unfavorably with the 10.0 grade equivalent score of the controls, it still is adequate for much useful reading. Furthermore comprehension, as gauged by the rather superficial questions on the Gray, was as good for the learning-disabled boys as for the controls for paragraphs up through 5th grade difficulty level. LD subjects showed, on average, no change in either verbal or performance IQ on the WISC, while controls registered a significant increase in performance IQ.

Learning-disabled boys were particularly deficient at diagnosis and remained so at follow-up on four WISC subtests thought to reflect information–manipulating skills: digit span, arithmetic, coding, and information. Neurological functioning, originally substantially deficient in the LD group, remained so at follow-up despite significant improvement. Scores on the 80 item neurological examination were lower for the learning-disabled boys at follow-up (age 14) then for the control boys at time of original diagnosis, according to the earlier report (Dykman, Peters, and Ackerman, 1973).

Attention was assessed by a series of increasingly complex reaction time tasks. Learning-disabled subjects overcame their earlier deficit on the simplest of these, but remained deficient on the more complex tasks which in general required inhibition of response to false signals or maintenance of attention in the presence of distraction. Anomalies in the intake and processing of simple information (pure tones) were indicated for some of the learning disabled boys by a detailed study of heart rate changes to tone onset.

Emotionally and behaviorally, the learning-disabled boys had a much higher frequency of problems than controls. Problems involving overt conflict with others (parents, teacher, community authorities) were however confined almost exclusively to the subgroup of the learning-disabled sample identified earlier as hyperactive. Eleven of 23 hyperactive learning disabled boys had significant conflicts of this sort, as compared with 3 of 39 hypo- and normo-active boys and one of 34 controls. Similar findings are reported for more systematic behavior ratings by parents and teachers. The hyperactive subgroup " . . . presented by far the greatest number of management problems for home and school" (Ackerman, Dykman, and Peters, 1977b, p. 579). Self-rating on the Minnesota Counseling Inventory indicated elevated ratings for nearly all scales by the LD boys, though the three activity-level subgroups showed some variation in precise patterns of self-reported problems.

In summary this carefully planned, comprehensive study shows persisting, but not overwhelming, deficits in learning skills along with similarly persisting deficits in attention and information processing. Behavior problems were strongly associated with hyperactivity in the learning disabled populations, but not with learning disability alone.

Adolescent Follow-Up of Hyperactive Children

Three groups of investigators have published two or more reports on the fate in adolescence of the child described or diagnosed as hyperactive in childhood. Weiss, Minde, and their collaborators at McGill (Montreal group) have reported on various subgroups of a cohort of 155 nonpsychotic, pervasively hyperactive children of normal intelligence referred to the psychiatric outpatient clinic of a pediatric hospital (Weiss, *et al.*, 1971, p. 409). Many, if not all of these children were initially treated with a drug or with two or more drugs in succession, but few were receiving any drug at the time of follow-up. A report on 37 of these children in late grades of elementary school (Minde, *et al.*, 1971) was summarized in the discussion on follow-up of hyperactivity in childhood, two other reports are summarized here, and another will be considered when we discuss predictive variables.

The second group concerned with hyperactive children as adolescents is that associated with Stewart (Mendelson, Johnson, and Stewart, 1971; Stewart, Mendelson, and Johnson, 1973). Stewart has used a procedure in designating children as hyperactive that is both reasonably objective and flexible. To be called hyperactive, a child must be overactive and distractible, and must have at least four other symptoms from a list of 35. Unlike the Montreal group, the Stewart group did not use control subjects.

A final pair of studies is that reported by Huessy (Huessy and Cohen, 1976; Huessy, et al., 1973, 1974). The two studies are on (evidently) nonoverlapping groups. One concerns a school-based cohort of 501 children followed via interim teacher ratings and an examination of school records together with final teacher ratings in 9th grade. The other study concerns patients for whom Huessy provided consultation services. These subjects were followed mainly via public records.

The Montreal group has set forth perhaps the most conclusive data on functioning of hyperactive children at adolescence, as they were able to get ratings and other scores on the same instruments at follow-up as at initial diagnosis. The Montreal group has presented two reports on their hyperactive children as adolescents, one presenting information on both cognitive and behavioral status of 64 subjects (Weiss, *et al.*, 1971), the other focusing more narrowly on behavioral changes in 91 subjects (Minde, Weiss, and Mendelson, 1972). Weiss and Minde (1974) summarized both of these reports and added more data on self-image. Both of these studies used control groups to provide comparative data for some of the measures on which "pre" data were not available.

In the Montreal studies test-retest data on the WISC showed that the hyperactive children actually had a small but significant increase in Full Scale and Verbal IQ scores. The authors attribute this to "practice effect" despite the lapse of five years and the fact that the performance IQ, ordinarily more subject to practice effect than the verbal IQ, did not increase. Average scores on the Lincoln Oseretsky test of Motor Development declined very significantly, from the 34 to the 14 centile. According to the authors this reflected the greater weighting of fine motor skills in the portions of the test taken by older children. Overall rate of EEG abnormalities in a subsample of 30 subjects remained constant at about 40% over the five-year period, though many individual children shifted from abnormal to normal classification and vice versa. Behavior ratings made during psychiatric interviews indicated substantial reductions in the "target symptoms" of hyperactivity, distractibility, aggressivity, and excitability over the five-year period. Scores on the Peterson-Quay Symptom Checklist also declined significantly for the 37 subjects on whom it was completed. However the subjects remained on average well above normative values on this scale; furthermore teacher ratings on behavior problems distinguished cases from classmates. These differences between hyperactive and nonhyperactive children remained after a 10-point difference in group IQ in favor of the controls was partialled out statistically. Perhaps most interesting in the behavioral picture was a subtle but evidently important shift in the quality of symptoms. Instead of displaying gross overactivity, the children seemed restless and fidgety in smaller ways. Distractibility, inability to concentrate and lack of persistence in working toward major goals over a larger period of time all were more evident to mothers than previously and emotional immaturity was the most common general complaint.

Cohen, Weiss, and Minde (1972) documented the persistence of impulsivity in a study of the performance of hyperactive adolescents on three tests requiring careful attention to visual detail: Matching Familiar Figures, the Embedded Figures test, and the Stroop Color Word test. Subjects were selected from the Montreal sample. On the first two of these tests, adolescent boys diagnosed about five years earlier as hyperactive had shorter latencies than controls matched on age, sex, and IQ. The hyperactive boys also had more errors on the MFF. None of the variables from the Stroop test differentiated the groups.

In the follow-up study of school performance (Weiss, *et al.*, 1971), academic achievement was evaluated only by school marks, teachers' ratings, and records of grade repetition and special class placements; no direct assessment of reading or arithmetic skills was made. Only 20% of the children were in the appropriate grade for age, and only 3 of 64 were doing above average work. All three of these were, interestingly enough, children who had had IQs above 125 and schizoid personality traits at diagnosis.

Emotionally many of the children seemed sad at follow-up, keenly aware of their failures and very pessimistic about any future success. This depressed mood was noted by the authors in some children considered carefree and happy-go-lucky by their parents. Hoy (reported in Weiss and Minde, 1974) further documented this lack of self-esteem. She matched 20 adolescents who had been hyperactive as children with 20 controls matched on age, sex, IQ, and SES. The hyperactives had lower scores on most aspects of the Davidson and Lang checklist and on Ziller's test of social ability with peers.

The functioning of these children was thus characterized by maintenance of average intellectual ability and some diminution in hyperactive traits. Nonetheless they were still plagued by monumental difficulties in school performance and in self-management. Interpretation of this seeming discrepancy between some improvement in behavioral functioning and good basic intelligence on the one hand versus persistence of major school performance problems on the other is hampered by lack of direct test information on academic skills. Is the persisting academic failure attributable to lack of mastery of reading, spelling and mathematics, or to inconsistent application of these skills to school assignments? The same question arises in relation to the poor social adjustment: Does the friendlessness (rated at 30% by mothers) or the antisocial behavior (given at 25% by the authors) reflect persistence of innate limitations on factors important in social empathy and cooperation, or is it a result of attitudes acquired as a result of earlier frustrations and crystallized into the self-concept in adolescence?

Mendelson, Johnson, and Stewart (1971) and Stewart, Mendelson, and Johnson (1973) present follow-up reports on general adjustment and self-description, respectively, in a group of about 80 adolescents who had been diagnosed as hyperactive two to five years earlier. Reports from mothers and from the adolescents themselves were the sources of information. No control group was used. Median and modal occupational status of the families was blue collar.

Mothers of these subjects, like those of the subjects in the Montreal studies, report improvement in hyperactivity per se; about half of the children were said to be markedly improved. Also like the Montreal mothers, those in this study reported persisting problems which were of somewhat different character than those initially cited by them. In this study however the shift was not so much to immaturity and distractibility as to antisocial types of behavior. Eighty-three percent were said to lie frequently, 66% to be incorrigible, and an incredible 34% were reported to have threatened to kill their parents. Fifty-nine percent had had at lease one contact with police, and 17% had had three or more police contacts. Also as in the Montreal studies, over half of the children had failed at least one grade in school. Some sense of the strain in the families is conveyed by the fact that 40% of the mothers had seriously considered sending their children away to military school or to Boys Town. However the child's behavior may not have been the only source of strain in the families: 22% of the fathers were said to be problem drinkers, 33% of the families had stepparents, and 14% of the families were currently broken by death or divorce.

Structured interviews with the children themselves were also conducted and the results reported in Stewart, Mendelson, and Johnson (1973). Two-thirds or more of the adolescents reported that they were quick tempered or irritable, that they lied and fought often, and were generally hard to raise. Sixty-two percent said they were disgusted with themselves. The adolescents' reports generally agreed with their mothers' reports about them, except that the adolescents generally reported much more acceptance by others, peers and adults, than their mothers did for them.

Thus Stewart's subjects, both by report of their mothers and by self-report, persist in the impulsivity, aggressiveness, and the failure to complete projects that characterize the hyperactive child syndrome. The agreement with the Montreal group in this regard is impressive as is the finding of substantial evidence of depressive reactions. It will be recalled also that Riddle and Rapaport (1976) found evidence of depressive reactions in about 15% of their subjects, mainly the older, or early adolescent members of their sample.

The final studies regarding adolescent outcome of hyperactivity are by Huessy and his collaborators. The first of these concerned the outcome of children seen in various settings by Huessy, Metoyer, and Townsend (1973, 1974) and treated with drugs for hyperactivity. Follow-up was by search of public records and by ratings and records from the schools. Ages of children at diagnosis and follow-up interval were highly variable, so that age at follow-up was even more so. Subjects ranged from 9 to 24 years at follow-up. Results published in two reports (Huessy, Metoyer, and Townsend, 1973, 1974) are hard to interpret because of the telegraphic style and lack of clarity as to which categories are mutually exclusive and which are overlapping in the listings presented. However the results appear to be consistent with those reported in indicating a high rate of academic and social maladjustment. Evidently at least 23 of 84 subjects were institutionalized at one time or another during the follow-up interval; only 25 of 77 had a "satisfactory" academic level; and only 37 of 77 had "satisfactory" relations with family. No direct assessments were made of the subjects themselves and no control group was available, so that neither the source nor the significance of the outcomes reported can be determined with any degree of precision.

The other study reported by Huessy and a collaborator (Huessy and Cohen,

1976) concerns a cohort of 501 second graders followed mainly via teachers' ratings and school records through ninth grade. At second, fourth, and fifth grades, the children were rated by teachers on an inventory designed by the authors to assess hyperkinesis. Questions on the instrument covered social maturity, neuromuscular development, academic performance, and general attitude and behavior. The total score, which was the basis for classification, would thus seem to reflect more than hyperactivity or the hyperactive child syndrome as usually defined. Nonetheless the authors report that the scores on their inventory had a correlation of .77 with the Conners Teacher Rating Scale.

The most deviant 20% of children at each rating were designated the high risk group, and the movement of children into and out of this high risk category at successive ratings was studied. At ninth grade social and academic adjustment of children who had been described one or more times as high risk were tallied. Children who had never been high risk served as controls, but no attempt was made to equate these controls on IQ (12 points higher), social status, or other factors. The data showed that those identified as high risk after second grade (that is in fourth or fifth grade) had a 35% risk of receiving ratings of poor social adjustment in ninth grade as compared with 7% for controls. Fifty percent of these high risk subjects were found to have repeated a grade as compared with 11% of the controls. However much of the grade repetition would probably have taken place before the fourth and fifth grade ratings were made and so may have influenced them.

This study would seem to show that a broad based rating measure completed by teachers can be a fairly powerful predictor. However it does not allow for determination of what dysfunctions in the child may account for this unfavorable chain of events. There is little evidence given which points specifically either to behavior traits typical of hyperactivity or to cognitive deficits typical of learning disability; instead both conditions would appear to be lumped together in the rating process.

Function and Status in Adulthood

Of the studies reporting data on adult functioning of ex-MBD children, those of Borland and Heckman (1976), Menkes, Rowe, and Menkes (1967), and of Laufer (1971) focus on behavioral attributes, while Rawson (1968), Silver and Hagin (1964), and Robinson and Smith (1962) report on skills related to learning.

Silver and Hagin (1964) presented one of the earliest follow-up reports on children diagnosed as having specific reading disability, not merely reading underachievement. They studied 24 children on whom they had extensive neurological and perceptual data, along with 11 controls who had received a diagnosis other than learning disability in the same Mental Hygiene Clinic. Follow-up interval was 10 to 12 years, when the subjects' ages would have averaged about 19. Many of the original tests were repeated, which makes the study valuable as a source of information about changes in functioning. Furthermore the authors divided their subjects into "organic" and developmental subgroups, permitting evaluation of outcome separately in two groups with presumably different etiologies. Results showed the pattern that has since become familiar. Learning disabled subjects showed significant improvement in some motor, visual, and visual-motor tasks, but still were inferior to controls. Median IQ (WAIS) became significantly lower in the learning disabled group than in the controls, although the groups had not differed initially. After taking IQ into account, the authors concluded that only 9 of the 24 cases were inadequate readers at follow-up. One may question the validity of "correcting" for a declining IQ in evaluating the outcome of a condition which may be the cause of the decline. This is rather like saying that malnourished children are not especially limited in playing basketball, given their short stature.

Silver and Hagin (1964) concluded that " . . . specific reading disability is a long-term problem in the life of an individual, the signs of which can be detected despite adequate educational, vocational and social functioning" (p. 101). However the authors did not provide data on the social or vocational adjustment of their subjects, an omission common in follow-up studies of learning disability. Nonetheless this study is most impressive, especially considering its early date, for the adequacy of its control group, the extensiveness of its follow-up evaluation, and its use of theory in structuring its procedures.

Rawson (1968) reports highly favorable adult outcomes for her 20 dyslexic boys from a private school, but acknowledges that her group was unusually intelligent at the outset and received exceptionally intensive and systematic remedial instruction. The average IQ of Rawson's 20 dyslexic boys on the Stanford-Binet was evidently about 122. The 36 non-dyslexic boys with whom Rawson compared the dyslexics had even higher IQs. The average IQ for all 56 boys was given as 131.

On follow-up Rawson found the dyslexics to have completed an average of 6.0 years of post high school education, actually somewhat more than the non-dyslexics. Eighteen of the 20 dyslexics were college graduates and 10 had advanced degrees. Occupationally all the dyslexics were employed if not in school. On Warner's 5-point scale of occupational status (on which 1 is the highest status) the dyslexics averaged 1.8 while the non-dyslexics were a little lower at 1.81. Eleven of the dyslexics had careers which ordinarily would be expected to demand very strong reading and writing skills: two were physicians, one a lawyer, two professors, two scientists, and four school principals or teachers. Only two were in laboring jobs, one a foreman and one a skilled laborer. No mention was made of adjustment difficulties in the dyslexics who were followed, before or after their school years. The extremely high level of achievement is of course most encouraging. It also raises the question: Just how do these successful adults cope with the great demands on them for reading and spelling? A number reported that reading and spelling were still difficult in adulthood.

Robinson and Smith (1962) followed up 44 ex-clients of the University of Chicago Reading Clinic after an interval of 10 years, relying primarily on interviews and questionnaires. These subjects, who had an average IQ of 120, reading retardation ranging from one to several grades, and a median age of 14 when seen at the clinic, were for the most part considered to be adequate readers as young adults. Thirty-three of 44 were reported by their parents to read as much as or more than average. Forty-one of the 44 were high school graduates and 27 were college graduates. Only one was out of school and out of work. No mention was made by the authors of behavioral or emotional problems in the later lives of these bright poor readers. Similarly benign outcomes were reported by Preston and Yarington (1967) for 50 ex-clients of the University of Pennsylvania Reading Clinic. These subjects, studied through follow-up interviews eight years after participation in the clinic, had an unusually wide range of IQ (53–123) and an average of 98. Subjects were at least two grades retarded in reading when they entered the clinic. Using population data as reference points, these authors found no elevation of dropout rates and only 4 of 50 unemployed and out of school. About 25% of those of college age were in college, and 12 of 21 who were employed had whitecollar jobs. Again no mention was made of emotional or behavior problems. Forty-six of the 50 subjects received remedial help in the clinic, but the authors made no attempt to relate type or amount of tutoring to outcome.

In a study which has been widely quoted, Menkes, Rowe, and Menkes (1967) reported on neurological and intellectual functioning as well as the gross social adjustment in adulthood of 14 individuals identified from clinic records as having both hyperactivity and learning disorder in childhood. Menkes, Rowe, and Menkes indicated that 8 of the 11 subjects studied in detail had definite evidence of neurological dysfunction at follow-up. Only 6 of the 11 had had definite signs of brain dysfunction at diagnosis. There thus seemed to be a trend toward worsening or at least crystallization of neurological symptoms, rather than resolution, in the intervening years. Four of 14 subjects were diagnosed as psychotic. Three of the 14 complained of restlessness and difficulty in sustaining attention even in watching a TV show. Signs of hyperactivity had reportedly disappeared in the other 11 patients. Thus the subjects as a group tend to become less overtly hyperactive and more obviously impaired in neurological tests. These trends would appear to raise questions about the neurological substrates of hyperactivity. IQ (Ammons Picture Vocabulary) averaged 88 at follow-up as opposed to 94 (Stanford-Binet) on the same 11 patients at time of original assessment (calculated by the present author from data tabulated in original). The meaning of this change is of course hard to assess, given the difference in tests used. The authors stress the changeability over time in IQ of MBD patients in both directions, pointing out that 7 of the 11 scores changed more than 10 points (5 decreases, 2 increases).

A rather high rate of persistence of hyperactivity seems implicit in Laufer's (1971) follow-up report on 66 hyperkinetic patients treated in his private practice. All were 15 years of age or older at follow-up and the mean age was just under 20 years. Only 27 (41%) of these 66 patients stated that their hyperactivity had disappeared. Other neuropsychiatric symptoms were rare however. Laufer reported that only 1 of 56 subjects providing information on the topic mentioned having had hallucinations, and only three described having had any seizures; incidence rates probably within expectation for an unselected population.

Borland and Heckman (1976) found that 10 of 20 men who had been diagnosed as hyperactive as boys still had three or more symptoms of hyperactivity at follow-up. In contrast only one of the brothers serving as controls had this many symptoms. Nonetheless the residual average of three symptoms (overall 20 cases) represented a highly significant decrease from the mean of eight symptoms reported for the same subjects on the same list at their time of original diagnosis.

These results conform closely in general outline to those reported for adolescents: behavioral symptoms of MBD decrease with age, but do not disappear entirely. In fact one gains the impression that the decrease in Borland and Heckman's subjects is not substantially greater than that documented in studies of adolescents. This raises the question as to whether improvement is less likely after, than during, adolescence—that is whether or not adolescence may represent a kind of "critical period" for development of controls over activity levels, attention span, impulses, and other behavioral aspects of MBD.

Life Adjustment in Adulthood

The four studies providing information about the adjustment and life circumstances of MBD children as adults (Laufer, 1971; Borland and Heckman, 1976; Rawson, 1968; Menkes, Rowe, and Menkes, 1967) presented rather widely divergent pictures of the gravity of the syndrome. On the bleak side Menkes, Rowe, and Menkes found that only 8 of 14 were self-supporting at follow-up and that 8 of 14 had been institutionalized at some time in their careers, including 4 who were institutionalized at time of follow-up, all with psychosis. Three of 14 had been institutionalized for delinquency or crime and one for retardation. These negative outcomes occurred despite the fact that only 3 of the 14 patients retained signs or symptoms related to hyperactivity itself.

A much more favorable picture is presented by Borland and Heckman's findings (1976). All 20 of the hyperactive subjects were working full time or were in college at an average age of 31. None was reported to have been imprisoned or institutionalized, though 4 of 20 were diagnosed as sociopathic. Only 2 pro-bands had been divorced, as had 2 in the control group, brothers of the probands. The major deficits obtaining in the hyperactive group were in the area of SES. The ex-patients entered the work force at lower status jobs than their brothers and had not eliminated the discrepancy by the time of follow-up, as both they and their brothers had risen in SES over the 10-year interval. The ex-patients actually worked longer hours than their brothers, possibly to avoid boredom and restlessness, though the men themselves cited need for income. The ex-patients had changed jobs more often than their brothers, again citing desire for advancement and more income; but they also admitted feelings of dissatisfaction with previous jobs because of the boring nature of the work and lack of appreciation by supervisors.

The relatively benign picture of the later social adjustment of the hyperactive child presented by Borland and Heckman (1976) is particularly interesting in view of the fact that fully half the men reported three or more persisting symptoms of hyperactivity, as compared with less than a quarter (3 of 14) in Menkes, Rowe, and Menkes (1967) who reported hyperactivity as a continuing problem. This relative freedom from hyperactivity was not enough to allow Menkes' subjects to achieve good adjustment, while the higher residual hyperactivity in Borland and Heckman's subjects did not prevent them from achieving an acceptable social position. And those men in Borland and Heckman's study who did have a larger number of persisting symptoms did not fare worse occupationally or diagnostically than those who reported fewer such symptoms: number of symptoms in adulthood did not relate to adjustment in adulthood. However this conclusion must be taken with considerable caution as the data could be seriously distorted by self-report bias. That this might be present is suggested by the fact that those men diagnosed as psychopathic tended to report fewer symptoms of hyperactivity and those who had sought psychiatric help tended to report more such symptoms. Those subjects who had not advanced on the job might well tend to be those who denied the presence of undesirable symptoms.

Laufer's (1971) follow-up data were less complete and lacked comparable information from controls. Nonetheless the general impression conveyed by his report is also more optimistic than that of Menkes, Rowe, and Menkes. Fourteen of 37 (19 or older) were in college or graduate school and 18 were employed, leaving only five as unemployed. None were in jail, though 16 of 55 reported having been in some kind of trouble with police. This latter figure is difficult to evaluate because of the absence of data on controls using the same criteria for "some kind of trouble with police," but it does seem somewhat higher than the usual rate given for arrests of teenagers and young adults.

Only 5 of 67 reported experimenting with marijuana or LSD; only 3 of 56 reported nonprescription use of stimulants. None reported habitual use of any drug, except alcohol; 4 of 50 reported excessive drinking. Three of 54 subjects had reported psychiatric hospitalization and 20 of 55 acknowledged getting psychiatric help as outpatients apart from and after their treatment for hyperactivity.

This study, based on a questionnaire returned by 66 of 100 ex-patients, would seem highly liable to underreporting of undesirable events and circumstances. In particular the reported rate of experimentation with street drugs seems very low for a group of adolescents and young adults, even in 1971.

Summary of Outcomes

Function

Despite all of the variability and imperfections of method, the studies reviewed show some consensus in results. They appear to agree that children diagnosed as MBD continue to show some impairment, at least in those functions initially assessed as deficient. On the average reading progress shown by reading-impaired children is much below normal expectation, when these gains have been measured via objective tests. Children diagnosed as hyperactive continue to be somewhat more active than the average child, and other symptoms in the hyperactivity syndrome become even more noticeable. Even Rawson's (1968) very bright and successful subjects reported residual difficulties in reading and spelling.

Reassessment of neuropsychological functions, while rare, showed reduced but still significant deficits in such variables as complex reaction time (Dykman, Peters, and Ackerman, 1973), figure-ground discrimination, and visual-motor skills (Silver and Hagin, 1964). Unfortunately these generalizations are limited by an essentially total lack of data on directly measured functioning of ex-MBD children beyond the age of 25 or so. Menkes, Rowe, and Menkes (1967) evaluated the general neurological condition of their cases at follow-up, but did not relate these results to actual ability to perform tasks important in adaptation to daily life. Also missing are long-term follow-up studies of behavior problems in children diagnosed originally as learning disabled, not hyperactive. Evaluation of emotional adjustment, when undertaken, rather consistently showed development of self-critical, even depressive reactions in some older children and adolescents with hyperactivity. The possibility that stimulant drugs administered over a long period of time may contribute to these mood changes apparently has not been studied.

Status and Adjustment

There appears to be good agreement that children diagnosed as either learning disabled or hyperactive have a great deal of difficulty subsequently in keeping up with their classmates in school. Several studies found only a minority of the diagnosed children in the appropriate grade for age at follow-up. Ratings of behavior adjustment of children diagnosed as hyperactive generally indicated major problems. The only study to collect data on adolescent behavioral adjustment of children diagnosed as having learning disability without hyperactivity (Ackerman, Dykman, and Peters, 1977a, 1977b) suggested strongly that behavioral adjustment is good in these cases. Parental concern about the present and future remained very high for both learning disabled and hyperactive children despite perceptions of some improvement by the parents in a large majority of cases.

In contrast to the agreement concerning the persistence of school problems, social and vocational adjustment after school years appeared highly variable from study to study. Menkes, Rowe, and Menkes (1967) found a high rate of institutionalization and a low rate of self-support in adult subjects; Rawson (1968) found extremely high levels of achievement and no dependency at all among her dyslexics. Borland and Heckman (1976) studied individuals of more modest social backgrounds and abilities, but nonetheless described a generally conventional pattern of adjustment among ex-hyperactive children. Even so they note an elevated rate of sociopathic personality (about 20% among their ex-patients), a finding consistent with that of Huessy, Metoyer, and Townsend (1973, 1974). Similarly, the Huessy studies (1973, 1974); Laufer (1971); and Borland and Heckman (1976) all report what seem to be elevated rates of later psychiatric contact among their ex-patients. Thus it seems safe to conclude that hyperactive children have an elevated risk of later emotional or behavioral problems, but that the impact of these problems on other aspects of the individual's life, such as marriage; work; and even the ability to remain out of an institution, depend on other, yet unknown, factors.

PREDICTION OF INDIVIDUAL OUTCOME

A wide variety of variables has been studied as possible predictors of outcome and an almost equally wide variety has been used as criteria of outcome. Here we shall look first at predictors of later academic functioning in learning-disabled and hyperactive children, and then consider predictors of later social and emotional status. In all instances we shall be considering prediction within groups of children diagnosed as having MBD. We will not consider correlations such as those presented by Rawson (1968), which are based on a combined sample of MBD and normal children. Such correlations primarily reflect differences between MBD and non-MBD children and do not help the person who is attempting to work out a prognosis for a child already diagnosed as MBD.

In discussing differences in outcome and their possible predictors we shall focus primarily on relationships documented statistically within the several studies. However we shall also consider, necessarily on a more impressionistic basis, the implication of the sometimes very large differences between studies.

Academic Achievement

Prediction from Intelligence

IQs and other scores derived from intelligence tests (primarily the WISC) have been tried as predictors of reading achievement and academic progress. Results have not been entirely consistent. Koppitz (1971), Muehl and Forell (1973), and Dykman, Peters, and Ackerman (1973) found IQs to predict school marks. Minde, *et al.*, (1971) likewise showed higher IQ to be associated with better academic outcome in their hyperactive groups, and also demonstrated that large discrepancies between performance and verbal IQs on the WISC were associated with poorer academic outcome. Muehl and Forell (1973) found that verbal IQ predicted reading test scores, while Hinton and Knights (1971) found all three WISC IQs to predict school marks and rate of progress through the school grades. The highly intelligent subjects in Rawson's study (1968) also had very high academic achievement in the later years, though their actual reading skills are unknown. Gottesman, Belmont, and Kaminer (1975) and Riddle and Rapaport (1976), on the other hand, found no relation between IQ and later reading achievement. Rourke and Orr (1977) found IQ to be a poor predictor of reading achievement in learning disabled subjects, but a fairly good predictor in normal controls. Yule (1973) presented data suggesting that brighter subjects with specific reading retardation had poorer subsequent achievement than duller subjects whose initial reading deficit was evidently based only on low general ability ("backwardness"). This would imply a negative correlation between IQ and later rate of academic learning. However Yule does not actually present such correlations and does not give absolute values of initial intelligence or achievement scores in the subgroups selected by his regression equation.

On balance it appears that higher intelligence does predict better academic achievement in children with MBD, though perhaps not as consistently as in normal children.

Prediction from Initial Reading Ability

Koppitz (1971), Campbell, Endman, and Bernfeld (1971), and Silver and Hagin (1964) all found reading level at diagnosis to predict reading achievement at follow-up; Riddle and Rapaport (1976) and Rourke and Orr (1977) failed to find such a relationship in learning disabled children. Hinton and Knights (1971) found reading level at diagnosis to predict later school marks. Thus the evidence appears to support the value of early reading level in the prediction of later progress. However it is important to differentiate the prediction of reading *gain* from the prediction of reading *level* at follow-up. Since reading level at follow-up in effect includes initial reading level (rarely does a child lose reading skills previously mastered) one would expect a positive correlation between initial and later reading scores if all children gained about the same amount. While gain scores have their complexities (Harris, 1963), it would seem important to devise a measure of reading progress which is not statistically tied to initial reading scores. None of the studies reviewed did this in any detailed or explicit fashion, although Rourke and Orr (1977) and Yule (1973) used initial reading scores as covariates in analyzing follow-up reading scores.

Prediction from Severity or Quality of MBD

Several investigators have attempted to differentiate kinds of MBD and to evaluate the prognostic significance of the several subcategories. Minde, *et al.*, (1971) classified information processing deficits as visual, verbal, or motor. They found that children with deficits in two or all three of these areas had more academic failure than those with a deficit in one or none. Hinton and Knights (1971) did not find a relationship between visual or motor skills considered separately and later school marks, though language and auditory skills were predictive.

In the study by Rourke and Orr (1977) different combinations of the 13 "underlining" tests of Doehring (1968) were effective in predicting reading scores four years later in retarded readers, while the WISC, ITPA, and initial reading test scores did not contribute further to accuracy of prediction.

The underlining subtests which best predicted outcome in retarded readers were those which required rapid discrimination of a particular geometric form or sequence of forms when these items were interspersed along with distractors on a page. Subtests involving selection of letters and syllables were not as consistently effective as those involving geometric or "gestalt" figures.

Predictions based on the general notion of organicity have had mixed results. Eaves and Crighton (1974) found that greater judged severity of MBD was associated with placement in a special class by the school. Silver and Hagin (1964) found that children with learning disabilities diagnosed as "organic" made slower reading progress than those with disabilities diagnosed as "developmental."

Gottesman, Belmont, and Kaminer (1975) failed however to find a relationship between degree of neurological impairment and reading level at follow-up; Muehl and Forell (1973) found no relation between EEG patterns and progress in reading. Campbell, Endman, and Bernfeld (1977) found hyperactivity and neurological signs at 4 to predict digit span at $7\frac{1}{2}$, but did not report findings regarding reading achievement.

Each of these studies used a different method of evaluating extent and/or kind of MBD. The results suggest that the precise method of making such assessments may be crucial to their predictive value. Methods which assess severity of dysfunctions attributable to MBD may have more promise than those which attempt to distinguish only their quality. The evident success of Doehring's underlining tests (Rourke and Orr, 1977) further suggests that fine details of an information processing task may be important in its validity as a predictor.

Prediction from SES

Muehl and Forell (1973) present data suggesting that learning disabled children of higher SES families achieved better reading outcomes than those of lower SES, but these authors did not control for IQ or other ability variables. Weiss, *et al.*, (1971) found no relation between school achievement and SES or rating of family functioning. Rawson (1968) and Buerger (1968) found impressive academic achievements in learning disabled children from high SES families, but did not actually measure reading level or study learning disabled children from lower SES families.

Prediction from Age

Age at diagnosis was considered by Muehl and Forell (1973), who found that children who were younger tended to show better progress, and by Gottesman, Belmont, and Kaminer (1975), who found essentially the opposite, that the children who were younger at diagnosis subsequently tended to lose more centile points on a reading test than older children.

Riddle and Rapaport (1976) found that older boys diagnosed as MBD had lower centile scores than younger boys on the mathematics section of the WRAT at follow-up, whereas the two groups had not differed at time of diagnosis. This implies that the older boys made less progress on mathematics in the two-year interval than the younger boys. These studies did not use comparable measures, and Gottesman, Belmont and Kaminer (1975) did not equate subjects on degree of reading retardation at diagnosis. Thus the question of age at diagnosis and subsequent progress remains very much an open one.

Treatment and Achievement

In several studies type and amount of treatment via one or more of several modes (drugs, psychotherapy, remedial education) were studied in relation to improvement in academic functions. Two of these studied the efficiency of drugs in promoting academic achievement. Weiss, *et al.*, (1975) found no difference in number of grades failed in children taking methylphenidate, chlorpromazine, or no drug for 1.5 to 5 years. However in an abstract Weiss, *et al.*, (1974) reported that 3 to 5 years of methylphenidate treatment produced improved school achievement as well as better emotional adjustment and lesser delinquency in children from families rated as functioning well before treatment was started. Riddle and Rapaport (1976) found no difference in academic achievement (WRAT scores) between a subgroup of 20 hyperactive boys who had been randomly assigned to methylphenidate for 2 years and their total group of 72 hyperactive boys, some of whom were on imipramine. Ackerman, Dykman, and Peters (1977a) found that medicated subjects improved less on achievement tests than nonmedicated subjects. However boys were assigned clinically, not randomly, to medication by their private physicians, and the medicated group proved to be more deficient initially on all four tests. All that can be said is that the medication did not succeed in eliminating this initial deficit. Thus it seems that drug treatment as currently practiced does not promote academic achievement, except possibly in children whose families can capitalize on the otherwise temporary benefits of the drug.

Several studies have looked at remedial educational efforts in relation to academic progress. Somewhat surprisingly however only one study was found in which longer term effects of a remedial program were evaluated through application of a controlled experimental design. Buerger (1968) compared 72 children who had received an average of 112 hours of special instruction in a school-operated reading clinic with 72 children of similar intellectual ability and reading deficit who did not receive such help. Follow-up interval averaged 5.6 years but the ages of subjects are not given. No difference in reading scores at follow-up was detected between the clinic and control groups, but the clinic group reported having had fewer adjustment problems. Unfortunately no information is provided as to the absolute levels of reading skill or mental ability in either group at diagnosis or at follow-up.

The immediate and later effects of an intensive summer reading program are described by Balow (1965). He found very rapid gains during the 10-week program itself, and evaluation two to four years later seemed to indicate somewhat more rapid subsequent gains in the tutored group than in an untutored group, though both groups progressed at a below average rate during this posttreatment interval. Minde, Weiss, and Mendelson (1972) tallied the amount of remedial help received by subjects of their study and found it unrelated to test scores at outcome. Muehl and Forell (1973) also found no relation between amount of remedial help (measured by number of semesters of attendance in a reading clinic) and reading test scores (assessed about five years after diagnosis).

Gottesman, Belmont, and Kaminer (1975) found no difference in rate of progress between children receiving reading clinic services in addition to regular class instruction and children not receiving such supplemental help. Both of these groups showed a slight increase in reading centiles at follow-up. On the other hand 38 children assigned to special classes or special schools declined substantially in reading centiles. This was attributed by the authors to the greater initial disability of the children assigned to special school programs. Ackerman, Dykman, and Peters (1977a) found that children who were most deficient in reading were given the most intensive remedial help, but nonetheless made the poorest progress. Confounding of treatment and initial deficit makes evaluations impossible.

Prediction of Status and Adjustment

Prediction from Intelligence

In the long-term study by Menkes, Rowe, and Menkes (1967) IQ was the only variable from the diagnostic work-up which predicted self-support status in adulthood. Few other studies have evidently looked at IQ as a predictor of adjustment in children with MBD, IQ being reserved it appears for the seemingly more logical application of predicting academic and cognitive outcome. Full scale WISC IQ was 1 of 12 variables which, used together in a discriminant analysis, significantly differentiated good and poor outcome groups in the Minde, Weiss, and Mendelson (1972) study. Weighting of individual variables in the predictive composite variable is not reported. However Weiss, et al., (1971) reporting on subjects from the same general sample, state that IQ considered separately, did not predict antisocial behavior at follow-up. Mendelson, Johnson, and Stewart (1971) found no difference in initial IQ between a group which showed overall behavioral improvement and a group which did not.

Prediction from Academic Achievement

No follow-up study reviewed attempted to relate differences in initial achievement per se to differences in adjustment at outcome. This is surprising in view of the oft repeated assertion that reading failure leads to delinquency and the common finding that institutionalized delinquents are several years retarded academically despite near-average IQs (Poremba, 1975).

Prediction from Severity of Initial Behavioral Symptoms

Weiss, et al., (1971) and Riddle and Rapaport (1976) both reported significant relationships between ratings of antisocial behavior at diagnosis and at follow-up.

However ratings of activity level did not predict antisocial behavior in either study, though they did predict later activity level in the Riddle and Rapaport (1976) study. Base line hyperactivity predicted peer rejection at follow-up in this latter study as well. By contrast ratings of hyperactivity obtained at follow-up did not correlate with concurrent peer rejection in this study. Evidently earlier hyperactivity presaged poor development of social skills. Mendelson, Johnson, and Stewart (1971) found no difference between generally improved and generally unimproved groups of hyperactive children in the occurrence of antisocial behavior at diagnosis.

In striking contrast, Ackerman, Dykman, and Peters (1977b), reported that earlier hyperactivity accounted for almost all of the conduct problems at age 14 in a sample of learning-disabled boys. Hypo-active or normally active boys had no more antisocial behavior at follow-up than those without learning disabilities. This is evidently the only study which has studied hyperactivity systematically as a prognostic sign in a learning-disabled population. The finding that hyperactivity, not learning disability per se, predicts later behavior problems would, if replicated, be highly important for theory and for practice. It would suggest that a learning disability, frustrating as it may be for the child, does not typically lead, in and of itself, to antisocial behavior. To complete the picture we need behavioral follow-up studies of hyperactive children who are free of learning deficits.

Prediction from Family Variables

Weiss, *et al.*, (1971) report that ratings of impaired mental health in parents and punitive discipline are associated with later antisocial behavior. Weiss and Minde (1974) mentioned a tendency for hyperactive children who are judged to have poor outcome after five years to have had lower SES, and poorer parent-child relationships at diagnosis than children with good outcomes.

In a later report Weiss, *et al.*, (1974) stated that a rating of family functioning predicted emotional adjustment and delinquency outcomes in their hyperactive children only in the group taking methylphenidate. Children had been on the drug for three to five years and were given a two-week drug holiday when the evaluations were made. Finally Weiss and Minde (1974) noted a tendency for changes in family functioning over the follow-up interval to parallel changes in the child " . . . families of good outcome children improved over five years while families of 'bad outcome' children are deteriorated" (p. 75). Mendelson, Johnson, and Stewart (1971) did not find relationships between family intactness or parent pathology and antisocial behavior, but did find that the father's own history of learning and behavior problems did predict antisocial behavior in his offspring. Social status of the family was not found by Menkes, Rowe, and Menkes (1967) to be related to self-support by adults who were hyperactive and learning disabled as children. Riddle and Rapaport (1976) were not able to find familial correlates of depressive symptoms in the hyperactive children they studied. Koppitz (1971) did find a higher incidence of family disorganization in learning disabled children who were emotionally disturbed enough to require referral for residential treatment, but it was not clear that this was a truly predictive relationship. In general relationships between family variables and socialization of children with MBD appear weaker than one might expect, given the generally consistent relationships between childrearing variables and antisocial behavior reported for children not known to have MBD. Of course the existing studies of these relationships in the MBD child and his family only scratch the surface.

Prediction from Treatment Variables

Consensus appears to exist that drug treatment has little impact on behavioral adjustment after cessation of medication. Laufer (1971); Huessy and Townsend (1973); Huessy, Metoyer, and Townsend (1974); and Minde, Weiss, and Mendelson (1972) all failed to find any relationship between length or kind of drug treatment and behavioral symptoms at follow-up. In fact Weiss and Minde (1974) concluded that drug treatment lasting longer than three years tends to be associated with poor outcome. However methylphenidate appeared to have beneficial behavioral effects in children from well-functioning families in the study by Weiss, *et al.*, (1974). It should be noted that these children had been off drug for only two weeks when the evaluations were made, so that the persistence of benefits is not assured even here.

Amount of counseling or psychotherapy also appeared generally unrelated to behavioral outcome. Mendelson, *et al.*, (1971), and Menkes (1967) found no outcome effects attributable to psychotherapy. Minde, Weiss, and Mendelson (1972) and Weiss and Minde (1974) reported no effect of psychotherapy on psychopathic symptoms, but possible beneficial effects on neurotic symptoms. This latter finding was not conclusive because psychotherapy tended to go to subjects high on neurotic symptoms, leaving only non-neurotic subjects to serve as controls. The treated neurotic children did improve significantly but there was no way to rule out maturation or time alone as the source of the improvement.

Summary of Predictive Effects

Prediction of the later adjustment and status of a child diagnosed as having MBD is highly uncertain at present. It is fairly safe to say that a child with an extremely high IQ, high social status, and intensive systematic educational efforts has a good prognosis both for academic achievement and vocational success. MBD children with more modest IQs and family backgrounds can lead generally conventional lives, albeit with a somewhat more hectic pace and lower SES according to the findings of Borland and Heckman (1976).

Over the shorter term at least, greater impairment of information processing capacities may predict poorer reading progress, and greater behavior problems initially may predict the same kinds of problems later. Punitive childrearing or disorganized family life also may predict later behavior problems in MBD children, as they do in children in general, but perhaps not as strongly.

In general prediction of outcome in the MBD child may be a more difficult problem than prediction for children in general. Partly this would stem from the restriction of the range of scores of almost all potential predictors which is implicit in the selection of children with MBD. However the problem may also be complicated by the generally more diffuse structure of abilities in the learning disabled child (Wallbrown, *et al.*, 1974). Thus each MBD child may face his own personal bottleneck, so that attempts to generalize statistically about deficits and treatment may be unproductive. Rourke and Orr's (1977) finding that rapid discrimination of various printed items (underlining tests) was predictive of later reading achievement in MBD children but not in normals, does suggest however that some commonality of deficit can be found for learning disabled children as a group. Nonetheless very large systematic studies will be required in order to put the various predictors in any sort of useful perspective.

CONCLUSIONS

What then shall we tell the parents of the MBD child? Or for that matter, the child himself? Sketchy as they are, the data appear consistent in indicating that he—and it is likely to be he rather than she if the child is selected as were those in the studies reviewed—will have a high risk of some lasting deficits in functioning. As regards adjustment, he has an exceptionally high risk, well above 50%, of repeating one or more grades in school, and, if he is hyperactive, an elevated risk of antisocial behavior. Beyond these generalizations, outcomes depend on the nature and extent of the cognitive and behavioral manifestation of MBD, the child's general intellectual level, and perhaps on the SES of his family. Number and kinds of information processing problems may be important in later reading progress.

If the child is fortunate enough to score at very high levels on intelligence tests, to have parents in a profession, and to attend a private school or a university-operated reading clinic, his prognosis for academic and vocational success is very good. This is true even though the child himself evidently is likely never to lose his feeling that reading and spelling are difficult for him.

At the other extreme, if the child has both learning and behavior problems, obtains a low (below 90) IQ, has a family of lower SES, and is subject only to the usual management efforts, prognosis for continued school failure is very high. Even with all of these negative factors however prognosis for vocational and life adjustment is evidently not totally gloomy. Risks of psychopathy, lowered SES, antisocial behaviors and psychiatric contact are elevated, but total social and vocational incapacitation are evidently not the rule, despite the findings of the small study by Menkes, Rowe, and Menkes (1967). However if the child has learning disability without hyperactivity, prognosis for continued freedom from behavior problems may be good, provided the results of Ackerman, Dykman, and Peters (1977b) hold up.

For the more nearly "average" MBD child with both cognitive and behavior problems, the parents can be told that in all probability they will notice some improvement in behavior, but not enough really to allay their anxieties about the child's future.

To the parents' pressing query, "What should we do?" the honest professional will have to admit his uncertainty, with apologies to the parents and inward imprecations at his colleagues and the funding agencies for the lack of more definitive information. While he can point to the success enjoyed by bright learning-impaired children in intensive remedial programs, he will have to add that no one knows what happens to equally bright learning-impaired children who do not receive such teaching. He can describe the effectiveness of stimulant drugs in limiting some disturbing behavior, but he cannot give assurances that these effects will outlast the administration of the drug, except possibly if there is an exceptionally stable and supportive family. To questions about counseling or psychotherapy, he would have to answer that it may be useful in reducing "internalized" personality problems, but that no methods. have been proven effective over the longer term for the more common "externalized" conduct problems.

What are the implications of the findings for future life history research in MBD? First, it is worth doing. Longitudinal research so far has indicated that childhood diagnosis of MBD has substantial long-term significance, but leaves many questions to be answered about the exact nature of MBD and reasons for its consequences.

Second, future studies should be more comprehensive. Behavioral and cognitive aspects of MBD should be studied separately and in interaction, all within a single prospective research design.

Third, IQ and social status should be controlled more tightly in future work. At present differences in outcome cannot always be related to difference in specific dysfunction, because the subjects also differ in general ability and family background.

Fourth, detailed study of the interaction of the child with MBD and his social and educational environment needs to be undertaken. At present life adjustment appears to get worse though some symptoms improve in some studies (for example Menkes, Rowe, and Menkes, 1967), while in others (Rawson, 1968) life adjustment is superb in adulthood even though reported symptoms persist. Especially intriguing is the evident impact of the hyperactive child on the behavior of his classmates and his apparent reduction of his teacher's tolerance for minor misbehavior by non-hyperactive children in the class (Campbell, Endman, and Bernfeld, 1977).

Cross-lagged panel designs (Campbell and Stanley, 1963) would be very useful in teasing out cause and effect relationships between the child's symptomatic behaviors and environmental events. Does school failure lead to aggressive behavior or does aggressive behavior predict later school failure?

Fifth, research on effectiveness of nonpharmacological intervention (remedial education, behavior management) needs to be pursued over a period of years, just as research on medication has. The latter has shown disappointing long-term efficacy despite seeming short-term benefits for activity level and some cognitive processes. Currently underway is a major effort by Educational Testing Service (Harris, 1976), with research funds from the federal government, to survey several hundred school districts with respect to effectiveness of special educational programs. It is intended to isolate a smaller number (about 30) for more intensive study of longer term effectiveness. Perhaps this effort will result in some more definitive information about effective long-term programs for various subtypes of children with reading problems. However it is not clear that the child who is an underachiever by virtue of MBD will be singled out for special attention in this study.

Finally it appears to this reviewer that a little more explicit reference to theory in the design of life history research in MBD would be profitable. It might help clarify and regularize the selection of subjects, the designation of control groups, the choice of measures and the interval of reevaluations. On the other hand it is recognized that theories, especially grand ones, can become obsolete before a longitudinal study is well underway. Therefore in designing research of this nature, one must also always keep one's eye on the enduring, real-life aspects of MBD which can make life so frustrating for the victims, their parents, and their teachers.

REFERENCES

Ackerman, P. T., R. A. Dykman, and J. E. Peters. "Learning-Disabled Boys as Adolescents." *Journal of the American Academy of Child Psychiatry*, 16(2), 296–313 (1977*a*).

Ackerman, P. T., R. A. Dykman, and J. E. Peters. "Teenage status of hyperactive and non-hyperactive learning disabled boys". *American Journal of Orthopsychiatry*, 47(4), 577–596, (1977*b*).

Balow, B. "The long-term effect of remedial reading instruction." *The Reading Teacher*, 18, 581–586, (1965).

Borland, B. L. and H. K. Heckman. "Hyperactive boys and their brothers." *Archives of General Psychiatry*, 33, 669–675, (1976).

Buerger, T. A. "A follow-up of remedial reading instruction." *The Reading Teacher*, 21(4), 329–334, (1968).

Campbell, D. T., and J. C. Stanley. "Experimental and quasi-experimental designs for research." Chicago: Rand McNally, 1963.

Campbell, S. B., M. W. Endman, and G. Bernfeld. "A three-year follow-up of hyperactive preschoolers into elementary school." *Journal of Child Psychology and Psychiatry*, 18, 239–249, (1977).

Cohen, N. J., G. Weiss, and K. Minde. "Cognitive styles in adolescents previously diagnosed as hyperactive." *Journal of Child Psychology and Psychiatry*, 13, 203–209, (1972).

Doehring, D. G. *"Patterns of Impairment in Specific Reading Disability."* Inidana University Press, Bloomington, Ind., (1968).

Dykman, R. A., J. E. Peters, and P. T. Ackerman. "Experimental approaches to the study of minimal brain dysfunction: A follow-up study." *Annals of New York Academy of Sciences*, 205, 93–108, (1973).

Eaves, L. C., and J. U. Crichton. "A five-year follow-up of children with minimal brain dysfunction." *Academic Therapy*, 10(2), 173–180, (1974–1975).

Gottesman, R., I. Belmont, and R. Kaminer. "Admission and follow-up status of reading disabled children referred to a medical clinic." *Journal of Learning Disabilities*, 8(10), 43–51, (1975).

Hammar, S. L. "School underachievement in adolescents." *Pediatrics*, 40(3), 373–381, (1967).

Harris, A. J. "Practical applications of reading research." *The Reading Teacher*, 29(6), 559–565, (1976).

Harris, C. W., ed., *Problems in Measuring Change*. Madison, Wis.: University of Wisconsin Press, 1963.

Hinton, G. G., and R. M. Knights. "Children with learning problems: Academic history, academic prediction, and adjustment three years after assessment." *Exceptional Children*, 38, 513–519, (1971).

Huessy, H. R., and A. H. Cohen. "Hyperkinetic behaviors and learning disabilities followed over seven years." *Pediatrics*, 57(1), 4–10, (1976).

Huessy, H. R., M. Metoyer, and M. Townsend. "Eight-ten year follow-up of children treated in rural Vermont for behavioral disorder." *American Journal of Orthopsychiatry*, 43(2), 233–238, (1973).

Huessy, H. R., M. Metoyer, and M. Townsend. "Eight-ten year follow-up of 84 children treated for behavioral disorder in rural Vermont." *Acta Paedopsychiatrica*, 40, 230–235, (1974).

Koppitz, E. M. *Children with Learning Disabilities: A Five Year Follow-up Study*. New York: Grune & Stratton, 1971.

Laufer, M. W. "Long-term management and some follow-up findings on the use of drugs with minimal cerebral syndrome." *Journal of Learning Disabilities*, 4, 518–522, (1971).

Mellsop, G. W. "Psychiatric patients seen as children and adults: Childhood predictors of adult illness." *Journal of Child Psychology and Psychiatry*, 13(2), 91–101, (1972).

Mendelson, W., N. Johnson, and M. A. Stewart. "Hyperactive children as teenagers: A follow-up study." *The Journal of Nervous and Mental Disease*, 153(4), 273–279, (1971).

Menkes, M. J., J. S. Rowe, and J. H. Menkes. "A twenty-five year follow-up study on the hyperkinetic child with minimal brain dysfunction." *Pediatrics*, 39(3), 393–399, (1967).

Minde, K., G. Weiss, and N. Mendelson. "A five-year follow-up study of 91 hyperactive school children." *Journal of the American Academy of Child Psychiatry*, 11, 595–610, (1972).

Minde, K., D. Lewin, G. Weiss, H. Lavigueur, V. Douglas, and E. Sykes. "The hyperactive child in elementary school: A 5-year, controlled followup." *Exceptional Children*, 38, 215–221, (1971).

Muehl, S., and E. R. Forell. "A followup study of disabled readers: Variables related to high school reading performance." *Reading Research Quarterly*, 9(1), 110–123, (1973–1974).

Poremba, C. D. "Learning disabilities, youth and delinquency: Programs for Intervention," in Helmer R. Myklebust, Ed., *Progress in learning disabilities, Vol. III*, pp. 123–149. New York: Grune & Stratton, 1975.

Preston, R. C., and D. J. Yarington. "Status of fifty retarded readers eight years after reading clinic diagnosis." *Journal of Reading*, 11(2), 122–129, (1967).

Rawson, M. B. *Developmental Language Disability: Adult Accomplishments of Dyslexic Boys.* Baltimore: Johns Hopkins University Press, 1968.

———— "Developmental dyslexia: Educational treatment and results," in M. B. Rawson and D. D. Duane, eds., *Reading, Perception and Language*, pp. 231–258. Baltimore: York Press, 1975.

Riddle, K. D., and Rapaport, J. L. "A 2-year follow-up of 72 hyperactive boys." *The Journal of Nervous and Mental Disease*, 162(2), 126–134, (1976).

Robins, L. N. "Problems in follow-up studies." *American Journal of Psychiatry*, 134(8), 904–907, (1977).

Robinson, H. M., and H. K. Smith. "Reading clinic clients—ten years after." *The Elementary School Journal*, 63(1), 22–28, (1962).

Rourke, B. P., and R. R. Orr. "Prediction of the reading and spelling performances of normal and retarded readers: A four-year follow-up." *Journal of Abnormal Child Psychology*, 5(1), 9–20, (1977).

Sameroff, A. J., and M. J. Chandler. "Reproductive risk and the continuum of caretaking casualty," in F. D. Horowitz, ed., *Review on Child Development Research*. Vol. 4, pp. 187–244. Chicago: University of Chicago Press, 1975.

Satz, P., D. Rardin, and J. Ross. "An evaluation of a theory of specific developmental dyslexia." *Child Development*, 42(6), 2009–2021, (1971).

Shelley, E. M., and A. Riester. "Syndrome of minimal brain damage in young adults." *Diseases of the Nervous System*, 33(5), 335–338, :1972).

Silver, A. A., and R. A. Hagin. "Specific reading disability: follow-up studies." *American Journal of Orthopsychiatry*, 34, 95–102, (1964).

Sleator, E. K., A. von Neumann, and R. L. Sprague. "Hyperactive children: A continuous long-term placebo-controlled follow-up." *Journal of the American Medical Association*, 229(3), 316–317, (1974).

Stewart, M. A., W. B. Mendelson, and N. E. Johnson. "Hyperactive children as adolescents: How they describe themselves.'' *Child Psychiatry and Human Development*, 4(1), 3–11, (1973).

Trites, R. L., and C. Fiedorowicz. ''Follow-up study of children with specific (or primary) reading disability,'' in R. M. Knights and D. J. Bakker, eds., *The Neuropsychology of Learning Disorders—Theoretical Approaches*, pp. 41–50. Baltimore: University Park Press, 1976.

Wallbrown, F. H., R. J. Wherry, J. Blaha, D. H. Counts. ''An empirical test of Myklebust's cognitive structure hypotheses for 70 reading-disabled children.'' *Journal of Consulting and Clinical Psychology*, 42(2), 211–218, (1974*b*).

Weiss, G., and K. K. Minde. ''Follow-up studies of children who present with symptoms of hyperactivity,'' in C. K. Conners, ed., *Clinical Use of Stimulant Drugs in Children*, pp. 67–78. Amsterdam: Excerpta Medica, 1974.

Weiss, G., E. Kruger, U. Danielson, and M. Elman. ''Long-term methylphenidate treatment of hyperkinetic children.'' *Psychopharmacological Bulletin*, 10(4), 34–35 (1974).

——— ''Effect of long-term treatment of hyperactive children with methylphenidate.'' *Canadian Medical Association Journal*, 112, 159–160, (1975).

Weiss, G., K. Minde, J. S. Werry, V. Douglas, and E. Nemeth. ''Studies on the hyperactive child. VIII. Five-year follow-up.'' *Archives of General Psychiatry*, 24, 409–414, (1971).

Yule, W. ''Differential prognosis of reading backwardness and specific reading retardation.'' *British Journal of Educational Psychology*, 43, 244–248, (1973).

PART THREE

Neural Substratum

CHAPTER 5

Theories of Brain Mechanisms in Minimal Brain Dysfunctions[1]

Herbert C. Lansdell

NATIONAL INSTITUTES OF HEALTH
BETHESDA, MARYLAND

INTRODUCTION

A handbook is usually constructed as a compendium of established fact and useful theory. The present handbook is somewhat different in that it emphasizes that the topic of minimal brain dysfunction is not a unitary disorder and also encourages doubt about the utility of the concept. The purpose of this chapter deserves more skepticism than most of the others. Theories of brain dysfunction to explain the aberrant behavior of children are very speculative. However there is no doubt that it is intriguing why some therapeutic effects have been obtained by providing "activating" drugs for those children deemed to be "hyperactive," most of whom are boys. Because of its importance, the question of how the regular ingestion of such drugs can "paradoxically" constrain some children to more normal levels with regard to amount of limb movement or general locomotion, or how such drug use can facilitate decorum, is of some embarrassment to contemporary biomedical and psychological sciences.

Much contemporary biomedical thought in the MBD field appears to be little more than myth or clinical superstition to some critics (Schmitt, 1975, 1976; Meier, 1976). Some skeptics think that regardless of what physiological and behavioral effects may be traced to the drugs, the effects are often irrelevant to the reasons of some educators or parents who seek to have the children medicated (Schrag and Divoky, 1975). That hypercritical view is not entirely beside the point. However some clinical conclusions are attaining respectability (Safer, 1978). There is probably sufficient evidence that the administration of methylphenidate (Ritalin) can significantly improve the ability of overactive boys to maintain attention on some laboratory tasks (Humphries, Kinsbourne, and Swanson, 1978; Everett, 1977; Sprague and Sleator, 1977). Though Ritalin and dextroamphetamine, another sympathomimetic drug, are not likely to improve school achievement scores (Rie, 1975, 1977; Rie and Rie, 1977; Rie, et al., 1976), they may, like the tranquilizer imipramine lead to less classroom disruption (Quinn and Rapoport, 1975; Waizer, et al., 1974). However there is a recent report that a dose of dextroamphetamine can improve scores of normal boys on cognitive tests (Rapoport, et al., 1978). The authors argue that hypotheses about biological de-

[1] I thank Karl Frank, Christy Ludlow, Ellen Silbergeld, Sandra Witelson and Theodore Zahn for helpful comments on parts of an early draft.

fects are not necessary to explain a beneficial drug effect, and that the effect has no diagnostic significance.

There are intelligent guesses about what is changed in the brains of the children by the drugs and why some parts of the brain may be assumed to work better with continual drug treatment. As scientific explanations, none of the guesses are satisfactory. The theories about MBD serve a purpose by helping to provide a foundation for guessing about the various neurophysiological events in these children's brains. However no theory can integrate both the chemistry of the therapeutic effects and the locus of the crucial changes in the young brain. Theoretical discussions might help develop interventions, either pharmacological, educational, or psychological, that are uniquely effective with given symptom complexes. They might help in understanding the processes underlying scholastic problems or the management of overactive children in the classroom and at home. The importance of this field is sufficient reason for surveying theories that attempt either to describe dysfunctional brain mechanisms or to provide reasons for the beneficial results.

For a good portion of children on these drug treatments, this chapter assumes that: (1) the resulting change in their behavior is in the direction of better school or home adjustment, if not "normalization," and (2) the useful change would not occur, or could not be maintained for long, with the administration of placebo pills. The neurophysiological speculation is more about the developing brain than about drug effects in later adolescence when beneficial changes may continue after the drug treatment stops. Before proceeding with the details of a survey of these issues, a brief outline of some modern ideas in anatomy, neuropharmacology, and functional characteristics of the young human brain will be provided.

ANATOMY, PHYSIOLOGY, AND CHEMISTRY

The Developing Brain

Well before birth the connecting neural pathways in the human brain have developed from the receptor surfaces to the midbrain structures and to the cortex, and from the cortical and subcortical cells out to the musculature and other effector organs. After the brain has developed all its nerve cell bodies, around the time of birth, the emergence of the complex coordinating activities of the central nervous system is largely dependent on how interconnections among neural cells develop and decay. Problem solving in the adult, and reflective thought and social adjustment, probably depend on the particular intricate relationships that have developed among the various cortical and subcortical groups of neurons.

In the first few weeks of life, after the majority of nerve cells are formed, a large portion die as a kind of discard group. Perhaps this phenomenon serves to insure that the connections which are formed later are better ones. There is a normal rate of loss of neural connections and of death of irreplaceable neural cells; these rates are probably accelerated during many forms of ill health. Ingrained personality characteristics and diminished rate of learning in older age are assumed to be related somehow to the cumulative loss of neural tissue and connections. Some neural cells are attacked by certain toxins and specific illnesses, and some are more susceptible than others to damage by febrile illnesses. For some extreme forms of dementia in childhood, progress has been made in describing the loss of connections and the abnormal shapes of some cell processes in the cortex (Purpura, 1975).

The size of the brain varies depending on genetic factors, nutrition, and other conditions of general health. The growth in size of mammalian brains after birth is relatively less than for other organs, which can grow new cells. Some of the increase in size of the brain is a result of enlargement of the cortical neural cells and their connections, but there is also growth and reproduction of glial cells, which are half the volume of the brain.

Rearing rodents in large, complex environments can accelerate the growth of cortical tissue and of some thalamic nuclei (Rosenzweig, 1976). These kinds of changes, particularly in the dorsal and posterior cortex, may be the reason why some handicaps are eliminated which otherwise would be incurred by rats reared in small cages and subjected to early damage to the anterior cortex of their brains (Lansdell, 1953; Smith, 1959; Will, Rosenzweig, and Bennett, 1976). Similarly for monkeys, Goldman (1976) has suggested that early exposure to test problems has a salutary effect on the scores obtained after frontal-lobe ablations in the adult.

In addition to providing some mechanical and nutritional support of neurons, the glial cells provide avenues for subtle chemical influences on brain function and can provide a more constant environment by "spatial buffering" (Grossman and Seregin, 1977). In experiments using rats the extent of early handling and environmental enrichment has been shown to affect the number of glial cells found in some cortical areas of the brain. The glial cells can affect both the number and the nature of the neural connections. This variation in input to the nervous system at the time of proliferation of the two main types of such cells, astrocytes and oligodendrocytes, may lead to permanent increases in either or both types of cell (Paterson and Leblond, 1977; Szeligo, 1977; Szeligo and Leblond, 1977). Szeligo speculates that perceptual elaboration tends to involve growth of oligodendrocytes more than astrocytes and the adaptation to handling tends to involve more the latter than the former.

The outer cortex of the brain of the larger mammals becomes wrinkled early in life as it gets fitted in place inside the skull. Convolutions develop in the embryonic cortex as it folds around its fiber connections, nerve tracts, and the fluid-filled ventricles. The major fissures of the human brain are consistent from one brain to another and in normal brains can be labeled with confidence; the boundaries of the frontal lobes and the anterior temporal regions are formed early and are usually clear to gross inspection. A recent report (Graham, et al., 1978) on how a baby without a cerebrum oriented and habituated at three to six weeks to sounds in the fashion of older normal infants, suggests that initially the cerebral structures can "interfere with or disrupt the activity of lower centers."

Different parts of the brain reach their adult form at different rates. An increasing amount of myelinization—the extent of development of a sheath around the axons of neurons to provide more rapid transmission—is commonly assumed to be correlated with the child's level of proficiency in locomotion and other coordinated aspects of bodily behavior (Adams and Victor, 1977). The myelinization of some parts, such as the large commissures and other intracortical fibers, continues up to 10 years of age, while the sheath for some of the major pathways leading to the spinal cord are stabilized before the end of the first year of life. In cases of Down's syndrome, Davison (1977) reports finding only half the expected amounts of myelin in cortical white matter.

There are individual differences in these developmental changes and they may be complexly related to parentage and external factors, such as nutrition and exercise. The form of the sulci are probably determined in part by the shape of the skull, which is affected, in part, by the birth process. Extreme deformation of the skull during delivery of a child can damage some parts of the brain to the extent that it will become manifest later as a neurological disorder.

Many morphological variations inside the brain probably have some bearing on psychological differences among people. The variations in how the different nerve fibers to the cord cross over in the midline of the medulla possibly have some relation to handedness and other asymmetries of motor skill (Yakovlev and Rakic, 1966). There is also a possibility that the presence of a band of tissue across the midline ventricle, known as the massa intermedia, might reflect something about a difference in the lateralization of cerebral function in the two-thirds of male brains that have this tissue (Lansdell and Davie, 1972).

Research into the morphology of the human brain and its variations is expensive and time consuming. However within a decade the new computerized, low-dosage X-ray scanning techniques should be safe for research with normal people and provide adequate visualization of the main fissures to enable research relating anatomical variation to the range of variation in traits.

Neural Pathways to and from the Brain

The main pathways from the distance receptors to the brain and from the brain out to the muscles, internal organs, and glands are insulated channels of neural activity. It used to be fashionable to emphasize that all selective input neural activity was similar and that the differentiation among the inputs was essentially in the terminal tissue in the brain. The main distinguishing features of visual and auditory systems are their types of cortex and the types of associated tissue, but there are also important differences in the pattern of neural activity in many input systems. For example pain pathways conduct slower than other input pathways. Much input activity also goes in parallel to noncortical structures. In some instances there are differences in the nature of feedback control over receptor orientation and level of adaptation at the receptor surfaces. Some degree of central neural adaptation also occurs in relation to variation in the general level of input neural activity.

The major input systems—vision, audition, and somesthesis—have large nuclei in the thalamus which have connections to the specialized parts of the cortex and to parts of the midbrain. The thalamic nuclei serve to "relay" information while modulating the neural activity. Distinct groups of nerve cell bodies make up nuclei in the thalamus, basal ganglia, limbic lobe, hypothalamus, and other parts of the "forebrain" and "midbrain."

The visual cortex has columns of cells and the relation of activity in these columns to types of visual input seems elaborate enough to handle many of the important features that constitute basic aspects of visual perception (Hubel, Wiesel, and Stryker, 1978). For example the direction of movement and the characteristics of the contours of objects seen by an organism have selective effects on various cells in the organism's visual cortex.

Experiments limiting the visual input in kittens or young rabbits have demonstrated later aberrations in the neurophysiological activity at the cortex (Grobstein and Chow, 1975).

Connections from the eye to subcortical structures also channel some patterned input; these systems are involved in the control of gaze and the blanking out of some cerebral activity during eye movements (Goldberg and Robinson, 1977). Analogous subcortical systems are involved during auditory and somesthetic reception and presumably are affected by the amount and forms of input activity.

Some of the intricate mechanisms of control over input function probably develop without regard to variations in normal rearing conditions, for instance convergence of the eyes as an aid in depth perception develops rapidly in the first few months after birth. And mammals develop several perceptual mechanisms— one interesting example is the tendency toward completion in the visual field, which enables them to deal accurately with the external world, although the input messages are modified by a variety of influences. There is no visual input from the retina in the area of the optic nerve, but there is a filling in of the visual field of view so that a person is ordinarily unaware that this input is missing. Individuals with field defects as a result of lesions of the visual system in the brain can also be unaware of the restricted input and show some completion (Teuber, 1975). As with most forms of color blindness, the phenomenon has to be demonstrated in test situations for an individual to understand the input limitation. In a loose sense there are other analogous differences that can be demonstrated in test situations, for instance people differ in their cardiac response or palmar resistance changes to startle situations. Other variations in the range and type of reactivity may become more evident to individuals upon listening to tape recordings and seeing movies of themselves. Chimps may not be capable of this self-recognition, although they can recognize themselves in a mirror and monkeys cannot.

The reticular substance of the brain (Figure 5–1) is a network of tissue in the core of the brain which is involved in providing a general activating function, and it is considered of importance in allowing a mammal to habituate to repetitive stimuli (Groves and Thompson, 1973). Barbiturates are assumed to have the sedative effect largely through effects on the reticular system, parts of which are clearly important in maintaining attention in continuous monitoring tasks (Mirsky and Orren, 1977). Lucas and Siegel (1977) using cats with implanted electrodes stimulated the reticular formation and demonstrated that the less excitable cats have lower thresholds for initiation of inhibition in the visual cortex. There are probably similar differences in human brain excitability.

The control of the fast-acting skeletal musculature by output systems of the brain is primarily through the "motor" cortex and nerve fibers to the spinal cord. This system is derived mostly from large pyramidal cells in the cortex and works in close concert with the "extrapyramidal," vestibular, and cerebellar systems. The muscle tone appropriate for the anticipated activity is controlled by the activity in these systems. The pyramidal tract neurons are thought to make the essential contribution to the presetting of spinal reflexes (Evarts, 1978; Evarts and Granit, 1976).

Although the cerebral cortex is essential for the execution of finely tuned acts of human skill, the tissue immediately in front of the central fissure is not the sole device for the execution of bodily movements. It is probably more in the nature of a crucial modulatory apparatus (Evarts, 1975). Some of the basal ganglia may profitably be conceived of as important as cortical tissue in keeping a person actively engaged in everyday coordinated activities. In particular the globus pallidus may be essential in the generation of slow voluntary movements and in the

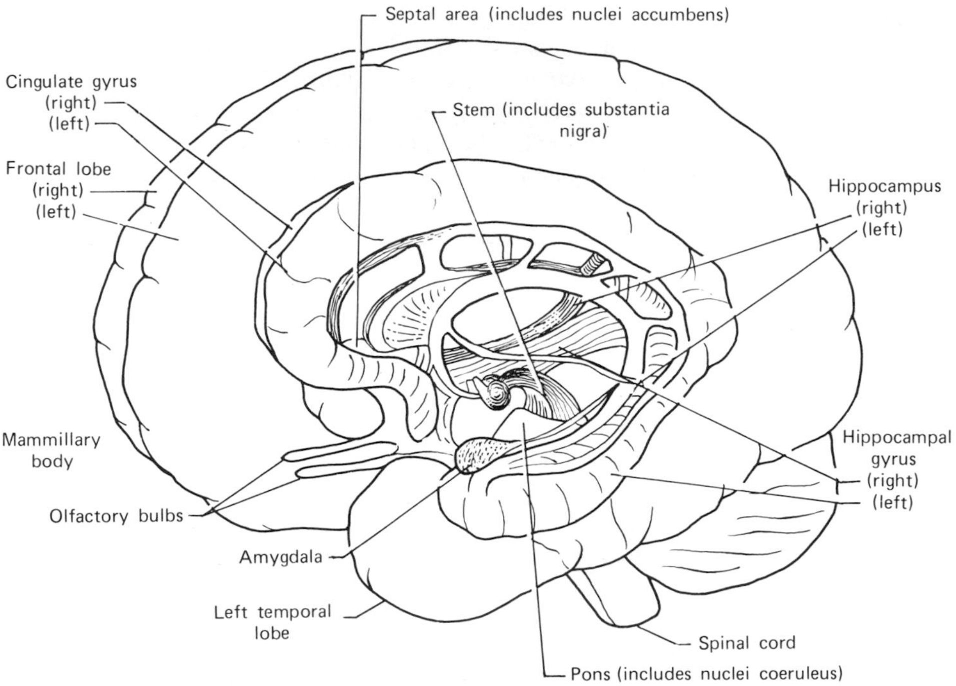

Figure 5–1.   Three dimensional drawing of the human brain viewed from the left side. It depicts the main structures of the limbic system, which surrounds the thalamus and basal ganglia. The major openings shown at each side contain thalamocortical projections, commissural and other intercortical fibers, the optic tract and ventricles. The more diffuse projection systems coming from the reticular formation in the pons also travel up through the thalamic tissue. A caudate nucleus, in front of the thalamus on each side, has a diminishing portion that parallels the hippocampus; the putamen and globus pallidus (also not shown) are adjacent to the caudate and lateral to the thalamus. (Adapted from Snyder, 1977.)

nonvisual control of limb movements (Hore, Meyer-Lohman, and Brooks, 1977).

The cerebellum, connected to the brain stem behind the cerebrum, is also involved in the control of limb movements through its connections to motor systems in the brain and spinal cord. Some kinds of incoordination are the result of cerebellar malfunction. However it is not likely that hyperkinesis will be traced in a significant portion of the children to a disorder in the cerebellum. Some forms of clumsiness can be attributed to cerebellar malfunction, but presumably should not be considered an essential neurophysiological feature of "hyperkinetic" children, except that some disruption of the optimal functioning of the basal ganglia may be involved.

Within each hemisphere longitudinal fibers connect portions of different lobes, and a variety of smaller fiber tracts connect tissue around different sulci. The largest band of connecting fibers within the brain, the corpus callosum, runs from one side to the other above the thalamus and it is interlaced with longitudinal fibers and the other main input and output pathways connected to the cortex. The corpus callosum serves to organize similar parts of the two halves of the brain in some manner that contributes to an individual's unity of behavior and action. Without the corpus callosum, either by congenital defect or surgical resection, there seems to be some separation of functions for the two hemispheres which can be revealed in specially contrived test situations where the input is limited to one hemisphere (for example flashes of perceptual material to either visual field for transmission to the contralateral hemisphere). This separation of functions is not readily apparent in such an individual's everyday activities, probably in part because the two hemispheres learn from each other continuously (LeDoux, et al., 1977). Two other large commissures through the thalamus also serve to connect activities on both sides. These and other structures serve to integrate in some degree the separated dorsal parts of the hemispheres in these patients (Teng, 1974). The lateralization of function to the two hemispheres will be described in more detail later.

Many of the longer fiber systems give off collateral connections to the tissue through which they pass. More diffuse pathways with more interconnections are found in the phylogenetically older parts of the brain such as the hypothalamus and the limbic lobes. The description of some of the subcortical structures that have been implicated in MBD will be described after considering some of the neurophysiological bases of transmission of information in neural structures. This neurophysiological interlude will also help provide a basis for understanding some of the slow modulating characteristics of the structures implicated in the modes of personality expression.

Synapses and Other Neural Junctions

Most of the neurons in the brain are usually transmitting nerve impulses, at least at a low rate, to other parts of the nervous system. Connections between the neurons are made at the various junctures or synapses, and most neurons in the brain have hundreds of synaptic connections. Undoubtedly the human brain continues to develop many of its internal connections up to early adulthood when it probably loses much of its plasticity in this respect.

Learning in the mature organism is assumed by contemporary neurophysiologists (for example Kandel, 1977) to involve alterations of existing pathways, that is mostly of the various types of synapses. It is probable that the exercise of an adult habit usually involves as much selective reduction of activity at many junctions as it does increased activity in some parts of the brain.

The synapses involve dendrites, processess that conduct nerve impulses toward nerve cell bodies and axons, processes which transmit nerve impulses to dendrites or axons of other cells, or to other nerve cell bodies. There are a variety of types of dendritic branching patterns, some short and sparse, some elaborate and a few millimeters long. Axons vary greatly in length, some extending even from the brain down into the spinal cord, while some hypothalamic cells do not even have axons.

The cell membranes at the cerebral synapses constitute "synaptic clefts," where chemical changes occur during the arrival of the nerve impulse. One main excitatory transmitter released at synapses is dopamine, which changes the permeability of the membrane to ions and causes other chemical changes. The nerve signal ends as the dopamine is either oxidized or absorbed. Another transmitter, acetylcholine, is the essential chemical that at some synapses causes the depolarization of the postsynaptic cell membrane; it is neutralized by cholinesterase. These and other neurotransmitters will be described later.

At many synapses inhibitory neurotransmitters are released and the cell membrane is made less subject to depolarization. This process usually entails a hyperpolarization. If the postsynaptic membrane changes are mostly excitatory, rather than inhibitory, and distributed in an appropriate area, then the next cell fires and sends an impulse along its axon. Changes at the axon hillock, where the axon exits from the cell body, are thought to be the major site of direct activation of the succeeding cell in a circuit. However the changes occurring at the dendritic membrane surfaces probably constitute the main locus for integrating the influences in most neural systems. This "integration" may include the summation of excitatory and inhibitory chemical and electrical influences, in relation to the status of internal factors which cause the axon to vary its frequency of firing.

Most dendrites have small branches or "spines" to which the other neurons abut. The number of spines and their shape in some parts of the brain can be affected by varying an animal's rearing conditions, for example Coss and Globus (1978) found that some fish brought up in social isolation had neurons in the midbrain with fewer and thinner dendritic branches than normal.

Not all neuronal activity is chemical and not all synapses are at the interface of axons and the next cell. Some dendrites are adjacent to each other but go to different cells, and even some axons when adjacent to each other, are assumed to have electrical influences on each other (Schmitt, Dev, and Smith, 1976). Some dendrites clearly have synapses with other dendrites. There are also neurons with synaptic effects on each other of a reciprocal nature, that is the facilitatory effect of one cell on another may be inhibited by the activity of the latter (Shepherd, 1978). In addition to electrical field effects, neural transmission can involve slow potential changes as a result of factors such as neural control over local blood circulation and hormonal changes. Furthermore recurrent loops of neural activity can develop which may be inhibitory (or excitatory) to other activity, including what occurs in inhibitory pathways. The number of different types of nerve cells in the human brain and the statistics on their distribution within the brain are still basic matters for future research. Systematic studies classifying the "types" of neural cells and their distribution could make a contribution to the understanding of mammalian brain function. At the moment it is more profitable for the researchers to concentrate on discovering connections, cell types, and new substances rather than on formal efforts at classification.

The kinds of information coming in from different types of receptors and going out in different output systems are differentiated primarily by the separate pathways used rather than by differences in the types of signals. Within the brain there are different modes of transmission apart from the differentiation by pathways. Many of the neurotransmitters have noteworthy concentrations in limbic and midbrain structures which are assumed to be the main sites of action of many drugs which have a distinct influence on behavior.

Functions of Limbic Lobe and Hypothalamus

A clear intention of the nineteenth century phrenologists, who claimed that variations in scalp and skull dimensions were related to psychological differences among people, was to provide an explanation of how brain characteristics determined various psychological functions. Neuroanatomists of a few decades ago probably had a similar intention when they parcelled out cortical areas according to subtle histological differences. With the advent of modern research into the large number of subcortical structures and their neurochemistry, there is now an opportunity for theorists to distribute some psychological attributes among these brain parts. The hazards of this type of basic theorizing are clear, even if a simple localizing of a process were often possible, as a physiological explanation of the system it has minimal value.

Within the midbrain and temporal lobes are the structures of the limbic system (see Figure 5–1). The limbic tissue has been called the paleomammalian brain by MacLean (1975). It has remained remarkably similar throughout mammalian forms (Jacobowitz and MacLean, 1978) and has been aptly termed as important for preservation of self and species, that is feeding, reproduction, and fighting. Except for olfaction and autonomic activities, connections of limbic structures with receptors and muscles are rudimentary in the mammal. None of the limbic tissue is as finely layered as the outer neocortical tissue of the mammalian brain.

The hypothalamus seems to serve as a link between the midbrain and limbic structures of the forebrain. It is directly affected by activity from the external receptors only in regard to olfaction. The hypothalamus contains cells that are important for the maintenance of fluid balance, body temperature, the regulation of blood glucose level, and other systems necessary for sexual responsiveness and reproductive activities. Cells in the hypothalamus are affected by other neural activities within the brain in addition to influences from substances circulating in the blood. The hypothalamus exerts considerable control over the pituitary gland beneath it, mostly by a special vascular system which carries the neurohormones to the gland (Schally, Kastin, and Arimura, 1977).

The main fiber tract in the hypothalamus is the medial forebrain bundle which interconnects a variety of nuclei along its course (Nauta and Haymaker, 1969). Disconnecting the anterior part of the bundle from the septal area leads to a hyperreactive rat which when touched attacks viciously for some weeks after the operation (Albert and Richmond, 1976).

The bundles of nerve fibers which course through the hypothalamus provide for some of the interaction among its systems. Of special interest is the nigrostriatal bundle, which, on each side, runs from a nucleus called the substantia nigra. This is behind the hypothalamus and is connected to the cerebellum, to the striatum within the frontal lobe. This pathway has been implicated in inhibitory effects on neural activity in frontal areas and regulatory effects of the striatum (Racagni, et al., 1977).

Various forms of experiments with surgical or chemical intervention in the hypothalamus of a rat can make it starve or overeat and, of course, has effects on other aspects of its behavior. Extirpation of different parts of the hypothalamus can make rats react differently to food substances (Ahlskog, Randall, and Hoebel, 1975). However it is not settled whether the overeating involves a change in some "satiety" system and whether failure to adjust intake can be understood in terms of the seeming "palatability" of food. There are also sex differences in the effects of hypothalamic lesions, with the changes being clearer in female rats than in male rats (Nance, 1976). The animals do not have greater or less motivation in the same sense that variations in duration of food deprivation in a normal rat produce changes in level of food motivation. Similarly the lesions that affect thirst motivation and salt preferences do not seem to be simple manipulations of normal motivation.

There should be little doubt that some kind of neural activity in the hypothalamus is an essential basis of normal hunger motivation, but it is far from clear how hypothalamic activity triggers the sequences of acts in locomotion toward a food goal or to water (Olds, 1977). Some experimental lesions in some parts posterior to the hypothalamus have produced rats that will eat, but often they will not proceed spontaneously to the food (Vanderhoof, 1978). Neurons in the striatum have recently also been implicated in hunger and thirst (Pettibone, et al., 1978).

In time it should be possible to understand better the changes that occur with obesity and anorexia, what cells in what neural systems have changed, what cellular changes constitute the metabolic and "motivational" aspects of such disorders. The reduced food intake following the administration of amphetamines can be understood as primarily an interference in these hypothalamic systems which have cells selectively responsive to the molecular configuration of some classes of drugs. However there is adaptation and differential learning depending on the mode of administration which complicates the story of anorexic drugs (Carey, 1978).

The amygdalae, inside the temporal lobes in the human brain, have been implicated in the regulation of sexual behavior, aggression, and other activities accompanied by emotional changes. They are connected to hypothalamic nuclei and connections with the frontal lobes have recently been described (Llamas, Avendano, and Reinoso-Suarez, 1977). Stimulation of parts of the limbic system can induce attacks which seem to be associated with internal changes like rage (Pinel, Treit, and Rovner, 1977; Gold, et al., 1977). However pinching the tail of a rat can cause it to duplicate some of the attack phenomena elicited by brain stimulation (Koob, Fray, and Iversen, 1976), and it is possibly better to interpret this as the result of general activation rather than some specific enraging effect. Aggressive and defensive sequences in behavior are not clear neurophysiologically and may remain so for some time until there is a better taxonomy of situations and lesion types (Marques and Valenstein, 1977). Even in rats the effects of drugs on attack and defense phenomena vary considerably with different subspecies and with differences in how the victim of the attack behaves (Sbordone and Garcia, 1977).

The hippocampus and the amygdala on each side of the brain are implicated in some fundamental processes that underly the ability to develop permanent memories from single exposures to stimuli, the initiation of habits or movement sequences, and possibly the maintenance of emotional "stability." Two of the more interesting areas of contemporary research on the functions of the hippocampus are those studies in which the cellular activity is related to where a rat is in a familiar maze (Orton, 1977), and studies in rabbits concerning what happens in some of its hippocampal cells just before a conditioned eye-blink type of response is learned (Berry and Thompson, 1978). It is not clear yet if the cellular activity can be said to be part of the actual circuits involved in conditioning or in spatial learning, or if the recorded activity is a manifestation of something crucial happening in other parts of the brain. Only recently have the neuroanatomical pathways from the hippocampus to frontal and other cortical areas and to the amygdala, been adequately described (Rosene and Van Hoesen, 1977). A recent review by Lopes da Silva and Arnolds, (1978) began, "Despite the large number of studies on all aspects of the hippocampus, the function of this structure is still an enigma" (p. 185).

Neurotransmitters and Drug Action

The various chemical substances that directly affect human behavior are generally assumed to have the site of action almost entirely at the synapses, or junctions, between neurons. At such sites neural circuits may be inhibited or made more prone to activity. The main neurotransmitter substances are contained in synaptic vesicles which burst at the surface when the nerve impulse occurs and the surface membrane is depolarized. These neurotransmitters affect the adjacent membrane of the next neuron, making a change in the probability that it will fire or not.

Other sites for chemical modulation of neural activity are possible, such as within the nerve cells where the propensity for firing may be increased or decreased, and where slower and less explosive changes than nerve firing may occur. Glial cells are also important loci of some drug effects. Although not involved in the actual propagation of nerve impulses, these cells are perhaps modulators of such activity.

Some of the hypothalamic cells secrete substances that serve in regulating the pituitary gland at the base of the brain. This secretory influence of the hypothalamus on the pituitary gland may be thought of as an extreme form of hormone-like effect by neurons. Unlike nerve firing, neurohormones have longer-lasting effects (Müller, Nistico, and Scapagnini, 1977). Guillemin (1977) has proposed the term "cybernins" for such classes of substances which often have, unlike hormones, local effects and multiple targets. Neurohumoral communication in the body extends beyond the brain and probably modulates synaptic activity in different ways, sometimes affecting presynaptic neurotransmitter production, sometimes postsynaptic activity (Barker, et al., 1978). Long-lasting neurohumoral effects are assumed to be acting on mechanisms for re-uptake of neurotransmitters (Barchas, et al., 1978).

Drugs, hormones, and neurotransmitters are assumed to act at what are called specific "receptor" sites, which are large molecules at the surface of the neural membrane. Substances which "bind" with their special receptor are thereby assumed to interfere with the ordinary level of neural activity wherever there are neurons with a good portion of the particular type of receptor. Some of the substances, after "binding," provoke the activity of other "second messengers" within the cell (Costa, 1976).

The main neurotransmitter substance at neural junctions outside of the brain is acetylcholine. It is not the main neurotransmitter within the brain; however its activity in cortical synapses is undoubtedly of significance.

One class of biochemical agents that is significant in affecting central neural activity, particularly in certain midbrain and limbic structures, is a group of "biogenic amines." They can be shown, in biochemical experiments, to affect transmission of impulses across the nerve junctions. Several nerve fiber systems have been described by the primary amine they display in histochemical studies.

One of the catecholamines, dopamine (DA), is said to involve several fiber systems, but mainly the neurons in a pathway from the substantia nigra in the hindbrain through the hypothalamus to the striated forebrain structures, the caudate nucleus, and the putamen.

There is a suggestion that after prolonged use of certain antischizophrenic drugs, which unfortunately often produce abnormal movements, the dopamine receptor sites in the corpus striatum may increase or become supersensitive (Burt, Creese, and Snyder, 1977). The nigrostriatal pathway is thought to be mainly inhibitory in effects on the basal ganglia. These parts of the basal ganglia inside the frontal lobes are described in Figure 5–1. There is some controversy however over whether the pathway has excitatory influences also on the caudate nucleus (Cooper, Bloom, and Roth, 1978; Cheney, Zsilla, and Costa, 1977; Moore and Bloom, 1978).

Besides this dopaminergic nigrostriatal pathway there are other parts of the brain where tracts or nuclei have this catecholamine formed (Costa, 1976). There is an important pathway from the substantia nigra to limbic nuclei and some cortical regions. Weak electrical stimulation of medial frontal cortex is rewarding to a rat, and direct measures of increased DA activity have been made in that area during the self-stimulation provided to the rat for pressing a bar (Mora and Myers, 1977).

Another catecholamine system is based on norepinephrine (NE) and is called adrenergic. Norepinephrine and epinephrine are metabolic products of dopamine. A nucleus in the brain stem reticular system called locus coeruleus is a major part of this system. The system is assumed to have widespread connections which can activate the brain, and rats will readily work for electrical stimulation of this nucleus. Lesions in the lateral hypothalamus, or chemical depletion of dopamine and noradrenaline from the brain, can produce a cataleptic rat which may cling to a wire mesh for several minutes, even when tested weeks after the damaging injection (Schallert, et al., 1978). Lesions of the locus coeruleus have been said to lead to "decreased nerve impulse flow" in DA neurons and also to increased sensitivity of DA receptors on neurons (Kostowski, et al., 1977).

A recent report of autopsies of four schizophrenics describes parts of the limbic system which had above-normal levels of NE (Farley, et al., 1978). However other data will be needed before the nature of the possible dysfunction in such patients is understood.

Antelman and Caggiula (1977) have described how diminished activity of NE-containing neurons may or may not facilitate DA-dependent activity. They argue that the stereotypy that occurs in rats from high doses of amphetamine acting on the DA-system is increased by NE depletion. Ettenberg and Milner (1977) however believe they have separated NE and DA effects in one type of experiment with rats lever pressing for electrical stimulation of the hypothalamus.

Another system is based on serotonin (5-hydroxytryptamine or 5HT) and is called serotonergic. The adrenergic and serotonergic systems are less localized perhaps than is the nigrostriatal dopaminergic system. Ellison (1977) has studied the effects of chemically disrupting cerebral levels of serotonin and NE. He showed differences depending on how familiar the rats were with the environment: with low NE and high 5HT levels the rats moved around more in an open field and seemed less fearful, as if affected by a tranquilizer; with the reverse imbalance the treated rats were more active than normal in the familiar colony cage and seemed to mimic the amphetamine effect. There is some controversy about how specific many of these chemical intervention techniques are since they can possibly affect several metabolic pathways rather than just one.

One of the most ubiquitous of the neurotransmitters in the brain, gamma-aminobutyric acid (GABA), is assumed to have the function of providing some inhibition of cortical activity (Tower, 1977). If it is shown to have widespread inhibitory effects, it may be a crucial factor in the orderly operation of some neural circuits involving the cortex. When injected into parts of the hypothalamus it can increase food intake (as can electrical stimulation), in the substantia nigra it can suppress it (Kelly, et al., 1977). DA may be an agent that releases GABA from the striatal pathway in the substantia nigra (Gale, Guidotti, and Costa, 1977).

Another substance that is also the subject of much contemporary research is monoamine oxidase (MAO). MAO and some other substances inactivate many of the amines and possibly regulate the amount of dopamine and other neurotransmitters in neural tissue. Various MAO-inhibiting substances act as antidepressants or mood elevators, possibly because, like amphetamine, they result in raising the level of norepinephrine and other amines at various places in the brain. Amphetamine inhibits MAO to some extent. Low amounts of MAO in the blood of normal people have been related to having high "ego strength" and high activity levels (Schooler, et al., 1978).

"Opiate-receptor" binding is prevalent in the limbic system, corpus striatum, and hypothalamus. The blocking of these receptor sites is assumed to be an essential aspect of the euphoric and analgesic effects of opiate drugs (Snyder, 1977). Some similar substances found in the pituitary gland, the enkephalins, are assumed to be important in normal inhibitory activity in limbic and other systems. They can have an analgesic effect when injected into a rat's brain near the middle of the hindbrain close to the cerebellum (Frenk, McCarty, and Liebeskind, 1978). Enkephalins have also been shown to have a protective effect with regard to the amnesia for foot shock produced by carbon dioxide anesthesia in rats (Rigter, 1978).

Because some of these potent peptide substances seemed to be endogenous mimics of the opiate, morphine, they were called "endorphins" (Pert and Gulley, 1977). Injected into the central nervous system in minute quantities, they can produce in rats temperature changes, shaking, or a catatonic state (Cooper, Bloom, and Roth, 1978). The probable sites of the neuromodulatory action of endorphins include the hypothalamus and limbic structures (Barchas, et al., 1978). When endorphins are injected into a part of the limbic forebrain called the nucleus accumbens they induce hypermotility in rats (Pert and Sivit, 1977). However in a test of the effects of naloxone, a substance that is inhibitory to endorphins in neurophysiological experiments, it failed to affect pain sensations in volunteers (Grevert and Goldstein, 1978). The matter has also become complicated in that different dosage levels of synthetic endorphins may have opposite effects under certain experimental conditions, and it is argued that more than one "receptor-type" exists for these substances (Frederickson, et al., 1978; Jacquet, et al., 1977).

There are other sequences or metabolic pathways of activity in neural tissue and in the surrounding medium, and brief disturbances in them can often be compensated for and without lasting damage. Persistent disruption of some of the metabolic pathways is now understood as the basis of a variety of rare neurological disorders (Cooper, Bloom, and Roth, 1978). Some of these are deficiency diseases in which there is an interference with the production of the substances which are essential for continuous healthy activity in important brain elements. In other diseases there is an accumulation of substances that damage brain tissue. At present none of these diseases are "MBD," nor are any distinguished primarily by hyperactivity without mental retardation. However it would seem likely that in future some small subgroups of so-called MBD children will be found to have specific biochemical abnormalities.

Hemispheric Asymmetry

The cortical tissue enables the mammal to perform more craftily than, but perhaps not as rapidly as, birds and amphibians do in response to typical environmental changes. This tissue of the primate brain has undoubtedly evolved in part as a component of some systems that are essential for the exercise of intellectual and complex social skills. The brains of the primates have become specialized in several ways in the different lobes and, although there are many histological distinctions which can be made between the tissue in the different lobes, as yet no meaningful difference has been discovered between the type of tissue found in human brains and that found in other primate brains. In the human brain, and probably in the brains of some other primates (LeMay, 1977; Yeni-Komshian and Benson, 1976), the two sides of the brain have become different from each other in some ways. It is not known yet whether hemispheric specialization involves different amounts of different types of tissue, but it is presently assumed to be more a cortical difference rather than one depending on subcortical differences (Whitaker and Ojemann, 1977; Reynolds, et al., 1978). One of the most important cortical differences in human brains is the slightly larger area on the top of the temporal lobe on the left side when compared with that on the right (Galaburda, et al., 1978).

This hemispheric asymmetry in anatomy and the tendency for lateralization of human cerebral function is well documented (Harnad, et al., 1977; Lansdell and Donnelly, 1977). From studies of people with neurological disorders, it has become obvious that the temporal and parietal areas on the left side of most human brains are specialized for the maintenance of ordinary language skills. There is some specialization of the right hemisphere in most people for certain nonverbal skills (Kimura, 1975; Jones-Gotman and Milner, 1977). The reasons for these phenomena, and for the exceptions in some people, are still obscure. There are many asymmetrical aspects to both surface features of the human body and the internal organs. The relation of brain asymmetry to hand preference for motor sequences, especially in regard to writing, is striking (Kimura, 1977). It seems likely that right-handedness was prevalent in our species before the advent of written language (Coren and Porac, 1977), however in recent times schools and parents have also exercised social pressure for right-handedness.

The slight expansion which has been observed on top of the left temporal lobe of many brains is assumed to be significant for the integrity of the important verbal skills. This type of asymmetry has also been reported for infant brains (Witelson, 1977a), however the asymmetry in neonates may not so often be as clearly in favor of the left hemisphere. In adults it has been possible to relate verbal activity with slight increases in blood flow in the left hemisphere (Ingvar and Philipson, 1977; Risberg, et al., 1975), and one might assume this hemispheric difference occurs almost from the beginning of speech. An initial predisposition toward use of tissue in the left hemisphere might, after years of verbal activity, lead to a clear anatomical asymmetry in the adult. But the relation between subsequent brain morphology and function may also be a relationship which develops largely independently of any specialized training to which the organism is exposed (Goldman, 1976).

About a quarter of normal brains have shown no left-right difference and it is not known whether such brains come from people who are less verbal than average or from people who tend to be ambidextrous. Furthermore the right side of the brain, not the left, in a small percentage of people serves the function of supporting speech mechanisms and the left side of their brains possibly serves to support ordinary right-hemisphere functions. The reason for this reversal in a normal healthy person is not clear. There are probably some rare people whose language functions are primarily dependent on right hemisphere integrity, although they are right-handed (Levy and Reid, 1978). It is likely that most left-handed people have the usual left-hemisphere support of verbal skills. Whether a person has left-handed relatives or not has been related to some features of lateralization of language functions, but there is some disagreement about the genetic mechanism underlying the phenomenon (Fennell, et al., 1978; Hicks and Kinsbourne, 1976).

In the case of individuals who have their left hemispheres damaged early in life, the demonstration that their speech and verbal skills depend on the integrity of their right hemispheres poses no mystery: the tissue on the right side of the brain was appropriated for the important verbal functions after the damage. This argument is based on the observed relation between the age at onset of neurological symptoms and decreasing level of verbal development (Lansdell, 1969). There is also speculation that some forms of developmental dyslexia may result in part from a brain not readily developing on either side some of the usual left-hemisphere functions (Witelson, 1977b).

The lateralization of noncognitive functions, such as tendencies toward extraversion or introversion, may also depend more on one hemisphere than the other, but adequate studies of lateralized personality phenomena are rare (Galin, 1977; Schwartz, Davidson, and Maer, 1975). There are reports of people showing noncognitive personality changes depending upon which side of the brain is injured, but there are many inconsistencies in the various reports (Galin, 1978). The neural systems involved in perceptual phenomena may not recover as quickly as those for verbal skills (Lansdell and Smith, 1975). It is likely that noncognitive functions have a different course of recovery after brain injury than cognitive skills. Intellectual systems may be more plastic than those involved in motivational or emotional phenomena.

Sex Differences in Hemispheric Asymmetry

Sex differences may have obscured results in some investigations of asymmetry in human brain function (Lansdell, 1973). There are studies which suggest that the brains of men tend to show clearer lateralization of function than the brains of women (Harris, 1978).

Witelson (1978) has studied the ability of children to recognize shapes which are palpated out of sight simultaneously with both hands; she found differences between the two hands in boys, but not in girls. Rudel, Denckla, and Hirsch (1977) have also reported sex-linked age differences in an investigation which compared the learning of Braille (in sighted subjects) with the left and right hands. In an investigation of relationships in college students between their hand posture for writing and scores on tachistoscopic tests of right-left differences in visual field efficiency for spatial and verbal material, Levy and Reid (1978) reported that females were less laterally differentiated than males. Levy and Levy (1978) have even found sex differences in which foot is longer.

Waber (1976) has shown that during adolescence there can be a relative lag in perceptual development in girls as compared to boys. She interprets these age-related differences as relevant to some of the reported sex differences in lateralization of brain function during development. We ordinarily assume a lag on the part of boys' brains rather than girls' brains with respect to the development of verbal skills. The implication of such studies of sex differences in specialization of the hemispheres could be that the female human brain develops earlier and does not usually become as lateralized in its verbal specialization (Hannay, 1976). Although there are sex-linked differences in developmental phases, they probably do not provide an adequate explanation of the final adult sex differences in asymmetry of cerebral function. Perceptual ("right-hemisphere") functions and verbal ("left-hemisphere") functions may in some degree be in competition with the adult brain (Lansdell, 1970; Smith, Chu, and Edmonston, 1977) and to some degree the two hemispheres learn from each other and cooperate (LeDoux, et al., 1977). These interhemispheric functions may be interrelated with gender.

There is no satisfactory theory to account for lateralization of human brain function let alone these differences in the lateralization. When future research succeeds in describing the histological and neurochemical differences between the hemispheres it could also provide clues regarding the nature of these sex differences.

NEURAL THEORIES OF CHILDHOOD MINIMAL BRAIN DYSFUNCTIONS

There are different types of neural theories in the field of MBDs dealing with different sets of symptoms and ranging from the primarily biochemical to the primarily neuroanatomical.

A neurologist needs little in the way of comprehensive theory of perception or of coordination to provide good diagnoses. A neurological diagnostician notices any impairments in reflexes, in vision and in several other input systems, and in various output systems. Other kinds of disturbance, such as sweating on one side of the body, hormonal changes, hiccups, and so on, can indicate various subcortical disorders. Sometimes changes in personality can indicate, along with other neurological symptoms, that certain kinds of diseases are likely, and it is perhaps too tempting to consider hyperkinetic or MBD children as having a specifiable lesion. Some writers (for example, Wender, 1975a; Shaywitz, Cohen, and Shaywitz, 1978) estimate that up to 10% of children may have the disorder. It would be surprising to find so many children with a common disorder manifesting itself in such a neurological syndrome. Of course many rare neurological disorders can be sensibly defined on a simple neural or biochemical basis without the extensive research that would be necessary for understanding the mechanisms determining the normal range of function.

For this discussion I have selected some of the more plausible ideas that have been proposed in recent years for certain therapeutic effects or for selected classes of MBD characteristics. They are the ideas which may help clinicians in the future deal with this problem. They may also help general theorists achieve greater agreement about the range of normal behavior that is to be encompassed by biochemical and neuroanatomical theory.

Dysfunctions in Monoamine Metabolism

Wender's book (1971) on MBD was important in structuring the contemporary concern for children with MBD. It was called a "new excursion into this murky territory" by one reviewer (Twitchell, 1971). Wender (1971) postulated an impaired function in inhibitory noradrenergic mechanisms that fail to keep an excitatory dopaminergic system at normal levels. In 1973 Wender speculated that rather than there being "altered structure—faulty wiring, so to speak," any genetic defect is likely to be an enzymatic deficit.

Wender (1975a, 1975b) continues to argue that children with MBD have certain changes in monoamine metabolism that are normalized by the therapeutic drugs. He thinks a considerable portion of the children have an inborn biochemical deficit. Familial association of some of the symptoms are well above chance expectancy (Nichols, Chen, and Pomeroy, 1978) and the strength of the association could be understood as genetic. Wender assumes that the drugs activate both inhibitory and excitatory systems and cause a better balance by having a greater effect on the inhibitory one. Recently Wender and Wender (1976) hinted of evidence that behavioral modification techniques used in conjunction with medication have not proven to be of additional value in helping the children. In research in which he participated at The National Institutes of Health (NIH) some differences in autonomic reactivity were found in carefully selected MBD children (Zahn, Little, and Wender, 1978), but these results do not distinguish a fundamental feature of an MBD disorder. Their results are important in demonstrating that "activating" drugs have little effect on autonomic phenomena in the MBD children.

Silbergeld and Goldberg (1976) have suggested that the hyperactivity found after lead poisoning of mice is analogous to MBD in children; in fact children with lead poisoning do often become hyperactive. But the time of development of the hyperactivity in the mice may not be early enough to be a good analogy. The authors assume that an increased monoaminergic activity is a major biochemical defect in a portion of hyperkinetic MBD children. More recently Silbergeld (1977) has argued for dysfunction of systems involving GABA (gamma-aminobutyric acid) and acetylcholine or other forms of cholinergic-aminergic interaction. Goldberg and Silbergeld (1978) in a recent survey have considered the problem of how the hypothesis of increased monoaminergic neurotransmission for hypermotility may account for the therapeutic effects of amphetamine: there could be decreases in cholinergic or GABAergic function among other dysfunctions.

Shaywitz and his colleagues (Shaywitz, Yager, and Klopper, 1976; Shaywitz, et al., 1976) claim that rats depleted of dopamine at birth later develop a transient prepuberal hyperkinesis and learning deficits. Shaywitz, Cohen, and Shaywitz (1978) have also studied the cerebrospinal fluid in six MBD boys and claim further evidence of DA-dysfunction in the brains of these volunteers. Kalat (1976) argued that their rat results were a special case of the more general phenomenon of a preponderance of norepinephrine (relative to other neurotransmitters). Shaywitz seems to ignore the possibility that serotonergic and cholinergic synapses may also be involved in the changes. McLean, Kostrzewa, and May (1977) have produced increases in activity with depletion of central norepinephrine and without known effects on neurotransmitters such as dopamine.

Sechzer (1978) has conducted some research with an animal model of a different type: kittens with their corpus callosum cut at birth. She demonstrated that amphetamine raised the level of activity in normal cats while reducing the hyperactivity in the operated cats (and even below normal at the higher doses). She does not conclude that MBD children have the same kind of brain damage, that would probably have been demonstrated by now if it had been the case. She suggests a "neuronal-reduction" theory for MBD, with drugs facilitating release of catecholamines to "augment the number of neuronal processes that participate in organized behavior."

Brase and Loh (1975) agree a balance may be involved in obtaining beneficial treatment, but suggest that 5-hydroxytryptamine-containing neurons (the serotoninergic system) is mainly involved in hyperkinetic behavior. Greenberg and Coleman (1976) have reported low blood serotonin in hyperkinetic brain-damaged children with mental retardation, but in a recent autopsy study (Coleman, et al., 1977) of a boy with an elevated blood level, the level in the brain tissue was found to be lower than in a control, comparison brain. Everett (1977) argues that because pemoline (Cylert), which is becoming popular in the treatment of hyperkinesis, has no effect on norepinephrine systems but increases dopamine turnover, only the latter system may be impaired in hyperkinetic children. However pemoline may well have some different effects from dextroamphetamine even though it may produce a comparable social effect. It is used essentially as a drug that is more convenient in being more long-lasting than others.

Developmental Deviations in the Brain

The observation that hyperactive boys and sometimes their parents show an above average incidence of certain minor physical anomalies, such as a high palate, can be taken to suggest that in an early stage of gestation some disruption in the development of neural tissue also occured (Rapoport and Quinn, 1976; Steg and Rapoport, 1975; Waldrup, et al., 1978). In some people the interruption could be ascribed to a genetic predisposition. It is conceivable that glial proliferation or the process of myelinization for some fiber tracts suffers disruption on these occasions, but this kind of anatomical speculation may not be amenable to checking for a long time.

Certain lines of investigation someday may help unravel the relationships between hazards for the fetus or the newborn and subsequent hyperactivity or other handicaps. Both statistical studies of children with impairments and animal studies with experimental lesions contribute clues to how the handicaps occur. Some substances which are commonly available may cause significant neural damage (Arnold, 1976). For example, hexachloraphene was once widely used as a soap with excellent disinfectant qualities until it was found in research with monkeys to be absorbed through the skin and cause neural damage. Its use in coping with diaper rash might have caused some children to suffer some minimal damage. Cigarette smoking during pregnancy is known to raise the probability that the offspring will suffer some neurological handicap (Nichols, Chen, and Pomeroy, 1978).

David (1978), in a preliminary report, has shown that use of a chelating agent to reduce the levels of lead in the blood to normal levels can help some hyperactive children. There is evidence that for some hyperactive children special diets to eliminate possible irritants can be helpful (Conners, 1978). In some cases the dietary regime may be providing a nonbiological family cohesion that comes into being as a result of the restructuring of family life necessary to follow a special diet; it may take many years of research to identify what may be significant food additives or components that are the source of some children's difficulties.

Rourke (1975) reported in his studies of normal and retarded readers that the gap in efficiency between them widened with age; the children were tested twice, at 8 and 12 years of age. There are other reports that suggest cognitive impairments may become more noticeable with age, and Benton (1973) suggested that the term "minimal" in MBD may be an underestimate of the extent of neuropathology. His argument is based on the considerable recovery usually found in investigations of the effects of lesions in infancy with experimental animals. In monkeys the recovery of climbing, walking, and manipulation of objects can be virtually complete after lesions made in the infant motor cortex. This is unlike the long-lasting disturbances found in adult animals with similar lesions. The good recovery is observed primarily in research dealing with locomotion and certain sensory discrimination tasks. But animals do not seem to recover as readily from subcortical damage received in infancy; it is commonly assumed that an organism will show greater resiliency after damage to cortical tissue than after damage to subcortical structures connected to the cortical tissue. It is also likely that young animals do not later recover function as readily when tested with tasks requiring more than simple sensory discrimination or motor phenomena (Goldman, 1976). Slow encroachment by a damaging process is not as deleterious as equivalent short-term damage; during the recovery from limited damage some factor is probably produced which accelerates the sprouting of axons during the later damage (Sheff, Bernardo, and Cotman, 1977).

Selective thalamocortical disorders involving the caudate nucleus and the frontal lobes could be a basis for certain kinds of MBDs (Pontius, 1973). Zambelli, et al., (1977) offer some suggestions in this vein from their studies of errors of commission in reacting to clicks and of evoked potentials in hyperactive children (some of whom had soft neurological signs). However their assumption that the frontal lobes are particularly important for such tasks involving attention is not accepted by others (Lansdell and Mirsky, 1964; Mirsky and Orren, 1977).

An occasional form of hyperactivity reported with adult monkeys after extirpations from the frontal lobes is a type of pacing that is possibly a "release" phenomenon, that is some tissue which inhibits such activity is destroyed. The pacing is probably not analogous to human hyperactivity. The activity is most often observed after damage to a particular sulcus in the frontal lobes; novel stimuli depress and familiar stimuli enhance the locomotion (Gross, 1963).

Human beings can also show good recovery in motor function after limited cortical damage in infancy, but early onset of convulsive seizures and other forms of early diffuse brain damage seem to be as devastating to human intelligence as similar adult disorders. Persistent seizures can lead to impairment in both cortical and subcortical function, perhaps affecting the latter less in terms of cognitive skills. The deleterious effect of early epilepsy at adulthood however may be because of the long-term cumulative effect of continual seizures (Dikmen, Matthews, and Harley, 1975).

After hemispherectomy (for extensive unilateral pathology), when there is only one hemisphere with cortical tissue, right or left, Dennis and Whitaker (1976) and Dennis (1977) argue that the subsequent ability to understand complex sentences depends on which hemisphere remains. They showed that patients with one hemisphere on the left side demonstrate a better development of speech and language than do patients with one hemisphere remaining on the right. This kind of result is consistent with a recent report that subtle impairments in sentence comprehension are shown by adults after they had good recovery from the type of brain damage that initially led to a gross speech impairment (Just, Davis, and Carpenter, 1977).

Gazzaniga (1973) subscribes to the notion that MBD children have a failure of dominance and suggests the possibility that training techniques to induce hemispheric "priority" could be helpful.

Witelson (1977b) argues that developmental dyslexia may be analogous to what conceivably would be the case with two hemispheres tending to function as "right" hemispheres and with neither as proficient as an ordinary left hemisphere with respect to reading. Her results suggest that dyslexic children do not have the usual asymmetric efficiency with regard to linguistic material presented either to the left or right visual field. The finding could imply that this disorder is a result of considerable brain dysfunction because it is generally assumed that early unilateral damage to a normal left temporo-parietal area can be followed by the development of language mechanisms in the corresponding tissue in the right hemisphere.

It has been argued that some behavioral disorders, rather than being mainly a congenital handicap, stem from the frustrations associated with some other problem such as dyslexia. Long-lasting perceptual impairments incurred by right hemisphere damage may not be as annoying as linguistic handicaps are to young people in the modern world. It has been argued that some left-handers, and perhaps others, seem to have bilateral speech functions in the brain (Milner, 1974), somewhat analogous perhaps to having two left hemispheres. Left-handed people can develop good verbal skills and relative perceptual limitations (Levy, 1976).

What limited forms of damage to the young brain will raise the probability that a child will have only "emotional" problems is not known. There are many children with obvious handicaps resulting from localized pathological cerebral functioning, for example, torsion dystonia and hemiplegia, who are pleasant, sociable youngsters and they cope with their special problems of school and family life. Children with Down's syndrome also may show neither hyperactivity nor persistent emotional problems.

Developmental Sexual Dimorphism

Goldman and her colleagues (1974) have shown that some impairments from early frontal lobe damage in monkeys can be fully revealed only after a period of growth; some deficits may be clear only in male and not in female monkeys.

Certain parts of the frontal lobes are assumed to develop earlier in the male monkeys (Goldman, 1975).

There is a temptation to draw an analogy between the difficulties the monkeys have with delayed response tasks and the impulsivity ascribed to many children with MBDs. However if the analogy were to be used, it would apply only to children who make errors while delaying their choices. There is no analogy to chimpanzees with frontal lobe damage. They do not become as disturbed by their mistakes as do normal chimpanzees. Witelson (1978) has reported results on tests of hemispheric lateralization which suggest that dyslexia in boys is different from that found in girls.

It is conceivable that a relative handicap with regard to verbal development could be relevant for an explanation of the slow adoption of adult systems of social controls by some boys. The greater incidence among boys of left-handedness, speech difficulties, and MBD may be related problems. If left-handedness were often the result of some minimal brain damage rather than a result of genetic predisposition, one might find that such boys tended to have the visuomotor handicaps found in cases of known left-hemisphere damage. This notion would not be helpful however in explaining the verbal superiority of some left-handed males (Levy, 1977). Suggestions have been made that MBD boys may be understood as showing some form of developmental lag; for example, Bodian and Wolff (1977) describe a manual asymmetry they found in dyslexic boys who were attempting complex tapping tasks. They consider the possibility that some delay has occurred in the boys' brains with respect to interhemispheric "cooperation."

Canalization of Arousal

Raskin (1977) and Campbell and Randall (1977) have experimented with rats 15 days old—at a stage of hypermotility. Examining the responses to either synthetic or real rat fur and other "surrogate" objects, they showed that the administration of amphetamine steepened the generalization gradient in a new environment. In other words the drug enhanced "attractive" stimuli for the rats when they were exposed to a new, activating environment. The authors suggest that some similar "canalization of arousal" might be relevant to understanding how hyperactive children are affected by therapeutic drug treatment and they encourage the idea of developmental lag in MBD. They suggest the canalization idea might help explain failures to show drug benefits when the children are maintained in overstabilized environments. Conners (1976) has expressed similar ideas about stimulant drugs increasing selective attention in MBD children. Douglas (1976) and Firestone and Douglas (1975) agree that many of the children have difficulty in sustaining attention. In a similar vein, they suggest that "hyperactive children may be overdependent on positive reinforcement."

Hyperactivity in children and hypomania in adults have a superficial similarity with regard to movement. There is also an interesting relation between the effects of the drugs used in treatment. Lithium has been used as a prophylaxis for manic-depressive patients; it attenuates amphetamine-induced euphoria; and in normal volunteers it appears to diminish interest in novel stimuli and to reduce initiative (Murphy, 1978).

Tecce, Savignano-Bowman, and Cole (1978) have described differences in event-related brain potentials in normal volunteers being studied for the effects of amphetamine and other stimulants. They suggest that MBD children who benefit from the drug (as compared with those who do not) can be said to be having distraction reduced and a narrowing of their attention. Barrett (1977) demonstrated recently that an administration of amphetamine could affect two trained monkeys, but not two relatively naive ones, so as to raise the rate of electric shocks to the tail which they received for failure to suppress lever pressing for food. Possibly the experienced monkeys became more engrossed with the food signals. Katz and Barrett (1978) confirmed that amphetamine increased response rate in another situation where the shocks were otherwise not reducing the food-getting response rate.

Matthysse (1977) notes that in normal animals long periods of visual fixation can occur with high doses of amphetamine and suggests that the behavior may be a result of increased activity in some subcortical dopaminergic nuclei which are connected to the parietal lobe. Cells in the parietal lobe can fire selectively, depending on some other features relevant to fixation (Mountcastle, 1978; Yin and Mountcastle, 1977), that is whether the stimulus is new or has some significance to the animal on the basis of training. How cortical tissue activates the mechanisms controlling gaze is still a puzzle (Goldberg and Robinson, 1977). The effect of activating drugs on this type of phenomenon in the parietal cortex has yet to be studied.

IMPLICATIONS OF NEURAL THEORIES OF MBDs

In the future some of the riddles in this field will be better explicated so that new practical ideas will emerge about what school and home problems can be handled safely with an astute combination of drugs and fuller understanding of the social situation. The major contributions will come from well-designed investigations to determine the main types of situations (Langhorne, et al., 1976) and the drugs that can be unequivocally relied on to have a high probability of helping parents or educators deal compassionately with their charges. Fortunately there is no indication that this form of early chemotherapy leads to a significant increase in later drug abuse (Beck, et al., 1975). The slight limitations of bone growth that can occur with the drugs seem to be overcome at adulthood. That such a delay should occur is not encouraging, since at times it does not occur with some forms of malnutrition.

Although the expansion of contemporary research in the field is encouraging, the practical contribution of contemporary neurophysiological theory could well remain negligible for many years with regard to professional therapeutic decisions. After more reliable facts have been developed about these children and their various difficulties, the theory will help to give some semblance of rationale. At present there is a clear need to avoid inadvertent encouragement of those who might discourse confidently about mechanism, without the reserve that comes with sophistication about biomedical research methodology.

The research demonstrating that the use of amphetamine can cause improvement in cognitive tasks (Rapoport, et al., 1978) and in speech (Ludlow, et al., 1977) in both hyperactive and normal boys need not discourage the administration of the drugs for some handicapped children. Possibly nearly a third of the children now labeled as MBD children need the benefit of medication for some of their school years. However Ludlow et al., (1978) have also observed greater drug benefit for language performance in the least active of their volunteer patients. This result implies an unfortunate limitation to the extent of drug benefits. Of course normal children should always be left without drug administration regardless of how small the risk in long-term administration of a drug. An encouraging report by Douglas has demonstrated some beneficial effects with a "cognitive training" program, with the children off medication (Douglas, et al., 1976).

The Dangers of Psychosurgery

In recent times there has been a danger that the reporting of plausible suggestions about brain mechanisms for a behavioral disorder might then lead a bold, innovative neurosurgeon to try to invent a procedure to correct the hypothetical neurological problem (Chavkin, 1978). Andy (1975) believes psychosurgery can be used in treating psychopathic behavior. In Japan and India, psychosurgery has been too readily used to deal with behavior disorders in children. Many of the children became obedient—some of them had the sole "neurological" symptom of being a nuisance (Lansdell, 1974). The danger of this type of attempt to produce docility by brain lesions is now small in the United States because of public criticism by concerned citizens and practitioners (Walker, 1977).

This contemporary concern resulted from a significant legal precedent and from the action of the United States Congress in chartering a commission to consider how to protect subjects of biomedical and behavioral research. Kaimowitz, a lawyer of the American Civil Liberties Union, intervened on behalf of a murderer in Detroit and thwarted a proposed experimental implantation of electrodes in this man who had once been violent. The prisoner was docile while incarcerated in an asylum for many years, and he was freed as a result of the legal action. This landmark decision brought together the issue of human rights and the justification for experimental physiological investigation of aberrant human behavior (Gaylin, Meister, and Neville, 1975). The National Commission for the Protection of Human Subjects of Biomedical and Behavioral Research was given the momentous task of investigating fetal research, psychosurgery, research on children and prisoners, and of formulating general ethical principles for biomedical and behavioral research with human subjects.

The Commission's reports on fetal research, psychosurgery, and research involving children and prisoners have been published (Ryan, 1975, 1977a, 1977b, 1978). Whether the Secretary of the Department of Health, Education, and Welfare (DHEW) and members of Congress will closely follow the Commission's recommendations on psychosurgery cannot be predicted. At the least psychosurgery on children in the United States is now likely to entail an explicit legal sanction and a careful review by research and institutional review boards. The elaborate restrictions will be unavoidable in major medical centers where the indirect power of the DHEW purse is great; ultimately the restrictions may encompass all hospitals if state legislatures follow the course of action taken in Oregon and Massachusetts. In time because of these precedents and the efforts of the World Health Organization, psychosurgical procedures on children in other countries may also be brought under better scrutiny. The Commission's other report on research with children provides suggested guidelines to encompass chemotherapy and "behavior modification" methods.

Areas for MBD Research

Basic research is needed to help understand the nature of the different possible brain variations and what types of variation constitute true "disorders." Neuroanatomical research, particularly when concerned with the range of normal variation, is almost prohibitively expensive. Anatomical research may help to answer a crucial question: why is the male brain more prone than the female brain to produce a person with some form of hyperactivity when the hyperactivity does not have extrinsic determinants? This problem may not be solved until more is learned about the basic sex differences in the subcortical areas of the human brain.

Basic research in the pharmacology of hypermotility is proceeding at a rapid rate and in time, as other features of behavior relevant to MBD-type of issues are better defined, the researchers will provide useful contributions to understanding of those features (Goldberg and Silbergeld, 1978).

There are still major problems in the search for the physiology of separate mechanisms, distinguishable from attentional or perceptual systems in the brain, which seem to power freely roaming children into locomotor or partial-body activity. As humans mature are there systems which are provided with a greater level of inhibitory impulses from the frontal lobes or basal ganglia or other parts of the brain? Or, is there rather a decrease with age in the activity in some other mechanisms?

A better physiological description is needed for the nature of attentional mechanisms postulated for the MBD child's seeming ability to focus on a task for longer periods during drug treatment—is it more neuronal firing of some type in circumscribed brain parts which can be said to be a general predisposition to orient, or to "canalize," or to have perceptual mechanisms "lock" onto certain types of events? Is any such "benefit" of the same quality in normal children? Devising such research in detail will require ingenuity and the concerted efforts of electrophysiologists, neuropharmacologists, and clinicians in an interdisciplinary program.

There is a difficulty in this field, as in many others, in relating social phenomena to brain functions. On the one hand the human brain is capable of psychological functions not found in other mammals, from rats to monkeys: Is it possible that facilitation of specifically human brain mechanisms accounts for much of the therapeutic change in social behavior as a result of medication? On the other hand school and home conditions in the modern world are clearly not environments for which there has been a significant amount of selection in our species: Is it possible that the drugs in some degree depress some functions that in almost all children are suppressed well enough by the socialization process in the school and the home?

There are also questions which are not of a biological nature, for example will the widespread use of the drugs reduce the number of useful rebels to appear in future generations? We should soon know much more about what happens to children labeled as having MBD when they become adults: What portion as adults have their energy provide a social advantage? What portion remain only with a personality difference?

SUMMARY AND CONCLUSIONS

This handbook argues that MBDs do not constitute a unitary phenomenon. This chapter has contributed to the argument by surveying some possible relationships between brain functions and socially aberrant behavior in youngsters. The inexplicable sex differences, the difficulties in relating the new neurochemistry to human social behavior, the primitive state of our understanding of how different pathways and nuclei in the brain could contribute to social learning, and several other puzzles may discourage the practitioner. In some respects the practical choice may be a matter of whether some children need a temporary advantage that is not an ethically sound treatment for normal children because of the risk of long-term changes. Practitioners have an unenviable task of judging what drug to use and how much. Let us hope that their task is not made much more difficult by our skepticism about the contemporary theorizing about what may be the relevant brain differences in the various types of MBD.

REFERENCES

Adams, R. D., and M. Victor. *Principles of Neurology.* New York: McGraw-Hill, 1977.

Ahlskog, J. E., P. K. Randall, and B. G. Hoebel. "Hypothalamic hyperphagia: dissociation from hyperphagia following destruction of noradrenergic neurons." *Science,* 190(4212), 399–401, (1975).

Albert, D. J., and S. E. Richmond. "Neural pathways mediating septal hyperreactivity." *Physiology and Behavior,* 17(3), 451–455, (1976).

Andy, O. J. "Thalamotomy for psychopathic behavior." *Southern Medical Journal,* 68(4), 437–442, (1975).

Antelman, S. M., and A. R. Caggiula. "Norepinephrine-dopamine interactions and behavior." *Science,* 195 (4279), 646–653, (1977).

Arnold, L. E. "Minimal brain dysfunction: A hydraulic parfait model." *Diseases of the Nervous System,* 37(4), 171–173, (1976).

Barchas, J. D., H. Akil, G. R. Elliott, R. B. Holman, and S. J. Watson. "Behavioral neurochemistry: Neuroregulators and behavioral states." *Science,* 200(4344), 964–973, (1978).

Barker, J. L., J. H. Neale, T. G. Smith, Jr., and R. L. Macdonald. "Opiate peptide modulation of amino acid responses suggests novel form of neuronal communication." *Science,* 199(4336), 1451–1453, (1978).

Barrett, J. E. "Behavioral history as a determinant of the effects of d-amphetamine on punished behavior." *Science,* 198(4312), 67–69, (1977).

Beck, L., W. S. Langford, M. MacKay, and G. Sum. "Childhood chemotherapy and later drug abuse and growth curve: A follow-up study of 30 adolescents." *American Journal of Psychiatry,* 132(4), 436–438, (1975).

Benton, A. L. "Minimal brain dysfunction from a neuropsychological point of view." *Annals of the New York Academy of Sciences,* 205, 29–37, (1973).

Berry, S. D., and R. F. Thompson. "Prediction of learning rate from the hippocampal electroencephalogram." *Science,* 200(4347), 1298–1300, (1978).

Bodian, N. A., and P. H. Wolff. "Manual asymmetries of motor sequencing in boys with reading disabilities." *Cortex,* 13(4), 343–349, (1977).

Brase, D. A., and H. M. Loh. "Possible role of 5-hydroxytryptamine in minimal brain dysfunction." *Life Sciences,* 16(7), 1005–1015, (1975).

Burt, D. R., I. Creese, and S. H. Snyder. "Antischizophrenic drugs: Chronic treatment elevates dopamine receptor binding in brain." *Science,* 196(4287), 326–328, (1977).

Campbell, B. A., and P. J. Randall. "Paradoxical effects of amphetamine on preweanling and postweanling rats." *Science,* 195(4281), 888–891, (1977).

Carey, R. J. "A comparison of the food intake suppression produced by giving amphetamines as an aversion treatment versus as an anorexic treatment." *Psychopharmacology,* 56(1), 45–48, (1978).

Chavkin, S. *The Mind Stealers.* New York: Houghton Mifflin, 1978.

Cheney, D. L., G. Zsilla, and E. Costa. "Acetylcholine turnover rate in N. accumbens, N. caudatus, globus pallidus, and substantia nigra: Action of cataleptogenic and noncataleptogenic antipsychotics." *Advances in Biochemical Psychopharmacology,* 16, 179–186, (1977).

Coleman, M., P. N. Hart, J. Randall, J. Lee, D. Hijada, and C. G. Bratenahl. "Serotonin levels in the blood and central nervous system of a patient with sudanophilic leukodystrophy." *Neuropädiatrie,* 8(4), 459–466, (1977).

Conners, C. K. "Learning disabilities and stimulant drugs in children: Theoretical implications," in R. M. Knights and D. J. Bakker, eds., *The Neuropsychology of Learning Disorders: Theoretical Approaches.* Baltimore: University Park Press, 1976.

Conners, C. K. "Effect of diet on hyperkinesis: Parental factors." (Paper presented at Hyperkinetic Behavior Syndrome Workshop, National Institute of Mental Health, Washington, D.C., June 16, 1978).

Cooper, J. R., F. E. Bloom, and R. H. Roth. *The Biochemical Basis of Neuropharmacology,* 3rd ed. New York: Oxford University Press, 1978.

Coren, S., and C. Porac. "Fifty centuries of right-handedness: The historical record." *Science,* 198(4317), 631–632, (1977).

Coss, R. G., and A. Globus. "Spine stems on tectal interneurons in jewel fish are shortened by social stimulation." *Science,* 200(4343), 787–790, (1978).

Costa, E. "Introduction to Part II. Second messengers: New vistas," in E. Costa, E. Giacobini, and R. Paoletti, eds., *First and Second Messengers—New Vistas.* Advances in Biochemical Psychopharmacology, 15, 267–272, (1976).

David, O. "Treatment of lead poisoning by chelating agent." (Paper presented at Hyperkinetic Behavior Syndrome Workshop, National Institute of Mental Health, Washington, D.C., June 16, 1978.)

Davison, A. N. "The biochemistry of brain development and mental retardation." *British Journal of Psychiatry,* 131, 565–574, (1977).

Dennis, M. "Cerebral dominance in three forms of early brain disorder," in M. E. Blaw, I. Rapin, and M. Kinsbourne, eds., *Child Neurology.* New York: Spectrum, 1977.

Dennis, M., and H. A. Whitaker. "Language acquisition following hemidecortication: Linguistic superiority of the left over the right hemisphere." *Brain and Language,* 3(3), 404–433, (1976).

Dikmen, S., C. G. Matthews, and J. P. Harley. "The effect of early versus late onset of major motor epilepsy upon cognitive-intellectual performance." *Epilepsia,* 16(1), 73–81 (1975).

Douglas, V. I. "Perceptual and cognitive factors as determinants of learning disabilities: A review chapter with special emphasis on attentional factors," in R. M. Knights and D. J. Bakker, eds., *The Neuropsychology of Learning Disorders: Theoretical Approaches*, pp. 413–421. Baltimore: University Park Press, 1976.

Douglas, V. I., P. Parry, P. Marton, and C. Garson. "Assessment of a cognitive training program for hyperactive children." *Journal of Abnormal Child Psychology*, 4(4), 389–410, (1976).

Ellison, G. D. "Animal models of psychopathology: The low-norepinephrine and low-serotonin rat." *American Psychologist*, 32(12), 1036–1045, (1977).

Ettenberg, A., and P. Milner. "Effects of dopamine supersensitivity on lateral hypothalamic self-stimulation in rats." *Pharmacology, Biochemistry, and Behavior*, 7(6), 507–514, (1977).

Evarts, E. V. "Activity of cerebral neurons in relation to movement," in D. B. Tower and R. O. Brady, eds., *The Nervous System*. vol. 1: *The Basic Neurosciences*, pp. 221–233. New York: Raven, 1975.

——— "Mediation of quick motor responses by motor cortex pyramidal tract neurons in the monkey." *Neuroscience*, 3(1), 95–98, (1978).

Evarts, E. V., and R. Granit. "Relations of reflexes and intended movements." *Progress in Brain Research*, 44, 1–14, (1976).

Everett, G. M. "Dopamine and the hyperkinetic child," in E. Costa and G. L. Gessa, eds., *Advances in Biochemical Psychopharmacology*, vol. 16, pp. 681–682. New York: Raven, 1977.

Farley, I. J., K. S. Price, E. McCullough, J. H. N. Deck, W. Hordynski, and O. Hornykiewicz. "Norepinephrine in chronic paranoid schizophrenia: Above-normal levels in limbic forebrain." *Science*, 200(4340), 456–458, (1978).

Fennell, E., P. Satz, T. Van Den Abell, D. Bowers, and R. Thomas. "Visuospatial competency, handedness, and cerebral dominance." *Brain and Language*, 5(2), 206–214, (1978).

Firestone, P., and V. Douglas. "The effects of reward and punishment on reaction times and autonomic activity in hyperactive and normal children." *Journal of Abnormal Child Psychology*, 3(3), 201–215, (1975).

Frederickson, R. C. A., V. Burgis, C. E. Harrell, and J. D. Edwards. "Dual actions of substance P on nocioception: Possible role of endogenous opioids." *Science*, 199(4335), 1359–1362, (1978).

Frenk, H., B. C. McCarty, and J. C. Liebeskind. "Different brain areas mediate the analgesic and epileptic properties of enkephalin." *Science*, 200(4339), 335–337, (1978).

Galaburda, A. M., M. LeMay, T. L. Kemper, and N. Geschwind. "Right-left asymmetries in the brain." *Science*, 199(4331), 852–856, (1978).

Gale, K., A. Guidotti, and E. Costa. "Dopamine-sensitive adenylate cyclase: Location in substantia nigra." *Science*, 195(4277), 503–505, (1977).

Galin, D. "Lateral specialization and psychiatric issues: Speculations on development and the evolution of consciousness." *Annals of the New York Academy of Sciences*, 299, 397–411, (1977).

——— "Lateralization of conversion symptoms—left side or dominant side—reply." *American Journal of Psychiatry*, 135(4), 509, (1978).

Gaylin, W. M., J. S. Meister, and R. C. Neville. *Operating on the Mind: The Psychosurgery Conflict*. New York: Basic Books, 1975.

Gazzaniga, M. S. "Brain theory and minimal brain dysfunction." *Annals of the New York Academy of Sciences*, 205, 89–92, (1973).

Gold, R. M., A. P. Jones, P. E. Sawchenko, and G. Kapatos. "Paraventricular area: Critical focus of a longitudinal neurocircuitry mediating food intake." *Physiology and Behavior*, 18(6), 1111–1119, (1977).

Goldberg, A. M., and E. K. Silbergeld. "Animal models of hyperactivity," in I. Hanin and E. Usdin, eds., *Animal Models in Psychiatry and Neurology*, pp. 371–384. New York: Pergamon, 1978.

Goldberg, M. E., and D. L. Robinson. "Visual mechanisms underlying gaze: Function of the cerebral cortex," in R. Baker and A. Berthoz, eds., *Control of Gaze by Brain Stem Neurons. Developments in Neuroscience*, vol. 1, pp. 469–481. New York: Elsevier/North Holland Biomedical Press, 1977.

Goldman, P. S. "Age, sex, and experience as related to the neural basis of cognitive development," in N. A. Buchwald and M. A. Brazier, eds., *Brain Mechanisms in Mental Retardation*, pp. 379–392. New York: Academic, 1975.

——— "Maturation of the mammalian nervous system and the ontogeny of behavior." *Advances in the Study of Behavior*, 7, 1–90, (1976).

Goldman, P. S., H. T. Crawford, L. P. Stokes, T. W. Galkin, and H. E. Rosvold. "Sex-dependent behavioral effects of cerebral cortical lesions in the developing rhesus monkey." *Science*, 186(4163), 540–542, (1974).

Graham, F. K., L. A. Leavitt, B. D. Strock, and J. W. Brown. "Precocious cardiac orienting in a human anencephalic infant." *Science*, 199(4326), 322–324, (1978).

Greenberg, A. S., and M. Coleman. "Depressed 5-hydroxyindole levels associated with hyperactive and agressive behavior: Relationship to drug response." *Archives of General Psychiatry*, 33(3), 331–336, (1976).

Grevert, P., and A. Goldstein. "Endorphins: Naloxone fails to alter experimental pain or mood in humans." *Science*, 199(4333), 1093–1095, (1978).

Grobstein, P., and K. L. Chow. "Receptive field development and individual experience." *Science*, 190(4212), 352–358, (1975).

Gross, C. G. "Locomotor activity following lateral frontal lesions in rhesus monkeys." *Journal of Comparative and Physiological Psychology*, 56(2), 232–236, (1963).

Grossman, R. G., and A. Seregin. "Glial-neural interaction demonstrated by the injection of Na+ and Li+ into cortical glia." *Science*, 195(4274), 196–198, (1977).

Groves, P. M., and R. F. Thompson. "A dual-process theory of habituation: Neural mechanisms," in H. V. S. Peeke and M. J. Herz, eds., *Habituation*, vol. 2: *Physiological Substrates*, Chap. 6. New York: Academic, 1973.

Guillemin, R. "Biochemical and physiological correlates of hypothalamic peptides: The new endocrinology of the neuron." 1976 *ARNMD Proceedings*. New York: Raven, 1977.

Hannay, H. J. "Real or imagined incomplete lateralization of function in females?" *Perception and Psychophysics*, 19(4), 349–352, (1976).

Harnad, S. R., R. W. Doty, L. Goldstein, J. Jaynes, and G. Krauthamer, eds., *Lateralization in the Nervous System*. New York: Academic, 1977.

Harris, L. J. "Sex differences in spatial ability: Possible environmental, genetic and neurological factors," in M. Kinsbourne, ed., *Asymmetric Function of the Brain*. Cambridge: Cambridge University Press, 1978.

Hicks, R. E., and M. Kinsbourne. "Human handedness: a cross-fostering study." *Science*, 192(4242), 908–910, (1976).

Hingtgen, J. N., and M. H. Aprison. "Behavioral and environmental aspects of the cholinergic system," in A. M. Goldberg and I. Hanin, eds., *Biology of Cholinergic Function*. New York: Raven, 1975.

Hore, J., J. Meyer-Lohmann, and V. B. Brooks. "Basal ganglia cooling disables learned arm movements of monkeys in the absence of visual guidance." *Science*, 195(4278), 584–586, (1977).

Hubel, D. H., T. N. Wiesel, and M. P. Stryker. "Anatomical demonstration of orientation columns in macaque monkey." *Journal of Comparative Neurology*, 177(3), 361–380, (1978).

Humphries, T., M. Kinsbourne, and J. Swanson. "Stimulant effects on cooperation and social interaction between hyperactive children and their mothers." *Journal of Child Psychology and Psychiatry*, 19(1), 13–22, (1978).

Ingvar, D. H., and L. Philipson. "Distribution of cerebral blood flow in the dominant hemisphere during motor ideation and motor performance." *Annals of Neurology*, 2(3), 230–237, (1977).

Jacobowitz, D. M., and P. D. MacLean. "A brainstem atlas of catecholaminergic neurons and serotonergic perikarya in a pigmy primate *(Cebuella pygmaea)*." *Journal of Comparative Neurology*, 177(3), 397–416, (1978).

Jacquet, Y. F., W. A. Klee, K. C. Rice, I. Iijima, and J. Minamikawa. "Stereospecific and nonstereospecific effects of (+)− and (−) −morphine: Evidence for a new class of receptors?" *Science*, 198(4319), 842–845, (1977).

Jones Gotman, M., and B. Milner. "Design fluency: The invention of nonsense drawings after focal cortical lesions." *Neuropsychologia*, 15(4–5), 653–674, (1977).

Just, M. A., G. A. Davis, and P. A. Carpenter. "A comparison of aphasic and normal adults in a sentence-verification task." *Cortex*, 13(4), 402–423, (1977).

Kalat, J. W. "Minimal brain dysfunction: Dopamine depletion?" *Science*, 194(4263), 450–451, (1976).

Kandel, E. R. "Neuronal plasticity and the modification of behavior," in E. R. Kandel, ed., *Cellular Biology of Neurons*, p. 2, vol. 1: *The Nervous System*, sect. 1, *Handbook of Physiology*, Chap. 29, pp. 1137–1182. Bethesda, Md.: American Physiological Society, 1977.

Katz, J. L., and J. E. Barrett. "Effects of d-amphetamine and ethanol on responding of squirrel monkeys on fixed ratio schedules of food presentation and stimulus shock termination." *Pharmacology, Biochemistry, and Behavior*, 8(1), 35–39, (1978).

Kelly, J., G. F. Alheid, A. Newberg, and S. P. Grossman. "GABA stimulation and blockade in the hypothalamus and midbrain: Effects on feeding and locomotor activity." *Pharmacology, Biochemistry, and Behavior*, 7(6), 537–541, (1977).

Kimura, D. "Cerebral dominance for speech," in D. B. Tower and E. L. Eagles, eds., *The Nervous System*, vol. 3, pp. 365–371. New York: Raven, 1975.

——— "Acquisition of a motor skill after left-hemisphere damage." *Brain*, 100(3), 527–542 (1977).

Koob, G. F., P. J. Fray, and S. D. Iversen. "Tail-pinch stimulation: Sufficient motivation for learning." *Science*, 194(4265), 637–639, (1976).

Kostowski, W., M. Jerlicz, A. Bidzinski, and M. Hauptmann. "Behavioral effects of neuroleptics, apomorphine and amphetamine after bilateral lesion of the locus coeruleus in rats." *Pharmacology, Biochemistry, and Behavior*, 7(4), 289–293, (1977).

Langhorne, J. E., J. Loney, C. E. Paternite, and H. P. Bechtoldt. "Childhood hyperkinesis: A return to the source." *Journal of Abnormal Psychology*, 85(2), 201–209, (1976).

Lansdell, H. "Effect of brain damage on intelligence in rats." *Journal of Comparative and Physiological Psychology*, 46(6), 461–464, (1953).

——— "Verbal and nonverbal factors in right-hemisphere speech: Relation to early neurological history." *Journal of Comparative and Physiological Psychology*, 69(4), 734–738, (1969).

——— "Relation of extent of temporal removals to closure and visuomotor factors."

Perceptual and Motor Skills, 31(2), 491–498, (1970).

—— "Effect of neurosurgery on the ability to identify popular word associations." *Journal of Abnormal Psychology*, 81(3), 255–258, (1973).

—— "Psychosurgery: Some ethical considerations," in S. Btesh, ed., *Protection of Human Rights in the Light of Technological Progress in Biology and Medicine*, pp. 264–275. Geneva: World Health Organization, 1974.

Lansdell, H., and J. C. Davie. "Massa intermedia: Possible relation to intelligence." *Neuropsychologia*, 10(2), 207–210, (1972).

Lansdell, H., and E. F. Donnelly. "Factor analysis of the Wechsler Adult Intelligence Scale subtests and the Halstead-Reitan Category and Tapping tests." *Journal of Consulting and Clinical Psychology*, 45(3), 412–416, (1977).

Lansdell, H., and A. F. Mirsky. "Attention in focal and centrencephalic epilepsy." *Experimental Neurology*, 9(6), 463–469, (1964).

Lansdell, H., and F. J. Smith. "Asymmetrical cerebral function for two WAIS factors and their recovery after brain injury." *Journal of Consulting and Clinical Psychology*, 43(6), 923, (1975).

LeDoux, J. E., G. L. Risse, S. P. Spinger, D. H. Wilson, and M. S. Gazzaniga. "Cognition and commisurotomy." *Brain*, 100(1), 87–104, (1977).

LeMay, M. "Asymmetries of the skull and handedness: Phrenology revisited." *Journal of the Neurological Sciences*, 32(2), 243–253, (1977).

Levy, J. "Evolution of language lateralization and cognitive function." *Annals of the New York Academy of Sciences*, 280, 810–820, (1976).

—— "Manifestations and implications of shifting hemi-inattention in commisurotomy patients." *Advances in Neurology*, 18, 83–92, (1977).

Levy, J., and J. M. Levy. "Human lateralization from head to toe: Sex-related factors." *Science*, 200(4347), 1291–1292, (1978).

Levy, J., and M. Reid. "Variations in cerebral organization as a function of handedness, hand posture in writing, and sex." *Journal of Experimental Psychology: General*, 107(2), 119–144, (1978).

Llamas, A., C. Avendano, and F. Reinoso-Suarez. "Amygdaloid projections to prefrontal and motor cortex." *Science*, 195 (4280), 794–796, (1977).

Lopes da Silva, F. H., and D. E. A. T. Arnolds. "Physiology of the hippocampus and related structures." *Annual Review of Physiology*, 40, 185–216, (1978).

Lucas, J. H., and J. Siegel. "Cortical mechanisms that augment or reduce evoked potentials in cats." *Science*, 198(4312), 73–75, (1977).

Ludlow, C. L., J. L. Rapoport, G. L. Brown, and E. J. Mikkelson. "The effects of dextroamphetamine on hyperactive and normal children's language behavior." (Paper presented at the Annual Convention of the American Speech and Hearing Association, Chicago, November 1977.)

Ludlow, C. L., J. L. Rapoport, C. B. Cardano, and E. J. Mikkelson. "Differential effects of dextroamphetamine on language performance in hyperactive and normal boys," in Knights, R. M. and D. J. Bakker, eds., *Rehabilitation, Treatment and Management of Learning Disorders*. Baltimore: University Park Press. [1978] in press.

MacLean, P. D. "Sensory and perceptive factors in emotional functions of the triune brain," in L. Levi, ed., *Emotions—Their Parameters and Measurement*. New York: Raven, 1975.

Marques, D. M., and E. S. Valenstein. "Individual differences in agressiveness of female hamsters: Response to intact and castrated males and to females." *Animal Behavior*, 25(1), 131–139, (1977).

Matthysse, S. "Dopamine and selective attention." *Advances in Biochemical Psychopharmacology*, 16, 667–669, (1977).

McLean, J. H., R. M. Kostrzewa, and J. G. May. "Behavioral and biochemical effects of neonatal treatment of rats with 6-hydroxidopa." *Pharmacology, Biochemistry, and Behavior*, 4(5), 601–607, (1976).

Meier, J. H. *Developmental and Learning Disabilities: Evaluation, Management, and Prevention in Children*. Baltimore: University Park Press, 1976.

Milner, B. "Hemispheric specialization: Scope and limits," in F. O. Schmitt and F. G. Worden, eds., *The Neurosciences: Third Study Program*. Cambridge: MIT Press, 1974.

Mirsky, A. F., and M. M. Orren. "Attention," in L. H. Miller, C. A. Sandman, and A. J. Kastin, eds., *Neuropeptide Influences on the Brain and Behavior*, 233–267. New York: Raven, 1977.

Moore, R. Y. and F. E. Bloom. "Central catecholamine neuron systems: Anatomy and physiology of the dopamine system." *Annual Review of Neuroscience*, 1, 129–169, (1978).

Mora, F., and R. D. Myers. "Brain self-stimulation: Direct evidence for the involvement of dopamine in the prefrontal cortex." *Science*, 197(4311), 1387–1389, (1977).

Mountcastle, V. B. "Columnar organization of the cerebral cortex," in F. O. Schmitt and F. G. Worden, eds., *The Neurosciences: Fourth Study Program*. Cambridge: MIT Press, 1978.

Müller, E. E., G. Nistico, and U. Scapagnini. *Neurotransmitters and Anterior Pituitary Function*. New York: Academic, 1977.

Murphy, D. L. "Animal models for mania," in I. Hanin and E. Usdin, eds., *Animal Models in Psychiatry and Neurology*, pp. 211–222. New York: Pergamon, 1978.

Nance, D. M. "Sex differences in the hypothalamic regulation of feeding behavior in the rat," in A. H. Riesen and R. F. Thompson, eds., *Advances in Psychobiology*, 3, 75–123, (1976).

Nauta, W. J. H., and W. Haymaker. "Hypothalamic nuclei and fiber connections," in W. Haymaker, E. Anderson, and W. J. H. Nauta, eds., *The Hypothalamus*, Chap. 4, pp. 136–209. Springfield, Ill.: Thomas, 1969.

Nichols, P. L., T.-C. Chen, and J. D. Pomeroy. "Minimal brain dysfunction: Familial associations." (Paper presented at the 86th Annual Convention of the American Psychological Association, Toronto, August 1978.)

Oke, A., R. Keller, I. Mefford, and R. F. Adams. "Lateralization of norepinephrine in human thalamus." *Science*, 200(4348), 1411–1413, (1978).

Olds, J. *Drives and Reinforcements: Behavioral Studies of Hypothalamic Functions*. New York: Raven, 1977.

Orton, D. S. "Spatial memory." *Scientific American*, 236(6), 82–98, (1977).

Paterson, J. A., and C. P. Leblond. "Increased proliferation of neuroglia and endothelial cells in the supraoptic nucleus and hypophysial neural lobe of young rats drinking hypertonic sodium chloride solution." *Journal of Comparative Neurology*. 175(4), 373–390, (1977).

Pert, A., and C. Sivit. "Neuroanatomical focus for morphine and enkaphalin-induced hypermotility." *Nature*, 265(5595), 645–647, (1977).

Pert, C. B., and B. L. Gulley. "The mechanism of opiate agonist and antagonist action," in L. Birnbaumer and B. W. O'Malley, eds., *Hormone Receptors*. New York: Academic, 1977.

Pettibone, D. J., N. Kaufman, M. C. Scally, E. Meyer, Jr., I. Ulus, and L. D. Lytle.

"Striatal nondopaminaergic neurons: Possible involvement in feeding and drinking behavior." *Science*, 200(4346), 1175–1177, (1978).

Pinel, J. P. J., D. Treit, and L. I. Rovner. "Temporal lobe aggression in rats." *Science*, 197(4308), 197–1089, (1977).

Pontius, A. A. "Discussion." *Annals of the New York Academy of Sciences*, 205, 61–63, (1973).

Purpura, D. P. "Dendritic differentiation in human cerebral cortex: Normal and aberrant developmental patterns." *Advances in Neurology*, 12, 91–116, (1975).

Quinn, P. O., and J. L. Rapoport. "One-year follow-up of hyperactive boys treated with imipramine or methylphenidate." *American Journal of Psychiatry*, 132(3), 241–245, (1975).

Racagni, G., F. Bruno, F. Cattabeni, A. Maggi, A. M. Di Giulio, M. Parenti, and A. Groppetti. "Functional interaction between rat substantia nigra and striatum: GABA and dopamine interrelation." *Brain Research*, 134(2), 353–358, (1977).

Rapoport, J. L., and P. O. Quinn. "Minor physical anomalies (stigmata) and early developmental deviation: A major biologic subgroup of 'hyperactive children'," in D. V. S. Sankar, ed., *Mental Health in Children*, vol. III. Westbury, N.Y.: PJD Publications, 1976.

Rapoport, J. L., M. S. Buchsbaum, T. P. Zahn, H. Weingartner, C. Ludlow, and E. J. Mikklesen. "Dextroamphetamine: Cognitive and behavioral effects in normal prepuberal boys." *Science*, 199(4328), 560–563, (1978).

Raskin, L. "Canalization of arousal in the neonatal rat: Effects of amphetamine on aggregation with surrogate stimuli." (Paper presented at the meeting of the Eastern Psychological Association, Boston, April, 1977.)

Reynolds, A. F., Jr., A. B. Harris, G. A. Ojemann, and P. T. Turner. "Aphasia and left thalamic damage." *Journal of Neurosurgery*, 48(4), 570–574, (1978).

Rie, E. D., and H. E. Rie. "Recall, retention, and Ritalin." *Journal of Consulting and Clinical Psychology*, 45(6), 967–972, (1977).

Rie, H. E. "Hyperactivity in children." *American Journal of Diseases in Children*, 129(7), 783–789, (1975).

Rie, H. E. "Psychology, mental health, and the public interest." *American Psychologist*, 32(1), 1–4, (1977).

Rie, H. E., E. D. Rie, S. Stewart, and J. P. Ambuel. "Effects of methylphenidate on underachieving children." *Journal of Consulting and Clinical Psychology*, 44(2), 250–260, (1976).

Rigter, H. "Attentuation of amnesia in rats by systemically administered enkephalins." *Science*, 200(4337), 83–85, (1978).

Risberg, J., J. H. Halsey, E. L. Wills, and E. M. Wilson. "Hemispheric specialization in normal man studied by bilateral measurements of the regional cerebral blood flow: A study with the 133–3e inhalation technique." *Brain*, 98(3), 511–524, (1975).

Rosene, D. L., and G. W. Van Hoesen. "Hippocampal efferents reach widespread areas of cerebral cortex and amygdala in rhesus monkey." *Science*, 198(4314), 315–317, (1977).

Rosenzweig, M. R. "Effects of environment on brain and behavior in animals," in E. Schopler and R. J. Reichler, eds., *Psychopathology and child development*. New York: Plenum, 1976.

Rourke, B. P. "Brain-behavior relationships in children with learning disabilities: A research program." *American Psychologist*, 30(9), 911–920, (1975).

Rudel, R. G., M. B. Denckla, and S. Hirsch. "The development of left-hand superiority for discriminating braille configurations." *Neurology*, 27(2), 160–164, (1977).

Ryan, K. J. "Report and recommendations: Research on the fetus." DHEW Publication

No. (OS) 76–127. Washington, D.C.: USDHEW, 1975.

—— "Report and recommendations: Psychosurgery." DHEW Publication No. (OS) 77–0001. Washington, D.C.: USDHEW, 1977a.

—— "Report and recommendations: Research involving children." DHEW Publication No. (OS) 77–0004. Washington, D.C.: USDHEW, 1977b.

—— "Report and recommendations: Research involving those institutionalized as mentally infirm." DHEW Publication No. (OS) 78–0006. Washington, D.C.: USDHEW, 1978.

Safer, D. J. "Drug treatments in child psychiatry," in L. L. Iversen, S. D. Iversen, and S. H. Eng, eds., *Handbook of Psychopharmacology*, vol. 11, *Stimulants*, Chap. 4, pp. 167–217. New York: Plenum, 1978.

Salamy, A. "Commissural transmission: Maturational changes in humans." *Science*, 200(4348), 1409–1411, (1978).

Sbordone, R. J., and Garcia, J. "Untreated rats develop 'pathological' aggression when paired with a mescaline-treated rat in a shock-elicited aggression situation." *Behavioral Biology*, 21(4), 451–461, (1977).

Schallert, T., I. Q. Whishaw, V. D. Ramirez, and P. Teitelbaum. "Compulsive, abnormal walking caused by anticholinergics in akinetic, 6-hydroxytryptamine-treated rats." *Science*, 199(4336), 1461–1463, (1978).

Schally, A. V., A. J. Kastin, and A. Arimura. "Hypothalamic hormones: The link between brain and body." *American Scientist*, 65(6), 712–719, (1977).

Schmitt, B. D. "The minimal brain dysfunction myth." *American Journal of Diseases of Children*, 129(11), 1313–1318, (1975).

—— "Minimal brain dysfunction myth." *American Journal of Diseases of Children*, 130(8), 901–902, (1976).

Schmitt, F. O., P. Dev, and B. H. Smith. "Electrotonic processing of information by brain cells." *Science*, 193(4248), 114–120, (1976).

Schooler, C., T. P. Zahn, D. L. Murphy, and M. S. Buchsbaum. "Psychological correlates of monoamine oxidase activity in normals." *Journal of Nervous and Mental Disease*, 166(3), 177–183, (1978).

Schrag, P., and D. Divoky. *The Myth of the Hyperactive Child and Other Means of Child Control*. New York: Pantheon, 1975.

Schwartz, G., R. J. Davidson, and F. Maer. "Right hemisphere lateralization for emotion in the human brain." *Science*, 190(4211), 286–288, (1975).

Sechzer, J. A. "The neonatal split-brain kitten: A laboratory analogue of minimal brain dysfunction," in J. D. Maser and M. E. P. Seligman, eds., *Psychopathology: Experimental Models*, pp. 308–333. San Francisco: Freeman, 1978.

Shaywitz, S. E., D. J. Cohen, and B. A. Shaywitz. "The biochemical basis of minimal brain dysfunction." *Journal of Pediatrics*, 92(2), 179–187, (1978).

Shaywitz, B. A., R. D. Yager, and J. H. Klopper. "Selective brain dopamine depletion in developing rats: An experimental model of minimal brain dysfunction." *Science*, 191(4224), 305–308, 1976).

Shaywitz, B. A., J. H. Klopper, R. D. Yager, and J. W. Gordon. "Paradoxical response to amphetamine in developing rats treated with 6-hydroxydopamine." *Nature*, 261(5556), 153–155, (1976).

Sheff, S., L. Bernardo, and C. Cotman. "Progressive brain damage accelerates axon sprouting in the adult rat." *Science*, 197(4305), 795–797, (1977).

Shepherd, G. M. "Microcircuits in the nervous system." *Scientific American*, 238(2), 92–103, (1978).

Silbergeld, E. K. "Neuropharmacology of hyperkinesis," in W. B. Essman and L. Vasselli, eds., *Current Developments in Psychopharmacology*, Chap. 8. New York: Spectrum, 1977.

Silbergeld, E. K., and A. M. Goldberg. "Hyperactivity," in A. M. Goldberg and I. Hanin, eds., *Biology of Cholinergic Function*, pp. 619–645. New York: Raven, 1976.

Smith, C. J. "Mass action and early environment in the rat." *Journal of Comparative and Physiological Psychology*, 52(2), 154–156, (1959).

Smith, M. O., J. Chu, and W. E. Edmonston, Jr., "Cerebral lateralization of haptic perception: Interaction of responses to Braille and music reveals a functional basis." *Science*, 197(4304), 689–690, (1977).

Snyder, S. H. "Opiate receptors and internal opiates." *Scientific American*, 236(3), 44–56, (1977).

Sprague, R. L., and E. K. Sleator. "Methylphenidate in hyperkinetic children: Differences in dose effects on learning and social behavior." *Science*, 198(4323), 1274–1276, (1977).

Stamm, J. S., and S. V. Kreder. "Minimal brain dysfunction: Psychological and neurophysiological disorders in hyperkinetic children," in M. Gazzaniga, ed., *Handbook in Neuropsychology*. New York: Plenum, 1978.

Steg, J. P., and J. L. Rapoport. "Minor physical anomalies in normal, neurotic, learning disabled, and severely disabled children." *Journal of Autism and Childhood Schizophrenia*, 5(4), 299–307, (1975).

Szeligo, F. "Quantitative differences in oligodendrocytes and myelinated axons in the brains of rats raised in enriched, control and impoverished environments." *Anatomical Record*, 187(4), 726–727, (1977).

Szeligo, F., and C. P. Leblond. "Response of the three main types of glial cells of cortex and corpus callosum in rats handled during suckling or exposed to enriched, control and impoverished environments following weaning." *Journal of Comparative Neurology*, 172(2), 247–264, (1977).

Tecce, J. J., J. Savignano-Bowman, and J. O. Cole. "Drug effects on contingent negative variation and eyeblinks: The distraction-arousal hypothesis," in M. A. Lipton, A. Dimascio, and K. F. Killam, eds., *Psychopharmacology: A Generation of Progress*, pp. 745–758. New York: Raven, 1978.

Teng, E. L. "Interhemispheric rivalry during simultaneous bilateral task presentation in commissurotomized patients." (Paper read at the 82nd Annual Convention of the American Psychological Association, New Orleans, September 2, 1974.)

Teuber, H. L. "Effects of focal brain injury on human behavior," in D. B. Tower and T. N. Chase, eds., *The Nervous System*, vol. 2: *The Clinical Neurosciences*, pp. 457–480. New York: Raven, 1975.

Tower, D. B. "Neurochemistry—one hundred years, 1875–1975." *Annals of Neurology*, 1(1), 2–36 (1977).

Twitchell, T. E. "A behavioral syndrome," review of *Minimal Brain Dysfunction* by P. H. Wender, *Science*, 174(4005), 135–136, (1971).

Vanderhoof, C. H. "The role of the cerebral cortex and ascending activating systems in the control of behavior," in E. Satinoff and P. Teitelbaum, eds., *Handbook of Behavioral Neurobiology*. New York: Plenum, 1978.

Waber, D. P. "Sex differences in cognition: Function of maturation rate." *Science*, 192(4239), 572–574 (1976).

Waizer, J., S. P. Hoffman, P. Polizos, and D. M. Engelhardt. "Outpatient treatments of hyperactive school children with imipramine." *American Journal of Psychiatry*, 131(5), 587–591, (1974).

Waldrop, M. F., R. Q. Bell, B. McLaughlin, and C. F. Halverson. "Newborn minor physical anomalies predict short attention span, peer aggression, and impulsivity at age 3." *Science*, 199(4328), 563–565, (1978).

Walker, S. *Help for the Hyperactive Child*. Boston: Houghton Mifflin, 1977.

Wender, P. H. *Minimal Brain Dysfunction in Children*. New York: Wiley, 1971.

Wender, P. H. "Some speculations concerning a possible biochemical basis of minimal brain dysfunction." *Annals of the New York Academy of Sciences*, 205, 18–28, (1973).

Wender, P. H. "A possible monoaminergic basis for minimal brain dysfunction." *Psychopharmacology Bulletin*, 11(3), 36–37, (1975a).

Wender, P. H. "The minimal brain dysfunction syndrome." *Annual Review of Medicine*, 26, 45–62, (1975b).

Wender, P. H., and E. H. Wender. "Minimal brain dysfunction myth." *American Journal of Diseases of Children*, 130(8), 900–902, (1976).

Whitaker, H. A., and G. A. Ojemann. "Graded localisation from electrical stimulation mapping of left cerebral cortex." *Nature*, 270(5632), 50–51, (1977).

Will, B. E., M. R. Rosenzweig, and E. L. Bennett. "Effects of differential environments on recovery from neonatal brain lesions, measured by problem-solving scores and brain dimensions." *Physiology and Behavior*, 16(5), 603–611, (1976).

Witelson, S. F. "Anatomical asymmetry in the temporal lobes: Its documentation, phylogenesis, and relationship to functional asymmetry." *Annals of the New York Academy of Sciences*, 299, 328–354, (1977a).

———— "Developmental dyslexia: Two right hemispheres and none left." *Science*, 195(4275), 309–311, (1977b).

———— "Sex differences in the neurology of cognition: Psychological, social, educational and clinical implications," in E. Sullerot, and C. Escoffier, eds., *La Fait Feminin*. France: Fayard, 1978.

Yakovlev, P. I., and P. Rakic. "Patterns of decussation of bulbar pyramids and distribution of pyramidal tracts on two sides of the spinal cord." *Transactions of the American Neurological Association*, 91, 366–367, (1966).

Yeni-Komshian, G. H., and D. A. Benson. "Anatomical study of cerebral asymmetry in the temporal lobe of humans, chimpanzees, and rhesus monkeys." *Science*, 192(4237), 387–389, (1976).

Yin, T. C. T., and V. B. Mountcastle. "Visual input to the visuomotor mechanisms of the monkey's parietal lobe." *Science*, 197(4311), 1381–1383, (1977).

Zahn, T. P., B. C. Little, and P. H. Wender. "Pupillary and heart rate reactivity in children with minimal brain dysfunction." *Journal of Abnormal Child Psychology*, 6(1), 135–147, (1978).

Zambelli, A. J., J. S. Stamm, S. Matinsky, and D. L. Loiselle. "Auditory evoked potentials and selective attention in formerly hyperactive adolescent boys." *American Journal of Psychiatry*, 134(7), 742–747, (1977).

PART FOUR

Determinants of Minimal Brain Dysfunctions

Chapters 6–9

CHAPTER 6

Genetic, Perinatal, and Constitutional Factors in Minimal Brain Dysfunctions

Mark A. Stewart

Charles Darwin in *On the Origin of Species* (1859) wrote, "Seedlings from the same fruit, and the young of the same litter, sometimes differ considerably from each other, though both the young and the parents have apparently been exposed to exactly the same conditions of life; and this shows how unimportant the direct effects of the conditions of life are in comparison with the laws of reproduction, of growth, and of inheritance; for had the actions of the conditions been direct, if any of the young had varied, all would probably have varied in the same manner."

Darwin reached his theory on the evolution of species by studying attributes of animals which were highly specific. Those exploring the origins of "minimal brain dysfunction" have tried to follow the same strategy as best they can. They have focussed on specific parts of MBD, such as hyperactivity and reading disability. Needless to say they are far from reaching any great new insight. In fact the reader will probably be disappointed at the state of knowledge on biologic origins of hyperactivity, which is the primary subject of this chapter.

Recent studies by Finucci, et al., (1976) and Foch, et al., (1977) have moved genetic determinants of reading disability from being an interesting possibility to a strong probability. Research on other aspects of MBD, such as enuresis or speech problems, has not gone beyond the stage of flirtation. This chapter is concerned with the controversial syndrome of hyperactivity, which is made up of abnormally high levels of activity and distractibility and aggressiveness. The syndrome affects about 5% of the population (Werner, et al., 1968) and is more common in boys than girls. It was first defined as a specific disorder by Laufer and Denhoff (1957), and has attracted a great deal of interest since then. This chapter will review research on possible biologic determinants.

FAMILY STUDIES OF HYPERACTIVITY

Morrison and Stewart (1971) interviewed the parents of 59 children who were hyperactive and distractible, had intelligence in the normal range, and did not have severe language or neurological dysfunctions. The authors wanted to discover what psychiatric symptoms the parents had experienced. They also interviewed a control group of parents whose children had been admitted to hospital for operations, such as appendectomies and herniorrhaphies. These control children matched the experimental subjects in age and sex. The investigators made psychiatric diagnoses on the parents using specific operational criteria. The main findings were that alcoholism was twice as common among the fathers of hyperactive children compared to the fathers of controls. Antisocial personality occurred in a few fathers and hysteria in a few mothers of the hyperactive children, but in none of the parents of controls. When these three disorders were combined they occurred significantly more often among subjects' parents compared with controls' parents (p< .01). Taking into account the histories of uncles and aunts, hyperactive children were twice as likely as controls to have a first or second degree relative with alcoholism (p< .025).

Morrison and Stewart (1971) also tried to determine whether parents had been hyperactive themselves as children. This retrospective diagnosis was made if a parent reported that he or she had been hyperactive, aggressive, or reckless as a child; had been involved in antisocial behavior at home or in school; and had suffered from distractibility, poor concentration, or learning difficulties for which there was objective evidence. Nine fathers and three mothers of the subjects had such a history compared with one father and one mother of the controls (a difference that was not significant). Twelve uncles and one aunt of the subjects also had such a history, while no uncle or aunt of the controls did. Combining the numbers for parents, uncles, and aunts did lead to a significant difference between the two sets of families (p< .001). Of the 14 parents (10 fathers and 4 mothers) who were diagnosed as having been hyperactive as children, 11 had a definite psychiatric illness as an adult. Five fathers were alcoholic; 1 was a sociopath; 1 had an unclassifiable disorder with chronic depressive, phobic, and compulsive symptoms; and 1 was a psychotic epileptic. One mother was depressed, 1 had been treated for bipolar affective disorder, and 1 was alcoholic and hysteric. The finding that of the 14 parents who were thought to have been hyperactive themselves, 11 had psychiatric disorders as adults, lent some validity to the restrospective diagnosis.

Cantwell (1972) investigated the families of 50 hyperactive children being seen in a clinic and 50 control children who were attending the same clinic for pediatric rather than psychiatric problems. He too found that alcoholism was twice as common among the fathers of hyperactive children compared to fathers of controls. Furthermore he found significantly more instances of antisocial personality among fathers and hysteria among mothers of subjects than among parents of controls. He also found significantly higher rates of alcoholism and antisocial personality in male second degree relatives of subjects, and similarly a higher frequency of hysteria among the female second degree relatives. The childhood histories of fathers and uncles suggested that hyperactivity had been commoner among the relatives of probands compared with controls.

Morrison and Stewart (1973) and Cantwell (1975) also studied the legal relatives of adopted hyperactive children and found that the prevalence of psychiatric disorders among them and the frequency with which they had behavior problems as children did not differ from the corresponding rates among relatives of control children. These negative studies were interpreted as arguing against the likelihood that hyperactivity was transmitted from parents to children through social factors such as modeling.

Borland Heckman (1976) found that behavior problems were more common among the children of 20 men who had once been treated in a child psychiatry clinic for hyperactivity than among the children of their brothers who had not been hyperactive. Two out of 8 sons of the ex-hyperactives were thought to be hyperactive themselves. Welner, et al., (1977) found that 11 of the 42 brothers of 43 hyperactive boys were affected themselves compared to 5 of the 54 brothers of control boys, but this difference only established a trend (p = .054).

Taken together these studies suggest that hyperactivity in children is associated with alcoholism in adult relatives, with antisocial personality in male relatives, and with hysteria in female relatives. The studies also suggest that fathers and uncles of hyperactive children may have been hyperactive themselves, but this conclusion is open to doubt because it is based on parents' memories of events which took place 30 years earlier.

Neither Morrison and Stewart nor Cantwell did their interviews blind, but if the former had a preconceived idea when they did their study, it was that they would find an unusual prevalence of bipolar affective disorder among relatives of hyperactive children. This turned out not to be true. Stewart and Morrison (1973) have reported data on affective disorder among relatives of hyperactive children. The incidence of bipolar affective disorder in natural parents of hyperactive children was much lower than figures reported for parents of patients with this type of affective disorder. Unipolar depression was more common among second degree relatives of hyperactive children than in the corresponding relatives of controls.

A serious shortcoming of the two main family studies is that neither included a control group of children attending a psychiatric clinic with problems other than hyperactivity. Emotional or psychiatric disorder is common among the parents of children attending such clinics; in fact this is a defining characteristic of children coming to a psychiatric clinic (Shepherd, Oppenheim, and Mitchell, 1971). Alcoholism is one of the commoner psychiatric disorders, affecting about 5% of men, and it is a disorder that tends to disrupt families and affect parents' ability to handle difficult children. There could well be a general association between alcoholism in fathers and children being patients in a psychiatry clinic, rather than a specific association with hyperactivity.

Other evidence suggests that hyperactivity may precede alcoholism. Jones (1968) followed subjects in the Oakland Growth Study into middle age and found that men who were drinking excessively were more likely to have been characterized as aggressive, talkative, noncompliant, and impulsive as adolescents. McCord and McCord (1960) found that boys who were alcoholic later in life were more likely to be rated as hyperactive, aggressive, and fearless than controls; their data came from a follow-up of subjects in the Cambridge-Somerville Youth Study. In a study of alcoholic adoptees, Goodwin, et al., (1975) found that these men were reported to have been hyperactive, truant, antisocial, aggressive, and disobedient as boys more often than nonalcoholic adoptees who formed a control group. A high proportion of the 14 alcoholic adoptees had biological parents who were alcoholic themselves, while there was no evidence of alcoholism among the biologic parents of the nonalcoholics. Finally Tarter, et al., (1977) have reported evidence that alcoholics with severe symptoms and an early onset of their disorder are more likely to have had some of the many symptoms of minimal brain dysfunction than alcoholics with late onset, psychiatric patients in general, or normal controls.

Direct Evidence of Genetic Influence

Cunningham, et al., (1975) compared a group of adolescent and young adult adoptees whose biologic parents had a psychiatric disorder with adoptees whose biologic parents were normal. The adoptees with disturbed parents had more often been treated for psychiatric disorders themselves, and a number of the male adoptees were diagnosed as having been hyperactive. Cadoret, et al., (1975) reported further findings from the same study. Hyperactive behavior in adoptees of either sex was associated with antisocial behavior in biologic parents. Nine of 22 adoptees with antisocial parents had a history of more than one type of hyperactive behavior, while this was true for only 5 of 37 adoptees whose parents had other psychiatric problems (p = .034). In a separate study Cadoret and Gath (1976; 1978) found that adoptees whose biologic parents were alcoholic had significantly more often been hyperactive than adoptees whose parents had other psychiatric disorders or adoptees whose parents were normal. There was also a trend to higher prevalence of hyperactivity among adoptees with antisocial parents. Unfortunately the numbers of affected adoptees in these studies were small. For example in the last study there were 16 adoptees whose biologic parents were alcoholic and 4 of these had a history of being hyperactive. In contrast only 6 of 97 adoptees whose biologic parents were normal had such a history. However when these studies are put together with evidence on the relatives of hyperactive children raised by their natural parents, the idea that alcoholism in adults is related to hyperactivity in children deserves to be taken seriously.

The adoptees studied by Cadoret et al., (1975) were separated from their natural parents at birth, and children in the two groups (those whose parents had a psychiatric disorder and those whose parents were normal) were matched on the time that they spent in foster care before being permanently adopted. The obvious social influences were therefore controlled. Questions which often cannot be resolved in such studies include the possibility that adopting parents knew the natural parents of their child had been antisocial and half expected him to follow suit. Another possibility is that the natural mother, being adolescent or poor, had a high risk pregnancy which affected brain development in the baby. Cadoret presents data which argue against the latter. Studies of adoptees, except the rare prospective one, also suffer from missing data on parents and children. On their own they may not be impressive, but linked to other studies they become powerful.

The study of half siblings of affected children may be the most direct way to discover genetic influence on children's behavior disorders. As far as the author knows only Safer (1973) has used this approach to finding the origins of minimal brain dysfunction. His probands were 17 children in foster care with these characteristics: short attention span (16), hyperactive (15), antisocial (14), and treated with amphetamine (12). Psychotic, retarded, and brain-damaged children were excluded, but 5 probands were epileptic. The siblings he studied were also in foster care. At least half the mothers were antisocial, alcoholic, or retarded, and the same was true of the fathers. Information on the 8 stepfathers was limited.

Safer's most interesting data concern the families of 5 probands who had both full and half siblings. Of the 9 full siblings, 7 were considered hyperactive, 5 had persistent behavior problems, 5 were diagnosed as having MBD, and 3 had been treated with amphetamine. The corresponding figures for the 14 half siblings were 2, 2, 0, and 0. Full siblings were significantly more often affected than half siblings. When the characteristics of all the full and half siblings of the 17 probands were compared there were significant differences between the groups on short attention span (9/19 full siblings versus 3/22 half siblings), behavior problems (10/19 versus 4/22) and diagnosis of MBD (9/19 versus 2/22).

Safer's findings (1973) are important in spite of the small size of the groups and the fact that the data were gathered from charts rather than systematic histories and examinations. Two serious gaps in the data weaken the conclusions. No information is presented on the homes in which the children were raised, natural or foster, so that we do not know whether social influences such as conflict between parents were equal for the two types of siblings. Neither is there information on the psychiatric state of stepfathers. When women remarry it is common for them to choose a second antisocial or alcoholic man. If the fathers of the half siblings were as deviant as those of the full siblings, the differences between the two sets of siblings could not be easily attributed to heredity. Finally the study of families as deviant as Safer's subjects should involve tests of paternity in order to verify the relationships between children.

It is interesting to note that while Welner, et al., (1977) found that a quarter of the brothers of hyperactive children from lower middle class families were hyperactive themselves, the proportion in Safer's full siblings was four out of five. The latter came from socially deviant families. Moreover their IQs were in the borderline range while Welner's subjects' IQs were in the average range. Since the prevalence of behavior problems is negatively related to intelligence (Rutter, Tizard, and Whitmore, 1970), concordance for such problems among siblings is likely to be greater when their IQs are lower.

Willerman (1973) asked mothers of same-sex twins to describe the twins on the Activity Level Questionnaire developed by Werry, Weiss, and Peters (Werry, 1970). Zygosity of the twins was determined through another questionnaire (Nichols and Bilbro, 1966). He got complete information on 93 pairs of twins whose age ranged from 1 to 14. The estimated activity level was the same for monozygotic (MZ) and dizogotic (DZ) boys but somewhat higher in DZ girls than MZ. The intraclass correlation for MZ boys (.94) was significantly higher ($p < .001$) than that for DZ boys (.60) and the same was true for girls. When the analyses were done separately for twins older and younger than 50 months the correlations for MZ twins were still higher than for DZ, but the difference among the older twins was less significant ($p < .05$ compared to $p < .001$ for the younger twins).

Willerman defined a twin whose score on the scale of activity was in the top 20% as hyperactive. Eight MZ pairs out of 54 contained at least one hyperactive; 16 DZ pairs out of 39 contained a hyperactive twin. Again the intraclass correlation for MZ twins (.70) was significantly higher than for DZ (.16, $p < .05$). A problem with these findings is the very low correlation for DZ twins and the surprisingly high proportion of DZ twin pairs (2 out of 5) that contained at least one hyperactive child.

Matheny, Dolan, and Wilson (1976) described the development of learning problems in 46 twins from a larger group enrolled in a longitudinal study. Compared to matched twins without such difficulties the affected twins were more active, less able to concentrate, and more labile in their emotions. Genetic influences for the apparent hyperactivity as well as the learning problems were suggested by greater concordance for identical twins than fraternal.

CONCLUSIONS

The studies that have been reviewed so far in this chapter suggest four conclusions:

1. There is a connection between hyperactivity in children and alcoholism, antisocial personality, and hysteria in their adult relatives.

2. Hyperactivity in childhood may predispose people to these psychiatric disorders of adult life.

3. Hyperactive children tend to have parents, uncles, and aunts who were hyperactive themselves and *vice versa.*

4. There is direct evidence for genetic determinants of hyperactivity.

Unfortunately each of the studies reviewed is either flawed by mistakes in design or limited by the small number of subjects involved. Looking at the work sceptically one would say that it has made the idea of heredity taking a part in the origins of hyperactivity respectable and the connection with adult psychiatric disorders an interesting lead.

FUTURE RESEARCH IN GENETICS

Everyone admits that the diagnosis of hyperactivity covers a varied group of children, but few researchers have divided their subjects, except into children with definite brain damage and without. Campbell, Erdman, and Bernfeld (1977) distinguished between "situational" hyperactivity and "true" hyperactivity. They used the former term for behavior problems which occurred only in the home and the latter for those occurring in school and home. "True" hyperactive children seemed to have a more serious problem and to be aggressive as well as overactive and distractible.

Aggressiveness, resistance to discipline, destructiveness, meanness, and anti-social behavior have generally been considered part of the behavioral syndrome of hyperactivity (Stewart, et al., 1966; Conners, 1970; Cantwell, 1975). That over-activity often goes with aggressiveness is clear from studies of various groups of children (Peterson, 1961; Collins, Maxwell, and Cameron, 1962; Wolff, 1971), but how often they are associated and how often they occur separately is not known. The fact of an association raises a hard question about research in this field. May aggressiveness, or some secondary symptom, be more significant than the primary symptom of hyperactivity? One study that shows this is so was reported recently by Loney, et al., (1976). These investigators found that aggressiveness was a powerful predictor of outcome in a large group of children with minimal brain dysfunction while overactivity was insignificant.

The studies reviewed earlier are open to the question whether the observed correlates of hyperactivity, for example alcoholism in relatives, are related to overactivity, to aggressiveness, or to another symptom. The present author is working on this question and has reported preliminary results (Stewart and Leone, 1978 in press). A blind family study of hyperactive boys who were also aggressive, resistant to discipline, and antisocial and of controls with other psychiatric disorders shows that this pattern is associated specifically with antisocial personality in fathers and not with alcoholism. It seems likely then that the association between antisocial personality and hyperactivity which appeared in the studies by Morrison and Stewart (1971) and Cantwell (1972) is actually an association with the combination of hyperactivity and aggressive, antisocial behavior. Further research will show whether hyperactivity is a necessary part of this association and what disorders, if any, are related within families to hyperactivity pure and simple.

With greater sophistication in classifying children's behavior problems we will surely develop clearer relationships between the disorders of children and their parents. It also seems certain that relating children's traits, singly or in clusters, to those of their parents will be as powerful an approach to the genetics of these disorders as relating diagnoses of children with those of parents.

TEMPERAMENT

If the behavior pattern named hyperactivity is hereditary to some extent, what is being inherited? It seems likely that stable tendencies in behavior such as activity level, responsiveness, and emotionality, or what has been called behavioral style, are genetically determined. Our ancestors in psychology, for example Robert Burton the author of *The Anatomy of Melancholy,* firmly believed in the inheritance of temperament. A typical statement by Burton is, "The character of the parents is transmitted to the children through the seed." Dog breeders have also taken this idea as established fact for centuries. To be more exact however it should be said that variation in temperament may be due to other biologic factors beside genetic, for example pre- or post-natal brain damage.

Thomas, Chess, and Birch (1968) were the first to study the relationship of temperament to the development of behavior problems in children followed from birth. They found that a group of traits (high reactivity, predominantly negative mood, irregularity of biologic rhythms, and low adaptability) which were identified in the first few years of a child's life predicted the development of "active" behavior problems between the ages of 4 and 10. The "active" symptoms overlapped somewhat with the syndrome of hyperactivity; all 34 children with these symptoms had unusually high levels of activity.

There is little hard evidence that children diagnosed as hyperactive at 8 or 9 were observably different from others in the first two to three years of life. Many investigators have reported that such children are described as babies as having been fussy, irritable, restless, and unable to sleep for long more often than control children, but this could be a case of interpreting the past in light of the present. Stewart, Thach, and Freidin (1970) followed up a group of 88 children who had attended an emergency room for accidental poisoning at an average age of 2.5. Six years later 22% of the boys (N=58) met criteria for the diagnosis of hyperactivity, a rate significantly higher than that found among controls or population surveys. Matheny, Brown, and Wilson (1971) found that in 49 pairs of twins who had had accidents in the first six years of life (mainly between one and four) there were significant differences between accident prone twins and their co-twins on behavior ratings made when they were one year old. The former were more active ($p < .001$), temperamental ($p < .01$) and inattentive ($p < .05$) than the latter. Besides supporting the idea of accident proneness these two studies suggest that some hyperactive children are observably different from their peers early in life.

Wilson, Brown, and Matheny (1971) have also published data from the Louisville Twin Study which bear more generally on the subject of temperament, but which may relate to hyperactivity. The data were derived from interviews with the mothers of 232 pairs of twins; the interviews were done regularly as the twins reached certain ages between three months and six years. The primary subject of this study was the emergence and persistence of differences between co-twins, but the authors also discovered trends in behavior which appeared early and were stable over time. They identified two main clusters of interrelated behaviors in one-year-old twins: temperament and sociability. The former included frequency and intensity of temper, irritability, crying, and demanding attention. The latter was made up of seeking affection, accepting people, and smiling. Attention span was negatively related to the first cluster. The two clusters remained relatively constant to the age of six years at least, and attention span continued to have a negative relation with the temperament cluster or specific items (temper frequency and demanding attention) until age five. Though level of activity was not part of the cluster, the combination of over-reactivity and impersistence does suggest a relationship between the temperament cluster and hyperactivity.

Bronson (1966) analyzed data from the Berkeley Guidance Study to discover central tendencies in the behavior of children from birth to the age of 16. Her primary data came from yearly ratings of behavior on 85 children as they grew from 5 to 16. The ratings were made by interviewers who got information from the children, parents, teachers, and others. Bronson constructed the central tendencies by finding which characteristics persisted over time and which had a high degree of generality, that is which were correlated with a number of other behaviors at each period. A brief summary of her painstaking and detailed work goes as follows. Three dimensions appeared, the first two of which (withdrawal-expressive and reactive-placid) were independent while the third (passive-domineering) was positively related to the first and negatively to the second. The main items in the first dimension were reserved-expressive, somber-gay, and shy-socially easy; among boys inactivity was one of the other behaviors related to this cluster. The second dimension comprised reactive-phlegmatic, explosive-calm, and resistive-compliant; secondary items for boys were emotional lability, quarrelsomeness, and frequent tantrums. Restlessness, showing off, and quarrelsomeness were negatively related to the third dimension (passive-domineering) in boys.

Bronson's (1966) reactive-placid cluster resembles the temperament cluster of Wilson, Brown and Matheny (1971) though it is derived from ratings on older children (5–16 in contrast to 1–16). Furthermore it is significantly correlated with the assertive direction of the third dimension. It therefore comes quite close at one pole to the pattern of hyperactivity, especially when the latter is defined to include aggressiveness and noncompliance, as it often is.

The relevance of the two studies to the subject of this chapter is that they establish stable trends in the behavior of children which can be related to the syndrome of hyperactivity. It is a reasonable possibility that a form of temperament underlies the syndrome which could be the behavioral genotype passed from one generation to another.

BRAIN DAMAGE AND INTERFERENCE WITH DEVELOPMENT OF THE BRAIN

There is no doubt that brain damage is sometimes associated with hyperactivity but whether this pattern of behavior is the most common correlate is a question that has not been settled. Graham and Rutter (1968) and Rutter, Graham, and Yule

(1970) have reported data from their epidemiologic studies in England which strongly support the idea that while psychiatric disorder is more common in brain-damaged children, the same range of disorders is seen in such children as in children whose problems are determined by psychological or social factors. Many clinicians in the United States believe, on the other hand, that hyperactivity is a specific sequel of brain damage in children. To some extent this disagreement seems to stem from different systems for classifying the problems of children. The pattern of behavior which is commonly diagnosed as hyperactivity in the United States falls primarily into the conduct disorder category of the English nomenclature, but also partly into the neurotic disorder category. It is distinctly possible then that both sides are right; hyperactivity may be the most common sequel to brain injury. It should be relatively simple to settle this question but so far the necessary research has not been dome.

The idea that hyperactivity and other aspects of minimal brain dysfunction have stemmed from perinatal stress has also been popular. A well-designed and large-scale prospective study has been carried out in the Island of Kauai, Hawaii. Werner, et al., (1968) followed at internals from birth 866 children, 90% of the live births on the island in 1955, as well as an additional 116 children born in 1956 who had moderate to severe perinatal complications. Data from the follow-up at 10 years show an effect of perinatal stress on intelligence and school placement, but no effect on the four emotional problems studied (chronic nervous habit, hyperkinetic symptoms, persistently withdrawn, and persistently overaggressive). In contrast emotional support at home and educational stimulation were strongly related to persistent aggressiveness and persistent withdrawal, but not to hyperkinetic symptoms.

Epidemiologic studies on perinatal stress necessarily lump many different factors together so that some specific factors operating at this time may be missed. A number of studies have suggested that babies born "small for dates" or with low birth weight are at risk for subsequent hyperactivity (Alden, et al., 1972; Drillien, 1973; and Francis-Williams and Davies, 1974). Neligan, et al., (1976) have published the most detailed investigation of the development of children "born too soon or too small." These authors followed from birth to age seven 141 children who were small for dates, 59 children who were born too soon, and 187 controls. Twins were excluded from the study. At age five and later, children born after a short gestation and the more extreme "small for dates" children scored significantly lower on intelligence tests than controls, but showed the same pattern of scores on subtests. Performance on other cognitive tests, for example the Illinois Test of Psycholinguistic Abilities, was also lower in the two test groups. Boys were affected more than girls, and there was evidence of an interaction between biologic factors and social class. The children's behavior was assessed by interviewing mothers, asking teachers to fill out questionnaires, and through several examinations; the assessments were carried out at ages five, six, and seven. In general ratings of both behavior and temperament showed more abnormalities among the test children than among the controls. Children born too soon and those who were very light for dates were more often hyperactive. This finding was most obvious from the psychiatric assessment which showed the two test groups to have a higher proportion of overactive, fidgety, and inattentive children.

Another stress which may lead to later hyperactivity is starvation in infancy (Klein, Forbes, and Nader, 1975). Studies on subclinical lead poisoning have produced contradictory results, some suggesting that intelligence is lowered and behavior altered while others find no such changes (David, et al., 1976; de la Burd'e and Choate, 1975; Lansdown, et al., 1974). Some types of meningitis may be followed by lowered intelligence and changes in behavior (Sell, et al., 1972; Feigin and Dodge, 1976) and the same is true for encephalitis. The question whether head injuries are followed by changes in behavior is complicated by the fact that many children who are injured in traffic accidents have been unusually active and impulsive before the injury (Hjern and Nylander, 1964; Craft, Shaw, and Cartlidge, 1972).

In a series of studies Waldrop and her colleagues have studied an association between minor physical anomalies and behavior problems in children. The anomalies include abnormal head circumference, epicanthus, hypertelorism, low seated ears, high arched palate, single palmar crease, and abnormalities of the fingers and toes. A full description is reported in Waldrop and Halverson (1971). Waldrop and Goering (1971) showed that hyperactive, impulsive, and disruptive behavior was associated with a higher than normal number of minor physical anomalies in boys of elementary school age, but this association was not found among girls. Recently Waldrop, Bell, and Goering, (1976) have reported that girls with inhibited behavior defined as including passivity, withdrawal, low level of activity, and chronic anxiety, have higher anomaly scores than outgoing and active girls. The mean IQ of the inhibited girls was 15 points lower than that of the outgoing girls and anomaly scores were negatively correlated with IQ and coordination.

Rosenberg and Weller (1973) failed to find an association between a high score on anomalies and behavior problems, but it is not clear whether they looked for the relationship in boys and girls separately. They did find that a higher than usual number of anomalies was related to lower verbal intelligence and to academic failure in first grade.

Quinn and Rapoport (1974) on the other hand found that the anomaly scores were positively correlated with ratings of hyperactivity in a group of 81 hyperactive boys. These investigators also found that high anomaly scores were associated with early onset of the child's problem, with a history of pre- and perinatal complications, and with fathers having a history of childhood hyperactivity themselves.

Steg and Rapoport (1975) studied the incidence of minor physical anomalies in a group of children on a general pediatric ward, a group who were attending a child guidance clinic for treatment of neurosis, a group of children with severe learning problems, and a group who were autistic or atypical children. The two last groups were in residential treatment centers. The more disturbed children had higher anomaly scores than children in the first two groups. The average IQ of the learning problem group was almost one standard deviation below average, while the neurotic children had IQs one standard deviation above the average. Presumably the autistic children had low IQs and it seems reasonable to expect the children on pediatric wards to have average intelligence; IQs were not available for either of these groups. It seems likely then that the two groups with the high scores on anomalies had lower intelligence.

These findings are intriguing. They suggest that genetic or environmental factors which interfere with the development of the fetus in the first three months of life may lead to hyperactive behavior in boys, to the opposite in girls, and possibly to other behavior disorders. Waldrop, Bell and Goering (1976) have shown by an analysis of covariance, that the association between anomalies and inhibited behavior of girls is independent of intelligence, but since the study involved children in a regular public school, the range of intelligence of the subjects was restricted. It is conceivable that the negative relationship between anomalies and IQ would become even stronger if retarded children were included. An earlier study (Smith and Bostian, 1964) showed that simple retardation is associated with higher than normal anomaly scores. The suspicion lingers that low IQ is the primary correlate of the anomalies rather than deviant behavior. Nevertheless these studies have opened an important new lead to the possible origins of hyperactivity and other disorders.

CONCLUSIONS

Research linking various stresses or signs of such stresses in the biologic environment of the fetus or young child to hyperactivity has the same shortcomings as the work done on possible genetic influences. Hyperactivity itself is defined loosely, subjects are selected in odd ways, arbitrary limits are put on the pool of subjects (for example by studying children in a particular range of IQ), boys are mixed with girls, and other possibly important variables are left uncontrolled. Nevertheless important facts have been discovered, for example the relationship of being born too soon or too small with lower intelligence and deviant behavior. Also for all its failings the recent research is more discriminating and better designed than the work done when MBD was in its infancy. We are learning.

Biologic research on the origins of hyperactivity is exciting. We have raised good meaty questions but so far have not answered any of them.

REFERENCES

Alden, E. R., T. Mendelkorn, D. E. Woodrum, R. P. Wennberg, C. R. Parks, and W. A. Hodson. "Morbidity and mortality of infants weighing less than 1,000 grams in an intensive care nursery." *Pediatrics*, 50, 40–49, (1972).

Borland, B. L. and H. K. Heckman. "Hyperactive boys and their brothers: *A* 25-year follow-up study." *Archives of General Psychiatry*, 33, 669–675, (1976).

Bronson, W. C. "Central orientations: A study of behavior organization from childhood to adolescence." *Child Development*, 37, 125–155, (1966).

Burd'e, B. de la, and McL. S. Choate. "Early asymptomatic lead exposure and development at school age." *Pediatrics*, 87, 638–642, (1975).

Cadoret, R. J., and A. Gath. "Biologic correlates of hyperactivity: Evidence for a genetic factor." (Paper presented at the annual meeting of the Society for Life History Research in Psychopathology, Ft. Worth, October, 1976 in S. B. Sells, ed., *Life History Research in Psychopathology* 6, City: Publisher, [1978] in press.

Cadoret, R. J., L. Cunningham, R. Loftus, and J. Edwards. "Studies of adoptees from psychiatrically disturbed biologic parents II. Temperament, hyperactive, antisocial, and developmental variables." *Journal of Pediatrics*, 87, 301–306, (1975).

Campbell, S. B., M. W. Endman, and G. Bernfeld. "A three-year follow-up of hyperactive preschoolers into elementary school." *Journal of Child Psychology and Psychiatry* 18, 239–249, (1977).

Cantwell, D. P. "Psychiatric illness in the families of hyperactive children." *Archives of General Psychiatry*, 27, 414–417, (1972).

———"Familial-genetic research with hyperactive children," in D. Cantwell, ed., *The Hyperactive Child*. Holliswood, N.Y.: Spectrum, 1975.

Collins, L. F., A. E. Maxwell, and K. Cameron. "A factor analysis of some child psychiatric clinic data." *Journal of Mental Science*, 108, 274–285, (1962).

Conners, C. K. "Symptom patterns in hyperkinetic, neurotic, and normal children." *Child Developemnt*, 41, 667–682, (1970).

Craft, A. W., D. A. Shaw, and N. E. F. Cartlidge. "Head injuries in children." *British Medical Journal*, 4, 200–203, (1972).

Cunningham, L., R. J. Cadoret, R. Loftus, and J. E. Edwards. "Studies of adoptees from psychiatrically disturbed biological parents: Psychiatric conditions in childhood and adolescence." *British Journal of Psychiatry*, 126, 534–549, (1975).

David, O., S. Hoffman, B. McGann, J. Sverd, and J. Clark. "Low lead levels and mental retardation." *Lancet*, 2, 1376–1379, (1976).

Drillien, C. M. "Biological and environmental determinants of early development," in *Proceedings Assn Res Nerv Ment Diseases*. Baltimore: Williams & Wilkins, 1973.

Feigin, R. D., and P. R Dodge. "Bacterial meningitis: Newer concepts of pathophysiology and neurologic sequelae." *Pediatric Clinics of North America*, 23, 541–556, (1976).

Finucci, J. M., J. T. Guthrie, A. L. Childs, H. Abbey, and B. Childs. "The genetics of specific reading disability." *Annals of Human Genetics*, 40, 1, (1976).

Foch, T. T., J. C. DeFries, G. E. McClearn, and S. M. Singer. "Familial patterns of impairment in reading disability. *Journal of Educational Psychology*, 69, 316, (1977).

Francis-Williams, J. and P. A. Davies, "Very low birthweight and later intelligence. *Developmental Medicine and Child Neurology*, 16, 709–728, (1974).

Goodwin, D. W., F. Schulsinger, L. Hermansen, S. B. Guze, and G. Winokur. "Alcoholism and the hyperactive child syndrome." *J Nervous Mental Disease*, 160, 349–353, (1975).

Graham, P. and M. Rutter. "Organic brain dysfunction and child psychiatric disorder." *British Medical Journal*, 3, 695–700, (1968).

Hjern, B., and I. Nylander. "Acute head injuries in children: Traumatology, therapy and prognosis." *Acta Pediatrica Scandinavica*, (Supplement 152), (1963).

Jones, M. "Personality correlates and antecedents of drinking patterns in adult males." *Journal of Consulting Clinical Psychology*, 32, 2–12, (1968).

Klein, P. S., G. B. Forbes, and P. R. Nader. "Effects of starvation in infancy (pyloric stenosis) on subsequent learning abilities." *Journal of Pediatrics*, 87, 8–15, (1975).

Lansdown, R. G., J. Shepherd, B. E. Clayton, H. T. Delves, P. J. Graham, and W. C. Turner. "Blood-lead levels, behavior, and intelligence: A population study." *Lancet*, 1, 538–541, (1974).

Laufer, M. W. and E. Denhoff. "Hyperkinetic behavior syndrome in children." *Journal of Pediatrics*, 50, 463–473, (1957).

Loney, J., J. E. Langhorne, Jr., C. E. Paternite, M. A. Whaley-Klahn, C. Broeker, and M. Hacker.' "The Iowa HABIT: Hyperkinetic/aggressive boys in treatment." (Paper presented at the annual meeting of the society for Life History Research in Psychopathology, Ft. Worth, October,1976 also in S. B. Sells, ed., *Life History Research in Psychopathology* 6, City: Publisher, [1978] in press.

McCord, W. and J. McCord. *Origins of Alcoholism*. Stanford, Cal.: Stanford University Press, 1960.

Matheny, A. P., Jr., A. M. Brown, and R. S. Wilson. "Behavioral antecedents of accidental injuries in early childhood: A study of twins." *Journal of Pediatrics*, 79, 122–124, (1971).

Matheny, A. P., Jr., A. B. Dolan, and R. S. Wilson. "Twins with academic learning problems: Antecedent characteristics." *American Journal of Orthopsychiatry*, 46, 464–469, (1976).

Morrison, J. R. and M. A. Stewart. "A family study of the hyperactive child syndrome." *Biological Psychiatry*, 3, 189–195, (1971).

———"The psychiatric status of the legal families of adopted hyperactive children." *Archieves of General Psychiatry*, 28, 888–891, (1973).

Neligan, G. A., I. Kolvin, D. M. Scott, and R. F. Garside. *Born Too Soon or Too Small.* Philadelphia: Lippincott, 1976.

Nichols, R. C., and W. C. Bilbro, Jr. "The diagnosis of twin zygosity. *Acta Genetica.* (Basel), 16, 265–275, (1966).

Peterson, D. R. "Behavior problems of middle childhood." *Journal of Consulting Psychology*, 25, 205–209, (1961).

Quinn, P. O., and J. L. Rapoport. "Minor physical anomalies and neurologic status in hyperactive boys." *Pediatrics*, 53, 742–747, (1974).

Rosenberg, J. B., and G. M. Weller. "Minor physical anomalies and academic performance in young school-children." *Developmental Medicine and Child Neurology*, 15, 131–135, (1973).

Rutter, M., P. Graham, and W. Yule. *A Neuropsychiatric Study in Childhood.* Philadelphia: Lippincott, 1970.

Rutter, M., J. Tizard, and K. Whitmore. *Education, Health and Behavior.* London: Longman, 1970.

Safer, D. J. "A familial factor in minimal brain dysfunction." *Behavior Genetics*, 3, 175–186, (1973).

Sell, S. H. W., W. W. Webb, J. E. Pate, and E. O. Doyne. "Psychological sequelae to bacterial meningitis: Two controlled studies." *Pediatrics*, 49, 212–217, (1972).

Shepherd, M., B. Oppenheim, and S. Mitchell. *Childhood Behavior and Mental Health.* New York: Grune & Stratton, 1971.

Smith, D. W., and K. E. Bostian. "Cogenital anomalies associated with idiopathic mental retardation." *Journal of Pediatrics*, 65, 189–196, (1964).

Steg, J. P., and J. L. Rapoport. "Minor physical anomalies in normal, neurotic, learning disabled, and severely disturbed children." *Journal of Autism and Childhood Schizophrenia*, 5, 299–307, (1975).

Stewart, M. A., and L. Leone. "A family study of unsocialized aggressive boys." *Biological Psychiatry*, 13, 107–118, (1978).

Stewart, M. A., and J. R. Morrison, "Affective disorder among the relatives of hyperactive children." *Journal of Child Psychology and Psychiatry*, 14, 209–212, (1973).

Stewart, M. A., F. N. Pitts, Jr., A. G. Craign, and W. Dieruf. "The hyperactive child syndrome." *American journal of Orthopsychiatry*, 36, 861–867, (1966).

Stewart, M. A., B. T. Thach, and M. R. Freidin. "Accidental poisoning and the hyperactive child syndrome." *Diseases of the Nervous System*, 31, 403–407, (1970).

Tarter, R. E., H. McBride, N. Buonpane, and D. U. Schneider. "Differentiation of alcoholics: Childhood history of minimal brain dysfunction, family history, and drinking pattern." *Archieves of General Psychiatry*, 34, 761–768, (1977).

Thomas, A., S. Chess, and H. G. Birch. *Temperament and Behavior Disorders in Children.* New York: New York University Press 1968.

Waldrop. M. F., and J. D. Goering. "Hyperactivity and minor physical anomalies in elementary school children." *American Journal of Orthopsychiatry*, 41, 602–607, (1971).

Waldrop, M. F., and Charles F. Halverson, Jr. "Minor physical anomalies and hyperactive behavior in young children," in J. Hellmuth, ed., *Exceptional Infant* v.2. New York: Brunner/Mazel, 1971.

Waldrop, M. F., R. Q. Bell, and J. D. Goering. "Minor physical anomalies and inhibited behavior in elementary school girls." *Journal of Child Psychology and Psychiatry*, 17, 113–122, (1976).

Welner, Z., A. Welner, M. A. Stewart, H. Palkes, and E. Wish. "A controlled study of siblings of hyperactive children." *Journal of Nervous Mental Disease*, 165, 110–117, (1977).

Werner, E., J. M. Bierman, F. E. French, K. Simonian, A. Connor, R. S. Smith, and M. Campbell. "Reproductive and environmental casualties: A report on the 10-year follow-up of the children of the Kauai pregnancy study." *Pediatrics*, 42, 112–127, (1968).

Werry, J. S. "Hyperactivity," in C. G. Costello, ed., *Symptoms of Psychopathology*, pp. 397–417. New York: Wiley, 1970.

Willerman, L. "Activity level and hyperactivity in twins." *Child Development*, 44, 288–293, (1973).

Wilson, R. S., A. M. Brown, and A. P. Matheny. "Emergence and persistence of behavioral differences in twins." *Child Development*, 42, 1381–1898, (1971).

Wolff, S. "Dimensions and clusters of symptoms in disturbed children." *British Journal of Psychiatry*, 118, 421–417, (1971).

CHAPTER 7

Nutrition, Injury, Illness, and Minimal Brain Dysfunction

Harold P. Martin

The medical literature is replete with data concerning the effect of illness, injury, and undernutrition upon the brain of the growing child. Most of that literature deals with the gravest consequences, that is death or severe brain damage. When one wishes to review the neurologic consequences of various illnesses, injuries, or nutritional disorders, one finds oneself pursuing the subspecialties of mental retardation; developmental disabilities; and neurology, covering such topics as cerebral palsy, seizure disorders, and mental retardation. Even in animal studies the researcher is usually interested in documenting anatomical or biochemical abnormalities of the central nervous system in the sacrificed animal. When neurologic function is assayed, gross deficits usually are measured, these would correspond to cerebral palsy or mental deficiency in the human. It is important to keep in mind the truism of developmental pediatrics: any disease, disorder, or condition that can seriously damage the brain or cause death through its effect on the central nervous system, in lesser degree can also result in less dramatic neurologic consequences. This author is clearly exposing his view of minimal brain dysfunction as one point on a spectrum of neurologic dysfunction with much in common with more severe entities, such as retardation, cerebral palsy, dementia, and possibly even infantile autism. It is postulated that the same mechanisms which can cause these more serious brain disorders (that is anoxia, hemorrhage, edema, inflammation, biochemical derangement) can also cause less severe disability with minimal dysfunction of the brain the final outcome. As a caveat, perhaps as our efforts are increasingly successful in preventing mortality or severe morbidity from following injury or illness or undernutrition, the frequency of minimal brain dysfunction may well increase.

It seems important to keep in mind the frequency of such potentially damaging problems of childhood. Illness is truly a part of life for the human, with the childhood years being especially vulnerable to repeated illnesses of an infectious nature. While the neurologic toll of many infectious diseases has been eliminated through active immunizations, upper respiratory illness occurs several times annually for the average infant and toddler. Perhaps even more relevant is the less capable physiologic response one notes with decreasing age. Imperfect temperature regulation, unstable metabolic homeostatis, and diminished general immunity to illness are the hallmarks of illness in the infant and young child. Injury too is ubiquitous in childhood. No human can grow to maturity without a series of minor falls and injuries. This ubiquity of injuries in childhood can be underlined by noting that accidents and injuries are the leading cause of death in the United States for all persons between 1 and 34 years of age (Chisolm 1968). Indeed most humans start their extrauterine life by a process rich with potential for cerebral trauma. Nutritional disorders are perhaps less commonly a part of normal childhood in this country. On an international perspective, calorie and protein inadequacy is gaining increasing prominence as a common state of childhood. Even in the United States, the frequency of undernutrition during the prenatal and neonatal years is clearly underestimated as affluence can easily lull one into a false sense of assurance. Thus this chapter does not deal with the rare and exotic conditions of man which can affect brain function, but with the frequent and common problems of childhood which can temporatily or permanently alter neurologic function.

One particularly interesting and fruitful area of research during the past two decades has come from interest in high-risk registries. The incredible growth of perinatology has accounted for much of our new knowledge in this area. Research and clinical practice have taken two different courses. One course has been to try to relate specific incidents, which are known to place infants and children at increased risk of neurologic damage, to ultimate outcome of children exposed to those risks. Prematurity, hyperbilirubinemia, vaginal versus caeserean delivery, and advanced maternal age are but a few of the literally thousands of high-risk events which prompted individual and collaborative studies of neurologic outcome. The more recent second thrust has attempted to correlate various "states" of the newborn or young infant to later neurologic function. In most of these instances, the state of the child was considered a reflection of neurologic status, and hence an indirect means of measuring the effects of illness, injury, or inadequate nutrition and growth. Perhaps the use of the APGAR (Apgar, et al., 1958) rating of newborns spurred this type of research as the physiologic status of the infant at one and five minutes of life have been used to classify various degrees of risk. More recently other measures of the child's behavior have been used (Brazelton, 1973; Prechtl and Beintema, 1964; Prechtl, 1972; Thomas, Chess and Birch, 1968) to alert the clinician to various degrees of neurologic and behavioral risk.

There have been difficulties and inconsistencies in attempting to link brain dysfunction to various early injuries, illnesses, and nutritional problems. Even infant behaviors, which are thought to reflect damage or immaturity of the central nervous system, may or may not persist in any individual child. For example Denhoff demonstrated in 380 children (Denhoff, 1973) a highly significant relationship between signs of hyperreactivity or hyporeactivity in infancy and learning difficulties at seven years of age. Chess and her co-workers however (Chess and Thomas, 1977) recently reported a follow-up of their 138 children assessed in infancy, now that the children are in adolescence. One is struck by the lack of predictability between the infant's neurologic and behavioral status and later, behavioral parameters.

The basis for such variability requires some comment. Many of these clinical follow-up studies suffer methodological problems, especially those studies of a retrospective nature. Additionally there is limited potential for comparability in many studies as differing and often inappropriate target behaviors are being used for correlational studies (Kalverboer, 1975). Some of these behaviors are too gross, while others are too heavily influenced by environmental factors to be utilized in relating early biologic processes to later neurologic function.

Two other critically important issues obfuscate many such studies and must be appreciated to understand adequately the relationship of minimal brain dysfunction to illness, injury, and nutrition. The first of these issues has to do with the interplay between environment and biologic events, which is taken up in some detail in Chapter 9. Some brief aspects of this interrelationship are essential however at this point. In 1964 Drillien's classic work on premature babies was published. This work involved a study of almost 600 prematures with follow-up data of an impressive magnitude up to age seven. It is essential to note that while, expectedly, birthweight correlated with eventual intelligence scores, the effect of social class was an equally potent factor. In the smallest of prematures, the developmental quotients varied quite remarkably according to social class. In social classes 1 and 2, there was an increase of 15.8 Developmental Quotient (D.Q.) points between ages 6 months and 48 months. In babies of the same birthweight in social class 3, there was an increase of only 2.5 D.Q. points. And in social class 4, there was a *drop* of 6.6 D.Q. points over this same time period. The Kauai study (Werner, Bierman, and French, 1971) demonstrated this same phenomenon. In this famous study perinatal high-risk factors were only significantly related to later neurologic function in the lowest socioeconomic classes by and large. So there is not a one-to-one linear relationship between early injuries, illnesses, or malnutrition and subsequent brain function. The effects of these problems are muted and modified by any number of factors which are closely related to social class.

The second issue is the importance of looking at a transactional model (Sameroff and Chandler, 1975) of child and parent. Caretaking behaviors can reinforce or act to change behaviors of the infant or the older child while these behaviors, in turn, affect the caretaking practices. Brazelton's work (Brazelton, Kislowski, and Main 1974; Brazelton, 1969) is largely predicated on just that concept, that is to help parents learn how to mute the neurologically based behavior patterns of difficult children. This is a circular reaction in fact. For the infant's behavior selectively modifies the adult's responses (Lewis and Rosenblum, 1974), indeed,:

Many parent behaviors are not spontaneously emitted in the service of educating the child, but rather are elicited by many of the child's own characteristics and behaviors. . . . Knowing only the temperament of the child, or knowing only child-rearing attitudes and practices of the parents would not allow one to predict the developmental outcome for the child. It would appear, rather, that it is the character of the specific transactions that occurred between a given child and his parents which determined the course of his subsequent development." [Bacon, 1977]

NUTRITION

The past 20 years have seen a tremendous surge of interest in the effects of various nutritional states. Of particular interest have been calorie and protein deficiencies and poor growth of the human during prenatal life. Despite the large amount of interest and research, some very basic questions remain unresolved. A major reason for this lack of clarity resides in the inability to study adequately various states of undernutrition in the human for obvious humane and ethical reasons. This has required an undue reliance on animal studies wherein the problem arises of extrapolation from differing species to the human. Studies in the human have had to be based almost exclusively on natural accidents or catastrophes and hence have been primarily retrospective in nature. It has been rare for the natural consequences of malnutrition to be studied in man.

It is because of this limited data base that one finds an unusually large number of review articles and compendia on undernutrition. Sometimes one gets the impression there are more review articles and books published on this subject than there are original studies. A few of these review articles are noted for the reader to seek out at his leisure (Canosa, 1975; Lloyd-Still, 1976a; Manocha, 1972; Martin, 1973; Prescott, Read and Coursino, 1975; Scrimshaw, 1968; Winick, 1976.) At this point it would seem in the interest of conciseness to summarize our state of knowledge regarding nutrition and its relationship to brain damage and dysfunction.

Animal studies have concentrated primarily on brain anatomy and biochemistry. Various types of inadequate diets are given to animals. After sacrificing them brain weight is found to be reduced as well as number of brain cells, DNA, cerebroside, and other biochemical entities. The results depend obviously on the type, duration, and severity of diet restriction. The effect of the diet restriction also depends on the age of the animal. The time of greatest neurologic deficit corresponds to the time of most rapid brain growth of the animal. This is an essential bit of information to know about the laboratory animal in question, as the rate of brain growth varies so considerably in different species. There seems no question that protein and calorie deficiency during periods of most rapid brain growth result in permanent changes in brain composition and probably in brain function. Brain function has been less well studied in animal research than brain composition. It is often by inference that the investigator assumes impaired neurologic function, although some studies of rather gross brain function have been accomplished. In those studies there has been corroboration that various functions, especially learning, are impaired in the animal undernourished during the critical period of rapid brain growth.

Parallel with this work clinical interest heightened in the 1960s in the human baby who was born with poor parameters of prenatal growth. Prior to that time small babies were assumed to be prematurely born babies. Lubchenco (1970, 1976) was one of the leaders in documenting gestational age of newborns. This advance has allowed considerable clinical research on the poorly grown infant, or the small gestational age (s.g.a.) baby. Studies of s.g.a. children are not strictly evaluations of nutritional status. There are many reasons why a fetus does not grow well. The pathological state which resulted in poor physical growth has its own effect on the developing fetal brain. For example chromosomal abnormality, prenatal infection, and placental insufficiency all result in poor prenatal growth, and each has its own potential for central nervous system damage on bases other than inadequate supply or utilization of nutrients by the developing baby. Yet s.g.a. babies are undernourished babies and, excluding some of the known causes of poor intrauterine growth, there remain a group of undergrown newborns who can be studied. They are at greater risk for neurologic disability through childhood.

Considerable growth of the brain of the human typically occurs during the first two years of extrauterine life. Since this is a critical period for brain development, there has been a focus on undernutrition during this time period. Children with marasmus, failure-to-thrive, and kwashiorkor have been studied and evaluated in several different cultures. With rare exceptions investigators have found these children to have physical and neurologic sequellae. Intelligence test scores or various scales of learning ability have been the primary neurologic function studied and deficiencies in mental abilities have been noted. What seems to be still unresolved is the exact cause and effect relationship between the nutritional deficiency and subsequent mental disability. As Latham noted (1974):

> The relative consistency of results does appear to prove the hypothesis that early severe malnutrition is associated with poorer scores on intelligence tests. . . . However, many authors go beyond this and imply that their research shows that malnutrition causes a retardation of intellectual development. The data do not seem to support this conclusion of cause and effect.

The lack of conviction as to the causality of undernutrition stems from a number of factors. Undernutrition does not exist in a vacuum, unassociated with other biologic and social factors. In some instances the child is undernourished because of neglect, raising the spectre of understimulation of cognitive development. In other instances poverty is a major factor of the undernutrition and other factors often associated with poverty, that is poor medical care, crowding, larger families, and so on, are known to affect intelligence and learning. Many of the studies of the relationship of early undernutrition to subsequent neurologic status have had inadequate or no control groups which might clarify these issues.

Despite these methodologic problems, most clinicians and researchers would not share Latham's reservations regarding the cause and effect relationship between undernutrition and intelligence in the human. Certainly the animal research all points to such a cause and effect relationship. Reviews of human studies with control groups (Lloyd-Still, 1976 *b*; Chase, 1973) also point to a long-term effect on neurologic integrity. Biochemical and structural assessment on a few autopsy studies of undernourished children further tends to support this view. Even clinically it has been pointed out that the behavioral symptoms of the malnourished child are similar to those resulting from somatosensory deprivation or neonatal hypoxia (Prescott, 1975). In this author's clinical experience and studies of undernourished, neglected, and physically mistreated children, the presence of early protein and calorie deficiency has played out in depressed intelligence and learning in a way that has seemed etiological (Martin, 1972, 1976; Chase and Martin, 1970).

Most of the clinical studies of humans have used intelligence test scores or other rather gross measurements of mental abilities. Fewer students have looked at neurodevelopmental functions more carefully and meticulously. Hence there are considerably less data relating undernutrition to minimal brain dysfunction. A review of the various tests which might well be utilized in studying children with undernutrition is available (Hurwitz, 1976). Despite the paucity of such refined measurements, there are *some* data which do suggest that minimal brain dysfunction is a likely consequence of early undernutrition. There has been documentation of deficiencies in various intersensory perceptual modalities, looking particularly at visual, auditory, and haptic perception (Birch and Leffard, 1963). Cross-perceptual modalities, sequencing, and language and reading skills were also assessed. Language skills have been looked at more carefully (Delicardie and Cravioto, 1975). Prescott has specifically addressed the issue of minimal brain dysfunction (Prescott, 1975), reviewing the relationship of various insults, including undernutrition to this syndrome. A few other studies have shown the effect of malnutrition on orienting responses (Winick, 1976) and the interplay between personality and cognitive factors (Klein and Adinolfi, 1975; Klein, et al., 1975).

One particularly neat study deserves a bit more attention as it addressed many of these issues (Hoorweg, 1976). Teen-age Ugandan children who had been malnourished in infancy and early childhood were assessed. Hence this study was a 10–15-year follow-up of early malnutrition. There is little reason to believe that these subjects were undernourished because of inattention by parents. Nor was there evidence that these were unique or unusual babies who engendered less care and nurturance. The battery of tests given these children was quite extensive. Nine different tests of cognition were used and described as well as a modified Lincoln-Oseretsky test. Assessments of behavior were also included. This allowed for a more careful analysis of specific cognitive and motor abilities, rather than lumping all such factors under the aegis of "intelligence." Perhaps the specific results of this study are not as important as the methodology and review of the literature. Hoorweg did find that there was a general impairment of intellectual abilities with reasoning and spatial abilities most affected, memory and rote learning intermediately affected, and language ability least affected. As had been noted (Richardson, et al., 1972) the previously malnourished children were more distractible, less cooperative, and presented more behavior problems. Motor tasks were also affected, especially those requiring simultaneous but independent activity of both hands and requiring lateral coordination and discrimination. Surprisingly, and perhaps quite pertinent in this study, was the finding that impairments in these subjects were related to the degree of *chronic* undernutrition at the time of the child's admission and not related to the severity of the *acute* undernutrition. These data certainly suggest disabilities in specific cognitive areas that are commonly found in the child with minimal brain dysfunction. Clearly there is a tremendous need for additional, similarly exacting studies of brain functions.

This same point was made in a much less sophisticated study by the author (Martin, 1975). A group of 232 children referred to a child development center for suspected developmental delays were used as the subjects. Nutritional data which any practicing clinician will have were gathered, that is mother's weight gain in pregnancy, history of any weight loss in the first trimester, child's birth weight, and the child's present height, weight, and head circumference. The subjects had rather complete developmental evaluations. The parameters of nutrition did not correlate with the child's intelligence quotient (IQ). However poor prenatal nutrition *did* correlate with the diagnosis of brain damage or dysfunction. This clinical study clearly showed that a single intelligence test score is much too gross a measurement to identify the short-and long-term consequences of undernutrition. As noted above it is behaviors such as attention span, perceptual abilities, activity level, orienting responses, attention to novel stimulae, speed of learning, and language skills which have been shown to be deficient in previously malnourished children. These of course are just those behaviors found to be deficient in children with minimal brain dysfunction.

The above review deals almost exclusively with the long-term effects of nutritional inadequacy. There is less documentation of the immediate and short-term effects of malnutrition. In 1950 there was the well-known study of volunteer students, showing that undernutrition did diminish mental capacities (Keys, Brazek, and Henschel, 1950). The recent practice of serving breakfast at school to children from lower socioeconomic groups stemmed from an awareness that hunger and marginal nutrition did affect learning. Data such as Sulzer's (Sulzer, Hanche, and Koenig, 1973) showed that current malnutrition decreases attentiveness, motivation, and resistance to fatigue. With iron deficiency Diamond (Ross Conference, 1970) is reported to have noted that females showed irritability, fatigue, and lassitude, all of which disappeared with iron therapy. What is suggested here is that even without long-term sequellae, inadequate nutrition may have an immediate short-term effect of presenting as minimal brain dysfunction. Clearly the child who is so handicapped, even without permanent central nervous system pathology, is seriously impeded in his academic learning. Clinical experience shows that such early impediments to learning may not be easily remediable, so that from a clinical standpoint, the disability may well have life-long effects cognitively and emotionally.

A summary of this literature on nutrition then might highlight the following. It is known that protein and calorie deficiency in early life (prenatally and in infancy) can result in permanent anatomical and biochemical changes in the brain (Read, et al., 1975; McKhann, 1975; Rose and Tanquay, 1975). Intelligence in undernourished humans is diminished. This diminution in intelligence and learning may be permanent and is probably related to the degree of chronic undernutrition, the timing of the malnutrition, and associated with family-social factors accompanying undernutrition. There is increasing evidence that minimal brain dysfunction results from undernutrition. Malnutrition at older ages in the human is less well studied, but there is evidence that there is a temporary diminution in mental abilities, attention span, activity level, and perseverance. Little has been noted regarding intervention. Several studies suggest that nutritional intervention and cognitive stimulation can and do make a difference in the ultimate cognitive abilities of the malnourished child. It should be clear that intervention directed at "acute malnutrition" alone is not sufficient. The cognitive deficits are more related to chronic malnutrition. In this country social and family factors will require intervention beyond provision of adequate protein and calories. The less drastic forms of deviant nutrition, that is mineral and vitamin deficiencies, have not been addressed in this review, but also require our attention.

Controversial Nutritional Issues

Many controversial nutritional issues have arisen regarding minimal brain dysfunction. The school of orthomolecular medicine has advocated the massive ingestion of vitamins for perceptual disorders, hyperactivity, and learning disorders (Hawkins and Pauling, 1973). There has been another camp of advocates of hypoglycemia as an explanation for any number of symptoms, including minimal brain dysfunction. More recently a special diet has been popularized (Feingold, 1975) which eliminates artificial flavors, coloring, and other additives in addition to salicylate-containing foods. The truth of the matter is that there have not been respectable clinical studies to assess the claims of such nutritional factors nor adequate studies of intervention based on these theories. The sparse reports one does find leave the reader disheartened and disillusioned. Most of the literature treats these controversial issues in a style that is anecdotal, lacking in controls, biased from the outset, and that reflects little more than personalized highly idiosyncratic experiences of the authors.

At least two factors seem to explain the resurgence of interest in dietary manipulation to "cure" these conditions. For one, the last decade has been marked by a
special orientation to "natural" foodstuffs, especially by adolescents and young
adults. Clearly much of this preoccupation with natural foods arose out of a
realistic and genuine awareness of the dangerous additives to which this society is
constantly being exposed. Part of the interest also stemmed from a wish to return
to a Walden-like pristine past. It seems to this author that the net result of this
food fadism is largely positive as citizens are demanding more meticulous concern
by producers regarding the chemical poisons used in production and processing of
our foods. There can be little doubt that there are some humans whose reaction to
specific food additives, whether allergy or idiosyncratic sensitivity, may play out
in any number of perplexing symptoms.

A second issue which seems germane is the historical search for simple answers
to conditions which are complex, chronic, and not curable by traditional means.
For example controversial and often illicit claims have been made for curative
approaches to cancer, arthritis, mental retardation. So why not minimal brain
dysfunction? Here is a condition which is not definable by etiology, seems almost
mystical in the innumerable masquerades it takes, and about which no scientist of
repute can offer very reassuring therapeutic recommendations. It causes a great
deal of heartache for children and their parents. Professionals who work with
such children easily become discouraged if not downright despondent. Naturally
enough there are efforts to hypothesize and test out nontraditional modes of
treatment. Unfortunately, as with most of these chronic incurable conditions,
there inevitably arise entrepreneurs of this human misery.

It would be easy and academically chic, but too glib, to dismiss these claims of
remarkable success for children with minimal brain dysfunction. One must naturally pause to consider each of these theories and claims as it arises. Clinicians
would be only too happy to find an inexpensive and simple dietary manipulation
which would alleviate the symptoms of minimal brain dysfunction. Practicing
clinicians and educators have no vested interest in children suffering the disabilities of this condition. The issue here is not one of supporting or disparaging these
nutritional theories. The issue is the paltry and inadequate data base on which
such claims are made. This is not merely a position of rigid academic insistence on
meticulous research design. Therapy, including nutritional manipulation, carries
some degree of biologic risk, considerable stress on parents, and the potential for
the consumer to focus entirely on the prescription, disregarding the other bioedu-
cational programs which carry some hope of help for the child. This is the same
identical concern that the prudent clinician has for the indiscriminate use of
medication for mood states or for hyperactivity. A healthy skepticism should
permeate the professional community regarding any unproven therapeutic approaches to this complex behavioral problem of childhood.

INJURY

Throughout recorded history the relationship between head injury and subsequent
alterations in cognition have been noted. Medical research has primarily focused
on the most serious sequellae of head injury, that is death and severe brain
damage. Yet in the experience of most children's physicians, the more common

experience is to find symptoms of minimal brain dysfunction following injury to a child's head. In a recent conference on the etiology of mental retardation, Angle pointed out that, "statistically, concussions, contusions and hemorrhages are an infrequent cause of severe retardation. Behavior and activity disorder, however, appear to be common even in mild injury..." (1970).

There is another whole body of literature concerning the effect of prenatal and perinatal injury. As the medical subspeciality of perinatology has flourished, more specific interventions have been discovered which can prevent such neurologic injuries. This not only includes injury from direct trauma to the newborn's head, but includes the injuries sustained by biochemical aberrations in the perinatal period (Battaglia, Meschia, and Quilligan, 1977; Goodwin, 1976). Most of this type of important data is not found in treatises on minimal brain dysfunction nor in the literature on injury, but scattered throughout perinatology, child development, and the basic science literature. The development of the concept of high-risk babies and high-risk registries in the United States and England over the past two decades has given impetus to truly remarkable gains in the prevention and treatment of injury to the newborn. In the introduction to the chapter, the problems of establishing linear relationships between early trauma and later neurologic function were noted. The immense mass of environmental conditions which can mute or intensify the effects of brain injury provide the researcher and the clinician with a most difficult task.

Any educated reader knows that injury to the brain can cause death, severe brain damage, and more commonly minimal brain dysfunction. This author was then left with a dilemma as what to review in this section which would not be completely redundant. Two aspects of injury were chosen for review. These two —accidents in children and nonaccidental trauma—were chosen because of their alarming frequency and their clinical importance.

Accidents in Children

Accidents are the leading cause of death in the United States for all children over one year of age (Chisolm, 1968). During the 1960s, accidents accounted for 25 to 30% of all deaths in the preschool child. Over 30% of preschool children sustain injuries *annually* which require medical attention or restricted activity. No one knows the exact morbidity of accidental injuries, but given the extremely high prevalence of accidental injuries, the estimation of the neurologic sequellae must be quite high. This seems an obvious arena in which to expend profitably our energies to prevent minimal brain dysfunction.

There are a number of avenues to pursue to lower the rate of accidents in children (Soman, 1974). One prime area is in the office of children's physicians. Anticipatory guidance for parents can greatly diminish injuries in childhood. Parents need to be forewarned of imminent dangers to their children and reminded of safety precautions which can diminish that risk. For example new parents especially need to be forewarned of the danger of their child falling from bed or couch before the baby learns to roll over. Stairway gates which toddlers cannot operate can prevent many head injuries, as 80% of fatal falls in infants result from the child falling from one level to another. Safety precautions in the home need to be taught. One efficient way is to produce written handouts for parents which need to be reinforced verbally by the child's doctor. Examples of items to be addressed include: locking up medicine cabinets, making household poisons unavailable to the child, using seat belts when children are in cars, teaching pedestrian safety to children, preventing of burns and inhalation of small objects, and practicing water safety. The American Academy of Pediatrics has materials which can be used in the physician's office or waiting room.

A second avenue for prevention of minimal brain dysfunction from injury requires local and national insistence on safety features in children's toys and clothes. In the present decade a number of quite dangerous toys have been taken off the market because of consumer concern and governmental pressure but, vigilance is still required by the populace. Paints containing lead continue to be found on children's toys and furniture. Dangerous toys and furniture continue to show up in the marketplace. With the recent increase in use of bicycles, pediatric groups have reached a point of encouraging use of helmets as the injury rate and sequellae from bicycle accidents is rapidly approaching that from motorcycles.

The bottom line concerning accidental injuries is rather simple. Injuries are exceedingly common in childhood. Injuries frequently result in brain damage. The majority of accidents and injuries to children can be prevented through community, family, and physician efforts. In addition to prevention of death and severe brain damage, there can also be a significant diminution in a major cause of minimal brain dysfunction.

Inflicted Injury

After accidents and perinatal injuries, the third major category of injuries which result in minimal brain dysfunction is nonaccidental trauma, also referred to as child abuse or the battered child syndrome. Public awareness and professional interest in child abuse only started in 1962 (Kempe, et al.) In the following decade the vanguard in this area produced legislation, public awareness, and social policy to deal with abusive parents. Professional interest also focused on divining the pathogenesis of child abuse. Personality profiles of abusing parents and the social conditions which foster such behavior were examined in some detail.

In the 1970s attention turned to effects on the child of being raised in an abusive home, that is the morbidity to the survivors. The pioneer in this field was Elizabeth Elmer who published the first follow-up data on abused children (Elmer, 1967; Elmer and Gregg, 1967). Of 50 abused children in the sample at follow-up, 12 were either dead or in institutions for the mentally retarded. Of the remaining abused children the morbidity was 88%, including various developmental delays. In Martin's follow-up studies (Martin, et al., 1974; Martin, 1976; Martin and Beezley, 1977) over 50% of his sample showed some neurologic abnormalities, of which 31% were functionally handicapping. Of 49 children given the Beery test of Visual-Motor Integration, 29 were scoring more than six months below their age level, while only 5 scored more than six months above their age level. Of children with a history of head trauma, 66% were scoring six or more months below age level. Over 25% of these abused children had school learning disabilities. Kline (1976) also reported that the frequency of placement in special education classes, including learning-disabled classrooms, was significantly greater for abused and neglected children than in the population of students who were not reported as abused or neglected. His review of 312 subjects suggested different outcomes for abused, neglected, and sexually molested children. The majority of abused children were below grade level in reading, mathematics, and spelling. Sexually abused youngsters showed even greater deficits in achievement, while neglected children were the least affected in academic progress.

MacKeith, while not looking at minimal cerebral dysfunction specifically, does speculate on the neurologic sequellae of abuse in England (1975). He points out that 50% of children with cerebral palsy and mental deficiency have no cause demonstrated. He speculates that abuse may account for 6% of new cases of cerebral palsy annually, 25% of new cases of serious mental deficiency, and for 20 times as many children with disturbed personality. If his figures are at all accurate, the number of children with minimal brain dysfunction from abuse must be even more remarkable as one would expect even larger numbers of children to suffer these sequellae than mental retardation or cerebral palsy.

The basis for such neurologic sequellae in abuse may seem obvious at first glance, as structural damage to the brain would seem the most common result of inflicted trauma. However there are potential causes of minimal brain dysfunction in the abusive environment other than the physical injury per se. Nutritional deficits are present in at least 30% of diagnosed child-abuse cases (Martin, 1972; Martin, et al., 1974).

Medical care of abused children has been shown to be less regular and meticulous than in a control group of children with accidental injuries (Gregg and Elmer, 1969). Neurologic disability in the abused child has also been shown to correlate with the social and family environment in which the child lives after abuse is diagnosed. Both psychiatric symptoms and neurologic dysfunction are more frequent in children subjected to family dysfunction, emotional rejection, frequent changes in foster homes, and uncertainty about future residence (Martin, et al., 1974; Martin, 1976).

I also point the reader to the provocative demonstration that the neurologic findings of an exaggerated startle, hyperreflexia, and increased muscle tone were secondary to an abusive environment and not secondary to structual central nervous system damage (Baron, Bejar, and Sheaff 1970). These findings quickly abated upon hospitalization. The point is that neurologic findings and behaviors consonant with a diagnosis of minimal brain dysfunction can be engendered by the social and family environment. This is particularly pertinent in the abused child, as the possibility of structural damage to the brain from injury can easily obfuscate the true basis of the minimal brain dysfunction syndrome in many of these abused and neglected children.

In clinical work at the National Center for the Treatment and Prevention of Child Abuse and Neglect in Denver, this problem of differential diagnosis is common. Abused and neglected children are seen with learning disabilities, perceptual-motor deficits, hypotonia, poor motor planning (dyspraxia), and a number of characterological traits which interfere with learning. While the exact genesis of these disabilities is rarely unequivocally clear, the improvement and clinical course of these children more often than not suggests an environmental etiology rather than structural brain damage.

The true incidence of child abuse cannot be reliably know. Nonetheless estimations of 1% of children being subjected to physical abuse appear to be supported in this country. A conservative estimate of neurologic morbidity of 35% in the survivors suggests a quite significant role that child abuse plays in the genesis of minimal brain dysfunction. This is particularly striking, inasmuch as child abuse should be a preventable syndrome. It is certainly a situation in which treatment and remediation for the abused child has proven to be successful (Martin, 1976). This necessitates the assessment of the neurologic, cognitive, and developmental status of the abused child. It also requires the inclusion, in intervention programs of child abuse teams, of treatment for the child's developmental disabilities.

ILLNESS

The subject of illness in children cannot begin to be adequately addressed in these pages. This is compounded by the paucity of data relating childhood illness to subsequent minimal brain dysfunction syndrome. Most childhood illnesses do not present with symptoms of a neurologic nature. At most, more obviously dangerous illnesses, such as meningitis and encephalitis, have been addressed with mortality in mind as well as severe brain damage in the survivors. Less dramatic forms of neurologic morbidity have not been extensively addressed in clinical research.

While many illnesses, especially infectious diseases, have been largely eradicated due to preventive measures such as immunization, illness is still quite common in childhood. As pointed out in our introduction, children have less sophisticated homeostatic mechanisms to deal with illness than adults. High fevers, metabolic disturbance from altered respiration, frequent vomiting and diarrhea in many illnesses, and hypoxia are common in sick children from almost any disease process. All of these have the potential for effecting brain chemistry and brain function. Symptomatological relief in sick children is largely geared to prevention of damage from these hazards of illness. It is hypothesized here that meticulous attention to these potential neurologic hazards will be adequately emphasized only if clinical research can demonstrate the degree of neurologic risks posed by these side effects of illness. The somatic disturbances in most childhood illnesses are not the *cause* of that illness and may be dealt with in cavalier fashion. For example, if an infant has an upper respiratory infection, or pneumonia, the primary therapeutic efforts of the clinician will be towards eradication of the offending infectious agent. Treatment of the fever, nausea, emesis, increased metabolic rate, and decreased hydration may be considered primarily in the context of making the child feel better. It is not clear at this point what the risks of these symptoms are to the neurologic integrity of the child. Epidemiologic and clinical research are sorely needed for this relationship to be understood. Only then will adequate impetus be given to preventive and treatment strategies.

Several years ago clinicians became aware of the remarkably high number of children with mumps or measles who had evidence of imflammation or infection of the central nervous system. This was detected by the routine examination of spinal fluid in children with these seemingly innocuous childhood diseases. Cellular and chemical changes in the spinal fluid offered evidence of a pathological process occurring within the nervous system. This was a major impetus to immunization efforts for these childhood illnesses. Similarly as the risks of brain damage from dehydration and acid-base imbalance became apparent, clinicians became much more intense in their treatment of these metabolic imbalances, regardless of the disease process which was causing them.

At this point then one can only state that the relationship between illnesses of childhood and manifestations of minimal brain dysfunction is inadequately understood. The potential for such sequellae from the most common and seemingly innocuous illnesses seems great. One ends by making a plea for such basic and clinical research to be increased.

SUMMARY

Nutrition, injury, and illness all play a prominent role in the genesis of minimal brain dysfunction. Because of inadequate data regarding the frequency of these problems, and only incomplete data regarding their relationship to minimal brain dysfunction, a clear picture of their role in the genesis of minimal brain dysfunction cannot be adequately portrayed. Data have been reviewed and reported in this chapter which show that undernutrition and injuries may frequently result in a clinical picture of minimal brain dysfunction. There is a clear need and role for prevention of this syndrome through accident prevention, treatment of the developmental disabilities of abused children, attention to childhood illness, and through assurance of an adequate diet for the pregnant mother and the young growing child. Some changes in clinical practice of medicine and in social policy as well as increases in clinical research are needed to decrease the incidence and severity of minimal brain dysfunction. Such preventive efforts seem quite pragmatically possible and feasible. The issues discussed in this chapter are common problems of childhood. The exciting challenge resides in the knowledge that something can be done in these areas to prevent and alleviate the symptoms of minimal brain dysfunction.

REFERENCES

Angle, C. "Preface," in C. Angle and E. Bering, eds., *Physical Trauma as an Etiological Agent in Mental Retardation*, pp. vii–viii. Washington, D.C.: U.S. Department of HEW, National Institutes of Health and Public Health Service, 1970.

Apgar, V., D. A. Holaday, L. S. James, I. M. Weisbrot, and C. Berrien. "Evaluation of the newborn infant: Second report." *Journal of American Medical Association.* 168, 1985 –1988, (1958).

Bacon, R. Lack of planning; Lack of care. Cambridge, England: 1977. [Unpublished paper.]

Baron, M. A., R. L. Bejar, and P. J. Sheaff. "Neurologic manifestations of the battered child syndrome." *Pediatrics,* 45, 1003–1007, (1970).

Battaglia, F., G. Meschia, and E. Quilligan, eds., *Perinatal Medicine: Review and Comments,* 2nd Edition. St. Louis: Mosby, 1977.

Birch, H., and A. Leffard. "Intersensory development in children." *Monograph Society of Research in Child Development,* 28 (5), 1–48, (1963).

Brazelton, T. *Infants and Mothers: Differences in Development.* New York: Delacorte, 1969.

――――*Neonatal Behavioral Assessment Scale.* Philadelphia: Lippincott, 1973.

Brazelton, T., B. Kislowski, and M. Main. "The origins of reciprocity: The early mother-infant interaction," in M. Lewis and L. A. Rosenblum, eds., *The Effect of the Infant on Its Caregiver.* New York: Wiley, 1974.

Canosa, C., ed., *Nutrition, Growth and Development: Modern Problems in Pediatrics* Basel, Switzerland: S. Karger, 1975.

Chase, H. P. "The effects of intrauterine and postnatal undernutrition on normal brain development," in F. de la Cruz, B. Fox, and R. Roberts, eds., *Minimal Brain Dysfunction*, 231–244 New York: New York Academy of Sciences, (1973).

Chase, H. P. and H. P. Martin. "Undernutrition and child development." *New England Journal of Medicine*, 282, 933–939, (1970).

Chess, S., and A. Thomas. "Temperamental individuality from childhood to adolescence." *Journal of the American Academy of Child Psychiatry*, 16 (2), 218–226, (1977).

Chisolm, J. J. "Accidents and poisoning," in Robert Cooke, ed., *The Biologic Basis of Pediatric Practice*, pp. 1591–1608. New York: McGraw-Hill, 1968.

DeLicardie, E. R. and J. Cravioto. "Language development in survivors of clinical severe malnutrition," in A. Chavez, ed., *Prognosis for the Undernourished Surviving Child*, pp. 322–329. Basel, Switzerland: S. Karger, 1975.

Denoff, E. "The natural life history of children with minimal brain dysfunction," in F. de la Cruz, B. Fox, and R. Roberts, eds., *Minimal Brain Dysfunction*, 188–205. New York: New York Academy of Sciences, (1973).

Drillien, C. M. *The Growth and Development of the Prematurely Born Infant*. Baltimore: Williams & Wilkins, 1964.

Elmer, E. *Children in Jeopardy*. Pittsburgh: University of Pittsburgh Press, 1967.

Elmer, E., and G. S. Gregg. "Developmental Characteristics of Abused Children." *Pediatrics*, 40, 596–602, (1967).

Feingold, B. F. *Why Your Child Is Hyperactive*. New York: Random House, 1975.

Goodwin, J. S., ed. *Perinatal Medicine: The Basic Science Underlying Clinical Practice*. Baltimore: Williams & Wilkins, 1976.

Gregg, G. S., and E. Elmer. "Infant injuries: Accident or abuse." *Pediatrics*, 44, 434–439, (1969).

Hawkins, D. and L. Pauling, eds. *Orthomolecular Psychiatry*. San Francisco: Freeman, 1973.

Hoorweg, J. C. *Protein-Energy Malnutrition and Intellectual Abilities*. The Hague, The Netherlands: Mouton, 1976.

Hurwitz, I. "Psychological testing in studies of malnutrition," in J. Lloyd-Still, ed., *Malnutrition and Intellectual Development*, pp. 81–101. Littleton, Mass.: Publishing Sciences Group, 1976.

Kalverboer, A. F. *A Neurobehavioral Study in Pre-school Children*. Lavenham, N. Y.: Lavenham, 1975.

Kempe, C. H., F. Silverman, B. Steele, W. Droegmueller, and H. Silver. "The battered child syndrome." *Journal of American Medical Association*. 181, 17–24, (1962).

Keys, A., I. Brazek, and A. Henschel. *The Biology of Human Starvation*. Minneapolis: University of Minnesota Press, 1950.

Klein, R. E. and A. Adinolfi. "Measurement of the behavioral correlates of malnutrition," in J. W. Prescott, M. S. Read, and D. B. Coursin, eds., *Brain Function and Malnutrition: Neuropsychological Methods of Assessment*, pp. 73–82. New York: Wiley, 1975.

Klein, R. E., B. M. Lester, C. Yarbrough, and J. P. Habicht. "On malnutrition and mental development," in A. Chavez, ed., *Prognosis for the Undernourished Surviving Child*, pp. 315–321. Basel, Switzerland: S. Krager, 1975.

Kline, D. F. "Educational and psychological problems of abused children." (Paper presented at First International Congress on Child Abuse and Neglect, Geneva, September 20, 1976.)

Latham, M. "Protein calorie malnutrition in children and its relation to psychological development and behavior." *Physiological Review*, 54(3), 541–565 (1974).

Lewis, M., and L. Rosenblum, eds. *The Effect of the Infant on Its Caregiver*. New York: Wiley, 1974.

Lloyd-Still, J., ed., *Malnutrition and Intellectual Development*. Littleton, Mass.: Publishing Sciences Group, 1976*a*.

Lloyd-Still, J. "Clinical studies on the effects of malnutrition during infancy on subsequent physical and intellectual development," in J. Lloyd-Still, ed., *Malnutrition and Intellectual Development*, pp. 103–159. Littleton, Mass.: Publishing Sciences Group, 1976*b*.

Lubchenco, L. "Assessment of gestational age and development." *Pediatric Clinics of North America*, 17, 125–146, (1970).

——The High-Risk Infant. Philadelphia: Saunders, 1976.

MacKeith, R. "Speculations on some possible long-term effect," in A. Franklin, ed., *Concerning Child Abuse*, pp. 63–68. London: Churchill-Livingstone, 1975.

McKhann, G. "Nutrition and the developing nervous system," in C. Canosa, ed., *Nutrition, Growth and Development: Modern Problems in Pediatrics*, vol. 14, pp. 75–82. Basel, Switzerland: S. Karger, 1975.

Manocha, S. L. *Malnutrition and Retarded Human Development*. Springfield, Ill.: Thomas, 1972.

Martin, H. P. "The child and his development," in Kempe, C. H. and R. E. Helfer, eds., *Helping the Battered Child and His Family*, pp. 93–114. Philadelphia: Lippincott, 1972.

—— "Nutrition—Its relationship to children's physical, mental and emotional development." *American Journal of Clinical Nutrition*, 26, 766–775, (1973).

—— Early malnutrition and developmental disabilities. University of Colorado Medical Center, Denver, 1975. [Unpublished study.]

—— *The Abused Child: A Multidisciplinary Approach to Developmental Issues and Treatment*. Cambridge, Mass.: Ballinger, 1976.

Martin, H. P., and P. Beezley. "Behavioral Observations of Abused Children." *Developmental Medicine/Child Neurology*, 19(3), 373–387, (1977).

Martin, H. P., P. Beezley, E. Conway, and C. H. Kempe. "The Development of Abused Children." *Advances in Pediatrics*, 21, 25–73, (1974).

Prechtl, H. "Strategy and validity of early detection of neurological dysfunction," in C. P. Douglas and K. S. Holt, eds., *Mental Retardation, Prenatal Diagnosis and Infant Assessment*, pp. 41–46. London: Butterworth, 1972.

Prechtl, H., and D. Beintema. *The Neurological Examination of the Full-Term Newborn Infant*. Lavenham, N. Y.: Lavenham, 1964.

Prescott, J. F. "Developmental neuropsychophysicis," in J. Prescott, M. S. Read, and D. B. Coursin, eds., *Brain Function and Malnutrition: Neuropsychological Methods of Assessment*, pp. 325–358. New York: Wiley, 1975.

Prescott, J., M. S. Read, and D. B. Coursins, eds., *Brain Function and Malnutrition*: Neuropsychological Methods of Assessment. New York: Wiley, 1975.

Read, M., JP. Habicht, A. Lechtig, and R. Klein. "Maternal malnutrition, birthweight, and child development," in C. Canosa, ed. *Nutrition, Growth and Development: Modern Problems in Pediatrics*, vol. 14, pp. 203–215. Basel, Switzerland: S. Karger, 1975.

Richardson, S. A., H. G. Birch, E. Grabie, and K. Yoder. "The behavior of children in school who were severely malnourished in the first two years of life." *Journal of Health and Social Behavior*, 13, 276–284, (1972).

Rose, G., and P. Tanguay. "Developmental neurophysiology," in J. Wortis, ed., *Mental*

Retardation and Developmental Disabilities, vol. 7, pp. 22–62. New York: Brunner/ Mazel, 1975.

Ross Conference in Pediatric Research. *Iron Nutrition in Infancy.* Ross Laboratories, November, 1970.

Sameroff, A. J., and M. J. Chandler. "Reproductive risk and the continuum of caretaking casualty," in F. D. Horowitz, ed., *Review of Child Development Research.* vol. 4, pp. 187–244. Chicago: University of Chicago Press, 1975.

Scrimshaw, N. S., and J. E. Gordon. *Malnutrition, Learning and Behavior.* Cambridge, Mass.: MIT Press, 1968.

Soman, S. *Let's Stop Destroying Our Children.* New York: Hawthorn, 1974.

Sulzer, J. L., W. J. Hanche, and F. Koenig. "Nutrition and behavior in head start children: Results from the Tulane study," in D. J. Kallen, ed., *Nutrition, Development, and Social Behavior,* pp. 77–106. Washington, D. C.: U. S. Department of HEW. Publication (NIH) 73–242, 1973.

Thomas, A., S. Chess, and H. G. Birch. *Temperament and Behavior Disorders in Children.* New York: New York University Press, 1968.

Werner, E., J. M. Bierman, and F. E. French. *The Children of Kauai: A Longitudinal Study from the Prenatal Period to Age Ten.* Honolulu: University Press of Hawaii, 1971.

Winick, M. *Malnutrition and Brain Development.* New York: Oxford University Press, 1976.

CHAPTER 8

Neuropathologic Factors In Minimal Brain Dysfunction

Abraham Towbin

In children with minimal brain dysfunctions, with hyperactivity and learning disabilities evident, the physical examination in many cases reveals distinct minor neurologic abnormalities, soft signs of organicity which reflect latent organic defects in the brain. In some instances there are slight motor impairments, incoordinations, abnormal reflexes, EEG changes. At times petit mal, other convulsive disease manifestations, or defects in vision, hearing, and other sensory changes are present. There is substantial evidence that the outward clinical symptoms as well as the soft neurologic signs are often related to perinatal brain injury, to lesions in the brain stemming from the fetal neonatal period.

Pertinent to this consideration are the questions: Is perinatal brain injury common? Do such injuries leave scars? Do such scars provoke neurologic dysfunctions? Are there other such neurologic syndromes, other similar clinical patterns analogous to minimal brain dysfunctions in children?

The pattern of minor neuropsychiatric sequels which occur in adults after cerebral injury is in many ways a facsimile of the pattern of minimal brain dysfunctions in children with a history of perinatal brain injury. Considered thus in the clinical-pathologic analysis of minimal brain dysfunction, three basic features of the syndrome are of significance: (1) the minimal nature of the symptoms, (2) the variability of the manifestations, and (3) the latency of the process.

MINIMAL NATURE OF THE SYMPTOMS

In many adults after traumatic intracranial injury—often after recovery from brief cardiac arrest with oxygen deprivation of the brain, commonly in adults surviving small strokes—clinically there appear subtle forms of neuropsychiatric disorders; minor signs and symptoms of a chronic nature, sensory-motor defects, often with involvement of affect and intellect appear; focal seizures, at times petit may occur. In such cases in adults, postmortem neuropathologic studies of the brain commonly reveal focal areas of remote damage, lesions having origin at the time of the injury, small scars, responsible for the clinical neurologic dysfunctions present during life.

Brain damage in the newborn may exercise similar effects. In the newborn, consequent to pregnancy complications and difficulties in delivery, the presence of brain damage is common (Yllpö, 1919; Schwartz, 1961; Towbin, 1970; Courville, 1971). Injury to the brain in the fetus and newborn is not an all-or-none process. Acute cerebral lesions present at birth are of a wide range of severity. Detailed anatomic-pathologic studies of the brain in fetuses and in infants dying in the postnatal period demonstrate that damage to the brain ranges from minor focal lesions to broad devastations leading to destruction of the cerebrum. In infants with perinatal injury that survive, with sublethal cerebral damage, the acute lesions, whether minor or extensive, gradually undergo "healing," leaving chronic lesions, scars, and cavitations. In the newborn, as in the adult, and as in the laboratory in experimental animals, there is essentially a direct correlation between the degree of brain damage present and the severity of the resulting functional disability: major lesions cause severe crippling of nervous system function; lesser lesions are responsible for lesser sequelant neurologic signs and symptoms. The conclusion is inescapable: minor lesions (minimal cerebral damage present in the newborn) contribute to the occurrence of sequelant minor functional disability, to manifestations of minimal brain dysfunctions.

Variability of the clinical pattern of minimal brain dysfunctions in children can be correlated pathologically with the diversity in distribution of damage that occurs in the newborn brain. In the fetus and newborn, all portions of the brain are vulnerable to injury, with some parts being biologically more susceptible than others with the site of injury varying with the gestational age. As in the adult and as observed in the laboratory in experimental animals the clinical abnormalities that develop following brain damage in the newborn depend on the specific location of the lesions in the brain. Perinatal damage to the cerebrum in the precentral region leads to motor defects; lesions in the frontal lobe are related to disorders of mentation; lesions at other sites result in corresponding defects in sensory or other functions and at times to manifestations of epilepsy.

Latency in the occurrence of clinical symptoms is common with brain damage in adults, with the outward effects being obscured, delayed, often surfacing months or years after the time of the brain injury. Analogously brain damage present in the newborn may remain latent, silent for years with neurologic signs and symptoms appearing later in childhood and adolescence as manifestations of minimal brain dysfunction.

The organic factor, perinatal brain damage, appears as the dominant etiologic mechanism in some cases of major as well as minimal brain dysfunction. For the most part, present-day clinical diagnostic refinements serve to separate the clearly organic from the group with neuroses, environmental deprivation, or other psychosocial conditions. Patently in a given case, more than one factor may be causal. Pertinent to this is the need clinically for a balanced perspective; a knowledge of organic substrates as well as other psychogenic mechanisms underlying minimal brain dysfunctions.

Historically the link between brain damage in the newborn and the consequent occurrence of cerebral dysfunction, mental retardation, cerebral palsy, and epilepsy, was recognized in the remote past. It was clearly enunciated in 1861 by Little in his classic report, "On the influence of abnormal parturition, difficult labor, premature birth, and asphyxia neonatorum, on the mental and physical condition of the child." As later stated by Knobloch and Pasamanick (1959) in their investigations of the cause-and-effect relationship between fetal-neonatal brain damage and sequelant nervous system disorders.

There is a lethal component of cerebral damage which results in fetal and neonatal deaths and a sublethal component which gives rise to a series of clinical neuropsychiatric syndromes depending on the degree and location of the damage.

Fetal and neonatal damage results not only in a *reduction* of cerebral function, but also in the *distortion* of such function. Focal injury to the cerebral cortex, leaving epileptogenic scars, results in convulsive disorders. The manifestations of cerebral palsy involve not only loss of motor function, paralysis, but also dyskinesia, athetosis—distorted motor function. Likewise, clinical attention is also being focused more precisely on the occurrence of behavioral disorders in cases with a history of perinatal complications. It is increasingly evident that perinatal cerebral injury may be reflected not only in a decrease in mental function, but also in abnormal function, psychopathy (Pasamanick, Rogers, and Lilienfeld, 1956; Taft and Goldfarb, 1964; Dalen, 1965; Rosen, 1969; Mednick, 1970; Garmezy and Steitman, 1974).

The sequels of perinatal cerebral damage thus form a syndromic tetralogy—mental retardation, cerebral palsy, epilepsy, and related psychopathy. That the symptomatic elements of this tetralogy are parts of a single clinical entity is embodied in the concept of the "brain-injured child," expressed in the broad studies of Strauss and Lehtinen (1947) and Strauss and Kephart, (1955). Pathologically the perinatal organic processes, the structural damage in the brain which provokes mental retardation, cerebral palsy, epilepsy, and related psychopathy—the causal lesions responsible for the clinical tetralogy—though varying in location in the brain, are anatomically of the same nature, cast in the same mold. Clinically one or more elements of the tetralogy may be evident in the same case; at times all four components appear. Children so afflicted should not be considered as having four different diseases. The mental, epileptic, and motor disturbances present, whether severe or minimal, are symptomatic expressions of a single pathologic process.

Neuropathology studies in cases of cerebral palsy and organic mental retardation, autopsy studies in the past, have defined the basic anatomic patterns of the chronic lesions occuring in these disorders (Towbin, 1955a, 1955b; Hallervorden and Meyer, 1956; Towbin, 1960; Malamud, et al., 1964). Two main forms of chronic cerebral lesions are recognized: *deep* cerebral lesions, scars and cavitations affecting the basal ganglia and neighboring structures at the core of the forebrain and *cortical* cerebral lesions, affecting mainly surface structures of the convolutions. The deep form of damage is the more frequent type. At times brain specimens show intermediate or mixed distribution of the lesions.

Although the anatomic pattern of cerebral damage in the chronic case material was well known in the past, the etiopathogenesis, the causal processes, long remained obscure. There were many misconceptions, some still persisting, that the chronic lesions causing cerebral palsy and mental retardation were due to obstetrical trauma, to physical "birth injury." Textbooks still appear with drawings showing the head of the half-delivered fetus being crushed by the obstetrician's forceps, implying that cerebral damage in the newborn is due to squashing of the brain.

Pathologists studying cases of cerebral palsy and mental retardation realized that the underlying causes could not be conclusively determined by analyses limited to studies of the chronic lesions. Such studies attempted to interpret the cause of the lesions at a time years or decades after incurrence of the injury. It was evident that the etiopathogenesis could be clarified only by studying the causal processes at their origin, by studying the antecedent fresh acute lesions imprinted in the fetal-neonatal period. However, in the neuropathology laboratory, the analysis of acute lesions in the human neonatal brain—soft and friable, often diffluent—presented technical difficulties which long remained insurmountable. Lacking adequate perinatal neuropathologic studies, the causes and effects of neonatal brain damage remained largely a matter of speculation. Clinically, likewise, a broad hiatus existed, a paucity of accurate information with regard to the long-term follow-up of infants with varying severity of manifest brain injury at birth.

Recognizing the need both for elucidation of these broad problems, the need for more valid information concerning perinatal brain injury and sequelant nervous system disability, extensive research programs have been undertaken in recent decades. In 1959 the National Institutes of Health formulated the Collaborative Perinatal Project (Collaborative Study of Cerebral Palsy, Mental Retardation, and Other Neurologic and Sensory Disorders of Infancy and Childhood, 1965). This study of 50,000 pregnant women and their offspring, with 15 medical centers across the country participating, correlated perinatal data with follow-up pediatric neurologic studies. Pathology studies carried out in the Collaborative Perinatal Project, postmortem investigation of the neonatal deaths, provided fundamental information defining the nature of organic perinatal brain damage and its neuropsychiatric sequels. In the laboratory, application of the required, highly complex technique of whole-brain serial histologic sectioning made possible the consistent preservation and analysis of acute focal lesions, even minimal lesions.

From neuropathologic studies in the Collaborative Perinatal Project and from other current investigations of fetal-neonatal disease (Norwood Project, 1970; Towbin, 1978), three relevant concepts have emerged:

1. Most cases of cerebral damage in the newborn are due to perinatal hypoxia. Many pathologic processes, complications of pregnancy and delivery, contribute to the development of hypoxia, inadequate oxygenation of the fetus and the newborn. Mechanical injury, mainly spinal cord and brain stem damage, is also common in the newborn, but of less significance than hypoxia (Towbin, 1969). A host of other neonatal central nervous system disorders—genetic, metabolic, infectious, and toxic processes —make their appearance and, although comparatively rare, these disorders often receive broader emphasis than the effects of hypoxia, the process that underlies the bulk of neonatal neuropathologic case material.

2. Two basic forms of perinatal hypoxic brain damage occur: *deep* cerebral damage, observed mainly in the premature fetus and newborn; *cortical* cerebral damage in the mature, at term. (Figure 8–1).

   The deep form of acute perinatal cerebral hypoxic damage is of more frequent occurrence than cortical damage. Significantly the high incidence of deep cerebral damage in the newborn correlates with the high incidence of deep lesions in the chronic case material, cases of cerebral palsy and related clinical disability.

3. The degree of brain damage is governed essentially by the intensity and duration of the perinatal hypoxic causal complication. Severe hypoxia

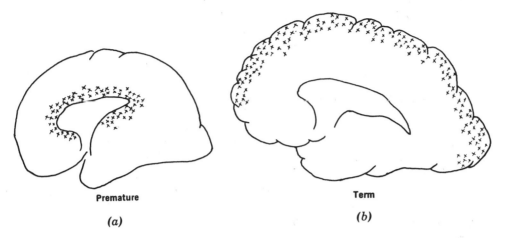

Premature   Term

(a)   *(b)*

Figure 8–1.   Two basic patterns of perinatal hypoxic cerebral damage related to gestational age. (a) In the premature, deep cerebral damage predominates with hemorrhagic infarctional destruction of periventricular germinal matrix tissue and adjoining structures. (b) At term, in the mature fetus and newborn, the cerebral cortex with subjacent white matter is the main site of hypoxic infarctional damage.

affecting the fetus and newborn may lead to necrosis of the cerebrum, to *in vivo* total destruction; in infants who survive, this results in hydranencephaly with the hemispheric walls reduced to a thin leathery sheet. Less severe hypoxic exposure leads to focal necrosis with resulting cavitation and scarring. Mild hypoxia results in cellular damage with patchy or diffuse neuronal loss.

Experimental studies investigating the effects of perinatal hypoxia in laboratory animals disclose findings essentially parallel to clinical and pathologic observations with human case material. Experimental animals exposed to varying degrees of perinatal hypoxia develop acute and chronic cerebral lesions of corresponding severity. Surviving offspring with chronic lesions manifest late sequels reflecting the degree of nervous system damage, disabilities ranging from major to minimal cerebral dysfunctions (Windle, 1968; Meyers, 1972).

NEUROPATHOLOGIC CORRELATION

Although studies of perinatal hypoxia applying to human case material lack the standard controls afforded in laboratory animal investigations, prospective studies, as in the Collaborative Perinatal Project, provide substantial bases for defining cause-and-effect patterns. In human studies, of fundamental importance is the application of direct anatomic-pathologic analyses based on autopsy material to demonstrate the sequential relationship between perinatal brain injury and the occurrence or residual chronic cerebral lesions which give rise to neuropsychiatric disabilities during life.

In defining this relationship it is requisite that (1) the acute forms of fetal-neonatal cerebral hypoxic damage, ranging from massive to minimal lesions be identified and correlated with (2) chronic lesions of corresponding severity, as found in cases of mental retardation, cerebral palsy, and other, lesser cerebral dysfunctions; (3) subacute case material the intermediate pattern of hypoxic damage present in fetuses and newborn who survive for a period after exposure to hypoxia is presented demonstrating the link between the acute and chronic forms (Towbin, 1969, 1970, 1971; Courville, 1971; Csermeley, 1972).

Acute Cerebral Hypoxic Damage

Figure 8–2 illustrates the intrinsic mechanism of visceral damage consequent to perinatal hypoxia, the formation of an acute hemorrhagic venous *infarction*. Pathologically an infarct is a localized portion of an organ, or an entire organ, rendered necrotic, devitalized *in vivo*, due to interference with local blood circulation, arterial or venous. With hypoxia, circulation through the venous system of the body gradually slows down; locally this stasis leads to occlusion of veins by the formation of blood clots, the process of *thrombosis*, with consequent infarction. Venous infarcts, far advanced, suffused with stagnant blood, give rise to local hemorrhage.

In varying degree all organs of the body are susceptible to infarctional hypoxic injury. In the fetus and newborn, focal and diffuse infarctional damage may occur not only in the brain, but also in the kidneys, adrenals, and in other structures. The brain however proves to be the most vulnerable, the most common target, and here with the most serious consequences.

The case in Figure 8–3 shows the basic pattern of acute cerebral hypoxic damage, deep cerebral infarction, present characteristically in the premature fetus

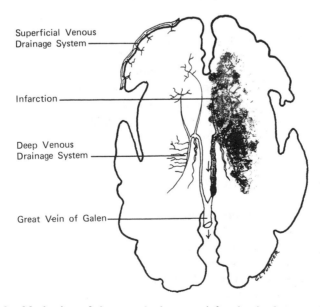

Figure 8–2.   Mechanism of deep cerebral venous infarction in the premature newborn. The deep cerebral vein on the right is dilated, distended with thrombus, *in vivo* blood clot. The corresponding deep portion of the cerebrum appears with confluent dark patches, areas of hemorrhagic infarction, portions of tissue devitalized and suffused with blood due to interference with local venous drainage. Deep venous channels in the premature brain prominently developed, in contrast to the rudimentary superficial cerebral veins. (A. Towbin, *American Journal of Diseases of Children*, 1970.)

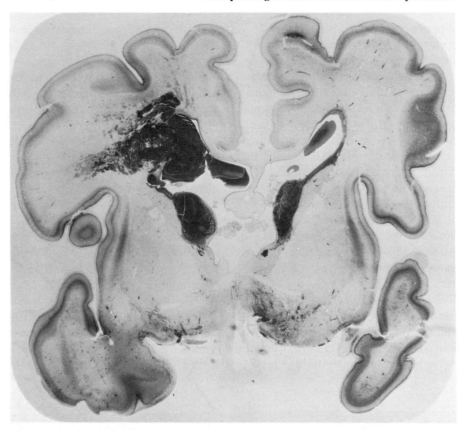

Figure 8–3.   Deep cerebral hemorrhagic infarction, characteristic pattern of acute hypoxic cerebral damage in the premature fetus and newborn. The area of infarction, deep in the upper portion of the left hemisphere, appears as dark confluent patches with infiltrating margins, obliterating the deep white matter and extending downward to involve the basal ganglia and germinal matrix tissue. On both sides the germinal matrix deposit is effaced, replaced by a hemorrhagic mound of infarcted tissue bulging into the lower part of the cerebral ventricles. The case history indicated premature delivery at 35 weeks gestation; the infant showed increasing generalized neurologic deterioration with death at 23 hours. (Case W–59, A. Towbin, *American Journal of Pathology*, 1968.)

and newborn. The main damage in this case, at the core of the cerebrum, in the upper portion of the left hemispheric wall, appears an island of dark tissue with irregular infiltrating margins, with the lesion obliterating portions of the periventricular white matter and extending to the basal ganglia and thalamus. The acute infarction in the fresh state, as at autopsy in this case, consists of structural debris and blood clot, devitalized tissue suffused with blood.

Chronic Cerebral Lesions

Figure 8–4 shows a corresponding cerebral lesion of chronic form, extensive deep cerebral damage pathologically the residue of a remote infarction stemming from birth. This chronic lesion was present at autopsy in the case of an eight-year-old child, clinically with multiple severe neurologic disabilities, with cerebral palsy, mental retardation, and epilepsy. The main lesion in this case is in the left cerebral hemisphere, in the deep periventricular region, with cavitation and scarring about the upper portion of the basal ganglia.

Another example of a chronic lesion, somewhat smaller, is shown in Figure 8–5. As in the previous case, the lesion involves the deep cerebral structures. The area of damage is smaller than that in Figure 8–4 and the clinical manifestations in this case were of a more moderate nature. The lesion, a remote infarction, forms a circumscribed cribriform seive-like scar occupying portions of the left basal ganglia and involves the corticospinal tract. (Brain section viewed anteriorly; lesion anatomically on the left.) The record indicated that at birth the infant was in poor condition, hypoxic. Postnatally the neurologic examination revealed hyperactive reflexes of the right arm and leg with partial paralysis which persisted. During childhood, mild mental retardation was evident, with behavior disorder and frequent periods of agitation. Death occurred at the age of 52 years due to causes unrelated to the nervous system. The neuropathologic findings at autopsy were concordant with the clinical neurologic dysfunctions present during life.

Figure 8–6 shows a focal chronic cavitary lesion, an area of remote cystic destruction with scarred margins, in the right frontal lobe of the cerebrum. (Brain section viewed anteriorly; lesion anatomically on the right.) The case history revealed a complicated birth, a twin delivery, with neonatal hypoxia; the other twin died soon after delivery. The surviving twin, who lived to the age of 42 years, showed varied neuropsychiatric symptoms, generally of moderate nature. In infancy he was noted to be mildly retarded. As a child he was withdrawn and in

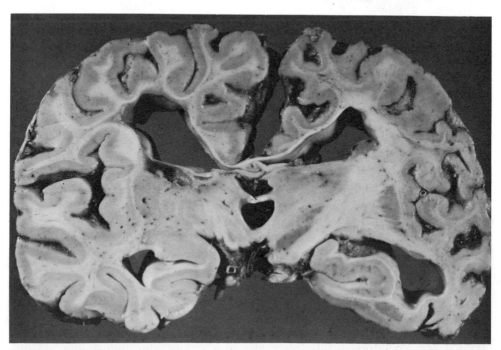

Figure 8–4. Chronic deep cerebral hypoxic damage, remote infarction, cavitation and scarring involving the basal ganglia on the left, with destruction and atrophy of the deep layers of white matter around the ventricles. Severe cerebral palsy in an eight-year-old child, with mental retardation and epilepsy. (Case CSH–10762, A. Towbin, *Archives of Pathology*, 1955b.)

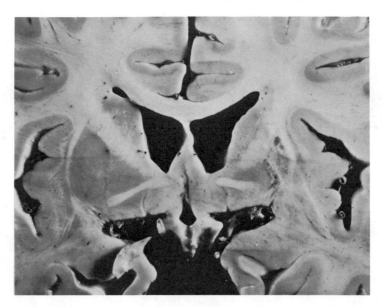

Figure 8–5.   Chronic deep cerebral hypoxic lesion, a circumscribed cribriform seive-like scar occupying portions of the left basal ganglia and adjoining corticospinal (motor) tract. (Brain section viewed anteriorly; lesion anatomically on the left side of cerebrum.) History of hypoxic birth with the infant in poor condition postnatally. Neurologic examination of the newborn revealed hyperactive reflexes of the right limbs, with partial paralysis which persisted. Mild mental retardation in childhood with behavior disorder, with periods of agitation. (Case CSS 10255, A. Towbin, *Archives of Pathology,* 1955*b*.)

adulthood became depressive. Neurologically there was slight left-sided spasticity with hyperreflexia and occasional focal seizures, reflecting the chronic lesion in the cerebrum.

Subacute Lesions

Pathologically the key to the interpretation of the chronic lesions, the scars and cavities shown in Figures 8–4, 8–5, and 8–6, lies in the study of subacute lesions found in cases with short-term survival, for weeks or months, after perinatal hypoxia. The lesions in these cases, presenting the transitional picture of subacute infarction, are an indispensible link in relating acute cerebral hypoxic damage to the chronic lesions found in mental retardation, cerebral palsy, and other sequelant cerebral disorders.

The subacute lesion represents a state of involution, the "healing stage." Unlike the acute lesion with its angry infiltrating appearance, the subacute lesion presents a reduced, more subdued, delineated pattern, usually with a firm grey-pink margin and a soft beige center. Microsocopic examination of these lesions reveals an active clean-up process, with the necrotic debris being removed by "scavenger cells." The center of the lesion is depleted, forming a cavity, or it is filled in from the margins with temporary "granulation tissue" and later this is transformed into scar tissue if survival extends to the chronic stage.

The subacute lesions vary in size and location and are associated with corresponding clinical manifestations during life. The area of damage may be massive,

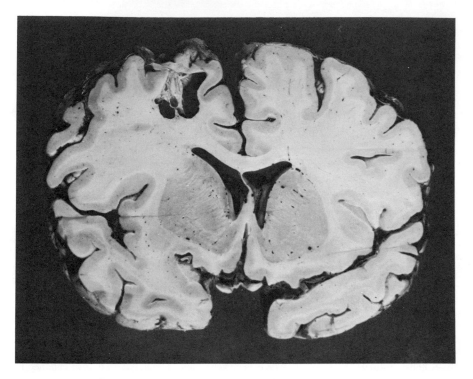

Figure 8–6.   Focal chronic cystic lesion with scarred margins, consistent pathologically with destruction due to remote hypoxic infarction. History of complicated hypoxic twin birth; other twin died postnatally. Section of cerebrum from surviving twin who lived to the age of 42 years. Moderate neuropsychiatric manifestations throughout life; mild retardation noted in infancy, withdrawn during childhood, depressive during adulthood. Neurologically showed slight left-sided spasticity and hyperreflexia, and had occasional focal epileptic seizures. (Brain section viewed anteriorly; lesion anatomically on the right side of the cerebrum.) (Case CSH 10544, A. Towbin, *Archives of Pathology*, 1955*b*.)

in the deep cerebral layers or cortex, with broad portions of necrotic tissue effacing formed structures; or the lesion may be small, minimal, appearing as a minute necrotic focus—an incidental finding in cases where death is due to other unrelated systemic disease.

Subacute infarctional damage may develop prenatally, in the fetus, or postnatally. Subacute lesions make their appearance in the brain prenatally in cases in which the intrauterine environment of the fetus is compromised by maternal illness or other disturbances in the maternal-placental-fetal complex. Subacute damage is found at autopsy in infants surviving for a period after a complicated hypoxic delivery and often in infants who die after protracted postnatal respiratory disorders.

In the following case, subacute cerebral damage accrued during intrauterine life due to maternal illness during pregnancy, with the fetus becoming debilitated, with the infant at birth already bearing far-advanced cerebral destruction.

Two months before the expected date of delivery the mother developed a severe respiratory infection and was hospitalized. Vaginal bleeding also occurred, indicative of a placental disorder. The pregnancy was maintained to term. In the delivery room, the newborn appeared "dysmature," malnourished; weight was

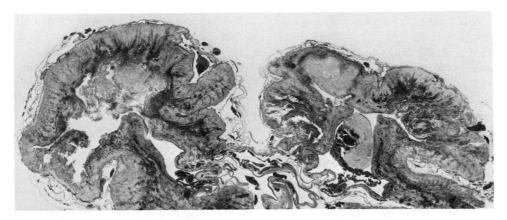

Figure 8–7.   Subacute hypoxic cerebral damage; deeply located infarctional damage incurred *irt utero* during premature period of fetal life. Confluent pale areas of necrotic infarcted tissue with irregular hemorrhagic margins; overlying cerebral surface layers, cortex and subjacent white matter, relatively preserved. The age of the subacute damage, pathologically about two months old, correlates with period of severe maternal illness during pregnancy. (Case T–1, A. Towbin, *American Journal of Diseases of Children,* 1970.)

2770 g, slightly over 6 pounds; the head and other parts were essentially of proportionate size. The infant lived 18 hours. At autopsy the brain appeared very small. The miniature cerebrum occupying the depths of the cranial cavity showed well-defined convolutions, giving the appearance of a collapsed loaf of braided bread. Brain weight was 130 g (average, 360 g). In the laboratory, studies of the whole-brain histologic sections of the brain indicated the nature of the destructive process within the cerbrum (Figure 8–7). While the surface layers of the cerebrum were relatively intact, the deep tissues involving most of the thickness of the hemispheric walls showed broad portions of pale necrotic infarcted tissue surrounded by dark hemorrhagic margins. The deep cerebral veins were filled with thromboses. Pathologically the cerebral lesions were subacute infarcts about two months old. This indicates that the damage, deep in the cerebrum, had its onset during intrauterine life at a time when the fetus was premature and corresponds in time to the onset of the mother's illness.

Other pathologists have reported the occurrence of similar subacute cerebral damage in young infants. Brand and Bignami (1969) described in detail the case of an infant born at 34 weeks gestation, who lived 8 weeks. The infant showed at autopsy softening and cavitations of the deep cerebral tissues. Another infant in this study, born at 30 weeks gestation, lived for 10 months and showed progressive scarring of the white matter deep in the cerebrum.

The clinical-pathologic relationship between early prenatal hypoxia and subsequent deep cerebral lesions—the effects of intrauterine hypoxia on the premature fetus—is demonstrated in reports by Neuburger (1935), Hallervorden (1949), and Bankl and Jellinger (1967). In the cases described, the fetuses were subjected to hypoxia months before birth during maternal attempts at suicide by asphyxia. Clinically in the offspring there were manifestations of mental retardation, motor disturbances, and other neurologic disabilities. Postmortem studies of these cases revealed extensive scarring and cavity formation in the deep white matter and in the basal ganglia.

When cases of subacute damage are taken into account, and when examples of acute cerebral hypoxic damage in the newborn and chronic lesions in cases of mental retardation and cerebral palsy are compared with the lesions placed side-by-side—the organic link, the evolution of the acute process to the chronic form, is clear. As noted the deep pattern of cerebral damage is the more frequent form in both the neonatal and chronic case material. That the acute deep cerebral damage characteristic of the premature newborn (Figure 8–3) closely resembles the common deep form of chronic cerebral damage (Figure 8–4) is evident not only as to the deep location, but also pathologically. Both lesions are infarcts differing only in the factor of time, one being acute, the other chronic.

The acute cerebral hypoxic damage described here, the local process of thrombosis, infarction, and hemorrhage, is the same as that which occurs in the adult with *stroke.* The acute hemorrhagic infarction in Figure 8–3 is comparable to the hemorrhagic lesions in the brain in adults with apoplectic stroke due to venous thrombosis (Kalbag and Woolf, 1967; Towbin 1973). The chronic lesion in Figure 8–4 is pathologically similar to lesions in the brain in adults who have survived remote strokes. Thus in a direct sense, clinically and pathologically, the hypoxic human fetus and newborn suffers stroke. If massive, this results in paralysis (cerebral palsy) or loss of other major cerebral function. Small strokes lead to minor cerebral dysfunctions.

In analyzing the perinatal pathologic case material, the identification of the acute, subacute, and chronic cerebral lesions as venous infarcts, while providing basic information, still left unanswered the question of pathogenesis, the underlying cause of the infarcts.

CAUSAL MECHANISMS

The causal mechanisms leading to the development of the acute cerebral lesions in the newborn remained a matter of speculation until the studies of the Collaborative Perinatal Project (1965).

These studies demonstrate that the acute infarctional damage that occurs in the brain and other organs with fetal-neonatal hypoxia is not a limited local phenomenon (Towbin 1968). The hemorrhagic infarcts represent the final segment in a series of pathologic systemic body processes which involve antecedent perinatal factors, processes which may have their origin before, during, or after birth. The development of the underlying processes leading to cerebral infarctional damage evolves through three stages, each precipitating the next:

1. *The hypoxic onset.* The hypoxia-producing complication—prenatally, intranatally, or postnatally—may have its origin in any of the components of the maternal-placental-fetal organization. Prenatally, fetal malnutrition and oxygen deprivation may be due to maternal illness and debility. The placenta, the oxygenating organ for the fetus, transferring oxygen from maternal blood to the fetal blood, very often is faulty, is functionally inadequate due to pathologic changes present, such as placental infarction or premature detachment of the placenta. At times the umbilical cord, the supply conduit between the placenta and the fetus, becomes compressed or knotted. These same complications may appear, often catastrophically, intranatally during labor and delivery. Frequently the hypoxic state initi-

ated prior to birth is extended postnatally, especially with prematures, resulting in the development in the infant of hyaline membrane disease, pneumonia, or other pulmonary complications.

Prolonged hypoxia imposed on the body, whether fetus, newborn, or adult, leads to weakening of heart function and then to failure of the blood circulatory system.

2. *Systemic circulatory failure.* The heart functions as a double-action pump, drawing out blood from the venous side of the circulation and propelling it forward into the arteries.

In the fetus and newborn, as in the adult, when the oxygen available to the body is inadequate, manifestly the tissue that suffers first is the constantly working, contracting heart muscle. The pump falters. Failure of the heart to pump out adequately the blood from the venous side of the circulatory system leads to venous engorgement, a stagnant back-log of blood in the veins of the body, congestive circulatory failure. This slowing and stasis of venous flow leads to local *in vivo* intravascular blood clotting, venous thrombosis, especially in the peripheries of the body, locally in the legs and intracranially, in the brain. Thrombosis causes infarction.

3. *Venous infarctional damage* (Figure 8–2). Interference with local circulation, stasis-thrombosis of veins (or arteries) of an organ or part of an organ, leads to corresponding tissue infarctional damage of varying severity, diffuse or localized. In the cerebrum the damage may be diffuse but of anatomically mild intensity, with selective neuronal depopulation of the cortex. In some cases with more severe hypoxic exposure, the entire thickness of the hemispheric wall may be rendered necrotic, total-organ infarction. More often, with local venous thrombosis affecting part of an organ, the infarction is focal, localized; the necrosis of the tissue is accompanied by breakdown of blood vessels, with consequent local bleeding— hemorrhagic venous infarction.

As previously noted, studies in the Collaborative Perinatal Project (Towbin, 1968, 1970) revealed that the infarctional damage in the newborn brain occurred in two basic forms, *deep* cerebral damage and *cortical* cerebral damage (Figure 8–1). The distribution pattern is related to the gestational age at the time of the hypoxic exposure. In the premature fetus and newborn at 25 to 35 weeks gestation, the hypoxic damage consistently is located in the deep cerebral strata, in the periventricular structures. In the mature fetus and newborn, acute damage in this deep location is relatively infrequent; as term approaches the cerebral cortex becomes the primary site of hypoxic injury. This specifity in location of the acute hypoxic damage—the predilection for deep cerebral structures in the premature and for the cortex at term—is not a random occurrence but is influenced by three biologic factors, all related to gestational age: presence or absence of germinal matrix tissue, the momentum of local organogenesis, and the level of development of local intracranial vascular elements.

Germinal Matrix

The germinal matrix is composed of residual deposits of embryonic tissue analogous to the germinal tissue that originally lines the neural tube, primitive tissue that persists until late in fetal life. The germinal deposits appear as thick pads of compact tissue deep in the cerebrum at the caudo-thalamic groove, dark mounds bulging from the hemispheric walls into the ventricles (Figure 8–8). The deposits of germinal matrix are depots of building material, *anlage* tissue required for the future formation of the basal ganglia and other deep neuronal assemblies as well as for the development of the cerebral cortex. The matrix tissue, soft and friable, is manifestly vulnerable to hypoxia and readily undergoes infarctional disintegration. Ordinarily as the fetus matures and histogenesis of the deep structures is completed, the germinal matrix is gradually used up. Consequently the occurence of acute infarctional damage in the deep cerebral tissue at term is uncommon.

Organogenesis

Organogenesis, the time during which visceral structure is undergoing active elaboration, is a period of manifestly increased vulnerability to hypoxia. During early fetal life, local organogenesis in the forebrain is most prominent in the deep structures where elaboration of neurohistologic elements from the deposits of germinal matrix is highly visible. The deep structures, undergoing rapid differentiation, are immediately susceptible to hypoxic infarctional injury. Later as the fetus nears term, as the germinal matrix becomes depleted, histogenesis at the core of the cerebrum declines and the momentum of organogenesis shifts to the cerebral surface where the cortex, maturing rapidly at term, becomes the main target of hypoxic injury.

Vascular Development

Vascular development, particularly the elaboration of venous elements, directly influences the occurrence of infarction in the fetal and neonatal brain. In the premature, coincident with active organogenesis, vascularization of the deep cerebral structures proceeds early, providing a broad venous bed for the occurrence of thromboses, fostering deep cerebral infarction (Figure 8–2). At term the cortex, previously essentially an avascular layer of tissue, rapidly undergoing differentiation, acquires a prominent venous drainage system. Thrombosis of the newly formed surface venous channels, the dural venous sinuses and tributaries draining the cerebral convolutions, results in cortical infarctional damage in the mature fetus and newborn.

MINIMAL CEREBRAL LESIONS

In the neuropathology laboratory, in perinatal studies in the past, efforts were confined mainly to gross anatomic analyses of large acute cerebral lesions in the newborn and to investigation of the resulting large chronic lesion in cases with severe mental retardation and cerebral palsy. Likewise, clinical efforts were occupied largely with the study of advanced forms of mental retardation, cerebral palsy, and other severe forms of cerebral disability stemming from birth. In recent decades however increasing attention has been focused on the importance of lesser forms of cerebral damage, with lesser sequels. Knoblock and Pasamanick (1959) in their clinical assessment of nervous system abnormalities consequent to perinatal brain damage concluded,

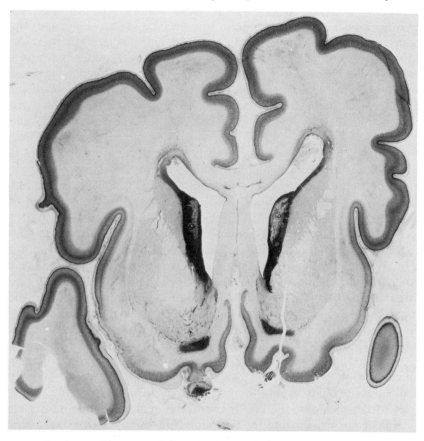

Figure 8–8.   Cerebrum of premature infant showing persisting germinal matrix tissue; the pad-like germinal deposits are deeply located, attached to the inner surface of the hemispheric walls, and bulge into the lower lateral portion of the ventricle space on each side. Matrix deposits show minimal hypoxic infarctional lesions, more pronounced on the right, appearing as irregular pale patches of necrosis; thromboses in small veins in the matrix. History of spontaneous delivery at 32 weeks gestation due to premature detachment of the placenta; infant lived 2 days. Autopsy revealed infarctional damage in other organs in addition to the brain. (Case W–73–61, A. Towbin, *American Journal of Pathology*, 1968.)

"We have found that these abnormalities range from the more obvious disabilities, such as cerebral palsy, epilepsy, and mental retardation, through the learning and behavior difficulties, such as reading disabilities, tics, and the behavior disorders of childhood, probably as a result of cerebral disorganization after minimal cerebral damage."

Accordingly it is of basic importance that attention be given pathologically to the study of minimal forms of cerebral damage present at birth. The common occurrence in the neonate of minimal lesions, latent cerebral damage, is not generally realized.

Minimal Deep Cerebral Lesions: Premature Newborn

Minimal hypoxic cerebral damage, small focal areas of infarction present in the deep deposits of germinal matrix, characteristic of the premature, is shown in Figure 8–8. On the right, the germinal matrix (the thick dark pad of tissue bulging from the inner aspect of the hemispheric wall into the ventricular space) shows a pale longitudinal patch of necrosis, infarctional damage, with a minute thrombus-filled vein at its center. The infant in this case, born at 32 weeks gestation with severe hypoxia due to premature separation of the placenta, lived 2 days.

In premature brains, in addition to lesions in the matrix deposits, small areas of necrosis may appear in the deep white matter around the ventricles, focal periventricular leucomalacia (leuco, white + malacia, softness), in the nature of microinfarcts (Banker and Larroche, 1962).

Minimal hypoxic lesions in the deep cerebral structures are of frequent occurrence in the premature, being evident at autopsy almost universally in infants at 7 months gestation (Yllpö, 1919; Arey and Anderson, 1965). In laboratory studies in the Collaborative Perinatal Project (1965), in postmortem examination of 140 premature newborn infants of 22 to 35 weeks gestation, deep cerebral infarctional damage of severe to moderate degree was present in 48% of the cases (Towbin, 1970). Significantly in the other 52% of cases, acute hypoxic changes of minimal form were present, often with the lesions scattered diffusely through the germinal matrix and adjoining deep cerebral tissue.

The natural growth and development of the fetal brain requires that the germinal matrix tissue be adequate and undamaged. Hypoxic damage in the germinal matrix and deep white matter, even though the lesions appear minute, imposes an irrevocable loss of *anlage* "building material" and an erosion of maturing tissue, creating a lasting handicap. These small acute infarcts are the precursors of subacute and chronic lesions.

Minimal subacute deep cerebral hypoxic lesions are common. As in the pathologic study of large lesions, the link between the minimal acute and the chronic lesions lies in demonstrating intermediate subacute lesions. In hypoxic premature infants who survive for periods of weeks or months and die of other intercurrent disease, at autopsy often there are evident small areas of tan softening in the deep periventricular tissues of the cerebrum near the basal ganglia at the site previously occupied by the germinal matrix deposits. Microscopically these are of subacute nature, granulation tissue with early scar formation and persisting hemosiderin (residual of hemoglobin pigment), elements present in the wake of past hemorrhagic infarctional damage (Towbin, 1971).

With prolonged survival, the small subacute lesions emerge as foci of minimal hypoxic brain damage—chronic scarring. In autopsy studies, in infants and children with a history of premature birth with perinatal hypoxia, as well as in adults, especially in case material from the neuropsychiatric hospital, there are at times present in the cerebrum, in the deep periventricular white matter and adjoining basal ganglia, small areas of cystic loculated scarring. Pathologically the pattern of damage here, small chronic lesions, is consistent with infarctional damage having origin remotely, in the fetal-neonatal period.

Minimal Cortical Cerebral Lesions: Term Newborn

In experimental studies with near-term pregnant monkeys subjected to asphyxia, the surviving offspring showed pronounced reduction in spontaneous activity and dexterity; examined after nine years survival, the brains of the animals showed substantial loss of cortical cerebral elements, most clearly evident in the precentral motor region (Windle, 1968).

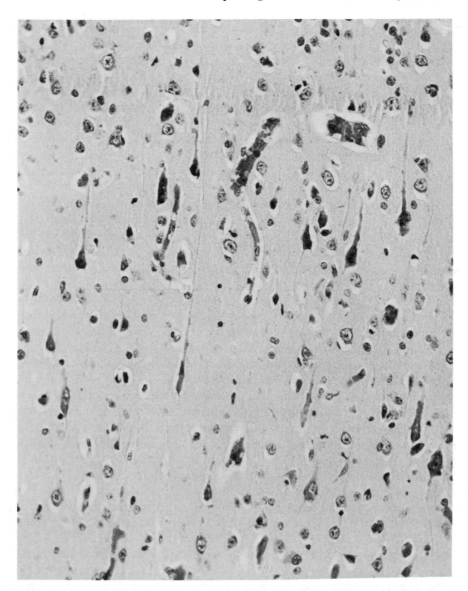

Figure 8–9.   Minimal cortical neuronal hypoxic cerebral damage. Section of precentral (motor) cortex. In the upper part of the illustration large pyramidal-shaped neurones (Betz cells) show acute hypoxic damage, appearing shrunken, deeply staining, with loss of fine architectural markings; in contrast nerve cells in the lower portion of the illustration are anatomically more preserved with nuclei and nucleoli well defined. From a term infant with respiratory depression, lived one day. (Case SMA 68–47, A. Towbin, *The Journal of the American Medical Association,* 1971.)

As evident in human acute perinatal case material, in the mature fetus and newborn, cortical cerebral damage may be diffuse or focal, patchy.

In diffuse cortical damage, with broad areas of the cerebrum affected, the brain externally appears swollen, congested, and often shows thromboses of superficial veins. Microscopically, distinctive changes are evident; the cortex becomes punctuated by shrunken, deeply staining neurones which appear singly or in clusters, as demonstrated in Figure 8–9 (a section of cortex from a one-day-old infant with respiratory depression). Some of the shriveled necrotic neurones are quickly wiped out by the oxygen deprivation; neighboring cells, appearing of similar caste and form, but having a higher threshold and proving more durable, remain unchanged and survive.

Parenthetically it should be recalled that, unlike the functional cells in the liver, kidney, and other basic organs, in the brain there is no regeneration of destroyed mature neurones; the deficit is permanent.

It is likely that the loss of mature neurones resulting from hypoxia is qualitative in nature. As in any population subjected to a noxious milieu, it is likely that with exposure to hypoxia, highly specialized members, the most differentiated cells, the prime neuronal elements, succumb first.

With diffuse cortical hypoxic neuronal loss, the cellular depopulation may be so lightly and evenly spread as to escape detection microscopically. A depletion of neurones up to 30% may go unrecognized even by experienced neuropathologists. Scholz has emphasized that posthypoxic neuronal loss such as this, diffusely distributed, although inconspicuous anatomically, may ultimately lead to significant cerebral disability (1956).

In the term fetus and newborn, with exposure to hypoxia somewhat protracted, the cortex may develop minimal lesions of focal, patchy form (Figure 8–10). In infants surviving, the small islands of damaged cortical tissue undergo "healing" leaving contracted scars of the cerebral convolutional surface. Such chronic hypoxic lesions may be associated with functional cerebral distrubances manifest in later life, as occurred in the following case example.

The case history indicated that the pregnancy was at term, that there was difficulty in delivery, and after prolonged labor, cesarian section was resorted to. The newborn was considered in good condition in the delivery room. The mother noted no abnormalities during infancy, but during early school years the child was described as "nervous" by her teachers; she was withdrawn from regular school because of emotional disturbances. She had difficulty in learning to read and was considered moderately retarded. She developed increasing personality changes, with periods of fantasy and delusions, and was institutionalized at 18 years of age with the diagnosis of schizophrenia. Physical examination revealed slight spasticity of the left extremities with hyperactive reflexes. She remained institutionalized; death occurred at age 42 years. At autopsy the cerebrum showed a circumscribed depressed contracted area of remote cortical infarction in the right frontal lobe (Figure 8–11). In this case, with history of hypoxia complications at birth, the cortical lesion provided the organic basis for the development of neurologic signs and behavioral disturbances elaborated during life.

MECHANICAL INJURY IN THE NEWBORN

The occurrence of direct mechanical injury in the fetus and newborn, though of much less importance than hypoxic damage, is of significance. Direct injury to the skull, fractures due to application of obstetrical forceps, once prominently portrayed, is in fact extremely rare. Intracranial hemorrhage, although more commonly due to hypoxic cerebral damage, may result from tearing of soft tissue

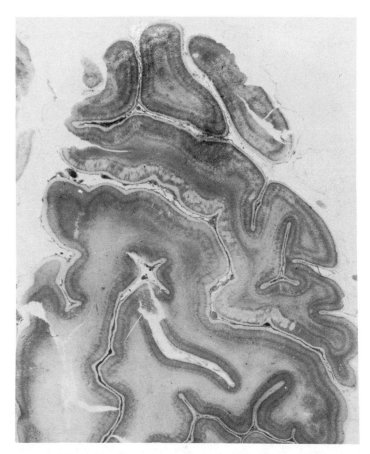

Figure 8–10.   Minimal cortical focal, patchy hypoxic cerebral damage. Section through frontal lobe convolutions; cortex well differentiated, with well-defined laminar architecture (term gestation). In the middle portion of the illustration the cortex shows patchy confluent pale areas of hypoxic infarctional necrosis. Mature stillborn infant; severe intrauterine hypoxia with fetal death prior to onset of labor due to retroplacental hemorrhage (premature detachment of placenta from uterine wall). (Case WM W –18, A. Towbin, *The Journal of the American Medical Association*, 1971.)

structures around the brain. Such hemorrhage proves to be essentially an all-or-none phenomenon, at times being responsible for fetal-neonatal death, but it is of relatively limited importance compared to hypoxia as a cause of chronic neurologic sequels.

The main form of physical trauma, as revealed in the Collaborative Perinatal Project investigations (1965), proves to be spinal cord and brain stem injury, incurred as the fetus is expressed through the birth canal and extracted at delivery (Towbin, 1969). This kind of injury is common in the newborn, present in over 10% of cases examined at autopsy. Such injury, with damage to vital regulatory centers in the brain stem and cord, may have direct effects, causing respiratory depression, and often results in stillbirth or death soon after delivery. Or the damaging effects may be indirect, the respiratory depression present leading secondarily to varying severity of cerebral hypoxic damage.

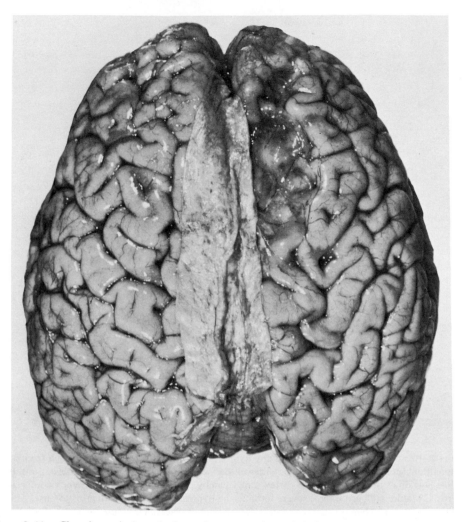

Figure 8–11.   Chronic cortical cerebral scarring, remote hypoxic lesion related to complicated birth. Right frontal lobe with circumscribed old infarction, depressed area of contracted distorted convolutions near the midline. The strip of dura on the surface of the cerebrum, lying midline between the hemispheres, contains the superior longitudinal dural sinus, the main channel for venous drainage of this surface of the cerebrum; the lower portion of this channel is patent, appearing as an irregular open trough gradually narrowing above; the upper part of this venous channel, adjoining the scarred convolutions on the right, is occluded by fibrous tissue, the consequence of a remote thrombosis. Brain specimen from an adult, 42 years old, with history of an hypoxic term delivery. Clinically with slight left-sided spasticity; moderate mental retardation and behavior problem in early life; schizophrenic manifestations in adulthood. (Case DA 69–59, A. Towbin, *The Journal of the American Medical Association*, 1971.)

SEQUELS OF PERINATAL NERVOUS SYSTEM INJURY: CLINICAL-PATHOLOGIC PATTERNS

Mechanical Injury

Direct injury to the brain stem with damage to cranial nerves may be the cause of hearing deficiency, disorders of deglutition, or imbalance in eye muscle function. Severe spinal injury may cause paraplegia from birth. Damage to the spinal cord may be less crippling, of minor degree, latent, the effects masked. As Ford (1966) has indicated, many cases of minor perinatal injury of the cord with mild impairment of neurologic function go unrecognized. Children with such disability, with this form of minimal neurologic dysfunction, are sometimes mistakenly considered to have "mild cerebral palsy" or are regarded as "clumsy children."

Hypoxic Injury

The late clinical manifestations of perinatal hypoxic brain damage are directly correlated with the gestational age at the time of incurrence of the damage and, correspondingly, with the location of the damage in the brain.

In the premature—in the newborn with extensive cerebral hypoxic injury, with destruction in the basal ganglia and other deep structures—in the immediate postnatal period the picture is that of total neurologic collapse, diffuse flaccid motor paralysis, with depression of respiration and other vital function. With less severe cerebral damage, in children that survive, varying severity of cerebral disabilities, sensory-motor paralyses, athetosis, and other dysfunctions that characterize cerebral palsy appear. The axiom applied clinically is, "Cerebral palsy is the disease of prematures." Thus children born prematurely, bearing deep cerebral lesions of minor degree, may present the *formes frustes* of cerebral palsy—tics, awkwardness, and other mild motor dysfunctions.

With severe prematurity, with hypoxia, there may be diffuse infarctional brain damage and subsequent disability in all spheres of cerebral function in children who survive. In very small prematures (1500 g or less), in addition to high incidence of cerebral palsy, 25% of those surviving have an I.Q. of 80 or less (Berendes, 1968).

In the mature newborn, the primary sign of hypoxic cerebral injury clinically is the occurrence of organized convulsive seizures which reflect cortical damage. Organized bodily seizures are essentially of cortical origin and do not occur until the cerebral cortex becomes mature, at term. (Accordingly seizures do not appear in the premature newborn.)

With severe cortical damage in surviving children the predominant cerebral sequel is mental retardation. Many of these children, with epileptogenic lesions imprinted in the cortex, have seizure disorders. Some affected children, higher level retardates, are extremely hyperactive with difficult behavior problems, manifestly psychotic. These late sequels that appear, defects in cerebral function, convulsive disease—whether of major or minimal form—specifically reflect cerebral *cortical* damage.

Predictably, cases with overlapping patterns occur with both deep and cortical damage manifest. With hypoxic damage diffuse, with all spheres of cerebral function compromised, the complete syndromic tetralogy—mental retardation, cerebral palsy, epilepsy, and psychopathy—appears.

Clinically and pathologically in the diagnosis of central nervous system disorders, there is need for more attention to be given to the perinatal history, to details concerned with complications of pregnancy and delivery. Regrettably in many cases the details of the pregnancy and birth records are vague, incomplete when information is sought retrospectively.

Latent neurologic effects of neonatal hypoxia are sometimes minimized or are overlooked clinically. Infants with hypoxic birth, with low Apgar score (indicating depressed neurologic, respiratory, circulatory function), particularly prematures, when examined during the first year have neurologic abnormalities in up to 10% of cases, apparently reflecting organic damage. However, in many cases, demonstrable neurologic abnormalities decrease or disappear by the age of four years. It has been implied that such infantile neurologic deviations are not of substantial importance, often being considered "functional" or "physiological." Indeed, if the infant is not carefully scutinized neurologically in his early years, the entire sequence escapes detection. The affected child, his original potential reduced, may grow up being "within normal limits," but not gifted. Or neurologic abnormalities may recur later in childhood or adolescence, surfacing as manifest cerebral dysfunctions.

The enigmatic occurrence of cerebral palsy, mental retardation, and related cerebral dysfunctions in cases with history of "uncomplicated gestation and delivery" requires comment. It should be emphasized that in some instances pathologic intrauterine processes occur that are damaging to the fetus, subjecting the fetus to varying periods of sublethal hypoxia, processes that are occult, silent, producing no maternal symptoms. In addition, relevant information, especially pathologic changes in the placenta portending future disability in the offspring, is commonly overlooked in the delivery room. In such cases, at birth, with no external manifestations immediately evident, the newborn who bears latent cerebral damage is pronounced "a good baby," but may subsequently develop cerebral palsy or other cerebral dysfunctions.

In assessing the effects of perinatal brain damage, it is evident that the prematurely born are especially vulnerable, at high risk. The high incidence of major as well as minor cerebral dysfunctions in children prematurely born is well documented (Lubchenco, et al., 1963; Harper and Wiener, 1965; Drillien, 1972; Churchill, et al., 1974). The premature are not merely "immature," but are born damaged, often. Premature labor is commonly preceded by vaginal bleeding and other clinical symptoms, the effects of pathologic changes in the placenta, such as infarction or premature separation of the placenta. These intrauterine processes often develop gradually, subjecting the fetus to varying severity of nutritional and oxygen deprivation in the period prior to delivery. Premature infants consequently often bear hypoxic damage, of major or minor extent, at the time of delivery. Additionally, in the premature, hypoxic brain damage initiated *prenatally* is frequently compounded, increased *postnatally* by the common complicating occurrence of hyaline membrane disease or other respiratory disorders during the first weeks after birth. Paradoxically, sophisticated present-day intensive care unit techniques manage to salvage a high precent of brain damaged premature newborn; however the ability to save the lives of these infants has outdistanced the medical capability to maintain the integrity of the cerebral structure. For the premature, deprived in utero, born before its time, organically rejected, unready and fragile, expressed through a physiologically unprepared, unrelaxed birth canal—sequelant cerebral dysfunction is an imminent threat.

Birth, whether premature or at term, is the most endangering experience to which most individuals are ever exposed. The perinatal period has a death rate greater than at any other time of life. The birth process, even under optimal, controlled conditions, is a potentially injurious, crippling event for the fetus. The processes of gestation and birth expose the fetus to many hypoxic and mechanical life-threatening complications. Biologically the components of the maternal-placental-fetal organization, expecially the oxygenating mechanisms, are delicately balanced, easily compromised. The hazards confronting the fetus mount to a climax during the hours of labor. At delivery the fetus is subjected to rapid, often turbulent, alterations in environment and is required to make complicated changes in circulation and respiration. For the fetus during its marginal existence *in utero* and as it is pistoned down the birth canal and separated, some degree of hypoxic and mechanical damage to the nervous system is inescapable.

Gestation and birth form thus an inexorable leveling mechanism. With the brain blighted at birth, the potential for cerebral function may be reduced from that of a genius to that of a plain child, or less. The damage may be slight; often the borderline between what is physiological and what is pathological is not distinct. Often the damage is imperceptible clinically; or it may spell the difference between brothers, one a dexterous athlete, the other an awkward child. Substantially, it is said, all of us have a touch of cerebral palsy, mental retardation, or other cerebral dysfunction, some more, some less—the endowment pathologically of gestation and birth.

REFERENCES

Arey, J. B., and G. W. Anderson. "Pathology of the newborn," in J. P. Greenhill, ed., *Obstetrics*, 13th ed. Philadelphia: Saunders, 1965.

Banker, B. Q., and J. C. Larroche. "Periventricular leukomalacia of infancy." *Archives of Neurology*, 7, 386–410, (1962).

Bankl, H., and K. Jellinger. "Zentralnervöse Schäden nach fetaler Kohlenoxydvergiftung." *Beitraege zur Pathologischen Anatomie und zur Allgemeinen Pathologie*, 135, 350–376, (1967).

Berendes, H. *Medical Tribune*, 9, 20, (1968). [Berendes quoted.]

Brand, M. M., and A. Bignami. "The effects of chronic hypoxia on the neonatal and infantile brain." *Brain*, 92, 233–254, (1969).

Churchill, J. A., R. I. Masland, A. A. Naylor, and M. R. Ashworth. "The etiology of cerebral palsy in pre-term infants." *Developmental Medicine and Child Neurology*, 16, 143–149, (1974).

Collaborative Perinatal Project: "Collaborative Study of Cerebral Palsy, Mental Retardation, and other Neurologic and Sensory Disorders of Infancy and Childhood." Research Profile No. 11. Public Health Service Publication No. 1370. Bethesda, Md.: National Institute of Neurological Disease and Blindness, NIH, (1965).

Courville, C. B. *Birth and Brain Damage*. Pasadena, Cal.: Margaret Farnsworth Courville, Publisher, 1971.

Csermely, H. "Perinatal anoxic changes of the central nervous system." *Acta Paediatrica Academiae Scientiarum Hungaricae*, 13, 283–299, (1972).

Dalén, P. "Family history, the electroencephalogram and perinatal factors in manic conditions." *Acta Psychiatrica Scandinavica*, 41, 527–563, (1965).

Drillien, C. M. "Aetiology and outcome in low-birthweight infants." *Developmental Medicine and Child Neurology*, 14, 563–584, (1972).

Ford, F. R. *Diseases of the Nervous System in Infancy, Childhood, and Adolescence.* Springfield, Ill.: Thomas, 1966.

Garmezy, N., and S. Streitman. "Children at risk: The search for the antecedents of schizophrenia. Conceptual models and research methods. Pregnancy and birth complications." *Schizophrenia Bulletin* No. 8, 28–30, (1974).

Hallervorden, J. "Über eine Kohlenoxydvergiftung im Fetalleben mit Entwicklungsstörungen der Hirnrinde." *Allgemeine Zeitschrift für Psychiatrie und Psychisch-Gerichtliche Medizin,* 124, 289–298, (1949).

Hallervorden, J., and J. E. Meyer. "Cerebrale Kinderlähmung," in F. Henke, O. Lubarsch, and R. Rössle, eds., *Handbuch der speziellen Pathologischen Anatomie und Histologie. Nervensystem,* vol. 13. part 4, pp. 194–282. Berlin: Springer-Verlag, 1956.

Harper, P. A., and G. Wiener. "Sequels of low birth weight." *Annual Review of Medicine,* 16, 405–420, (1965).

Kalbag, R. M., and A. L. Woolf. *Cerebral Venous Thrombosis.* New York: Oxford University Press, 1967.

Knobloch, H., and B. Pasamanick. "Syndrome of minimal cerebral damage in infancy." *The Journal of the American Medical Association,* 170, 1384–1387, (1959).

Lubchenco, L. O., F. A. Horner, L. H. Reed, I. E. Hix, D. Metcalf, R. Cohig, H. C. Elliott, and M. Bourg. "Sequelae of premature birth." *American Journal of Diseases of Children,* 106, 101–115, (1963).

Little, W. J. "On the influence of abnormal parturition, difficult labour, premature birth and asphyxia neonatorum on the mental and physical condition of the child especially in relation to deformities." *Lancet,* 2, 378–380, (1861).

Malamud, N., H. H. Itabasi, J. Castor et al, "An etiologic and diagnostic study of cerebral palsy." *Journal of Pediatrics,* 65, 270–293, (1964).

Mednick, S. A. "Breakdown in individuals at high risk for schizophrenia: Possible predispositional perinatal factors." *Mental Hygiene,* 54, 50–63, (1970).

Meyers, R. E. "Two patterns of perinatal brain damage and their conditions of occurrence." *American Journal of Obstetrics and Gynecology,* 112, 246–276, (1972).

Neubuerger, F. "Fall einer Intrauterinen Hirnschädigung nach Leuchtgasvergiftung der Mutter." *Beitraege zur Gerichtlichen Medizin,* 13, 85–95, (1935).

Norwood Perinatal Project: "Profile of research program." Project Protocol Publication No. 2. Norwood, Mass.: Department of Pathology and Department of Obstetrics and Gynecology, Norwood Hospital, (1970).

Pasamanick, B., M. E. Rogers, and A. M. Lilienfeld. "Pregnancy experience and the development of behavior disorder in children." *American Journal of Psychiatry,* 112 (2), 613–618, (1956).

Rosen, E. J. "Behavioral and emotional disturbances associated with cerebral dysfunction." *Applied Therapeutics,* 11, 531–543, (1969).

Scholz, W. "Die nicht zu Erweichung führenden unvollständigen Gewebsnekrosen (Elektive Parenchymnekrose)," in F. Henke, O. Lubarsh, R. Rössle, eds., *Handbuch der Speziellen Pathologischen Anatomie und Histologie: Nervensystem,* vol. 13, part 1, pp. 1284–1325. Berlin: Springer-Verlag, 1956.

Strauss, A. A., and N. C. Kephart. *Psychopathology and Education of the Brain-Injured Child,* vol. II. New York: Grune & Stratton, 1955.

Strauss, A. A., and L. A. Lehtinen. *Psychopathology and Education of the Brain-Injured Child,* vol. I. New York: Grune & Stratton, 1947.

Schwartz, P. *Birth Injuries of the Newborn: Morphology, Pathogenesis, Clinical Pathology and Prevention.* New York: Hafner, 1961.

Taft, L. T., and W. Goldfarb. "Prenatal and perinatal factors in childhood schizophrenia." *Developmental Medicine and Child Neurology,* 6(1), 32–43, (1964).

Towbin, A. "Pathology of cerebral palsy: I. Developmental defects of the brain as a cause of cerebral palsy." *Archives of Pathology*, 59, 397–411, (1955a).

———"Pathology of cerebral palsy: II. Cerebral palsy due to encephaloclastic processes." *Archives of Pathology*, 59, 529–552, (1955b).

———*The Pathology of Cerebral Palsy*. Springfield, Ill.: Thomas, 1960.

———"Cerebral intraventricular hemorrhage and subependymal matrix infarction in the fetus and premature newborn." *American Journal of Pathology*, 52, 121–139, (1968).

———"Latent spinal cord and brain stem injury in newborn infants." *Developmental Medicine and Child Neurology*, 11, 54–68, (1969a).

———"Mental retardation due to germinal matrix infarction." *Science*, 164, 156–161, (1969b).

———"Central nervous system damage in the human fetus and newborn infant." *American Journal of Diseases of Children*, 119, 529–542, (1970).

———"Organic causes of minimal brain dysfunction." *The Journal of the American Medical Association*, 217, 1207–1214, (1971).

———"Syndrome of latent cerebral venous thrombosis: Its frequency and relation to age and congestive heart failure." *Stroke*, 4, 419–430, (1973).

———"Obstetrical factors in fetal-neonatal visceral injury." *Obstetrics and Gynecology*, 52, 113–124, (1978).

Windle, W. F. "Brain damage at birth." *The Journal of the American Medical Association*, 206(9), 1967–1972, (1968).

Yllpö, A. "Pathologish-anatomische Studien bei Frühgeborenen." *Zeitschrift für Kinderheilkunde*, 20, 212–432, (1919).

CHAPTER 9

Environmental Interaction in Minimal Brain Dysfunctions

Emmy E. Werner

The present chapter will integrate and critically evaluate a number of studies published during the last decade, or still in progress, which have examined the role of postnatal environmental factors among the determinants of behavior commonly subsumed under the "minimal brain dysfunction" syndrome (MBD), in infants, children, and adolescents.

THE MULTIFACETED CONCEPT OF MBD

The problems attending the definition(s) of the concept of MBD have been examined at length in Chapter 1. Studies reviewed in this chapter tend to refer to the definition of the U. S. Department of Health, Education, and Welfare's task force on terminology and identification (Clements, 1966) and deal with children:

of near average, average or above average general intelligence, with certain learning or behavioral disabilities, ranging from mild to severe, which are associated with deviations of functions of the central nervous system. These deviations may manifest themselves by various combinations of impairment in perception, conceptualization, language, memory, and control of attention, impulse or motor functions. . . . [pp. 9–10].

This definition is strictly behavioral. More often than not it is based on information provided by parents and/or teachers and a medical/developmental history, suggestive of central nervous system (CNS) impairment. Only a minority of the children so designated show clearly abnormal EEG's or neurological signs of brain damage.

While a clustering of variables, such as hyperactivity, impulsivity, and underachievement is generally assumed, multiple measures of these constructs are seldom utilized and intercorrelations are almost never reported. Recently Nichols, Chen, and Pomeroy (1976) examined the associations among MBD symptoms in a nonclinic sample of 34,556 seven year olds from the Collaborative Perinatal Project. Four major factors, representing *school achievement* (reading/spelling—IQ discrepancy), *hyperactivity/impulsivity,* *"socio-emotional" immaturity,* and *minor neurological signs* were derived. Most children with problems in one area did not have problems in other areas. The risk of problems in one area however increased up to two times for children with problems in another area.

As this review will show, the role of environmental interaction effects among the determinants of minimal brain dysfunctions has not yet been adequately studied in human populations; in turn, the MBD concept has often been applied to childhood learning and behavior disorders that appear to have no demonstrated organic base.

SOURCES OF EVIDENCE

Prospective Studies

The role of environmental interaction in minimal brain dysfunctions has only been examined in a few prospective studies in the United States and Europe. In the United States cohorts of children were followed longitudinally from the perinatal period through infancy, childhood, and/or adolescence, allowing for comparisons at sensitive time periods between children with and without CNS impairment. Prospective research permits the selection of subjects with early characteristics implicated in the etiology of childhood behavior and learning disorders subsumed under the MBD syndrome, such as perinatal risk factors, prematurity, and social conditions. Longitudinal studies have however to deal with the technical problems of maintaining a sample over a considerable length of time and making certain that sample loss is not related to independent variables. The studies cited in this section have managed to do this with low attrition rates.

The Collaborative Perinatal Project

The largest of the longitudinal studies, the *Collaborative Perinatal Project* (CCP), was conducted by the National Institute of Neurological and Communicative Disorders and Stroke (NINCDS). Its population was selected from some 50,000 women registering for prenatal care in 12 university medical centers in mainland United States. Of the women 45% were white, 47% were black, and the rest a variety of other ethnic groups, mostly Puerto Rican. Representatives of many disciplines followed the women during pregnancy and delivery and examined more than 40,000 children from birth through eight years. Published results and studies in progress have focused on the interaction effects of prenatal and early postnatal environmental variables on outcome in the neonatal period, infancy, and at four and seven years (Broman, Nichols, and Kennedy, 1975; Broman, 1977; Nichols, Chen, and Pomeroy, 1976; Nichols, 1977a, 1977b; Niswander and Gordon, 1972).

Among the most recent analyses are a series of studies dealing with MBD (the association among symptoms, perinatal complications, behavior in infancy) and the early development and family characteristics of low achievers (LA) with full scale IQs of 90+ on the WISC, and reading/spelling achievement test scores (on the WRAT) more than one year below grade placement.

The Kauai Longitudinal Study

The prospective study covering the widest range is the *Kauai* longitudinal study. At 1, 2, and 10 years a team of pediatricians, psychologists, public health and social workers examined the interaction effects of perinatal stress and quality of environment on the physical, cognitive, and social development of some 1,000 children—the cohort of 1955 births and a selected sample of "high" risk 1956 births on this Hawaiian island (Werner, et al., 1967; Werner, et al., 1968; Werner, Bierman, and French, 1971). The 18 year follow-up of the 1955 cohort (some 660 children) has now been completed (Werner and Smith, 1977). The children are of Japanese, Filipino, Hawaiian, and mixed Oriental-Polynesian descent and represent a wide socioeconomic status (SES) range.

On the basis of some 60 conditions occurring during prenatal, labor and delivery, and neonatal periods, each infant was initially scored on a four-point scale for severity of perinatal complications. Among the cohort of 1955 births, 56% had no perinatal complications, 31% had mild complications, 13% had moderate complications, and 3 % showed severe complications. By age ten, 3% of the time sample had been diagnosed as probable MBD and referred to a learning disability (LD) class, because of serious reading and communication problems (in spite of WISC IQs in the average or above average range), visual-motor impairment, hyperactivity, and difficulty in attention and concentration. Only one out of five in this group had physical evidence of organicity on pediatric-neurologic examinations, but low birth weight and other perinatal complications were found among nearly half of the LD children.

The Johns Hopkins Study of Premature Infants

In the Johns Hopkins Study approximately 400 low birth-weight and full-term infants were followed from birth to 12–13 years of age. Examinations were conducted at 3–5 years (Harper, Fischer, and Rider, 1959); 6–7 years (Wiener, et al., 1965); 8–10 years (Wiener, 1970; Wiener, et al., 1968); and 12–13 years (Wiener, 1968). The investigations substantiated the association of pre-term birth with increased cognitive, perceptual-motor, and learning problems, but also documented significant interaction effects of social class and maternal attitudes.

The Edinburgh Study of Premature Infants

An important European study is Drillien's (1964) longitudinal follow-up of 595 babies in Edinburgh, Scotland, that analyzed the interaction effects of *both* obstetric and environmental stress on low birth-weight babies. One third of the total sample weighed 4.5 lbs. or less at birth; one third were between 4.5 lbs. and 5.5 lbs.; and one-third weighed 5 lbs. 9 oz. or more. Children were examined at home at half-year intervals between 6 and 18 months and at yearly intervals between 2 and 5 years, and teachers' behavior ratings were obtained at 6–7 years.

The Groningen Study

In Holland, Prechtl and his collaborators have followed several subgroups of infants "at risk" of minor brain dysfunctions and normal controls (Prechtl, 1963; Kalverboer, Touwen, and Prechtl, 1973) from birth through preschool age. These children were randomly selected from the hospital population of full-term newborns in Groningen and were examined by standard neurological examinations. Subgroups of hyperexcitable children and normal controls were observed in their homes in the first year and the mother-child interaction monitored. Fifty-eight babies with abnormal signs on the neonatal examination and 53 normal babies were seen in follow-ups between 18 months and 4 years and maternal behavior was recorded; 147 four to five year olds, half with minor neurological dysfunctions in the neonatal and preschool period and diagnosed as hyperexcitable, hypotonic, or apathetic; the others without suspect signs were observed at play in a nursery school.

Studies of Clinic Populations

There exists a handful of studies of selected samples of children admitted to child guidance or outpatient psychiatric clinics which have examined the role of environmental factors in the MBD syndrome, either at the time of admission in middle childhood and/or as predictors of (good/poor) outcome in follow-ups in adolescence. These studies suffer from a number of methodological shortcomings, that is selection bias, lack of appropriate controls, and often high attrition rates at follow-up. They tend to focus on the *hyperactive child syndrome* with (secondary) behavior problems (with or without additional MBD symptoms). For example hyperactive children (N: 54–83) admitted to the outpatient department of the St. Louis Children's Hospital appear to have been selected on the basis of a *history* of being hyperactive, and distractible, but without associated cognitive, language, reading, coordination, or neurological dysfunctions (Morrison and Stewart, 1971; Mendelson, Johnson, and Stewart, 1971; Stewart, Mendelson, and Johnson, 1973). In contrast hyperactive children (N: 64–91) admitted to the outpatient psychiatric clinic of the Montreal Children's Hospital had a wide variety of minor neurological, behavioral, and cognitive signs of MBD, though their intelligence was in the normal range (Weiss, et al., 1971; Minde, Weiss, and Mendelson, 1972).

An additional series of cross-sectional studies, dealing with different time samples of MBD children admitted to the Child Development Clinic of the University Hospital of Iowa City have been published by Alley and Solomons (1971) and Paternite, Loney, and Langhorne (1976). Relationships among (primary and secondary) symptomatology, socioeconomic status and parenting styles were examined for 113 hyperkinetic (HK)/MBD boys from intact families. Primary symptoms were hyperactivity, fidgetiness, inattention, impulsivity, negative affect, excitability, irritability, and lack of coordination. Secondary symptoms were aggressive interpersonal behavior, no impulse control, and self-esteem deficits.

Studies of Children in Special Education Programs

With one notable exception studies of learning disabled (LD) or educationally handicapped (EH) children enrolled in special education classes suffer from similar methodological shortcomings as the studies of MBD children admitted to clinics: lack of comparability of definitions, selection bias, and absence of appropriate controls. Probably the most carefully designed study in this group that focuses on environmental determinants was undertaken by Owen, et al., (1971) in Palo Alto, California. A total of 304 Ss, 76 quartets of children (mean age: 10 years) and their parents made up the sample. Included were 76 EH children (2% of the population of the school district) and their same-sex sibling, and 76 matched academically successful children and their same-sex sibling. A child was considered "educationally handicapped" if she or he had a significant discrepancy between ability and school achievement (1.5 to 2 years below grade level expectancy in reading and/or spelling, with a full scale IQ of 90 or above on the WISC). Among this group were 17 (approximately 20%) who showed abnormal findings on medical-neurological examinations and medical history data.

At the same time, Koppitz (1971) completed a five-year follow-up of 177 children who had been enrolled between the ages of 6 and 12 years in an LD program in New York City. A child was considered to have a learning disability if his school achievement was more than one year below his mental age and he could not profit from attendance in a regular public school class, despite normal intellectual potential and a lack of gross motor impairment. More than 90% of this LD group were also hyperactive. Koppitz analyzed *both* the medical and developmental history and the social background at the time of admission and their relationship to outcome five years later.

From the University of Arkansas' Medical Center comes a report on family structure and family relations of 31 LD/MBD boys and 22 normal controls, first seen between the ages of 8 and 12 years and followed at age 14 years by Dykman, et al., (1973). The diagnosis of LD was based on school and parents' reports and actual or impending failure in reading, spelling, and arithmetic, in spite of normal intelligence. Each subject received a special neurological examination and his EEG was monitored.

Experimental subjects in cross-sectional studies were either drawn from special schools (Denhoff, 1973), special classes (Touliatos and Lindholm, 1974) or from normal classroom settings (Clarkson and Hayden, 1972) and ranged in age from 5 through 10 years (K–grade 5). Only the last study included neurological evaluations of children rated hyperactive by their teachers.

A NOTE ON THE ASSESSMENT OF ENVIRONMENTAL VARIABLES

Most of the studies examining the role of environmental interaction in children "at risk" for or with MBD symptoms have dealt with global status variables, such as social class, parental income, employment, education, or parental (usually maternal) medical and psychiatric history. The impact of these environmental variables has been most often considered singly without much attention to interaction and multiplier effects.

Only a few of the prospective studies and the intervention studies with high-risk infants have dealt with environmental *process* variables and have utilized behavior observations of caregiver-child interactions in free play or in response to an experimental situation in the hospital, at home, or in school.

The impact of the family environment has usually been demonstated through indirect methods with heavy emphasis on recall (with its attending problems of reliability) via parental (usually maternal) interview; parent attitude research inventories, such as the one by Schaefer and Bell (1958); and reports of child-rearing practices by the mother.

Within the family the contribution of the father has been infrequently assessed, though his influence may be crucial in the development of a syndrome that afflicts mostly boys. Least attention has been paid to the role of siblings and other relatives.

In addition to the relative lack of specific observations of the transaction process between the child "at risk" or with MBD signs and caregivers within his family, the role of the extrafamilial environment, that is peers, teachers, and cultural (especially sex role) expectations as well as the impact of the physical environment (open space versus enclosure, crowding) have rarely been explored. This, in spite of the fact that the MBD syndrome is behaviorally defined as a lack of acceptable behavior in school, with peers, or as inappropriate expression of motor activity.

THE EVIDENCE

I shall first examine the accumulated evidence on status variables that appear to make a persistent impact on the behavior of children "at risk" for or with signs of MBD *across their whole developmental history.* I shall then review the scattered evidence on environmental process variables, that is specific caregiver dimensions that appear to facilitate or impede the development of a constitutionally vulnerable child at sensitive time periods.

Socioeconomic Status

The studies reviewed here have yet to produce a predictive variable more powerful than social status and family characteristics of the caretaking environment. In our follow-up studies at ages 2, 10, and 18 years on the island of Kauai (Werner, Bierman, and French, 1971) there was a significant interaction between the effects of SES and perinatal complications which produced the largest deficits for the most disadvantaged children. The short- and long-term impact of SES appeared more powerful than the residual effects of perinatal complications, except for a small group of children with moderate and severe perinatal stress. Ten times more children had learning and behavior problems related to the effects of a poor environment than to the effects of perinatal complications.

As early as age 20 months, these interaction effects were seen in several ways:

1. Children growing up in (upper) middle class homes who had experienced the most severe perinatal complications had mean scores on the Cattell Infant Intelligence Scale (at this age largely a measure of sensorimotor development) almost comparable to children with *no* perinatal stress who were living in lower SES homes.
2. The most developmentally retarded children (in physical, intellectual, and social maturity) were those who had both experienced the most severe perinatal complications and who were also living in the poorest homes.
3. Social status differences provided for a greater difference in mean Cattell scores (37 points) for children who had experienced severe perinatal stress than did perinatal complications for children living in favorable environments.

By age 10, postnatal environmental influences were even more powerful:

1. Children with and without severe perinatal stress who had grown up in (upper) middle class homes both achieved mean PMA IQ and factor scores (including reading, verbal, spatial, perceptual, and numerical factors) well above the average (Werner, Simonian, and Smith, 1967).

2. PMA IQ scores were seriously depressed in children of low social status, particularly if they had experienced severe perinatal hazards.
3. The family's SES showed significant associations with the type of behavior that is usually subsumed under the MBD syndrome, that is language problems, perceptual problems, reading problems, and overaggressive behavior.

Three out of four children considered in need of placement in a LD class came from low SES homes (Werner and Smith, 1977). However among the youth in this time sample who had delinquency records between the ages of 10 and 18 years, a significantly higher proportion of (upper) middle class than of lower class adolescents had been diagnosed at birth as having "chronic conditions probably leading to MBD" (that is anoxia, prematurity, and other obstetrical complications).

The prevailing impact of SES at birth and at school age on children "at risk" or with MBD symptoms has also been documented by Broman (1977) who reports from the CPP on a subgroup of the syndrome, children with significant discrepancies between (normal) IQ and (poor) reading/spelling achievement (LA). A comparison of the LAs with academically successful controls, matched by IQ and race, showed that indices of SES prior to birth and at age seven were more strongly related to low achievement than Apgar scores, obstetrical complications, and neurological soft signs at age seven (though the latter were significantly more frequent among both black and white underachievers than among IQ matched controls).

In Drillien's (1964) study, an interactional effect, favoring the most advantaged babies of high birth weight was evident at age four. Term babies living in higher SES homes performed better than pre-term babies reared in comparable SES homes. However, very low birth-weight infants (3.5 lbs.) were at less of a disadvantage in better-off homes than very low birth-weight babies living in poor homes. By the ages of five to seven years, few pre-term children from middle class homes had problems in school, except when birth weight had been below 3.5 lbs., while in poor homes there was a marked excess of children with learning problems in all birth weight categories.

In the Johns Hopkins Study, pre-term babies whose IQs rose rather than declined from the three to five years to the six to seven years period, all grew up in upper social status homes (Wiener, Rider, and Oppel 1963).

Studies of children in special education programs and/or referred to outpatient guidance (psychiatric) clinics report significant associations between SES and two symptom groups subsumed under the MBD syndrome, hyperactivity and behavior problems. Among 85 children attending a special school for MBD children (Denhoff, 1973), nonhyperactive children came from higher social class families, were clumsier, had less adequate speech and language related abilities and more right/left discrimination problems than their peers. Hyperactive MBD children had parents in lower social classes, weighed less at birth and had a greater number of emotional problems than their nonhyperactive peers.

In a time series of 113 HK/MBD boys (mean age 8.2 years), seen initially for outpatient evaluation at the Child Psychiatry Service of the University of Iowa (Paternite, *et al.*, 1976), the primary symptom of hyperactivity did not vary as a function of SES, but SES related differences emerged for secondary symptoms, that is aggressive interpersonal behavior, impulse control, and self-esteem deficits.

In a series of follow-up studies of hyperactive MBD school children seen as outpatients at Montreal's Children's Hospital no significant SES differences were found upon initial referral, but low SES status (interacting with a positive history of CNS damage and initial hyperactivity) was a significant predictor of poor outcome in a follow-up study five years later when the children ranged in age from 11 to 17 (mean 13.4) Minde, Weiss, and Mendelson (1972).

Likewise in her follow-up of 177 LD children, Koppitz (1971) found that a child's social background was more closely related to his progress five years after entry into the special education program than his diagnostic label (MBD) or his medical/developmental history.

Two comprehensive reviews of the influence of social class on child development (Deutsch, 1973) and socialization (Hess, 1970) remind us however that social class is not a unitary variable, but an aggregate (Deutsch, 1973). This aggregate appears to subsume not just fixed structural features of a social system (power, prestige, access to information and services) but other environmental features which influence behavior and which are not necessarily a part of the SES system.

The external configuration of the physical and social environment shows both between and within social class variations, probably more so than do expressed values (Hess, 1970). This includes persistent differences in physical condition, space, resources in the home, the display of order and routine as against disorder and unpredictability, and in children's exposure to physical and verbal exchanges that occur between adults and between adults and children.

The Physical Environment

There are only a few tantalizing clues about the impact of the physical environment on the behavior of children "at risk" for developmental retardation or with MBD symptoms. Reinforcement theorists have maintained that hyperactivity for example is a function of the contingencies that the child meets in his environment (Bower and Mercer, 1975) and Cruickshank and his associates (1961) stress that restructuring the environment should be an important aspect of educational intervention in brain-injured and hyperactive children. Yet little systematic research has been done on the effect of the *physical* environment on the development of MBD children. A study of home environments for 30 infants at increased risk for MBD (15 of whom were attending a day-care intervention program and 15 who were not) showed significant differences between high-risk groups and 30 control infants from the general population (matched by age, sex, and parity) in the organization of the environment, the availability of appropriate toys, and opportunity for variety (Ramey, et al., 1975). The possible effects of a barren physical environment can only be inferred from the findings of a study which employed videotaped observations of free-field behavior: Kalverboer and associates (1973) report that among 4-5-year-old Dutch children, boys with "soft" neurological signs of MBD (and hyperactivity or hypotonicity/apathy) showed more inconsistency in motor activity and play behavior in "sensory depriving" and "nonmotivating" situations (that is alone in an empty room without a variety of toys) than did boys who were neurologically intact. The neurologically impaired preschool children showed a significant drop in visual exploration from the first to the second encounter in an empty room, a change that was not found in the neurologically intact children.

Crowding may also seriously restrict opportunities for self-initiated exploration, an important antecedent of achievement motivation: Broman (1977) for example reports significant differences in housing density prior to birth and in number of people in the household at age seven between both black and white LD children and IQ and race matched controls from the CPP.

Parental Malaise

A number of prospective and retrospective follow-up studies with special school and clinic samples have shown an interaction effect between parental illness and behavior problems among children "at risk" for or with MBD symptoms, that is independent of social class. The mother's illness appears to make a more important impact on attachment behavior in the preschool years, the father's illness or deviancy may contribute to antisocial behavior in middle childhood and adolescence (Rutter, 1974).

Drillien (1964) found that stress due to incapacitating and chronic mental or physical ill health of the mother gave a more accurate rating of environmental factors than using social grade. In her longitudinal study, the difference in incidence and type of behavior problems (between birth and two; and two and five years) between the small prematures and the mature controls was more obvious where there had been this type of environmental stress.

Serious mental or physical illness of one or both parents, chronic disability of one or both parents (for example blindness, deafness, severe crippling by arthritis or alcoholism) was one of four significant predictors of poor outcome (for example hospitalization) among school-age children in the LD program followed by Koppitz (1971) five years later.

Poor mental health of parents was also found to discriminate between hyperactive youth seen at Montreal's Children's Hospital (Weiss, el al., 1971) who became delinquent in adolescence from those who did not. No other initial evaluation predicted antisocial behavior better.

Morrison and Stewart (1971) report a high prevalence of sociopathy, hysteria, alcoholism, and affective disorders (bipolar and depression) in *both* mothers and fathers of children with the hyperactive syndrome that differentiated them significantly from controls admitted to the St. Louis Children's Hospital for surgery. In their follow-up at 12 to 16 years, the more antisocial youth were likelier to have a father who had been arrested several times or who had mental health problems (Mendelson, Johnson, and Stewart, 1971). Morrison and Stewart (1971) note that these findings could lend themselves to either an environmental or genetic interpretation of the origin of the hyperactive child syndrome; they stress however that, regardless of etiology, an ill parent will teach the child by example (modeling) or by selectively reinforcing active behavior.

Father Absence

Prolonged absence of the father, either because of desertion, divorce, separation, or extended service in the military has been found to be associated with learning and behavior problems in children who showed MBD symptoms. This association in both the CPP and the Kauai longitudinal study appeared across a wide range of SES and ethnicity and underscores the important, but neglected, role of the father in child development (Lynn, 1974).

The debilitating effects of father absence was demonstrated in two ways: (1) a

higher proportion of LD/MBD children when matched with academically successful controls for age, IQ, SES, or race were found to come from homes where the
father was absent at birth (Broman, 1977) or in early childhood (Drillien, 1964;
Broman, 1977) and (2) the likelihood that children diagnosed as LD/MBD would
develop serious behavior problems in middle childhood or adolescence, requiring
either hospitalization (Koppitz, 1971) or more than six months of (outpatient)
treatment in a mental health clinic, was significantly increased when there was
prolonged absence of the father in early childhood (Werner and Smith, 1977).

Family Stability and the Emotional Climate of the Home

In a number of longitudinal studies of children "at risk" for MBD, because of
perinatal complications or prematurity as well as in cross-sectional and follow-up
studies of children with learning disabilities or the hyperactivity syndrome, ratings of family instability were found to contribute significantly to developmental
retardation in infancy and to serious learning and behavior problems in childhood.

In the Kauai longitudinal study we evaluated family stability by using information from home interviews postpartum and at one and two years that gave evidence of family cohesiveness or upheaval. The correlation between SES and
family stability ratings was low (r .21). But the difference in mean Cattell IQs
around age two between children who had experienced severe perinatal stress,
but were growing up in a (very) stable early family environment (94), and those
with severe perinatal complications growing up in an unstable early family environment (77), was nearly as dramatic as that found for SES (Werner, Bierman,
and French, 1971).

Among children who at birth had been diagnosed as having "chronic conditions
probably leading to MBD" the highest proportion with serious mental health
problems, at age 10, came from homes that were (very) unstable in early childhood. In contrast the rates of serious mental health problems among children at
increased risk for MBD at birth were much smaller for those who had grown up in
stable homes. The rates were comparable to those of children without perinatal
complications.

Interaction effects between family stability, obstetrical complication, and low
birth weight were also documented by Drillien (1964). She divided her families
into those providing a relatively stable environment in the preschool period and
those where the child had been subjected to instability of a degree which might be
expected to affect behavior. At six to seven years teachers rated children of all
birth weights who had been subjected to severe preschool (two to five years)
familial stress as exhibiting more adverse behavior. The effect was most marked
with the low birth-weight babies who had additional perinatal complications.

That children within the same family can be differentially susceptible to disorganization and instability in their home, with a child with MBD symptoms more
vulnerable to this type of stress, has been demonstrated by Owen, et al., (1971).
Families with EH children were more disorganized and less stable than control
families of academically successful children of the same social class. Disorganization and instability were especially marked among families of EH children with
abnormal findings on medical-neurological examinations. Owen, et al., (1971)
speculate that the presence of a neurologically handicapped child within the family increases the probability that the parents will be less able to organize and
structure the home environment and that worry and anxiety will contribute to

emotional instability. They also note that this lack of stability had a much more detrimental effect on the EH child who lived in a different emotional climate than his same-sex sibling.

Among children in normal classroom settings (Clarkson and Hayden, 1972) the presence of a disturbance or disruption in the family seems to increase the likelihood of hyperkinetic behavior, even in the absence of sequelae of neurological damage, especially in the 8 to 10 year range.

The emotional climate and the stability of the family (or lack of it) has also been found to be among the most discriminating predictors of good/poor outcome in follow-ups in adolescence of children with learning disabilities by Koppitz (1971) and of youth with the hyperactivity syndrome by Minde and associates (1972).

Caregiver-Child Interaction

Data on caregiver interactions with children considered at increased risk for MBD (pre-term infants with obstetrical complications) or showing MBD sysptoms come from naturalistic observations in prospective studies of "high risk" infants. They also come from reported child-care practices in cross-sectional and follow-up studies of children with learning disabilities and the hyperactivity syndrome (with or without soft neurological signs). There are very few data on *paternal* child-rearing practices except in middle childhood; transactions between the mother and the MBD child however have been documented from the neonatal period through the school years.

Mother-Neonate Interaction

The diminished contact that mothers have with prematurely born infants may actually diminish the attachment the mother feels toward her new-born baby (Klaus and Kennell, 1970). When mothers of pre-term infants were compared with mothers of full-terms as to their style of contact in the initial meetings, mothers of pre-terms were more tentative in their physical contact and showed less eye-to-eye contact. Increasing the opportunity for early contact with their pre-term neonates in the hospital changed their care-giving styles. Mothers who had been allowed contact during the first 5 days showed many more intervals of cuddling and more en face intervals than mothers separated for 20 days. These differences in maternal behavior persisted and were observed at home one month after discharge.

Residence in hospital nurseries in isolettes may deprive the pre-term infant of proprioceptive stimulation (Solkoff, et al., 1969) and reciprocal stimulus feedback experiences (Siqueland, 1973). Studies of increased handling of prematurely born babies in the nursery show more sustained attention at four months of age (Korner, 1973; Powell, 1974; Siqueland, 1973), more advanced gross and fine motor activity at seven to eight months (Solkoff, et al., 1969), and increased infant test scores at one year (Scarr-Salapatek and Williams, 1973).

Mother-Infant Interaction

The earliest observations of mother-infant interaction in the home that correlated with neurological status have been reported by Beckwith (1978, in press); Beckwith, et al., (1976), and Prechtl (1963).

Among a cohort of prematurely born infants at the UCLA nursery, caregiver-infant interactions were assessed through naturalistic observations in the home at 1, 3, 8, 12, and 24 months. The new-born neurologic score related significantly and negatively with the proportion of time the mother-infant pairs spent in social interaction in the home. Infants who scored at greater neonatal risk were held more sensitively for a greater proportion of their awake time.

Prechtl and associates followed a small group of Dutch infants with abnormal signs on neonatal neurological examinations. The babies in this group were hyperkinetic, cried more than normal, and showed sudden changes of state, from being drowsy and difficult to arouse to being wide awake, crying, and difficult to pacify. Nearly all of their responses were exaggerated and had a low threshold. During home visits at 3, 6, 9, and 12 months the infant-mother interactions were compared with that of a neonatally normal control group. The mothers, as early as 3 months, perceived their neonatally abnormal babies as "temperamental," became overanxious and disquieted, and blamed themselves for mishandling their infants. The results of the PARI showed a significantly higher "approval of activity of the child" and a greater "fostering of dependency" among the mothers of neonatally abnormal than mothers of normal infants.

In the Kauai longitudinal study, at one year a significantly higher proportion of mothers of infants who were later to become learning disabled characterized their offspring as "*not* cuddly, *not* affectionate [and] *not* good natured; fretful" than control mothers from the same SES and ethnic group. A significantly higher proportion of mothers of infants who later were diagnosed as learning disabled were rated as "erratic" or "worrisome" by observers in the home; more control mothers were described as "energetic," "patient," and "happy."

By two, children who later became learning disabled were characterized significantly more often by both mothers and observing psychologists as "awkward," "distractible," "fearful," "insecure," "restless," "slow," and "withdrawn." Controls were more often characterized as "alert," "calm," "quiet," and "responsive." Mothers whose offspring were later to become learning disabled were described in their interactions with their toddlers as "careless," "indifferent," or "overprotective"; control mothers as "kind, temperate," "matter-of-fact," and "content." Apparently a vicious cycle between a "non-rewarding" infant and an increasingly frustrated mother had begun in the first year of life and became aggravated in the second year (Werner and Smith, 1977).

Mother-Child Interaction in the Preschool Years

Drillien's (1964) study shows a significant interaction effect between (low) birth weight, (low) SES, and (adverse) maternal handling between birth and two and between two and five years on children's behavior problems in the preschool and early years.

In high SES homes mishandling was more often observed when birth weight had been 4.5 lbs. or less. This was due to an excess of overanxious and overprotective mothers. In poor working class homes adverse handling most often took the form of physical neglect, permissive, or variable attitudes. There was an increase in incidence and severity of both early (preschool) and later (school-age) behavior problems with adverse maternal handling of low birth-weight infants. Hyperactivity was most common in children of two to five years of age who had either been treated without any control at all or with variable control.

Children subjected to permissive and variable attitudes, physical neglect, and absence of discipline (most common among low SES mothers of low birth-weight infants) showed an excess of hyperactivity, at both preschool (two to five years) and school age (six to seven years). Children of overanxious, overprotective mothers (most common among high SES mothers of low birth-weight babies) showed a marked excess of behavior disturbance in the preschool period, but no more disturbance in school than those whose handling in infancy and the preschool years had been satisfactory.

Parental Interaction in the Middle Childhood Years

At this age distinctions have been made in some studies between parental interaction patterns that relate to control of impulse and affect and caregiving practices that relate to intellectual functions and school achievement. A few investigators have also taken a look at the role of the father in transactions with his school-age MBD child.

In the Kauai longitudinal study (Werner, et al., 1968; Werner, Bierman, and French, 1971) ratings of the educational stimulation and emotional support provided by the home were made at age 10 by a clinical psychologist, based on standardized home interviews.

To rate emotional support, we examined the information on interpersonal relations between parents and child, on kind and amount of reinforcement used, on methods of discipline and ways of expressing affection and approval, and on opportunities provided for satisfactory sex role identification.

Educational stimulation was rated by considering the opportunities provided by the family for enlarging the child's vocabulary; the intellectual interests and activities in the home; the values placed by the family on education; the work habits emphasized in the home; the availability of learning supplies, books and periodicals; and the opportunities for exploration of the larger environment.

By age 10 educational stimulation ratings of the home were found to correlate more closely with the children's achievement problems (reading, perceptual, and language) than did measures of SES. Ratings of emotional support in the home differentiated better than the other environmental dimensions between children with and without serious behavior problems at age 10. Among children judged to have chronic conditions possibly leading to MBD at birth, both (very) low educational stimulation ratings and (very) low ratings of emotional support—between 2 and 10 years—led to a significant increase in the proportion of children in need of long-term (6 months) mental health services by age 10. A significantly higher proportion of LD children than SES matched controls at age 10 came from homes rated (very) low in educational and (very) low in emotional support (Werner and Smith, 1977).

In the Johns Hopkins Study of Premature Infants, a modification of the PARI was used to rate the mother's tendency to ignore her child, her emotional involvement with the child, her use of fear in controlling the child, her intellectual interests and achievement striving, and the degree of positive relation between mother and child. Though social class provided the largest component to measures of intellectual functioning, maternal attitudes also contributed and had more influence than (low) birth weight at 12 to 13 years (Wiener, 1968).

In contrast to the predominantly lower class and non-Caucasian children participating in the Kauai and Johns Hopkins studies, the EH children studied by Owen, et al. (1971) came from a privileged suburban university community and did not differ from their academically successful controls in social or economic background. Yet there were significant differences between EH parents and control parents in their perceptions and attitudes toward their children's behavior, their affectional warmth, and their pressure for educational accomplishment.

The EH children were considered by both their mothers and fathers to have more serious problems than either their same-sex siblings or the academically successful controls and their parents worried more about them. Mothers perceived their EH child as having less verbal ability, less impulse control, less ability to structure and organize the environment and more anxiety than control children and same-sex siblings. Mothers of EH children: (1) were more annoyed by them than were mothers of control children and (2) tended to withold affection if the child, in their judgment was irresponsible and disorganized.

Fathers of EH children noted differences in perseverance (in and out of school), motor coordination, impulse control, and anxiety between their EH children and control children. They also noted differences in verbal ability between the EH child and same-sex sibling, but they tended to show less insight into the behavior of their EH children than did fathers of control children. EH children tended to lose the affection of their fathers if they were apathetic or worried, lacked concentration, or could not control their impulses, whereas their fathers did not seem to be affected by these same traits in their same-sex sibling.

Differences between mothers and fathers in expectancies and responsiveness to the needs of their minimally brain-injured children have been reported by Touliatos and Lindholm (1974). They compared 16 middle class families with 8 to 13 year old MBD children (diagnosed on the basis of both medical examinations and psychological tests and enrolled in special education classes) with 16 families with normal children, matched for age, sex, birth order, and education of the father. The mothers of MBD children appeared to have lower expectancies for independence and achievement than mothers of normal children, there were no differences among fathers. Fathers of minimally brain damaged children were more rewarding and less punishing in their reactions to their children's behavior than the fathers of normal children. There were no differences between the mothers.

Paternite, Loney, and Langhorne (1976) have shown that parenting variables were better predictors of secondary behavior problems in hyperkinetic MBD boys than was SES. For the symptom aggressive interpersonal behavior, the most significant seven predictors were: father's love-hostility, spouse-reported "mother's short temper" mother's consistency, spouse-reported mother's shortcomings, self-reported "mother's easygoing," and mother's autonomy-control. For the symptom impulse control deficiency, three predictors resulted: mother's consistency, father's placidity, and mother's short temper. The four significant predictors for the symptom self-esteem dificits were: father's consistency, selfreported "mother's strictness," mother's firmness, and spouse-reported "mother's too easygoing" variables.

Parent-Child Interactions in Adolescence

Several follow-up studies of hyperactive and LD children with associated MBD symptoms have demonstrated the long-term effect of parental variables on (good/ poor) outcome in adolescence.

In their follow-up at age 14, Dykman, Peters, and Ackerman (1973) found that the greatest difference between LD children and controls was in the proportion of those who reported problems in family relations. Among hyperactive clinic Ss, an assessment of initial mother-child relationship and child-rearing practices discriminated significantly between good and poor outcome groups in adolescence (Minde, Weiss, and Mendelson, 1972.)

In the 18 year follow-up of the Kauai longitudinal study (Werner and Smith, 1977) family involvement outweighed involvement with friends for a significantly higher proportion of LD children than (SES matched) control cases. In spite of this "turning into one's own family," more LD youth than controls saw both their mothers and fathers as nonsupportive, opposed, disagreeing, or uninterested in their plans, fathers more so than mothers. Fathers emerged as less understanding and less concerned and appeared to influence their offspring less. Youth who had improved by age 18 (only 1:4) tended to have higher ratings of emotional support in their family than those who did not improve.

More of the improved LD cases found their mothers easy to talk to and viewed them as supportive of their ideas and plans, treating their offspring as separate individuals worthy of respect. More of the improved LD cases also reported that both their mothers and their fathers were consistent in enforcing family rules.

Siblings and Birth Order Effects

Little is known about the effects of siblings on the behavior and development of children "at risk" for or with MBD signs. The Owen, et al., (1971) family study indicates that same-sex siblings of EH children have a higher incidence of attention, perceptual, and achievement problems than academically successful controls. While these findings may suggest that a genetic factor is involved in the transmission of specific learning disabilities in families, the investigators also noted that parents treat the EH child more negatively than his same-sex sibling.

Birth order may be an intervening variable that ought to be more closely investigated. In a study of caregiving behavior and early cognitive development in "high risk" infants, Cohen and Beckwith (1977) found that everyday transactions with pre-term infants with and without siblings begin to diverge after the first month.

First-born premature infants received more responsive care and stimulation from the mother than a later-born child as well as social transactions from others in the family. Although the late born pre-term infants had siblings nearby, the interactions they and others provided in the first year of life (between 3 and 8 months) did not compensate in frequency for the decreased attention of the mother.

Extrafamilial Influences: Peers and Teachers

There is a huge gap in our knowledge of how peer and teacher models affect the behavior of a child with MBD symptoms. The exceptions are some studies of observational learning: (1) Caspo (1972) has demonstrated that the cognitive style of impulsive learning disabled children has been modified by peer models and (2) Yando and Kagan (1968) have reported that impulsive first-grade children had more of a tendency to be influenced by reflective teachers than reflective children were by impulsive teachers.

Cultural Expectations

This is an area to which little attention has been paid in research on environmental interaction with MBD, especially in a multi-ethnic and pluralistic society, such as the United States.

In their longitudinal and cross-sectional studies of temperament and development among normal infants (born without obstetric complications) in New York City, Thomas and Chess (1977) have noted differential cultural tolerance of and susceptibility to the child's level of activity, excitability, intensity, and threshold of frustration between native middle class New York parents and lower working class Puerto Rican immigrant parents. The middle class native born New Yorkers were greatly concerned over any evidence of "deviant" behavior, even in early infancy, had high educational and career expectations for their children, and emphasized early accomplishment of self-care activities with structured feeding and sleep schedules. The Puerto Rican parents tolerated behavioral deviations more easily, had more modest goals for their children, and did not press for early self-care achievement. One wonders how much more powerfully these differential cultural expectations would affect the caregiver transaction pattern with a child who is vulnerable because of CNS impairment.

One wonders also whether discrepancies in behavioral and achievement standards between minority and majority cultures in the United States have contributed to the greater current popularity of the MBD diagnosis in this country, in contrast to more homogenous European countries where more precise diagnosis into specific disability groups has been advocated, especially by British investigators (Rutter, Graham, and Yule 1970).

Sex Differences and Sex Role Expectations

Few transactions between children diagnosed as having MBD symptoms and their environment have been analyzed separately for boys and girls. Yet we are dealing with a syndrome which afflicts four to eight times more boys than girls and which is almost defined behaviorally as failure of a child to live up to prevailing sex-role stereotypes (the clumsy, sensitive, withdrawn boy; the reckless, defiant, impulsive girl).

Data from the Kauai longitudinal study seem to indicate that boys who are "at risk" or show MBD symptoms are more vulnerable to the effects of environmental deprivation than girls with the same predisposing conditions. There were no sex differences in the proportion of surviving boys and girls at age 2 who had been exposed to moderate and severe perinatal complications (Werner, Bierman, and French 1971). There were however significant sex differences in the effects of environmental factors operating in infancy (SES at birth; family stability between birth and 2) and in childhood (educational stimulation and emotional support in the home between 2 and 10 years) that led to a differential rate of poor outcomes at 10 (that is need for long-term remedial education, long-term mental health care, and delinquency) for the "high-risk" boys more than for the "high-risk" girls. Twice as many boys as girls were considered in need of placement in a learning disability class by age 10. Interestingly enough improvement rates of diagnosed (hyperactive) LD cases between the ages of 10 and 18 favored the boys: none of the LD girls had improved by age 18, but 40% of the boys did. It may take additional environmental stress and a display of more aberrant behavior to arrive at an MBD diagnosis for a girl than for a boy. Once the label sticks however it becomes a more significant predictor of serious mental health problems in young adulthood for women than for men (Werner and Smith, 1977).

We are not aware of comparable data from other studies that have analyzed environmental interaction effects separately for MBD boys and girls, but there is ample evidence in the literature of normal child development of sex differences in early mother-child interaction (Moss, 1967), in parental correlates of cognitive abilities and achievement motivation, (Honzik, 1967; Maccoby and Jacklin, 1974) and in response to stress (Rutter, 1974). Sex differences in the context of hyperactivity over time have been reported by Battle and Lacey (1972) in a nonclinical sample from the Fels longitudinal study followed from birth to adulthood. Mothers of highly active males were critical, disapproving, not affectionate, and severe in their punishment in childhood. None of these maternal behaviors related to activity level in females. While there was high peer involvement for active children of both sexes, males were rejected and females accepted by other children. Achievement striving in the intellectual-academic area was negatively associated with activity for males, positively associated for females. Thus it appears as if boys, more than girls, are stressed by punitive maternal caregiving practices in response to their activity level and that the consequences of a high activity level on social and intellectual life are more negative for boys than for girls.

SUMMARY AND CONCLUSIONS

The contributions that the muddled concept of "minimal brain dysfunctions" has made to diagnosis and treatment of childhood and learning disorders have been questioned in many chapters of this handbook. Taking the role of the devil's advocate, I would suggest at least one positive impact of the so-called "MBD syndrome." It has forced researchers and clinicians in the behavioral sciences to face up to the bi-directionality of child-caretaker effects. The MBD concept itself may be soon discarded, it is hoped, as a consequence of systematic studies that will determine whether the domain of mixed behavioral and neurologic childhood disabilities belongs to one global syndrome or whether they will be classified separately according to differences in etiology, functional significance, and response to therapeutic intervention as Wolff and Hurwitz (1973) have advocated. The evidence presented makes me impulsive enough to predict an early demise of the MBD syndrome, but a resurrection of the symptoms. What I hope will survive is a renewed appreciation of the role of individual differences in constitution and coping mechanisms that is being fostered by the recent outpouring of research on the effects of the infant on his caretaking environment (Beckwith, 1976; Harper, 1975), on the origins and contributions of temperament to normal human development and childhood disorders (Thomas, Chess, and Birch, 1968; Thomas and Chess, 1977), and on children's resiliency in the face of great physical and psychological stress, long noted by those engaged in longitudinal research.

The studies reviewed in this chapter, though beset with methodological flaws, have impressed me with two persistent patterns that cut across children of different ages, races, socioeconomic levels and cultures, both in clinic and nonclinic populations. The first gives hope: For the minority of children currently diagnosed as MBD who are vulnerable—because of genetic predisposition or biological insult in the pre-, peri-, and early post-natal periods—a supportive environment in infancy, early and middle childhood can ameliorate or suppress the consequences of impairment to the CNS. The second creates concern: A highly disordered and nonsupportive environment can convert the majority of children presently labeled MBD into what Sameroff and Chandler (1975) have called "caretaking casualties," even in the absence of any demonstrable organic CNS impairment. Discriminant function analysis by Broman, Nichols, and Kennedy (1975), Minde, Weiss, and Mendelson (1972), and Werner and Smith (1977) have all shown that the best (though moderate) predictions of outcome could be made when measures of the neurological integrity of the child and an assessment of his activity level and sensorimotor integration were combined with social status and parental caretaking variables.

From the sketchy evidence available on the course of development of "high risk" children and from studies of normal child development, one can only speculate how specific clusters of environmental variables interact to create or modify the expressions of subsets of MBD symptoms. An initial (biochemical) impairment may well be related to greater variability in arousal level (Sroufe, 1975) and conditionability (Wender, 1971) that lead to the problems in control of attention and activity demonstrated in neonatal neurological examinations. Attention and motor control deficits may be suppressed or accentuated in infancy by physical handling and visual and auditory stimulation, especially in low birth-weight children with perinatal complications. Problems with control of motor activity might develop into behavior perceived by the caretaker (mother or teacher) as hyperactive if there is adverse maternal handling of the toddler, that is when in a crowded home parental control is variable or too permissive and there is an absence of routine and structure.

Antisocial behavior and "socio-emotional immaturity" appear to be the consequence of bond-disruption or bond-distortion in the preschool and early school years when intrafamilial relationships are full of discord, hostility, or lack affection. Specific learning disabilities seem to arise in response to perceptual and language (de)privation or overload. The absolute amount of stimulation seems less important than distinctiveness and meaningfulness of the stimulation to the child.

Father-absence or a deviant parent model appears to contribute to the likelihood of delinquency in adolescence. There is finally a persistent thread that seems to pull the different subsets of the MBD syndrome (soft neurological signs, hyperactivity-impulsivity, socioemotional immaturity, school achievement problems) together. Belonging to the culture of poverty increases the original risk of exposure to perinatal stress as well as the likelihood of serious consequences in childhood and adolescence because of the cumulative impact of both physical privation and psychosocial stress.

Why then in the face of such overwhelming odds might one choose hope instead of despair when contemplating the fate of "high risk" infants in an adverse postnatal environment? The hope lies in the evidence of a number of longitudinal studies of nonclinic populations that have documented the course of human development from birth to maturity. In all the risk categories reviewed (prenatal and perinatal pathology; parental characteristics; and other inter- or extra-familial environmental factors) it is possible to identify large numbers of children who, though subjected to these influences, develop normally. Sameroff and Chandler

(1975) have argued forcefully that the human organism appears to have been programmed by the course of evolution to produce normal developmental outcomes under all but the most adverse circumstances. Given the self-righting tendencies of Homo sapiens, malfunctions in the transaction between environment and child can be interrupted at a number of sensitive time periods and leave options for intervention. Thus we have repeated opportunities to peel back the multiple layers of adversity that threaten to envelop the vulnerable child.

The evidence reviewed and the questions raised in this chapter should hold out enough challenges for us to continue the search for specific patterns of transactions between caregiver and child, both within the family and larger social context, which make a discrete impact on the affective and cognitive development of "high risk" boys and girls and to show how amenable they are to change. Along the way we may discover, as did Piet Hein in *Grooks I,* that:

> Problems worthy of attack
>   prove their worth
>   by hitting back.

REFERENCES

Alley, G. R., and G. Solomons. "Minimal cerebral dysfunction as it relates to social class." *Journal of Learning Disabilities,* 4, 246–250, (1971).

Battle, E. S., and B. Lacey. "A context for hyperactivity in children over time." *Child Development,* 43, 757–773, (1972).

Beckwith, L. "Caregiver—infant interaction as a focus for therapeutic intervention with human infants," in R. N. Walsh and W. T. Greenough, eds., *Environments as Therapy for Brain Dysfunction.* New York: Plenum, 1976.

———"Caregiver—infant interaction and the development of the risk infant," in T. Tjossem, ed., *Intervention Strategies for High-Risk Infants and Young Children.* Baltimore: University Park Press. [1978] in press.

Beckwith, L., S. E. Cohen, C. B. Kopp, A. H. Parmelee, and T. G. Marcy. "Caregiver—infant interaction and early cognitive development in preterm infants." *Child Development,* 47, 579–587, (1976).

Bower, K. B., and C. D. Mercer. "Hyperactivity: Etiology and intervention techniques." *Journal of School Health,* 45, 195–201, (1975).

Broman, S. H. "Early development and family characteristics of low achievers." (Paper presented at the 14th International Conference of the Association for Children with Learning Disabilities, Washington, D.C., March 1977.)

Broman, S. H., P. L. Nichols, and W. A. Kennedy, *Preschool IQ: Prenatal and Early Developmental Correlates.* Hillsdale, N.J.: Earlbaum, 1975.

Caspo, M. "Peer models reverse the 'one bad apple spoils the barrel' theory." *Teaching Exceptional Children,* 5, 20–24, (1972).

Clarkson, F. F., and B. S. Hayden. "Relationship of hyperactivity in a normal class setting with family background factors and neurological status." *Proceedings of the 80th Annual Convention of the American Psychological Association,* 7, 559–560, (1972).

Clements, S. D. *Minimal Brain Dysfunction in Children—Terminology and Identification.* Public Health Service Publication No. 1415. Washington, D.C.: U.S. Department of HEW, 1966.

Cohen, S., and L. Beckwith. "Caregiving behaviors and early cognitive development as related to ordinal position in pre-term infants." *Child Development,* 48, 152–157, (1977).

Cruickshank, W. M., F. A. Bentzen, F. H. Tatzeburg, and M. T. Tannhauser. *A Teaching Method for Brain Injured and Hyperactive Children.* Syracuse: Syracuse University Press, 1961.

Denhoff, E. "The natural life history of children with minimal brain dysfunction." *Annals of the New York Academy of Sciences,* 205, 188–205, (1973).

Deutsch, C. P. "Social class and child development," in B. M. Caldwell and H. N. Ricciuti, eds., *Review of Child Development Research,* vol. 3. Chicago: University of Chicago Press, 1973.

Drillien, C. M. *The Growth and Development of the Prematurely Born Infant.* Edinburgh and London: E. S. Livingstone, 1964.

Dykman, R. A., J. E. Peters, and P. T. Ackerman. "Experimental approaches to the study of minimal brain dysfunction: A follow-up study." *Annals of the New York Academy of Sciences,* 205, 93–108, (1973).

Harper, L. V. "The scope of offspring effects from caregiver to culture." *Psychological Bulletin,* 82, 784–801, (1975).

Harper, P. A., L. V. Fischer, and R. V. Rider, "Neurological and intellectual states of prematures at three to five years of age." *Journal of Pediatrics,* 55, 679–690, (1959).

Hess, R. D. "Social class and ethnic influences on socialization," in P. H. Mussen, ed., *Carmichael's Manual of Child Psychology,* 3rd ed., vol. II. New York: Wiley, 1970.

Honzik, M. P. "Environmental correlates of mental growth: Prediction from the family setting at 21 months." *Child Development,* 38, 337–364, (1967).

Kalverboer, A. F., B. C. Touwen, and H. F. R. Prechtl. "Follow-up of infants at risk of minor brain dysfunction." *Annals of the New York Academy of Sciences,* 205, 173–187, (1973).

Klaus, M. H., and J. H. Kennell. "Mothers separated from their newborn infants." *Pediatric Clinic of North America,* 17, 1015–1037, (1970).

Koppitz, E. M. *Children with Learning Disabilities—A Five-Year Follow-up Study.* New York: Grune & Stratton, 1971.

Korner, A. F. "Early stimulation and maternal care as related to infant capabilities and individual differences." *Early Child Development and Care,* 2, 307–327, (1973).

Lynn, D. B. *The Father: His Role in Child Development.* Monterey, Cal.: Brooks/Cole, 1974.

Maccoby, E. E., and C. N. Jacklin. *The Psychology of Sex Differences.* Stanford: Stanford University Press, 1974.

Mendelson, W., N. Johnson, and M. A. Stewart. "Hyperactive children as teenagers: A follow-up study." *The Journal of Nervous and Mental Disease,* 153, 273–278, (1971).

Minde, K., G. Weiss, and N. Mendelson. "A five year follow-up study of 91 hyperactive school children." *Journal of the American Academy of Child Psychiatry,* 11, 595–610, (1972).

Morrison, J. R., and M. A. Stewart. "A family study of the hyperactive child syndrome." *Biological Psychiatry,* 3, 189–195, (1971).

Moss, H. A. "Sex, age, and state as determinants of mother-infant interaction." *Merrill Palmer Quarterly,* 13, 19–36, (1967).

Nichols, P. L. "Minimal brain dysfunction: Associations with perinatal complications." (Paper presented at the Biannual Meeting of the Society for Research in Child Development, New Orleans, March 1977*a.*)

———"Minimal brain dysfunction: Associations with behavior." (Paper presented at the

85th Annual Convention of the American Psychological Association, San Francisco, August 1977b.)

Nichols, P. L., T-C. Chen, and J. D. Pomeroy. "Minimal brain dysfunction: The association among symptoms." (Paper presented at the 84th Annual Convention of the American Psychological Association, Washington, D.C., September 1976.)

Niswander, K. R., and M. Gordon, eds. *The Collaborative Perinatal Study of the National Institute of Neurological Diseases and Stroke: The Women and Their Pregnancies.* Philadelphia: Saunders, 1972.

Owen, F. W., P. A. Adams, T. Forrest, L. M. Stolz, and S. Fisher, "Learning disorders in children: Sibling studies." *Monographs of the Society for Research in Child Development,* 36, (4), Serial No. 144, (1971).

Paternite, C. E., J. Loney, and J. E. Langhorne. "Relationships between symptomatology and SES-related factors in hyperkinetic/MBD boys." *American Journal of Orthopsychiatry,* 46, 291–301, (1976).

Powell, L. F. "The effect of extra stimulation and maternal involvement on the development of low birth-weight infants and on maternal behavior." *Child Development,* 45, 106–113, (1974).

Prechtl, H. F. R. "The mother-child interaction in babies with minimal brain damage (a follow-up study)." in B. M. Fess, Ed., *Determinants of Infant Behavior,* vol. II. New York: Wiley, 1963.

Ramey, C. T., P. Mills, F. A. Campbell, and C. O'Brien, "Infants' home environments: A comparison of high risk families and families from the general population." *American Journal of Mental Deficiency,* 80, 40–42, (1975).

Rutter, M. *The Qualities of Mothering: Maternal Deprivation Reassessed.* New York: Jason Aronson, 1974.

Rutter, M., P. Graham, and W. Yule. *A Neuropsychiatric Study in Childhood.* Clinics in Developmental Medicine, Nos. 35/36. Philadelphia: Lippincott, 1970.

Sameroff, A., and M. J. Chandler. "Reproductive risk and the continuum of caretaking casualty," in F. D. Horowitz ed., *Review of Child Development Research,* vol. 4, 187–244. Chicago: University of Chicago Press, 1975.

Scarr-Salapatek, S., and M. L. Williams. "The effects of early stimulation on low birth-weight infants." *Child Development,* 44, 94–101, (1973).

Schaefer, E. S., and R. A. Bell, "Development of a parental attitude research instrument." *Child Development,* 29, 339–361, (1958).

Siqueland, E. R. "Biological and experimental determinants of exploration in infancy," in L. J. Stone, H. T. Smith, and L. B. Murphy, eds., *The Competent Infant,* 822–823. New York: Basic Books, 1973.

Solkoff, N., S. Yaffe, D. Weintraub, and B. Blase. "Effects of handling on the subsequent development of premature infants." *Developmental Psychology,* 1, 765–768, (1969).

Sroufe, L. A. "Drug treatment of children with behavior problems," in F. D. Horowitz, ed., *Review of Child Development Research,* vol. 4, 367–377. Chicago: University of Chicago Press, 1975.

Stewart, M. A., W. B. Mendelson, and N. E. Johnson. "Hyperactive children as adolescents: How they describe themselves." *Child Psychiatry and Human Development,* 4, 3–11, (1973).

Thomas, A., and S. Chess. *Temperament and Development.* New York: Bruner/Mazel, 1977.

Thomas, A., S. Chess, and H. G. Birch. "*Temperament and Behavior Disorders in Children.*" New York: New York University Press, 1968.

Touliatos, J., and B. W. Lindholm. "Influence of parental expectancies and responsiveness on achievement motivation of minimally brain-injured and normal children." *Psychological Reports*, 35, 395–400, (1974).

Weiss, G., K. Minde, J. S. Werry, V. Douglas, and E. Nemeth. "Studies on the hyperactive child. VIII. Five-year follow-up." *Archives of General Psychiatry*, 24, 409–414, (1971).

Wender, P. H. *Minimal Brain Dysfunction in Children.* New York: Wiley, 1971.

Werner, E. E., J. M. Bierman, and F. E. French. *The Children of Kauai: A Longitudinal Study from the Prenatal Period to Age Ten.* Honolulu: University Press of Hawaii, 1971.

Werner, E. E., K. Simonian, and R. S. Smith. "Reading achievement, language functioning and perceptual-motor development of 10 and 11 year olds." *Perceptual and Motor Skills*, 25, 409–420, (1967).

Werner, E. E., J. M. Bierman, F. E. French, K. Simonian, A. Conner, R. S. Smith, and M. Campbell. "Reproductive and environmental casualties: A report on the 10-year follow-up of the children of the Kauai pregnancy study." *Pediatrics*, 42, 112–127, (1968).

Werner, E. E., K. Simonian, J. M. Bierman, and F. E. French. "Cumulative effects of perinatal complications and deprived environment on physical, intellectual and social development of preschool children." *Pediatrics*, 39, 490–505, (1967).

Werner, E. E., and R. S. Smith. *Kauai's Children Come of Age.* Honolulu: University Press of Hawaii, 1977.

Wiener, G. "Scholastic achievement at age 12–13 of prematurely born infants." *Journal of Special Education*, 2, 237, (1968).

————"The relationship of birth weight and length of gestation to intellectual development at ages 8 to 10 years." *Journal of Pediatrics*, 76, 694–699, (1970).

Wiener, G., R. V. Rider, and W. Oppel. "Some correlates of IQ changes in children." *Child Development*, 34, 61–67, (1963).

Wiener, G., R. V. Rider, W. Oppel, L. K. Fischer, and P. A. Harper. "Correlates of low birth weight: Psychological states at 6–7 years of age." *Pediatrics*, 35, 434–444, (1965).

Wiener, G., R. V. Rider, W. Oppel, and P. A. Harper. "Correlates of low birth weight: Psychological states at 8 to 10 years of age." *Pediatric Review*, 2, 110–118, (1968).

Wolff, P. H., and I. Hurwitz. "Functional implications of the minimal brain dysfunction syndrome." *Seminars in Psychiatry*, 5, 105–115, (1973).

Yando, R. M., and J. Kagan. "The effect of teacher tempo on the child." *Child Development*, 39, 27–34, (1968).

PART FIVE

Effects of Minimal Brain Dysfunctions

Chapters 10–14

CHAPTER 10

Muscular Control and Coordination in Minimal Brain Dysfunctions

Alexander R. Lucas

To discuss muscular control and coordination in the context of their relationship to minimal brain dysfunctions poses many difficulties. Three among these stand out:

1. Motor functions are the result of complex neurophysiologic mechanisms mediated by an exceedingly complicated central and peripheral nervous system of the human.
2. The concept of minimal brain dysfunction is at best an ill-defined controversial one of questionable validity.
3. Study of the relationship between complex functions and an ill-defined concept cannot lead to clear, valid generalizations.

Thus any conclusions to be drawn run the risk of being erroneous and oversimplified. These obstacles perhaps make the discussion a futile task.

As to the first difficulty the physiologist, John Eccles, expressed the opinion that "the human brain . . . is without any qualification the most highly organized and the most complexly organized matter in the universe" (1977). In most individuals this complex brain functions in an amazingly effective, efficient, and predictable manner. There is however much that can go wrong with this complex mechanism. None of us has achieved the full potential with which he was genetically endowed; all of us have been subjected to some biologic insults which can lead to impairment of function. These insults occur prenatally, perinatally, and postnatally. Interpersonal and social experiences can also impair the quality of functioning or permit a nearly optimal developmental unfolding of capacities and talents. While some of these influences leave discernible scars of an anatomic or psychologic nature, most often our complexly organized and plastic brain compensates for these injuries so that their effects cannot be detected even with highly sophisticated methods of neurologic and psychologic assessment. Some functional impairments are detectable. These may involve relatively simple skills (motor abilities) or complex manifestations of sensory, perceptual, and integrative functions (such as reading ability). When impairments are identified it may be possible to describe them in terms of particular brain functions, but it is often difficult to date the time of their origins or to attribute them to specific causes.

Much space and time have been devoted in professional journals and at debates at many conferences to discussion of the second difficulty, the concept of minimal brain dysfunction (Knobloch and Pasamanick, 1959; Clements and Peters, 1962).

To reiterate the entire debate is unnecessary as the arguments for and against the concept have been amply summarized in several reviews (Pond, 1960; Paine, 1962; Bax and MacKeith, 1963; MacKeith, 1963; Gomez, 1967; Wender, 1971; Gross and Wilson, 1974; Schmitt, 1975).

Fortunately the editors selected the plural term "minimal brain dysfunctions" rather than "minimal brain dysfunction" to imply that many forms of dysfunction are subsumed under the term. It is misleading to suggest that minimal brain dysfunction, or worse yet MBD, is a specific disease or disorder with specific symptomatology. There are as many dysfunctions as there are functions of the human brain. Children with particular dysfunctions differ markedly one from another. It is much more useful to identify the particular functions which are impaired (Gomez, 1967). The adjective "minimal" poses great difficulties in definition. These concepts will be discussed below.

Certain assumptions will be made in this chapter: there are children who have demonstrable brain damage; there are other children who have minor degrees of brain abnormality affecting one or more functions, and these abnormalities may be difficult to demonstrate because of the absence of clear localizing neurological signs.

As to the third difficulty, the relationship between motor functions and minimal brain dysfunctions elucidating the relationship is the central task of this chapter. Put in another way one may ask, "What is characteristic about motor performance in children with minor brain dysfunctions?" The question may be answered by stating, "It depends on the particular child and on his or her particular dysfunction." It might be most judicious simply to state that some children with brain dysfunction have disorders of motor control, but that there is no consistent correlation between motor dysfunction and minimal brain dysfunctions. Children should be evaluated as individuals and their abilities and particular areas of dysfunction assessed. Nonetheless there has been an ill-advised tendency to classify together children who have in common a particular characteristic, such as hyperactivity or clumsiness. Such categorizations may satisfy our need for structure but they may lead to the erroneous conclusions that these children are similar to one another in ways other than the described characteristic. When "brain damage" is substituted for "minimal brain dysfunction" the semantic problems are largely resolved. If one then asks, "Do some children with brain damage have motor disorders?" the answer is an unequivocal, "Yes" To the question, "Do *all* children with brain damage have motor disorders?" the answer is an equally unequivocal, "No!"

MUSCULAR CONTROL AND COORDINATION

As long ago as in the Middle Ages it was thought that mental faculties could be localized in the cerebral ventricles. At the beginning of the nineteenth century the anatomist Gall asserted that human faculties are located in particular areas of the brain. He developed a phrenological chart used to determine individual differences by observing prominences of the skull. Gall's localization of faculties and mental qualities such as aggressiveness, love of life, loyalty, and ambition had little basis in fact.

Before the end of the nineteenth century Broca and Wernicke identified specific areas of the cortex which were associated with the expressive and sensory aspects of speech. Continued clinical-pathological correlation of cerebral cortical lesions led to the mapping and localization of function of the cerebral cortex. While elementary physiologic functions, such as cutaneous sensation, vision, hearing, and movement could accurately be represented in clearly defined areas of the cortex, Hughlings Jackson decried the concept of complex mental processes must be approached from the standpoint of levels of organization rather than of their localization in particular areas of the brain (Luria, 1973).

Anatomic Basis

The control of muscles involves five levels in the central nervous system: the cerebral cortex, the basal ganglia, the cerebellum, the brain stem, and the spinal cord. Impulses coming from motor areas in the frontal lobes ultimately travel through the brain stem and to the spinal cord whence spinal nerves transmit them to the muscles of the body.

There are excitatory and inhibitory mechanisms within the brain stem that project to the spinal cord, which in turn are influenced by the cerebellum, basal ganglia, and cerebral cortex. Direct projections from the cerebral cortex to the brain stem and spinal cord make up the pyramidal system of the corticobulbar and corticospinal tracts. Indirect projections to motor nuclei by way of the cerebellum and basal ganglia and the brain-stem excitatory and inhibitory centers comprise the extrapyramidal system. The pyramidal system is primarily excitatory and is largely responsible for control of the head, neck, and limb muscles. The extrapyramidal system is concerned with timing and coordination of muscle groups and with the modulation of muscle tone. Lesions in these systems result in paresis (weakness) or paralysis of muscle groups (Gardner, 1975).

The cerebellum is involved in coordinating the timing of activity in muscle groups, both in postural and locomotor mechanisms. In doing so it enhances muscle tone. It receives information from peripheral receptors and from motor and sensory regions of the cerebral cortex. It carries out its functions primarily through brain-stem inhibitory and excitatory mechanisms, which it modifies. Disorders of the cerebellum are manifested chiefly as hypotonia, difficulties in timing, defects in coordination of muscular activity, balance, and ataxia.

The basal ganglia are especially important in inhibitory mechanisms, in the suppression of muscle tone, and in the coordination of muscle groups. They have an important role in complex muscular activities including locomotion and associated movements. Diseases of the basal ganglia have signs such as increased muscle tone, rigidity, and dyskinesias or abnormal involuntary movements (Gardner, 1975).

The old concept of the nervous system held that there are centers subserving specific functions, such as the processing of sensory information and the control of movement. It was assumed, on the basis of some supporting clinical data, that if one center was damaged or obliterated, that function would be impaired or lost. During the past 100 years it was learned that matters are much more complex, with anatomically separate areas being functionally interdependent and hierarchies of nerve fibers being necessary for simple and complex acts.

Neurons or nerve cells transmit information from one point to another by means of electrochemical impulses. The single long fibers arising from neurons are axons which transmit the information. Within each brain center nerve cells give rise to dendrites, short branching strands that terminate in the vicinity of the nerve cell.

In addition to macrocircuits composed of axons transmitting information from one brain to another, there are microcircuits made up of dendrites in the form of feedback loops. These microcircuits are concerned with synaptic excitation, inhibition, and with sequences of these activities. Thus the nervous system is built up of hierarchies of functional units of increasing scope and complexity. The traditional concept of the single neuron receiving information from its dendrites and sending it on through its axon is only one type of functional unit within these hierarchies. Recent findings suggest that a single neuron comprises many functional units with its synaptic relations. And each neuron is but a small component of larger functional units made up of multineuronal assemblies. At the highest level of organization such functions as perception, memory, learning, and complex behavioral acts require the coordination of many centers (Shepherd, 1978).

Neurochemical Basis

At the cellular level the transmission of neuronal impulses is based on electrophysical and biochemical changes mediated by chemical messengers known as neurotransmitter substances. They serve to excite or inhibit the postsynaptic cell. "Normal brain function depends on the integration of the synthesis, storage, release, and inactivation of neurotransmitters localized in different brain structures and pathways (Cohen and Young, 1977)." The neurotransmitters include acetylcholine and the catecholamines dopamine, norepinephrine, and epinephrine. The indoleamine serotonin and an amino acid, GABA, also function as neurotransmitters. There are undoubtedly many other neurotransmitter substances, some putative and others not yet identified. Cyclic adenosine monophosphate (AMP) and prostaglandins are also involved in synaptic transmission. All are essential for normal brain function and some have been implicated in certain neurological and psychiatric diseases. Abnormal neurotransmitter function has been implicated in some movement disorders. There may be derangements in the levels of these substances or in their metabolism which affects movement and coordination (Siegel, et al., 1976).

Neurophysiologic Mechanisms

Movement begins in the human fetus only a few weeks old. Flexion and extension of the limbs occur and automatic movements such as swallowing begin. At birth automatic movements necessary for survival such as respiratory and swallowing movements occur regularly. The skeletal movements are not yet very complex or purposeful. From these simpler movements postural control is acquired to overcome gravity effects and chain reactions become important in the development of complex movements and the determination of the pattern of movements. Finally infants acquire an awareness of their movements and the ability to control them.

The last step requires sensorimotor integration. Afferent stimuli from joints, tendons, muscles, and skin are interpreted by the brain and result in modification of the limb movement. In addition to kinesthetic stimuli, visual, auditory, and tactile sensorimotor links develop to provide information which reveals the results of movements and enables the brain to modify the position of movements.

These sensorimotor links occur quite early in infant development. In order to perform skilled movements quickly, precisely, and smoothly, all the neurological chain reactions and the sensorimotor links must be intact (Holt, 1975).

Developmental and physiological aspects of neuromuscular control have been reviewed in more detail in a monograph on movement and child development (Connolly, 1975; Harrison, 1975; Holt, 1975; Wyke, 1975).

Movements are voluntary or automatic. Each motor act, even a simple one, picking up an object, involves complex muscular interaction. Volitional control of movement, how learning occurs, and how practice maintains and improves performance, are as yet not well understood. Eccles (1977) suggested that there is a sequence of events akin to computer programming. It originates with the *idea.* The *plan*, or *program* is established in the association cortex, basal ganglia, and thalamus, and is *executed* through the nervous pathways from the motor cortex to the muscles. Somato-sensory feedback mechanisms to the motor cortex continually modify and modulate the movement. Eccles maintained that trained movements are largely preprogrammed, whereas exploratory movements are imperfectly programmed, being provisional and subject to continous revision. The somato-sensory loop to the motor cortex provides for the reporting back of corrective information in accord with learned skill. The total movement, a smooth, highly integrated performance, may be accomplished in only a split second. In the carrying out of the skilled movements, there is an immense integration of neuronal activity in interacting dynamic loops. Most movements are complex, almost automatic, patterns with volition often having only an initiating role (Eccles, 1977).

NORMAL CHILDREN

Patterns of movement in children are influenced by their age, individual variability, talent, and environmental influences.

Age

From the simplest movements which begin in the early weeks of embryonic life, neuromuscular development progresses in a predictable manner as a function of age (Mittelmann, 1960; Wyke, 1975). Increasingly complex fine and gross motor skills are acquired as the infant and child progress through developmental stages (Gesell, 1940; Gesell and Ilg, 1946; Knobloch and Pasamanick, 1974). The unfolding of progressively more complex skills proceeds in predictable sequences with characteristic patterns evident at each stage. Children of one to two years of age experiment freely with their newly learned motor skills when given the opportunity (Freud and Burlingham, 1944).

The second and third year of life constitute the period of most rapid development of motor skill. Motility is one of the most important avenues for exercising such functions as mastery, integration, reality testing, and control of impulses (Mittelmann, 1954).

At certain stages children are characteristically active. The 11-year-old for example, as described by Gesell, Ilg, and Ames, looks as follows:

He wriggles with great versatility. He twists, bounces, and moves all over the chair, swings a foot across the arm, retracts his legs, knocks his knees together, bends over and pulls at his shoes. Concurrently he grimaces, cocks his head, and interjects comments and bursts of laughter. His activity embraces the whole body, extending from head to foot. Yet the movements are not "nervous" in quality or import. It is as though the entire psychomotor system of the 11-year-old was richly supplied with sparking facilities.

His activity, especially when he is in any way confined, is so constant that one almost becomes seasick watching him. He bounces up and down in the chair. He rocks back and forth. He pushes the chair around on the floor if the floor covering allows. Suddenly he will jerk his head or whole body forward, tipping his chair with him. Or he will wave his arms over his head and clasp his hands on his head. He stretches. His hands seem to be in constant activity. [1956]

The motor and coordination skills tested on neurological examination—standing, running, balance, hopping, standing on one foot, standing on toes, standing on heels, spontaneous movements, coordinated acts, rapid alternate movements —all develop with age. Rutter and his co-workers emphasized the importance of relating the findings of the neurological examination to the age and developmental level of the child. They pointed out that this concept has not always been fully appreciated by clinicians and ignorance of it has contributed to the confusion surrounding the interpretation of minor and soft neurological signs (Rutter, Graham, and Yule, 1970). Schmitt asserted that soft signs represent transient phenomena which disappear with age (1975). This contention was confirmed by Rie and Rie and their co-workers in a study of 80 learning disabled children. They found that the primary determinant for the majority of soft neurological signs is chronological age and that the signs do tend to disappear with age (Rie, et al., 1978).

Individual Variability

Although the sequence is predictable and there are typical patterns at each age, there is much variability in motor behavior among children of the same age. The studies of Thomas, et al. (1963, 1977) and their co-workers have emphasized behavioral individuality in childhood. They have focused in their long-term longitudinal study on temperamental differences in childhood. The temperamental characteristics which make up the behavioral style of children are determined by a combination of hereditary, prenatal, paranatal, and early life experiences. Children vary markedly in their innate activity levels with some being highly active and restless, while others are sluggish and sedentary. These characteristics, although modifiable, tend to persist for the most part throughout childhood (Thomas, et al., 1963; Thomas and Chess, 1977).

Just as children differ from each other in their level of activity, they vary in their dexterity and in their motor and coordination skills. Some have excellent fine motor or gross motor abilities while others are maladroit. Children who possess a particular type of motor skill do not necessarily become proficient in others. Thus graphic skills, the finger coordination required to play the piano, and gross muscular coordination required for sports are quite independent of each other. Teachers of first graders appreciate that learning readiness varies markedly among 6-year olds. In just such a way does motor readiness vary. Some children take longer because of a slower rate of neuromuscular development. But just as some children never learn to read well, some will never be motorically adept.

Talent

Talent is a natural capacity or gift which can be developed by practice. Some children are motorically talented while others are not. The talent may involve the propensity for coordinated fine motor tasks or for gross body movements. Combined with other talents, for rhythm, timing, and sense of pitch, it can make a child a capable musician. The way in which the talent develops depends on practice. Skill or technical proficiency is the result of persistent practice. Without talent no amount of practice will make the child into an accomplished pianist or violinist.

The talented artist needs good perceptual appreciation as well as fine motor coordination skills. A different kind of talent is seen in the successful dancer or diver involving the integration of timing, coordination of muscle groups, and position sense in space, functions carried out by the cerebellum and vestibular system.

Some children have a notable lack of talent for motor acts but this lack does not preclude high intelligence, good learning capacity, or other talents. Moreover a child may be inept in certain motor tasks, yet be highly skilled in others. A boy with multiple body tics, who all his life had been very poorly coordinated, taught himself as a teenager to play the piano well, thereby revealing an unknown talent (Lucas, Kauffman, and Morris, 1967).

Environmental Influences

It has been emphasized that technical proficiency at any task comes only with sufficient practice. Motor skills can be trained and improved. This is as well understood by physical therapists who work with handicapped children as by those individuals who nurture their own talents.

Lack of opportunities for motor activity, restraint, and immobilization can interfere with the rate of motor development or impair the quality of movements. Among the many causes of hyperactivity, Ross and Ross included reactions to environmental and social stressors. When certain children are stressed by environmental pressures, they become restless and overactive (Ross and Ross, 1976). Overstimulation as well as lack of consistency and structure in the child's environment can lead to hyperactivity.

Levy observed overactivity in consequence of hampered freedom of locomotion when children were forcibly restrained or immobilized by a plaster cast (Levy, 1944). When children have the freedom to express their motor urge in a group nursery, they do so without hesitation (Mittelmann, 1954). This behavior was vividly described for toddlers of one and two years of age (Freud and Burlingham, 1944):

The greatest event in the child's life is his new ability to move freely and to control his movements, an ability which progresses quickly from crawling to walking, running, climbing, jumping, and is continued with the handling and moving of objects, as pushing, pulling, dragging, carrying, etc. . . . Toddlers in their own homes remain in their cribs, or strapped to a pram, or at best confined to the narrow space of a playpen, at a period when in a nursery like ours they cover miles in a continual movement about their room. Some children at this period for a while disregard all toys and show little interest in their companions; they behave as if they were drunk with the idea of space and even of speed; they crawl, walk, march and run, and revert from method of locomotion to the other with the greatest of pleasure.

Mittelmann (1954) described motility as an urge akin to basic drives or instincts; a close relationship exists between motility and emotions because motor experience evokes emotion and certain emotions are accompanied by particular motor patterns. He distinguished five kinds of motor phenomena in early childhood:

1. Random movements of infants.
2. Affectomotor patterns that accompany emotional reactions such as joy, fear, rage, or depression.
3. Well-organized rhythmic patterns, rocking and bouncing, termed "autoerotic."
4. Skilled motor activity involving posture, locomotion, and manipulation.
5. Motor phenomena that are indispensable elements of the function of certain organs, such as sucking or eating.

While children tend to be more active at some ages than at others and boys are characteristically more active than girls, environmental expectations and tolerance play an important role in determining what is considered overactive. Macfarlane and co-workers in studying normal children between the ages of 21 months and 14 years found that nearly one-third of the boys and one-fifth of the girls were described as excessively active (Macfarlane, Allen, and Honzik, 1954). An even larger number, nearly half of the children age 6 to 12 years, were described by their mothers as overactive in a study by Lapouse and Monk (1958). The child's emotions and the influences of environment are closely interrelated, then, with motility.

BRAIN DAMAGE IN CHILDREN

Damage means loss due to injury or harm. Clearly there are children who have sustained harm to their brains and who have incontrovertible manifestations of this damage. The damage may be structural involving actual tissue loss or there may be physiologic impairment of function. The pre-Jacksonian concept held that anatomically discrete areas of the brain housed functions such as movement, speech, vision, hearing, and cognition. While there are areas of key importance to motor and sensory function in the cerebral cortex, it has become evident that the integral activity of many structurally separate areas is necessary for particular functions to occur. Thus the organization of anatomically contiguous units; anatomically separate units connected by nervous pathways; and metabolic systems, with receptor sites located in different areas of the central nervous system which are selectively sensitive to neurochemical changes, are all involved in particular motor, sensory, and other behavioral functions.

Multiple Influences

Brain damage in children varies with respect to its cause; the location and extent of injury; type, duration, and rate of damage; and the developmental stages at which the injury occurs (Birch, 1964). Specific isolated functions may be impaired or a wide variety of functions affected in a child with diffuse, generalized brain damage.

Multiple Forms

Just as the normal physiologic functions the brain are multiple and diverse, the effects of damage to the brain can take on an almost endless variety of forms. The complexity of the brain; the enormous variability among individuals in physiologic, intellectual, and emotional functions; the varying forms of damage; and the influences of environment account for the differences.

Brain damage in children is generally classified on the basis of the impaired functions. Thus there are children with motor disorders, intellectual impairment, communication disorders, sensory and perceptual deficits, and convulsive disorders. The disorders may occur singly or in combination, and children with such dysfunction may manifest behavioral disorders varying in form and severity.

The diversity of brain damage and the uniqueness of each child make it impossible to describe a typical pattern of associated behavior problems. Certain behaviors including hyperactivity, short attention span, distractibility, mood oscillation, high impulsivity, and perseveration have nonetheless been implicated as frequently accompanying brain damage. Strauss, Werner, and Lehtinen popularized the notion that brain damage in children resulted in a specific cognitive and behavioral syndrome (Strauss and Werner, 1941; Strauss and Lehtinen, 1947). Subsequent writers emphasized the lack of specificity of such a syndrome, and stressed the importance not only of organic but also of environmental influences in determining the behavior of brain-damaged children (Bender, 1949; Bradley, 1957; Eisenberg, 1957; Graham and Rutter, 1968; Chess, 1972).

Birch differentiated what he termed the *fact* of brain damage—actual anatomic or physiologic alteration—from the *concept* of brain damage—a behavioral syndrome assumed to arise from damage. The fact of brain damage refers to pathologic alterations in the nerve tissue of the brain. The functional consequences of such an anatomic or physiologic change are quite diverse. They range from the absence of discernible functional alteration to complete paralysis, amentia, and death. The concept, "the brain-damaged child," Birch pointed out, does not necessarily apply to all children who *in fact* have brain damage—those with cerebral palsy, hemiplegia, mental deficiency from hydrocephalus, and epilepsy as a result of cortical scarring. Rather it has been used to designate a certain pattern of behavioral disturbance including hyperactivity impulsivity, short attention span, and emotional lability (Birch, 1964). Whether any or all of these symptoms are directly attributable to tissue damage or to the brain-damaged child's reaction to his environment is still subject to dispute.

Minimal Conditions

The terms "minimal brain damage" and "minimal brain (cerebral) dysfunction" have confusing semantic connotations. The definitions of these terms are necessarily vague and imprecise. This has led neurologists and pediatricians to vary greatly in their application of the terms to children (MacKeith, 1963). To psychiatrists, psychologists, and educators the connotations have become even more disparate.

Minimal means "the least attainable or possible." It is therefore an unfortunate choice of qualifier for damage or dysfunction. If brain damage is truly minimal, then it is of no consequence. It could readily be compensated for and it should be impossible to detect. On the other hand tissue damage of considerable magnitude in certain parts of the brain connot be detected by neurological examination or psychological tests. There is no convenient line of demarcation between what is minimal and what is more than minimal. The adjectives "mild," "moderate," and "severe" lend themselves much more readily to quantitative description of impaired function.

The term "minimal brain damage" has been used, like brain damage, to signify both a fact and a concept. Whether it can be a fact is open to semantic dispute. Knobloch and Pasamanick (1959) first used the term "minimal cerebral damage" to emphasize that there is a continuum of damage in infants ranging from severe to those which are undetectable. More recently the terms have indiscriminately been applied to slight forms of damage to the brain, but more often to designate the consequences presumed to arise from slight damage or physiologic malfunction. "Minimal brain dysfunction" most often has been used to connote a concept as in "the MBD child" (Wender, 1971). Just what this concept is however is particularly unclear as the intended meaning varies greatly among those who use this designation. Many who use the term seem themselves uncertain of its meaning. Dysfunction means impaired function of an organ. Used appropriately then the term should describe malfunctioning of the brain (the result) and should not suggest cause or the state of anatomic integrity. But what is *minimal* dysfunction? And which function? The term became popular because many workers did not wish to use the pejorative label "brain *damaged*" which would project the specter of severity and permanence. Yet these same users of the term were generally organically oriented and wished to attribute responsibility for the disorder to the central nervous system of the child rather than to environmental, interpersonal influences.

Wender (1971) stated that minimal brain dysfunction is the single most common disorder seen by child psychiatrists. In describing what he terms "MBD children," he states that they manifest dysfunction in motor activity and coordination; attention and cognitive function; impulse control; interpersonal relations, particularly dependence-independence and responsiveness to social influence; and emotionally. He identifies a broad range of distinct etiologies—organic brain damage, genetic transmission, intrauterine variation in biological development, fetal maldevelopment, and even psychogenetic determinants (deviant psychological experience). When used to describe such a wide range of clinical symptoms and such thoroughly encompassing causes, the term does not clarify understanding of a condition but obfuscates. Lauretta Bender commented, tongue in cheek, that, "It may be safely assumed that any preadolescent child in a child guidance clinic may be put in the category of MBD until proved otherwise" (Bender, 1975). Gomez (1967) correctly pointed out that the introduction of the diagnostic labels "minimal cerebral dysfunction" and "minimal brain damage" represented a backward step in nosology and that their use leads to maximal neurologic confusion.

Historically the notion of linking the brain-damaged child with a behavioral syndrome had clinical utility in distinguishing children with "something wrong with their brain" from those who had "something wrong with their psychosocial experience." In the generation prior to the 1950s, environmental determinism had become the dominant force in psychiatric and psychological thinking (Thomas and Chess, 1977). Overzealous adherents of the psychoanalytic movement suggested that all children's behavior problems could be traced to faulty parenting, early emotional traumas, and unconscious conflicts. Learning theorists on the other hand attributed all behavioral deviations to learned responses. It became important to recognize that the ready scapegoat, the mother, was not in all instances to blame, but that in many cases abnormal brain function and temperamental differences among children contributed significantly to manifest behavior. The designation "brain-damaged child" was an appropriate label for children with recognized brain lesions and associated behavioral problems. Children with milder central nervous system deficits were then labeled as having "minimal brain dysfunction" in an attempt to spare them and their parents the brain-damage appelation. Unfortunately the term began to be used more and more generally to describe children with all types of dysfunction regardless of cause. Perhaps some of the present generation of psychiatrists have overenthusiastically identified what they presume to be organic factors in their eagerness to embrace the biomedical model.

RELATIONSHIP BETWEEN MOTOR DYSFUNCTION AND BRAIN DISORDERS

Clearly there are some disorders of brain function in children which are associated with motor dysfunction or incoordination. These constitute some of the classic neurologic disorders of childhood, among which are the motor disorders commonly known as cerebral palsy and the movement disorders. Specific abnormalities of motor function and coordination on neurological examination localize the origin of these disorders to the cerebral cortex, the basal ganglia, or the cerebellum. The etiology of many of these disorders is known. Structural damage to the brain may have resulted from physical trauma, infection, toxins, or metabolic derangements. Some are static and some are progressive disorders. Evidence from the neurologic examination of children with these disorders leaves no doubt as to the presence of and location of damage in the brain. While such children may have intellectual, sensory, perceptual, and emotional impairment, many do not. Children with cerebral palsy may be intelligent and without learning impairment, while there are others who have both motor disturbances and mental retardation.

Other children, in whom the motor signs are not definite or severe enough to make the neurological diagnosis, have minor motor disorders variously labeled as "clumsy" (Walton, Ellis, and Court, 1962; Illingworth, 1963), and "congenitally maladroit" (Ford, 1973). Other designations such as developmental apraxia (Walton, Ellis, and Court, 1962), choreiform syndrome (Prechtl and Stemmer, 1962) and developmental clumsiness (Reuben and Backwin, 1968) have also been used. As most of these terms imply, the poor motor abilities of these children should be regarded as physiologic variants or as developmental immaturities rather than signs of underlying brain pathology. Yet these children tend to be singled out, particularly if they have learning or behavioral problems. When both conditions occur in a child, it is often assumed that there is a causal relationship. This assumption is not necessarily warranted. Significant associations were not found between choreiform movements of the type described by Prechtl and Stemmer and reading disability, psychiatric disorder, neurological abnormality or pregnancy complication (Rutter, Graham, and Birch, 1966).

What is the research evidence to support the assumption that there is a relationship between motor dysfunction, brain disorder, and learning problems? A number of investigators have studied children utilizing multivariate analysis in an attempt to relate the motor findings of the neurological examination to information from the medical history, the presenting complaint, the behavioral problems, and the results of the neurologic examination, the electroencephalogram, and the psychological examination. Some have attempted to find correlations among indicators objectively rated. Others have used diagostic terms such as minimal brain dysfunction, encephalopathy, and organicity to which to relate these specific findings. Problems in definition of diagnostic terms (Bax and MacKeith, 1963), as well as the differing measures taken and the heterogeneity of groups of children studied, makes comparison of the several studies difficult.

An investigation of 70 school children (59 boys and 13 girls) attending the first three grades of school was carried out by Lucas, Rodin, and Simson (1965). The children were identified by classroom teachers as presenting behavioral or learning problems. The complaints leading to referral included antisocial behavior (N=12), withdrawn behavior (N=12), hyperactivity—impulse control problem (N=27), speech disturbance (N=5), learning problems other than reading disability (N=35), reading disability (N=12), emotional immaturity (N=12), and muscular dyscoordination (N=6). Neurological dysfunction was seen as reflecting:

1. Actual structural damage to the nervous system on an anatomic basis.
2. Derangements in bioelectrical circuits.
3. Defects in the integration of physiologically functional units of the nervous system.
4. Developmental lags.
5. Familial patterns of neurological integration.

It was pointed out that a wide range of variation exists in the development and maturation of the nervous system in children.

Information obtained from the neurological history, family history, neurological examination, electroencephalogram, psychiatric interview, and psychological examination, was coded and correlated. Correlation coefficients for a large number of associations were analyzed.

The complaint of hyperactivity-impulse control problem correlated at better than the 1% level of statistical significance with overactivity on examination, poor general muscular coordination, talkativeness, long duration of chief complaint, and disruptiveness during examination, and there was a negative correlation with chief complaint of learning problems other than reading disability.

The complaint of emotional immaturity correlated at better than the 1% level of statistical significance with chief complaint of muscular dyscoordination. Difficulty of the mother during pregnancy correlated with poor general muscular coordination and several items of impaired functioning on the neurological examination. Birth difficulty correlated with problems on the Bender Gestalt Test.

An association was identified between hyperactive-impulse behavior and minor abnormalities on the neurological examination. Lack of correlation between items of abnormality on the neurological examination and the chief complaint of muscular dyscoordination suggested that poor muscular coordination, as described by school and parents, was a manifestation of general immaturity of the child rather than a demonstrable coordination difficulty on examination. Findings suggested that earlier insults to the central nervous system during pregnancy may manifest themselves mostly in disturbances of the maturational process involving the phylogenetically older extrapyramidal motor system, while the later insults at the time of birth may result in disturbances that are more of a cortical nature, leading to perceptual-motor difficulties (Lucas, Rodin, and Simson, 1965).

Since correlation coefficients give only the strength of the relationship between two variables, it was of interest to determine whether groups of variables could be demonstrated to have significant relationships on the basis of some common denominator. For this purpose, the data were subjected to factor analysis. Fifty variables with the highest correlation coefficient were selected from the correlation matrix. By the principal axis method and varimax rotation, nine factors were extracted and identified. Factor 1 dealt with the dimension of muscular coordination and amount of motor movement. In this factor motor activity appeared as an essentially independent phenomenon. Difficulty during the pregnancy, although appearing in the factor, contributed only to a very small degree. Factor II represented intelligence or underlying sensory preception and integration. Factor III related to age. Factor IV dealt with the electroencephalogram and stood mostly by itself, not highly related to any of the other measures. Factor V represented developmental hyperactivity dating from the first year of life. Factors VI, VII, and VIII dealt with dimensions of motor development, performance IQ, and aspects of gross muscular coordination. Factor IX on antisocial behavior suggested that antisocial behavior is as a rule not the result of organic cerebral disturbances.

Rodin, Lucas, and Simson (1964) concluded that:

1. Muscular dyscoordination manifested in the neurological examination as a factor by itself.
2. Electroencephalographic abnormalities are a factor by themselves.
3. Both muscular dyscoordination and electroencephalographic abnormalities tend to show some relationship to disturbances in the pregnancy, but the relationship is not very strong.
4. Antisocial behavior is not the result of brain injury.
5. A combination of different insults to the central nervous system and the developing personality structure appears to be responsible for the clinical symptomatology rather than one single cause.

Rutter, Graham, and Yule, drawing from their experience in the extensive Isle of Wight epidemiologic study, came to the conclusion that there is a significant association between the hyperkinetic syndrome and evidence of neurological abnormality or brain damage. On the other hand they stated that most brain-damaged children are not overactive and that many overactive children show no evidence of brain damage (1970).

In a study of a group of 100 children with learning and behavioral problems, clinically heterogeneous, referred for suspected "minimal brain dysfunction,"

Kenny and Clemmens (1971) found no significant relationship between neurological examination findings, electroencephalogram, and diagnosis. They questioned the value of neurological screening for such children.

Werry and co-workers studied 20 hyperactive children (18 boys and 2 girls) ranging in age from 6 to 12 years in comparison with neurotic and normal controls. The aim was to compare the frequency of neurological, electroencephalographic, and perinatal abnormalities in these groups. The hyperactive children showed significantly more neurological abnormalities, principally an excess of soft signs reflecting sensory motor incoordination, but no differences in major neurological signs, electroencephalographic abnormalities, or medical history. It was hypothesized that chronic hyperactivity in children of normal intelligence is a disorder discrete from neurosis and is probably an organic syndrome, most likely a biological variant (Werry, et al., 1972).

Shaffer and co-workers expressed the opinion, based on objective measurements taken from boys with and without a conduct disorder and with and without associated brain injury, that overactivity is a function of psychiatric disturbance rather than of an abnormality of the central nervous system (Shaffer, McNarmara, and Pincus, 1974).

Two studies on 10- and 11-year-old children failed to distinguish those with learning disabilities from normally achieving children on the basis of soft neurological signs. Adams and co-workers compared learning disabled fourth graders with a control group for incidence of selected neurological signs (Adams, Kocsis, and Estes, 1974). Stine and co-workers, in examining 10- and 11-year-old children found correlation between certain neurological signs and observed classroom behavior, but no one-to-one relationship between the neurological sign and a particular form of behavior (Stine, Saratsiotis, and Mosser, 1975).

Rie, et al. (1978) examined 80 children (56 boys and 24 girls) with a mean age of 8 with learning problems in order to study the relationship among signs on neurological examination, hyperactivity, and the diagnosis of organicity. Test scores, age, sex, individual soft neurological signs, and total number of soft signs were subjected to factor analysis. Within the learning disabled group:

1. The number of neurological soft signs did not predict organicity.
2. Hyperactivity and organicity were not interrelated.
3. So-called neurological signs tended to disappear with age.
4. Neurological signs requiring complex responses incorporating motor functions along with sensory-processing functions were the most predictive of organicity.

These investigators identified two types of organicity relating to different perceptual/conceptual processes. One was described as having to do with the inability of the individual to perceive his environment visually and subsequently to replicate that perception motorically or conceptually; the other reflected the inability to translate verbal cues into conceptual symbols for purposes of synthesis and/or recall, toward either motor responses or verbal responses. They concluded that motor coordination is a very poor indicator of either hyperactivity or organicity in a group of learning disabled children. They emphasized the importance of relating findings to the age and developmental level of the child.

CLINICAL IMPLICATIONS

What are the clinical and educational implications of this information? Does dyscoordination (dyspraxia) suggest the presence of brain damage in a child? By no means. Is poor motor performance a reliable predictor of learning problems? Does early screening for motor coordination skills in public school identify the child who will develop learning disabilities? The answer to these questions is "No." There is ample evidence that preschool children and early elementary school children differ greatly in the rates of their motor development. At a given age there is much variability in motor performance. Moreover for a particular child there are often discrepancies among the rates at which motor, language, and social and adaptive skills are progressing. For many children the inability to perform certain motor tasks at a given age is a reflection of a slower rate of development or developmental lag. Given time these children will catch up. Other children are innately more clumsy and will remain so all their lives.

Should the classroom teacher be concerned about the clumsy, awkward child? Not if the child is functioning well academically and socially. Motor coordination skills are relatively simple neurological functions often operating independently of other neurological functions. More complex motor tasks of course require of the child a certain level of intelligence in order to comprehend and execute the task. Academic skills such as oral and written language, reading, and arithmetic require a still more complex integration of sensory, perceptual, cognitive, and motor functions. Prediction of academic difficulties on the basis of isolated dysfunctions before integrated functions have developed is unsound. It is still best to observe the child's acquisition of reading and other academic skills and to base conclusions about learning problems on actual performance.

The experienced clinician, physician or psychologist, familiar with children will be able to make valid interpretation of certain behavioral characteristics including motor, sensory, perceptual, cognitive, and emotional. On the basis of the total evaluation of the child, deviation in one or more of these areas may suggest the presence of normal variation, brain disorder, or reaction to the environment.

CONCLUSIONS

The human brain is a highly complex mechanism organized in a hierarchical structure of many levels and complexly integrated circuits and subcircuits. Motor, sensory, perceptual, cognitive, and emotional functions are independent capacities which can be observed, measured, and studied in isolation. Coordinated acts and learning tasks require the integrated action of these functions. Children may show dysfunction in one or more areas to a greater or lesser degree. Some children have difficulty with the integration of functions. There is a multiplicity of causes, ranging from genetic and organic to environmental and experiential, which influence the development of these difficulties.

Motor function progresses in a predictable, yet individually variable, manner throughout the development of the child and becomes more refined as the central nervous system matures. Mass action gives way to increasingly exact motor skills. There is much variability among individual children in their activity level and in patterns of neurological integration and skillfulness. Individual children develop at differing rates and vary in their motor skills. Damage to the central nervous system at various levels can cause reversion to more primitive modes of functioning. The locus, extent, duration, and type of damage will result in different syndromes of brain dysfunction. The damage may be so slight as to be not detectable, may produce clinical dysfunction of a mild sort, or it may lead to severe clinical disturbances of function. Hyperactivity is one kind of motor expression with numerous causes, organic and environmental. Differences in muscular control and coordination among children are based upon many types of mechanisms. Individual variability should not be overidentified as pathologic. The complexities of the human brain, differences in age, temperamental individuality, and differing environmental experiences among children result in an unending and refreshingly unique combination of characteristics which is each individual child.

REFERENCES

Adams, R. M., J. J. Kocsis, and R. E. Estes. "Soft neurological signs in learning-disabled children and controls." *American Journal of Diseases of Children*, 128, 614–618, (1974).

Bax, M. C. O., and R. C. MacKeith. "Minimal brain damage—A concept discarded," in R. MacKeith and M. Bax, eds., *Minimal Cerebral Dysfunction*, Little Club Clinics in Developmental Medicine, No. 10, pp. iv–v. London: Heinemann, 1963.

Bender, L. "Psychological problems of children with organic brain disease." *American Journal of Orthopsychiatry*, 19, 404–415, (1949).

——— "The prescription of treatment for children," in D. X. Freedman, and J. E. Dyrud, eds., *American Handbook of Psychiatry*, 2nd ed., p. 69. New York: Basic Books, 1975.

Birch, H. G. "The problem of 'brain damage' in children," in H. G. Birch, ed., *Brain Damage in Children: The Biological and Social Aspects*. Baltimore: Williams & Wilkins, 1964.

Bradley, C. "Characteristics and management of children with organic brain damage." *Pediatric Clinics of North America*, 4, 1049–1069, (1957).

Chess, S. "Neurological dysfunction and childhood behavioral pathology." *Journal of Autism and Childhood Schizophrenia*, 2, 299–311, (1972).

Clements, S. D. and J. E. Peters. "Minimal brain dysfunctions in the school-age child." *Archives of General Psychiatry*, 6, 185–197, (1962).

Cohen, D. J. and J. G. Young. "Neurochemistry and child psychiatry." *Journal of the American Academy of Child Psychiatry*, 16, 353–411, (1977).

Connolly, K. "Movement, action and skill," in K. S. Holt, ed., *Movement and Child Development*, Clinics in Developmental Medicine, No. 55, pp. 102–110. London: Heinemann, 1975.

Eccles, J. C. *The Understanding of the Brain*, 2nd ed. New York: McGraw-Hill, 1977.

Eisenberg, L. "Psychiatric implications of brain damage in children." *Psychiatric Quarterly*, 31, 72–92, (1957).

Ford, F. R. *Diseases of the Nervous System in Infancy, Childhood, and Adolescence*, 6th ed., pp. 59–60. Springfield, Ill.: Thomas, 1973.

Freud, A., and D. T. Burlingham. *Infants without Families*, pp. 14–15. New York: International Universities Press, 1944.

Gardner, E. *Fundamentals of Neurology*, 6th ed. Philadelphia: Saunders, 1975.

Gesell, A. *The First Five Years of Life*. New York: Harper, 1940.

Gesell, A., and F. L. Ilg. *The Child from Five to Ten*. New York: Harper, 1946.

Gesell, A., F. L. Ilg, and L. B. Ames. *Youth: The Years from Ten to Sixteen*, pp. 68, 73–74. New York: Harper, 1956.

Gomez, M. R. "Minimal cerebral dysfunction (maximal neurological confusion)." *Clinical Pediatrics*, 6, 589–591, (1967).

Graham, P., and M. Rutter. "Organic brain dysfunction and child psychiatric disorder." *British Medical Journal*, 3, 695–700, (1968).

Gross, M. D., and W. C. Wilson. *Minimal Brain Dysfunction*. New York: Brunner/Mazel, 1974.

Harrison, A. "Components of neuromuscular control," in K. S. Holt, ed., *Movement and Child Development*, Clinics in Developmental Medicine, No. 55, pp. 34–50. London: Heinemann, 1975.

Holt, K. S. "How and why children move," in K. S. Holt, ed., *Movement and Child Development*, Clinics in Developmental Medicine, No. 55, pp. 1–7. London: Heinemann, 1975.

Illingworth, R. S. "The clumsy child," in M. Bax and R. MacKeith, eds., *Minimal Cerebral Dysfunction*, Little Club Clinics in Developmental Medicine, No. 10, pp. 26–27. London: Spastics Society, 1963.

Kenny, T. J., and R. L. Clemmens. "Medical and psychological correlates in children with learning disabilities." *Journal of Pediatrics*, 78, 273–277, (1971).

Knobloch, H., and B. Pasamanick. "Syndrome of minimal cerebral damage in infancy." *Journal of the American Medical Association*, 170, 1384–1387, (1959).

————, eds. *Gesell and Amatruda's Developmental Diagnosis*, 3rd ed. Hagerstown, Md.: Harper & Row, 1974.

Lapouse, R., and M. Monk. "An epidemiologic study of behavior characteristics in children." *American Journal of Public Health*, 48, 1134–1144, (1958).

Levy, D. M. "On the problem of movement restraint." *American Journal of Orthopsychiatry*, 14, 644–671, (1944).

Lucas, A. R., P. E. Kauffman, and E. M. Morris. "Gilles de la Tourette's disease: A clinical study of fifteen cases." *Journal of the American Academy of Child Psychiatry*. 4, 700–722, (1967).

Lucas, A. R., E. A. Rodin, and C. B. Simson. "Neurological assessment of children with early school problems." *Developmental Medicine and Child Neurology*, 7, 145–156, (1965).

Luria, A. R. *The Working Brain*. New York: Basic Books, 1973.

MacKeith, R. "Defining the concept of 'minimal brain damage'," in R. MacKeith and M. Bax, eds., *Minimal Cerebral Dysfunction*, Little Club Clinics in Developmental Medicine, No. 10., pp. 1–9. London: Heinemann, 1963.

Macfarlane, J. W., L. Allen, and M. P. Honzik. *A Developmental Study of the Behavior Problems of Normal Children between Twenty-One Months and Fourteen Years*. Berkeley: University of California Press, 1954.

Mittelmann, B. "Motility in infants, children and adults: Patterning and psychodynamics." *Psychoanalytic Study of the Child*, 9, 142–177, (1954).

————"Intrauterine and early infantile motility." *Psychoanalytic Study of the Child*, 15, 104–127, (1960).

Paine, R. S. "Minimal chronic brain syndromes in children." *Developmental Medicine and Child Neurology*, 4, 21–27, (1962).

Pond, D. "Is there a syndrome of 'brain damage' in children?" Cerebral Palsy Bulletin, 2, 296–297, (1960).

Prechtl, H. F. R., and C. J. Stemmer. "The choreiform syndrome in children." Developmental Medicine and Child Neurology, 4, 119–127, (1962).

Reuben, R. N. and H. Bakwin. "Developmental clumsiness." Pediatric Clinics of North America, 15, 601–610, (1968).

Rie, E. D., H. E. Rie, S. Stewart, and S. R. Rettemnier. "An analysis of neurological soft signs in children with learning problems." Brain and Language, 5 (4), (1978).

Rodin, E., A. Lucas, and C. Simson. "A study of behavior disorders in children by means of general purpose computers," in K. Enslein, ed., Data Acquisition and Processing in Biology and Medicine, vol. 3, pp. 115–123. London: Pergamon, 1964.

Ross, D. M., and S. A. Ross. Hyperactivity: Research, Theory and Action. New York: Wiley, 1976.

Rutter, M., P. Graham, and H. G. Birch. "Interrelations between the choreiform syndrome, reading disability and psychiatric disorder in children of 8–11 years." Developmental Medicine and Child Neurology, 8, 149–159, (1966).

Rutter, M., P. Graham, and W. Yule. A Neuropsychiatric Study in Childhood, Clinics in Developmental Medicine, Nos. 35/36. London: Heinemann, 1970.

Schmitt, B. D. "The minimal brain dysfunction myth." American Journal of Diseases of Children, 129, 1313–1318, (1975).

Siegel, G. J., R. W. Albers, R. Katzman, and B. W. Agranoff. Basic Neurochemistry, 2nd ed. Boston: Little, Brown, 1976.

Shaffer, D., N. McNamara, and J. H. Pincus. "Controlled observations on patterns of activity, attention, and impulsivity in brain-damaged and psychiatrically disturbed boys." Psychological Medicine, 4, 4–18, (1974).

Shepherd, G. M. "Microcircuits in the nervous system." Scientific American, 238, 93–103, (1978).

Stine, O. C., J. B. Saratsiotis, and R. S. Mosser. "Relationship between neurological findings and classroom behavior." American Journal of Diseases of Children, 129, 1036–1040, (1975).

Strauss, A. A., and L. E. Lehtinen. Psychopathology of the Brain-Injured Child. New York: Grune & Stratton, 1947.

Strauss, A. A., and H. Werner. "The mental organization of the brain-injured mentally defective child." American Journal of Psychiatry, 97, 1194–1203, (1941).

Thomas, A., and Chess, S. Temperament and Development. New York: Brunner/Mazel, 1977.

Thomas, A., S. Chess, H. G. Birch, M. E. Hertzig, and S. Korn. Behavioral Individuality in Early Childhood. New York: New York University Press, 1963.

Walton, J. N., E. Ellis, and S. D. M. Court. "Clumsy children: Developmental apraxia and agnosia." Brain, 85, 603–612, (1962).

Wender, P. H. Minimal Brain Dysfunction in Children. New York: Wiley-Interscience, 1971.

Werry, J. S., K. Minde, A. Guzman, G. Weiss, K. Dogan, and E. Hoy. "Studies on the hyperactive child—VII: Neurological status compared with neurotic and normal children." American Journal of Orthopsychiatry, 42, 441–451, (1972).

Wyke, B. "The neurological basis of movement. A developmental review," in K. S. Holt, ed., Movement and Child Development, Clinics in Developmental Medicine, No. 55, pp. 19–33. London: Heinemann, 1975.

CHAPTER 11

Perceptual Organization and Minimal Brain Dysfunctions

Ira Belmont

There is considerable disagreement regarding the accuracy, meaning, and value of diagnosing or classifying children as having minimal brain dysfunction. This is clearly evident from a reading of the various contributions to a conference of MBD held at the New York Academy of Sciences in 1972 (de la Cruz, et al., 1973). The present chapter however is not directly concerned with the designation of children as MBD, hyperkinetic, learning disabled, perceptually hadicapped, central processing dysfunctioned, and so on, though the most effective treatment is ultimately dependent upon correct diagnosis. Correct diagnosis of the same child may be different depending upon differing professional responsibilites and goals (Gallagher, 1960, 1966). Rather our starting point is the fact that the different terms are applied more or less to the same failing children. Therefore no matter what the classification used, this chapter will consider possible deficits subsumed under "perceptual disorders" in school children. This strategy has been chosen since, if there are specific perceptual disorders associated with MBD, per se, they have been inadequately described (Wender, 1971; Gross and Wilson, 1974). No attempt will be made to cover systematically the large extant literature on children with proven or presumed brain injury since this has been more than adequately done (for example Diller and Birch, 1964; Birch, 1964*b*; Chalfant and Scheffelin, 1969). Nor is it assumed that the classifications MBD, brain injured, learning disabled, and so on, necessarily refer to the same set of children. While such an impression may be gained from some sources (Clements, 1966; Chalfant and Scheffelin, 1969; Clements and Peters, 1973), others (Wender, 1971; Gross and Wilson, 1974) suggest the partial, though large, overlap among children so designated.

PERCEPTUAL DISORDERS AND SCHOOL FAILURE

Successful adaptation to the demands of school is frequently critical for a child's present and future adjustment to life. We are therefore taking educational performance as the point of departure for approaching issues of perceptual functioning in children. Moreover learning to read is given major consideration because it is the most important task facing the young school age child; it has indeed received more attention than any other aspect of education (Gibson and Levin,

1975). Since the work done in this and related areas is vast, only selected studies which exemplify certain issues will be presented.

The view that perceptual and/or perceptual-motor dysfunction underlies reading failure is widespread. This claim rests first on the contention that the early reading task is, on the face of it, in large part perceptual; learning to read requires the separate processing as well as the integration of visual and auditory information. The argument for perceptual disorders is particularly persuasive for the early stages of reading. For example, visual discriminations and differentiations must be made among shapes (letters) some of which are similar in form (n and h) and among the same shapes which are in different positions (m and w) or are mirror images of each other (b and d). Also visual analysis and synthesis together with appropriate visual-motor directional patterns (scanning) are required for word identification and sequential reading. Sound-symbol relations (auditory-visual linkages) must be learned, that is, what the learner sees must become equivalent to what he hears. The failure to establish these relatively simple perceptual functions when semantic requirements are made easy, it is argued, is in contrast to already well-developed complex language skills possessed by the children involved.

Testing for Perceptual Deficiencies

A second basis for the claim of impaired perceptual functioning as underlying reading failure is poor performance on standardized perceptual and/or perceptual-motor tests. A number of these tests and related remedial procedures have their origin in work done with children who were, or were presumed to be, brain-injured (Strauss and Lehtinen, 1947). While the question of whether these children were in fact brain injured has become a moot point, the original developmental flavor of the approach, as shown in the work of Heinz Werner, has been retained and applied to the normal as well as the special school setting. It is contended that failure to profit from initial reading instruction is due to perceptual immaturity or maldevelopment and that a course of perceptual and perceptual-motor traning can be effective in preventing or reducing initial reading failure. Leading examples of this approach are the diagnostic and remedial programs developed by Kephart (1960), Cruickshank, et al. (1961), and Frostig and Horne (1964). The programs are based on the assumption that the ability to acquire primary reading skills is dependent upon the possession of specific perceptual-motor and perceptual competencies (Kephart, 1960; Frostig, 1968; Cruickshank, 1972). While each program uses a unique set of terms and has a unique set of procedures they are similar in general conception, focusing on the development of:

1. Relevant visual, auditory, tactile, and kinesthetic-motor organization within a context of reduced environmental stimuli (Cruickshank, 1972).

2. Eye-motor coordination, figure-ground perception, perception of shape constancy, perception of position in space, and perception of spatial relations (Frostig, 1968).

3. Movement integration and awareness, perceptual development through matching with motor awareness, and intersensory organization (Kephart, 1960).

These programs include material which is thought to be useful for improving perceptual memory, planning, attention, and sequencing behavior. They regard perceptual and perceptual-motor developmental progressions as precursors of the development of the more complex levels of language, thought, and symbolic functions. (See Myers and Hammill, 1976, for other perceptual and motor intervention programs.)

Other Widely Used Perceptual Tests

Probably the best known single instrument used to tap perceptual deficiencies in children is the Bender Visual Motor Gestalt Test (1938) which derives from a merging of psychiatry and gestalt psychology. The test's reputation rests not only on briefness and simplicity of administration, but also on its relative strength compared to other single instruments to predict early reading failure (de Hirsch, Jansky, and Langford, 1966). To increase objectivity in measuring performance, scoring systems have been devised, the best known (for children) being that developed by Koppitz (1964) for ages 5 to 10 years. The Koppitz system calls for scoring the quality of certain details and general features of each of the nine designs, including as major aspects rotations, perseverations, distortions, and failures of integration. The total error score is then compared to age-related norms for determining inadequacy of overall performance. However, while good test performance tends to be related to reading success, poor performance is related to either poor or good reading performance. Moreover the test may yield false negatives for children above the age of 8 years and is of questionable value for the socially disadvantaged (Welcher, et al., 1974).

Another design-copying test, Benton's Revised Visual Retention Test (1974), is now receiving increased attention for use with children. It contains 3 equivalent forms, each with 10 designs. The designs and the sequence of presentation were planned to tap systematically certain features of visual perception, visual memory, and visuoconstructive abilities. Scoring is done in two ways, an overall score of number correct and an error score. For the latter each design is scored systematically for specific kinds of errors: omissions (and additions), distortions, perseverations from previous designs, rotations, misplacements, and size errors. Children's norms are currently based on relatively few cases and could use further development.

In fact design-copying tests of all kinds have proliferated, as separate tests or as parts of batteries, indicating the diagnostic value placed upon them by educators and psychologists. For other perceptual and perceptual-motor tests see Anastasi (1968), Satz and Friel (1973), Reitan and Davison (1974), Smith (1975), Lerner (1976).

The well known Illinois Test of Psycholinguistic Abilities (ITPA) (Kirk, McCarthy and Kirk, 1968), while not regarded as a test of perceptual functioning, should be mentioned here since 8 of its 12 subtests refer specifically to visual or auditory operations. It has subtests for visual, as differentiated from auditory, reception, association, closure, and sequential memory. The separate testing of these four abilities by each of the two perceiving systems (auditory and visual) implies that there are different sensory mechanisms for similar general task requirements. Thus if the separate subtests tap different kinds of abilities, then the operation of the specific skills must be managed by different sense systems. In addition to the abilities already mentioned, verbal expression, grammatic closure, manual expression, and sound blendings are evaluated. The test results, as planned by the authors, are then used to construct individual programs of remediation based on the pattern of success and failure in the various abilities and sense modalities.

It should be mentioned that another testing source commonly used to diagnose perceptual disorders is the finding of a large discrepancy between (higher) verbal IQ and (lower) performance IQ score on those intelligence tests which permit the differentiation (for example that Wechsler Intelligence Test for Children).

Perceptual Dysfunction and MBD

When perceptual and other school-related functions are examined from an educational viewpoint, failing children in the normal range of intelligence are most frequently regarded as having specific learning disabilities (SLD). SLD is a term as unspecific as MBD (for example see Federal Register, 1976). However from a medical viewpoint many of the same children are termed MBD with SLD seen as a consequence, an indicator, or subtype of the condition. Despite the close relation between the two classifications, deep concern has been shown and detailed attention given to the perceptual functioning of children labeled SLD, while most frequently only brief reference is made to such functioning in MBD children (Wender, 1971, 1975). The difference in approach is probably related to differences between educational and medical diagnostic and treatment responsibilities.

It is true that studies of the effects of drugs on MBD children have included large batteries of tests among which are perceptual and perceptual-motor tests. Yet test performance after medication is most often interpreted not as reflecting changes in specific perceptual or language or cognitive functions—the work of Butter and Lapierre (1974) is a rare exception—but rather as reflecting changes in some general quality, such as attention (Douglas, 1974; Dykman, et al., 1974) or "learning" ability (Sprague and Sleator, 1977) with the concept of attention deficit being the most prominent view. Serious questions are now being raised regarding the usefulness of such general concepts for understanding deficiencies in MBD children. Gittelman-Klein and Klein (1975) have argued that when pre- to post-drug performance on specific tests are examined the concept of unitary attention deficit is unsubstantiated since some attention-related performances change while others do not. In fact Rie, et al., (1976a, 1976b) have found few reliable improvements in any specific psychological function, perceptual and perceptual-motor included, as measured on the tests used. Nor did they find improvements in school achievement or "learning." It is becoming clear that more attention to the specifics and details of psychological, including perceptual, functions is required before a clearer picture can be gained of the effects of medication on school achievement, if any. In this regard we might want to contrast drug-related results with those produced by perceptual training.

The Effectiveness of Perceptual Training

In recent years perceptual remediation has been offered to many MBD-like children in order to improve their reading skills. The question of the value of such remediation has been the subject of much experimentation. Unfortunately most of the studies suffer from poor design (for critiques of design see Belmont and Birch, 1974; Myers and Hammill, 1976). Despite this there is sufficient evidence to

permit the conclusion that perceptual and perceptual-motor intervention programs do not result in improved reading (Robinson, 1972; Myers and Hammill,
1976). At best the children exposed to the programs tend to improve on the kinds
of tasks on which they were originally tested and trained, but as a group they do
not show the expected improvement in reading. It is important to note that the
strategies underlying the diagnostic tests and remedial programs derive for the
most part from untested hypothetical generalizations. They do not derive from a
detailed analysis of the acquisition of reading skills as a learning task nor the
related perceptual competencies and learning sets, which must be developed for
learning to read (Belmont, 1974). It is therefore not surprising that available
evidence has not shown any of these methods to be generally successful in reducing reading failure and facilitating the acquisition of reading skills.

In this regard Vellutino and his associates (1977) argued that not only are the
currently used perceptual and perceptual-motor preventive and remedial programs ineffective, but also they are simplistic, incorrectly conceived, and premature applications of the original (and controversial) developmental theories (those
of Piaget, Werner, and Strauss) on which they are based. While there is an
accumulating body of work, including their own, which suggests that linguistic
deficiencies, not strictly perceptual ones, underlie reading failure Vellutino, et al.,
(1977) opt for a more practical approach to diagnosis and remediation. At this
point in time remedial programs that are based on formal reading instruction per
se cannot be ignored since no special programs, including the little studied linguistic and language training programs, have been proven to be particularly effective.

To date then perceptual dysfunctions, have generally been defined as the failure
to achieve a minimum, norm-based score on perceptual or perceptual-motor tests,
which derive from untested generalizations concerning normal and aberrant perceptual functioning.

PERCEPTION, MULTIPLE SYNDROMES, AND DEVELOPMENT

The failure to develop broadly effective perceptual intervention programs does
not permit the conclusion that perceptual functions per se are intact in MBD (or
SLD) children. It does permit the conclusion expressed by Vellutino, et al., (1977)
that the current approaches taken to perceptual training may be simplistic and
incorrectly conceived. We are not considering at this time the possibility that the
remedial programs are generally ineffective because of uncorrectable deficiencies
or lags in the failing children.

Two major issues relating to the classification of MBD children require consideration prior to discussing perception per se. The first concerns the possibility that
there are multiple syndromes of specific disorders, now subsumed under the
general classification MBD, which require separate and primary attention. The
second is a developmental issue, the probability that there are age-related changes
in specific deficiencies shown by MBD children.

Different Syndromes of MBD Children

It is quite clear that MBD cannot be considered as a unitary disorder. The variety
of patterns of disorder exhibited by MBD and SLD children suggests that different syndromes of specific disorders exist (Benton, 1975; Senf, 1973). In particular

this should follow if, as some believe, brain damage is involved, which of course has not been proven. Depending upon the location, size, and nature of the lesion and age sustained, there should be a number of different MBD syndromes (Birch, 1964; Benton, 1973; Conners, 1973). These syndromes may include different kinds of perceptual deficit and perhaps none in some constellations of disorder.

Little work has been done to search for different syndromes, but what exists is suggestive. Two studies are presented which may serve as examples of ways of exploring for possible syndromes. Denckla (1972), based on an extended neurological examination of two hours for each of 190 private patients, indicated that certain clusters or symptom complexes appear to emerge from the list of 10 most frequent signs of minimal brain dysfunction. She found that about 30% (N=57) of the children could be divided into easily recognizable clusters of signs and 70% (N=133) showed an unclassifiable mixture. The first subgroup included 29 (15% of 190) children, mainly boys, who were classified as having specific language disability. These children, failing in reading and spelling, showed a pattern of inadequacy on repetition, sequencing, memory, language, motor, and other tasks —all requiring rote functioning. While often labeled as perceptually impaired, the basis of their poor performance Denckla argued is not perceptual, but rather an aphasic-like rote-related disorder. The second group, termed specific visuo-spatial disability, consisted of 9 (5% of 190) children who were at least average in reading and spelling, were poor in arithmetic, and seriously inadequate in writing and copying, and were all socially emotionally maladjusted. The third group were said to manifest a dyscontrol syndrome and included 19 (10% of 190) children who had poor motor and impulse control, were behaviorally immature, and normal in language and perceptual functioning. Denckla claimed that it is the last group which is helped by drugs. Neurologic findings per se were not reported.

In the second study Mattis, French, and Rapin (1975) reported on 113 children and young adults, 8 to 18 years of age, who were referred to a medical clinic for learning and/or behavior problems. They were administered a large battery of standard and special psychological tests, a reading test (Wide Range Achievement Test), and an extensive neurological examination. Based on the neurological examination and the reading test, three subgroups were formed:

a. 53 brain-injured poor readers, 2 or more grades below expected level.

b. 29 nonbrain-injured poor readers (same criterion).

c. 31 brain-injured adequate readers.

Two major findings emerged: the first was that no systematic relation was found between poor reading and a diagnosis of brain injury; the second finding is relevant to the issue of syndromes. The poor readers were separable into three distinct dysfunctional groups based on psychological test performance, independent of whether they were brain-injured or not. They were:

a. A language-disordered (anomic) group.

b. A group exhibiting articulatory and graphomotor incoordination.

c. A group showing visuospatial perceptual disorder.

The purpose of presenting the two studies was not to compare findings since there are undefined differences in population and in tests used as the basis of differentiating groups. Rather the studies suggest the value and necessity of searching for subtypes of MBD and SLD children. They offer the possibility that not all, but only certain subgroups of disordered children manifest perceptual disorders. A weakness in the reports however is the failure to include an analysis by age.

Age-Related Deficiencies or Lags

On the basis of what is generally known about growth and development, we are compelled to argue that a developmental orientation is essential when considering perceptual and perceptual-motor dysfunctions or lags in children of different ages. In this light it has been suggested that there are different age-related problems underlying school failure in the different grades. Belmont and Birch (1966) considered the possibility that early reading failure may be related to depressed perceptual and performance skills, whereas later reading failure is probably related to language deficiencies.

A similar developmental view has been elaborated by Satz and Sparrow, (1970). In essence they theorize that early reading failure reflects a maturational lag in perceptual-spatial and cross-modal integration (sensori-perceptual skills), while later failure is based on delayed development of language and formal operations (conceptual-linguistic skills). They are testing these hypotheses using a large battery of selected tests in an anterospective study now reported through its sixth year (Satz, et al., 1978). A series of analyses done on an annual basis and across longer periods of time as well as new predictive studies derived from the original work have considerably strengthened the hypothesis. In addition to pursuing multiple goals regarding prediction, remediation, and underlying process over age, this work is now moving towards a consideration of perceptual-conceptual-linguistic relations, a direct result of the developmental approach taken.

One issue considered by Satz, et al., (1978), the consistency of reading performance over the grades, may require reconsideration. They pointed to the relative consistency shown particularly by poorest (severe) and best (superior) readers over the years. In comparing performance over two points in time (grades two and five) they may have have overestimated stability in level of performance. If the analysis had included the intervening years, then more (perhaps considerable) inconsistency would have been revealed. Relative instability was shown to be the usual pattern in an epidemiological, longitudinal study by Belmont and Belmont (1978) which examined annual performance across the first six grades. Many children who showed similarity in level of performance in two grades did not show such consistency when the other four grades were included. Four different performance patterns were found:

1. Only a very small proportion of the children consistently failed over all grades.
2. A small proportion showed developmental lag, failing in the early years and performing adequately later (slow starters or late bloomers).
3. An equally small proportion were adequate early, but failed in later years.
4. Most of the children who failed in one grade or another fluctuated in performance over the years, alternating idiosyncratically year by year between failure and average reading.

It was suggested that many of the last-described children are in the (low) normal range of functioning with temporary periods of retardation or backwards in reading. If the same kinds of patterns over time seen by Belmont and Belmont (1978) are found to be characteristic of the children in the study by Satz, et al., (1978) then some revision may be necessary in the latter's view of the frequency of occurrence and of the persistence of developmental lag.

The most productive approach to the question of studying perceptual dysfunctions that may be characteristic of MBD children then probably requires as a context: (1) a search for different syndromes of disorder, or lag, at given ages and (2) a search for changes over time in the nature of given disorders or lags.

NEEDED: NEW APPROACHES TO THE STUDY OF PERCEPTUAL DYSFUNCTION

The failure to develop generally effective perceptual training programs and the tendency to rely on nonqualitative, norm-based perceptual-motor test scores as indicators of perceptual handicap calls attention to the need for developing new approaches to the study of perceptual dysfunction. Such study must be a prelude to the development of more rational remedial procedures. For such an endeavor it is important to be reminded of both the complexity of perception and the intertwined nature of perceptual and other functions. What follows is one, hopefully useful, approach to the study of perceptual dysfunction derived from sources having similar underlying conceptualizations.

Definition of Perception

Even a brief review of the literature on perception will produce a variety of definitions of perception. For our purposes we are presenting a definition which contains the essential elements common to most of them. Perceiving can be regarded as a process of extracting information from the environment (Gibson, 1969). This implies that it is an active process of searching for, selecting, and organizing stimuli from the immediate surroundings and that these occur in relation to specific purposes or tasks. Perception includes a variety of processes, such as discrimination, differentiation, recognition, recall, analysis, synthesis, set (expectation or anticipation), attention, motivation, creating hypotheses and testing (verifying) them against the task requirements. Moreover the processes involved in searching and selecting necessarily include motor components, the sequential organization of perceptual-motor patterns related to the task (Birch and Lefford, 1967; Luria, 1973).

Perception and Interacting Systems

No test, school task, or other situation involves single qualities per se, such as perception, or language, or personality, and so on. Rather the behavior we observe is the product of a complex set of interacting systems, no one of which operates by itself. This view suggests that while there is unique processing by the separate sense systems (vision, audition, kinesthesis, and so on), they operate conjointly. Moreover these interacting sensory systems are themselves interacting with other systems, for example linguistic, language, motivational, memory,

planning, goal orienting, motor, and so on, all in relation to the specific requirements of given tasks and within the context of socially determined expectations.
The operation and development of any given system is therefore determined not
only by its part in person-environment interactions but also by the influence of the
systems upon each other. The study of the organization and development of each
of these systems then requires more than an approach which considers the functioning of each of these subsystems by itself. Rather the specific contribution of a
particular subsystem to behavior cannot be directly observed and at best can only
be deduced by abstracting common elements from a variety of behaviors (Luria,
1966,1973).

Perception per se cannot then be directly tested or observed. For example
perceptual tests may include verbal instructions and/or responses. In such instances deficient or unusual responses may reflect verbal inadequacies, perceptual
inadequacies, or failure of verbal-perceptual interaction. Further, when tests require the conversion of percepts (for example what one sees or touches) into
verbal equivalents, the process appears to be different from the reverse demand,
that is when verbal information is to be converted into percepts. Aspects of these
different processes were illustrated, for example in Rorschach studies (Birch and
Belmont, 1964; Belmont, Belmont, and Birch, 1969) which focused not on personality characteristics but on perceptual and verbal functioning. In the initial free
association phase of the test, the subject was asked to look at and then say what
he saw in the inkblots. This was regarded as a visual recognition-verbal task in
which self-determined percepts are produced and then converted into words communicated to the examiner. In the second, inquiry phase of the examination, the
subject was asked to specify the parts of each response as seen in the inkblot.
This required that the subject analyze his percepts; it was regarded as indicating
visual-analytic ability. In the final, testing-of-limits phase of the test, the subject
was asked if he was able to see selected objects (so-called "populars") which
were suggested by the examiner. This required the subject to alter his perception
to fit a verbal suggestion and was termed verbal-visual in its demand.

The possible value of interpreting the findings within the framework of interacting systems may be illustrated by some of the results reported in a study of 8-to
10-year-old educable, mentally subnormal children (Belmont, Belmont, and
Birch, 1969). First, the subnormal children were not passive in responding to the
open-ended, complex stimulation patterns, but rather were as reactive as normal
children in initiating their own organizations of the inkblots (visual-verbal level;
total number of spontaneous responses). However they tended to use single
words in reporting their percepts and gave little embellishment in contrast to
normal children who tended to use more extended and organized verbalizations
(phrases and sentences). Thus a combination of equal perceptual responsivity and
unequal language usage was shown. Second, the subnormal children tended to do
very poorly in analyzing their percepts; this was characterized by active, gross
inaccuracies and distortions in analysis, not apparently related to the use of
simpler language. Thus though actively involved, they were frequently unable to
isolate one feature of the percept and then another while at the same time maintaining the appropriate relationship of each part to the total gestalt. Moreover the
subnormal children were less capable than the normals of modifying their perceptions when verbal suggestions were offered (poorer response on verbal-visual
level). Subnormal children may therefore be less able to profit from verbal instruction when visually presented material is to be learned. Such interpretation is

relatively general and will require more precise analysis of perceptual and verbal elements. However it illustrates an approach and, for what it is, requires cross-checking with other similarly defined tasks and responses.

Perceptual-Motor Tasks and Interacting Systems

The same task-analytic approach may help to define interrelated psychological systems involved in, for example the Bender Gestalt (design copying) Test. Frequently serious errors of interpretation are made by the examiner regarding children's performance on this test. When a child fails to reproduce the figures accurately, it is commonly said to reflect deficient visual perception. If the figure is drawn at a different angle from the model, the child is said to be unaware of spatial position or unable to perceive it accurately. If two figures in the model are not interrelated accurately in the drawing, then the child is said to be deficient in perceiving spatial relations among objects. To begin with such interpretations fail to differentiate between perceptual and perceptual-motor functioning. This was demonstrated by Birch and Bortner (1962), who examined cerebral-palsied children, and by Zach and Kaufman (1972), who studied kindergarten children. The former study, using the block design subtest of the Wechsler Intelligence Scale for Children, and the latter, using the Bender-Gestalt test, showed that many children who failed to reproduce the model accurately were capable of selecting the failed items correctly in a multiple choice situation. Thus visual recognition of spatial position, of spatial relations, and of design forms was shown to be intact in these children. While visual discrimination may be deficient in some, we should be aware that other functions may be deficient. This can lead to incorrect perceptual-motor performance on the Bender-Gestalt.

In addition to intact visual discrimination, adequate drawing involves an organized pattern of sequential action which requires "perceptual analysis, perceptual synthesis and perceptual-motor organization" (Birch and Bortner, 1962, p. 104). These aspects of performance require elaboration. To begin with essential features of the figure must be separately considered (analyzed) and also reconstructed in relation to each other (synthesized). These appear to be two separate processes (Birch and Lefford, 1963). For accurate reproduction these two processes probably are in constant alternating interaction. Moreover this dual visual process must be coordinated with the required action pattern. The latter entails yet another perceptual process involving kinesthesis. Copying is a visually guided motor act, it requires that kinesthetic information, which derives from the action, be constantly and dynamically interrelated with the visual direction of movement. Thus ongoing intersensory organization of the relevant sense information is required, one (visual) guiding, the other (kinesthetic) organizing patterns of motor sequences; the kinesthetic system prepares and monitors appropriate changes in muscle tension related to the necessary succession of movements. The visual-kinesthetic combination must therefore, be dynamically related to the motor system per se.

Failure to copy adequately then may have as its basis functional deficiencies of the visual or kinesthetic system separately, integrational failure between these afferent systems, defective interaction between the visual-kinesthetic complex and the motor system, as well as failure of the motor system per se. It may even be that these subsystems are potentially adequate but are undeveloped in, for example the disadvantaged child who has had insufficient experience with or paid insufficient attention to this kind of task and has not yet developed generalized perceptual-motor patterns necessary for successful copying. This possibility is suggested by the work of Held (1965). They demonstrated the critical role of kinesthetic-tactile experience and practice in the development of visually guided behavior. Visual experience alone, without action and its kinesthetic component, was insufficient for the development of skilled movement. In this connection another series of investigations (Braine, 1978) is pertinent. One aspect of her work suggests that rotations of the model when drawn by young children may in part represent not failure in the appreciation of spatial orientation, but rather an attempt to present the figure in what is considered to be the correct upright position. The work suggests that spatial orientation should also be investigated relative to the meaning of rotations produced by deviant children.

Failure in copying designs may also be related to higher level functions. Visual and kinesthetic reception, analysis, synthesis, and integration may be essentially adequate but subsystems for planning, programming, verifying, and correcting performance may be faulty. Thus, for example inadequate planning or inadequate regulation of the act of copying may be other causes of misplaced or distorted drawings.

The foregoing analysis of perceptual-motor performance suggests that there may be any one or a number of specific and varied bases for failure. This view is consonant with Luria's concept of "complex functional systems" (1966; 1973, especially pp. 43–101). The particular subsystems postulated in this chapter as underlying Bender-Gestalt test performance were derived from a hypothetical task analysis. Yet it may be that the relatively high predictive value of the Bender-Gestalt test results from the breadth of the different functions it taps. If this is true, then the narrow interpretation that it reflects perceptual ability misdirects attention to what may actually be deficient. If the test is to point to particular deficiencies for remedial purposes, then considerably more study of Bender-Gestalt performance is needed to define the variety of disorders, deviances, and developmental lags that are inherent in the failures it elicits.

In this regard Benton's Visual Retention Test (1974) and Smith's Symbol Digit Modalities Test (1973) represent advances in test construction in that they permit increased differentiation of deficient processes. Each of the 10 designs in Benton's test and their order of presentation permit one to study specific kinds of visuoconstructive failure shown by a given child or adult. These include: the nature of omissions, distortions, perseverations, rotations, misplacements, and size errors. Moreover the use of equivalent forms and different task requirements (copy from a model; draw from memory) extend the usefulness of the test. The test permits more accurate specification of the nature of the perceptual-motor failure and a comparison of current perceptual-motor ability with perceptual-motor memory. Smith's coding test requires the child (or adult) to relate specific numbers to given, randomly presented, repeated simple geometric figures, both by writing the numbers in appropriate boxes under the figures and by verbal response. In addition to estimating general performance by use of norms, the child's perceptual-verbal writing skill can be contrasted with perceptual-verbal oral skill which may help in separating writing from speech difficulties. These tests represent a needed new orientation as well as steps toward improved diagnosis and perhaps remedial procedures.

Perception and the Development of Directed Action

All perceptual and perceptual-motor tests for children have norms based on age, obviously recognizing the developmental character of skills and abilities. However Birch and Lefford (1967) argued that there is no systematic account of the normal mechanisms subserving the development of perceptually guided motor performance, so that it is difficult or impossible to determine what alterations of underlying process occur in deviant children. They then offered three related hypotheses connecting the development of organized and directed action to changing patterns of organizing perceptual (afferent) information over age. The hypotheses conceptualize three simultaneously developing, interacting processes of afferent control of directed action:

1. A shift with increasing age from dominance of proximoceptor (tactile) to teloreceptor (visual) control systems.

2. A tendency with increasing age for directed action to be subserved by multisensory rather than unisensory patterning.

3. A tendency with increasing age for directed action to be based on increased intrasensory (within sense system) differentiation and definition.

The first hypothesis was not tested in their study. However a shift from tactile to visual dominance in performance was shown to have occurred between the ages of five and seven years in two other studies (Kaufman, et al., 1973; Rafael, 1975). This finding depends upon the equating of tasks across sense modalities.

As predicted from the second hypothesis Birch and Lefford (1967) found an increasing ability with age to integrate sensory information deriving from different sense systems. This result, in a different form, was also found by Kaufman, et al., (1973). Relative to the last hypothesis, Birch and Lefford found that increased intrasensory differentiation did occur with age. However it was not possible in their study to examine whether there was coordinated development of the hypothesized perceptual processes, although the changes did co-occur in time (between the age range of five to eight years). Nor was it possible to relate directly the improved perceptual functioning and the improved motor (design-copying) ability shown by the children. Thus only beginning steps have been taken to test the complicated set of ideas outlined. Yet the developmental hypotheses conceptualized by Birch and his colleagues focus attention on the need not only for studying the underlying processes of directed action, but also to do so on a developmental basis to permit an understanding of age-based differences in perceptual dysfunctions.

Perception and Reading

The relation between perception and language is the subject of considerable debate and controversy both in its practical application (Myers and Hammill, 1976) and in its theoretical formulation Young and Lindsley, 1970; Kavanagh and Mattingly, 1972). A central issue is whether the reception and expression of speech involves general perceptual functions or whether it involves unique perceptual (linguistic) features related only to language (Liberman, et al., 1967). There is evidence to support both views. This chapter however does not enter the controversy. It briefly refers to certain experimental perceptual approaches to studying reading disorders which have achieved prominence and which may ultimately lead to more rational remedial procedures. General reviews of perceptual studies related to reading can be found in Gibson (1969), Vernon (1971) and Gibson and Levin (1975).

Probably the most systematic and comprehensive experimental program for studying the reading process in recent years has been conducted by Gibson and her co-workers (1975). However since this work dealt with normal developmental features of reading processes, it has had as yet relatively little impact on fields directly related to learning disorders. For example no mention of Gibson's work is made in two recent major works on the subject (Lerner, 1976 and Myers and Hammill, 1976). Since an understanding of normal processes is necessary for an understanding of deviancy, it would be profitable to extend Gibson's work to the study of reading disorders. This perceptually related work includes studies of the normal course of achieving the ability to discriminate features of letters (straight versus curved, open versus closed, horizontal versus vertical versus diagonal, spatial position) when they are contained in letter-like forms, learning salient versus irrelevant features for letter identification, grapheme-phoneme (writing-listening) correspondences, and the convergence of meaning for words and pictures, among others. Gibson's (1975) position regarding perception and reading is instructive,

Reading is a cognitive process . . . it starts with perception, it requires perceptual learning of many things, and it ends up as a conceptual process, a tool for thinking and learning that can take the place of first hand experience. [P. 3]

In a different vein Birch brought to reading his view that adaptive behavior is the result of the development of organized patterns of functional relations within and among sensory systems (Birch and Bitterman, 1951; Birch, 1954). He revived interest in conceptualizing reading acquisition as establishing functional equivalences between the auditory and visual systems (Birch and Belmont, 1964). The latter study and others from the same laboratory provided data which was interpreted as demonstrating general failure in auditory-visual integration among retarded readers. The work of other investigators produced both agreement and other interpretations which suggested that some other deficiency (failure in attention, in memory, in response to seriality) and not auditory-visual processes per se account for failure in reading (Freides, 1974). More recently Rudel and Denckla (1976) argued from their data that,

the difficulty of the process for the young child or retarded reader does not depend upon the integration of information from two sensory modalities but rather on the translation of serial information into spatial information. [P. 176]

Concurrently in an attempt to explore the general usefulness of the sensory integration model for reading, Belmont (1974) attempted a detailed hypothetical analysis of the early reading task using that model. He postulated a variety of task requirements and related competencies in terms of intrasensory requirements (separate visual and auditory analyses, discriminations, differentiations and syntheses regarding letters and words), intersensory requirements (often conflicting rules of analysis and synthesis for sound blending relative to reading), and sensory-motor search patterns (variety of scan patterns with controlled head, neck, and eye movements). Further experimental work is clearly needed to clarify the processes involved. In this work the question of conflicting processes in interacting systems is a most important area of study (Liberman, et al., 1967) as is the isolation of systems in disordered children (Belmont, et al., 1967).

In the course of resolving the different interpretations, it seems critical that the populations studied must be more carefully defined and contrasted. The basis for poor reading must certainly vary and there are probably subpopulations having different disorders or lags which result in reading failure, note that many poor readers in the Birch and Belmont study (1964) showed normal auditory-visual performance. Care must be exercised when relating findings across studies. Rudel and Denckla studied children referred to a pediatric neurologist and as a group they are probably similar to clinic populations, whereas Birch and Belmont studied school populations of poor readers. Clinic and school populations of failing children should be differentiated since they differ in many ways. Clinic populations include many multiply handicapped children who are often chronically failing readers (Gottesman, Belmont, and Kaminer, 1975). School populations of poor readers in contrast include far fewer multiply handicapped children and many children who show varying patterns of achievement over the years which include failure only at times and adequate reading at other times (Belmont and Belmont, 1978).

However remedial help to currently failing children cannot wait for the future experimental resolution of what underlies failure. While such experimentation will over time contribute to the development of more rational remedial procedures, a practical approach to current practices would seem to be the best course. This was also the conclusion drawn by Vellutino, et al., (1977) who suggested that the concept of maximum transfer proposed by Ferguson and Gagné be used. The essence of the concept is to "focus upon performance and task variables in units that most closely approximate the skill to be learned" (p. 383); these units are based on a hierarchical ordering of transfer skills. This position is not far removed from that of Bateman (1969) and Chen (1969) among others, who in disagreeing with the use of perceptual intervention programs argued that the best way to prevent failure is to provide more and better formal reading instruction.

PERCEPTUAL MODES OF THOUGHT

The final section of the chapter is devoted to a general issue in the education of children. Probably the dominant view in our educational system today is that thought is mediated by language. Certainly reading is the central subject in the early grades and reading failure is so critical because of the later reliance on printed matter for instruction. However it is probable that other major modes of thought exist which can be used systematically to further the education of children. Some who think so have pointed to the example of Albert Einstein who apparently used predominantly visual and kinesthetic modes of thought in his creative work. The example of this great scientist has recently been brought to the attention of those interested in educational problems by Patten (1973) who reported on Einstein's early difficulty with language and later struggle to use it for communicating his ideas. According to Einstein,

The words of the language, as they are written or spoken, do not seem to play any role in my mechanism of thought. The psychical entities which serve as elements in thought are certain signs and more or less clear images which can be "voluntarily" reproduced and combined . . . this combinatory play seems to be the essential feature in productive thought —before there is any connection with logical construction in words or other kinds of signs which can be communicated to others. The above mentioned elements are, in my case, of visual and some of muscular type. Conventional words or other signs have to be sought for laboriously only in a secondary stage, when the above mentioned associative play is sufficiently established and can be produced at will as reported by Patten (1973): [P. 417]

It could be argued that Einstein was unaware of his use of language in thinking. While that is possible, the major role played by his sense systems and his struggle to convert into language what he knew perceptually is dramatic.

There is other than anecdotal evidence for this point of view. Ferguson (1977), a professor of history and curator of technology, provides historical, sociological, and biographical evidence for the existence of nonverbal, visual thinking as the major method underlying invention and learning in the mechanical field. In reviewing the use of major technical manuscripts and books over the last 500 years, he found that the most effective, longest used, and influential of them transmitted technical information mainly through drawings, charts, plates, and pictures which were developed into formal, complex, and varied systems of representation. He also reports the experiences of numbers of inventors who indicated the visual and manual nature of their thinking, and visual mental construction of the final product before actually building the machine. Ferguson concluded that,

Much of the creative thought of the designers of our technological world is nonverbal, not easily reduced to words; its language is an object or a picture of a visual image in the mind. [P. 835]

This work suggests that different people use different methods of thinking, some using language, others perception as a dominant mode depending upon individual style and the task requirements. It suggests further that the relation between language and perceptual modes of thinking requires systematic study and application to the classroom. Moreover there may be a considerable amount of educational material which can be taught through perceptual means while a poor reader is in the process of learning to read. More broadly it can be argued that we should use whatever means are possible to teach a child while helping him learn to read.

Implied here is that the processes of perceiving and understanding the world of objects and their relations may be of a very different sort from those involved in other kinds of perception-related tasks, such as learning to read. If so, then an additional dimension of perceptual functioning must be included in the study of those MBD children who may manifest perceptual disorders.

REFERENCES

Anastasi, A. *Psychological Testing*, 3rd ed. New York: Macmillan, 1968.

Bateman, B. "Critique of Cohen, S. A. 'Studies in visual perception and reading in disadvantaged children'." *Journal of Learning Disabilities*, 2, 506–507, (1969).

Belmont, I. "Requirements of the early reading task." *Perceptual and Motor Skills*, 38, 527–537, (1974).

Belmont, I., and L. Belmont. "Stability or change in reading achievement over time: Developmental and educational implications." *Journal of Learning Disabilities*, [1978] in press.

Belmont, L. and H. G. Birch. "The intellectual profile of retarded readers." *Perceptual and Motor Skills*. Monograph Supplement 6–V22 (1966).

——"The effect of supplemental intervention on children with low reading readiness scores." *Journal of Special Education*, 8, 81–89, (1974).

Belmont, I., L. Belmont, and H. G. Birch. "The perceptual organization of complex arrays by educable mentally subnormal children." *Journal of Nervous and Mental Disease*, 149, 241–253, (1969).

Belmont, I., H. G. Birch, and L. Belmont. "The organization of intelligence test performance in educable mentally subnormal children." *American Journal of Mental Deficiency*, 71, 969–976, (1967).

Bender, L. *A Visual Motor Gestalt Test and Its Clinical Use*. Research Monographs No. 3. New York: American Orthopsychiatric Association, 1938.

Benton, A. L. "Minimal brain dysfunction from a neuropsychological point of view," in F. F. de la Cruz, B. H. Fox, and R. H. Roberts, eds., *Minimal Brain Dysfunction*, pp. 29–37. New York: New York Academy of Sciences, 1973.

——Revised Visual Retention Test. New York: Psychological Corporation, 1974.

——"Developmental dyslexia: Neurological aspects," in W. J. Friedlander, ed., *Advances in Neurology*, vol. 7, pp. 1–47. New York: Raven, 1975.

Birch, H. G. "Comparative psychology," in F. L. Marcuse, ed., *Areas of Psychology*, pp. 446–447. New York: Harper, 1954.

——"The Problem of 'Brain Damage' in Children," in H. G. Birch, ed., *Brain Damage in Children. The Biological and Social Aspects*, pp. 3–12. Baltimore: Williams & Wilkins, 1964*a*.

——"A selective bibliography on brain-damaged children," in H. G. Birch, ed., *Brain Damage in Children*, pp. 132–199. Williams & Wilkins, 1964*b*.

Birch, H. G., and I. Belmont. "Functional levels of disturbance manifested by brain-damaged (hemiplegic) patients as revealed in rorschach responses." *Journal of Nervous and Mental Disease*, 132, 410–416, (1961).

Birch, H. G., and L. Belmont. "Auditory-visual integration in normal and retarded readers." *American Journal of Orthopsychiatry*, 34, 852–861, (1964).

Birch, H. G., and M. E. Bitterman. "Sensory integration and cognitive theory." *Psychological Review*, 58, 355–361, (1951).

Birch, H. G. and M. Bortner, "Perceptual and perceptual-motor dissociation in cerebral palsied children." *Journal of Nervous and Mental Disease*, 134, 103–108, (1962).

Birch, H. G. and A. Lefford. "Intersensory development in children." *Monographs of the Society for Research in Child Development*. 28, Serial No. 89, (1963).

——"Visual differentiation, intersensory integration and voluntary motor control." *Monographs of the Society for Research in Child Development*. 32, Serial No. 110, (1967).

Braine, L. G. "A new slant on orientation perception." *American Psychologist*, 33, 10–22, (1978).

Butter, H. J., and Y. D. Lapierre. "The effect of methylphenidate on sensory perception and integration in hyperactive children." *International Pharmacopsychiatry*, 9, 235–244, (1974).

Chalfant, J. C., and M. A. Scheffelin. *Central Processing Dysfunctions in Children: A Review of Research*. NINDS Monograph No. 9, NIH, Bethesda, Md.: U.S. Department of HEW, 1969.

Clements, S. *Minimal Brain Dysfunction in Children—Terminology and Identification*. National Institute of Neurological Diseases and Blindness, Monogram No. 3, NIH. Bethesda, Md.: U.S. Department of HEW, 1966.

Clements, S., and J. E. Peters. "Psychoeducational programming for children with minimal brain dysfunctions," in F. F. de la Cruz, B. H. Fox, and R. H. Roberts, eds, *Minimal Brain Dysfunction*, pp. 46–51. New York: New York Academy of Sciences, 1973.

Cohen, S. A. "Studies in visual perception and reading in disadvantaged children." *Journal of Learning Disabilities*, 2, 498–503, (1969).

Conners, C. K. "Psychological assessment of children with minimal brain dysfunction," in F. F. de al Cruz, B. H. Fox, and R. H. Roberts, eds., *Minimal Brain Dysfunction*, pp. 283–302. New York: New York Academy of Sciences, 1973.

Cruickshank, W. M. "Some issues facing the field of learning disability." *Journal of Learning Disabilities*, 5, 380–383, (1972).

Cruickshank, W. M., F. Bentzen, F. H. Ratzebury, and M. Tannhauser. *A Teaching Method for Brain Injured and Hyperactive Children*. Syracuse: Syracuse University Press, 1961.

Cruz, F. F. de la, B. H. Fox, and R. H. Roberts, eds., *Minimal Brain Damage*. New York: New York Academy of Sciences, 1973.

Denckla, M. B. "Clinical syndromes in learning disabilities: The case for splitting vs lumping." *Journal of Learning Disabilities*, 5, 401–406, (1972).

Diller, L., and H. G. Birch. "Psychological evaluation of children with cerebral damage," in H. G. Birch, ed., *Brain Damage in Children*, pp. 27–43. Baltimore: Williams & Wilkins, 1964.

Douglas, V. I. "Differences between normal and hyperkinetic children," in C. K. Conners, ed., *Clinical Use of Stimulant Drugs in Children*, pp. 12–23. Amsterdam, The Netherlands: Excerpta Medica, 1974.

Dykman, R. A., P. T. Ackerman, J. E. Peters, and J. McGrew. "Psychological tests," in C. K. Conners, ed., *Clinical Use of Stimulant Drugs in Children*, pp. 44–52. Amsterdam, The Netherlands: Excerpta Medica, 1974.

"Federal Register, Proposed Rulemaking, Education of Handicapped Children," vol. 41, No. 230. U.S. Department of HEW, (Nov. 29, 1976).

Ferguson, E. S. "The mind's eye: Nonverbal thought in technology." *Science*, 197, 827–836, (1977).

Freides, D. "Human information processing and sensory modality: Cross-modal functions, information complexity, memory and deficit." *Psychological Bulletin*, 81, 284–310, (1974).

Frostig, M. "Education for children with learning disabilities," in H. R. Myklebust, ed., *Progress in Learning Disabilities*, vol. 1, pp. 234–266. New York: Grune & Stratton, 1968.

Frostig, M., and D. Horne. *The Frostig Program for the Development of Visual Perception*. Chicago: Follett, 1964.

Gallagher, J. J. *The Tutoring of Brain Injured Mentally Retarded Children*. Springfield, Ill.: Thomas, 1960.

———"Children with developmental imbalances: A psychoeducational definition," in W. M. Cruickshank, ed., *The Teacher of Brain-Injured Children*, pp. 23–43. Syracuse, N.Y.: Syracuse University Press, 1966.

Gibson, E. J. *Principles of Perceptual Learning and Development*. New York: Appleton-Century-Crofts, 1969.

———"Reading for some purpose," in J. F. Kavanagh and I. Mattingly, eds., *Language by Ear and by Eye*, pp. 3–10. [Keynote Address], Cambridge: MIT Press, 1975.

Gibson, E. J., and H. Levin. *The Psychology of Reading*. Cambridge: MIT Press, 1975.

Gittleman-Klein, R. and D. F. Klein. "Are behavioral and psychometric changes related in methylphenidate-treated, hyper-Children?'' *International Journal of Mental Health*, 4, 182–198 (1975).

Gottesman, R., I. Belmont, and R. Kaminer. "Admission and follow-up status of reading disabled children referred to a medical clinic." *Journal of Learning Disabilities*, 8, 642–650 (1975).

Gross, M. B., and W. C. Wilson. *Minimal Brain Dysfunction*. New York: Brunner/Mazel, 1974.

Held, R. "Plasticity in sensory-motor systems." *Scientific American*, 213, 84–94 (November 1965).

Hirsch, K. de, J. J. Jansky, and W. S. Langford. *Predicting Reading Failure*. New York: Harper, 1966.

Kaufman, J., I. Belmont, H. G. Birch, and L. J. Zach. "Tactile and visual sense system interactions: A developmental study using reaction time models." *Developmental Psychobiology*, 6, 165–176, (1973).

Kavanagh, J. F., I. G. Mattingly, eds. *Language by Ear and by Eye. The Relationships between Speech and Reading*. Cambridge: MIT Press, 1972.

Kephart, N. C. *The Slow Learner in the Classroom*. Columbus, Ohio: Merrill, 1960.

Kirk, S. A., J. J. McCarthy, and W. D. Kirk, *The Illinois Test of Psycholinguistic Abilities*, Revised Edition. Champaign: University of Illinois Press, 1968.

Koppitz, E. *Bender-Gestalt Test for Young Children*. New York: Grune & Stratton, 1964.

Lerner, J. W. *Children with Learning Disorders*, 2nd ed. Boston: Houghton Mifflin, 1976.

Liberman, A. M., F. S. Cooper, D. P. Shankweiler, and M. Studdert-Kennedy. "Perception of the speech code." *Psychological Review*, 74, 431–461, (1967).

Luria, A. R. *Higher Cortical Functions in Man*. New York: Basic Books, 1966.

———*The Working Brain. An Introduction to Neuropsychology*. New York: Basic Books, 1973.

Mattis, S., J. H. French, and I. Rapin. "Dyslexia in children and young adults: Three independent neuropsychological syndromes." *Developmental Medicine and Child Neurology*, 17, 150–163, (1975).

Myers, P. I., and D. D. Hammill. *Methods for Learning Disorders*, 2nd ed. New York: Wiley, 1976.

Patten, B. M. "Visually mediated thinking: A report of the case of Albert Einstein." *Journal of Learning Disabilities*, 6, 415–420, (1973).

Rafael, J. "Tactile-visual relations in lower class children" (Ph.D. diss., Yeshiva University, 1975).

Reitan, R. M., and L. A. Davison, eds., *Clinical Neuropsychology: Current Status and Applications*. Washington, D. C.: Winston, 1974.

Rie, H. E., E. D. Rie, S. Stewart, and J. P. Ambuel. "Effects of methylphenidate on underachieving children. *Journal of Consulting and Clinical Psychology*, 44, 250–260, (1976a).

———"Effects of Ritalin on under-achieving children: A replication." *American Journal of Orthopsychiatry*, 46, 313–322, (1976b).

Robinson, H. M. "Perceptual training—Does it result in reading improvement?," in R. C. Auckerman, ed., *Some Persistent Questions on Beginning Reading*, pp. 135–150. Newark, Del.: International Reading Association, 1972.

Rudel, R. G., and M. B. Denckla. "Relationship of IQ and reading score to visual, spatial and temporal matching tasks." *Journal of Learning Disabilities*, 9, 169–178, (1976).

Satz, P. and J. Friel. "Some predictive antecedents of specific learning disability: A preliminary one year follow-up,'' in P. Satz and J. J. Ross, eds., *The Disabled Learner*, pp. 79–98. Rotterdam, The Netherlands: Rotterdam University Press, 1973.

Satz, P. and S. S. Sparrow. ''Specific developmental dyslexia: A theoretical formulation,'' in Dirk J. Bakker and Paul Satz, eds., *Specific Reading Disability. Advances in Theory and Method*, pp. 17–40. Rotterdam, The Netherlands: Rotterdam University Press, 1970.

Satz, P., H. G. Taylor, J. Friel, and J. M. Fletcher. ''Some developmental and predictive precursors of reading disabilities: A six year follow-up,'' in D. Pearl and A. Benton, eds., *Dyslexia: An Appraisal of Current Research*. Washington: National Institute of Mental Health, 1978.

Senf, G. M. ''Learning disabilities.'' *Pediatric Clinics of North America*, 20, 607–640, (1973).

Smith, A. ''Symbol Digit Modalities Test.'' Los Angeles: Western Psychological Services, 1973.

———''Neuropsychological testing in neurologic disorders,'' in W. J. Friedlander, ed., *Advances in Neurology*, pp. 49–110. New York: Raven, 1975.

Sprague, R. L., and E. K. Sleator. ''Methylphenidate in hyperkinetic children: Differences in dose effect on learning and social behavior.'' *Science*, 198, 1274–1276, (Dec. 23, 1977).

Strauss, A. A., and L. Lehtinen. *Psychopathology and Education of the Brain-Injured Child*. New York: Grune & Stratton, 1947.

Vellutino, F. R., B. M. Steger, S. C. Moyer, C. J. Harding, and J. A. Niles. ''Has the perceptual deficit hypothesis led us astray?'' *Journal of Learning Disabilities*, 10, 375–385 (1977).

Vernon, M. D. *Reading and Its Difficulties*. Cambridge: Cambridge University Press, 1971.

Welcher, D. W., K. W. Wessel, E. D. Mellits, and J. B. Hardy. ''The Bender-Gestalt Test as an indicator of neurological impairment in young inner-city children.'' *Perceptual and Motor Skills*, 38, 899–910, (1974).

Wender, P. H. *Minimal Brain Dysfunction in Children*. New York: Wiley, 1971.

———''The minimal brain dysfunction syndrome.'' *Annual Review of Medicine*, 26, 45–62, 1975.

Young, F. A. and D. B. Lindsley, eds. *Early Experience and Visual Information Processing in Perceptual and Reading Disorders*. Washington, D.C.: National Academy of Sciences, 1970.

Zach, L. J., and J. Kaufman. ''How adequate is the concept of perceptual deficit for education?'' *Journal of Learning Disabilities*, 5, 351–356, (1972).

CHAPTER 12

Effects of MBD on Learning, Intellective Functions, and Achievement

Ellen D. Rie

INTRODUCTORY COMMENTS

Because a logically conceived and scientifically defined syndrome of minimal brain dysfunction has yet to emerge, present theoretical formulations, empirical data, and institutional practices require reexamination. Once again it becomes necessary to specify precisely behaviors regarded as unique sequelae of neural defect to distinguish them from behaviors of other etiologies. Presently the diagnosis of minimal brain dysfunction is presumptive as little empirical evidence exists to argue for a cause and effect relationship. Even less is known about the effects of neural defect on learning, intellective functions, and achievement. Yet these latter constructs comprise some of the most significant functions of the human brain.

In this chapter an attempt will be made to present a rationale for the study of learning, intellective functions, and achievement in relationship to minimal brain dysfunctions and to review what little pertinent data are available.

In emphasizing that the transformation of experience into memories involves complex and multiple brain functions, the distinguished English neurologist, Ritchie Russell (1959), suggested that the basis of cortical organization is an interaction between neuronal activities and experience, each exerting a profound influence on the other. He conceptualized an act of behavior as the work of elaborate neuronal connections innervated and conditioned by one's environment. More simply Luria (1961) in an address to the American Orthopsychiatric Association stated that mental activity is stimulated by the interaction of the child with the adult, and that "inner activity" is enhanced through linguistic acquisition.

While it is generally acknowledged that inherent cortical dispositions limit the level of integration of experience and that skill development in intact humans is substantially dependent on the nature of experience, less is known regarding the impact of environmental events on cortical morphology and physiology. By citing animal and human studies J. McV. Hunt (1969) stressed the point that anatomical or structural maturation of the nervous system can be affected by environmental influences. This theoretical position, albeit largely unexplored, renders the nature-nurture controversy simplistic and the mind-body dichotomy artificial. An account of behavioral and psychologic phenomena as reciprocal interactions between manifest external events and morphophysiological processes is suggestive of the possibility that pathological environments can alter the physical state of cerebral tissue as well as the biochemistry of the brain.

If it is true, as Russell (1959) attested, that the establishment and complexity of reliable neuronal pathways are dependent on the availability of reliable and complex experience, one might speculate that the ontogenetic development of neuronal cells does not occur in isolation but in response to some stimulating event.

That the substance and actions of neural mechanisms may not be fixed or predetermined but flexible and responsive to multiple environmental impingements (Rosenzweig, 1976) complicates both the definition and the diagnosis of minimal brain dysfunctions. In addition to the distinction between neurogenic and psychogenic determinants of behavior, it becomes necessary to distinguish between neural defects resulting from trauma, illness, or genetic determinants and those resulting from impoverished or aversive experiences.

Current explorations of evoked potential, arousal level, monoamine metabolism, acetylcholine operations, neuropeptide influences, and oxygen level as exciting as they may be as bases for the study of brain functions, do not and cannot provide a comprehensive analysis of behavior if treated as phenomena independent of the potential constraints imposed on the human brain by its surroundings. Thus the search for a morbid anatomy as the final proof of cortical dysfunctions would appear unduly restrictive. Multiple factors including genetic predispostions, physiological anomalies, and psycho-social-cultural impingements, as well as blatant damage or lesion may affect the programming of a sensory experience. In this vein minimal brain dysfunctions may be viewed as a neural insult especially as it occurs at the cortical level. It would seem reasonable to explore the premise that some children may have difficulties with the accuracy of their perceptions, with the establishment of good memories, and with the processing of ideas primarily because of a faulty mechanism in the central nervous system.

There is evidence from studies of demonstrable brain damage in humans and animals that higher level mental processing can be affected by trauma to the brain. Memory and learning have been studied extensively in brain damaged subjects (Lashley, 1963; Luria, 1966). More recently Rutter (1977) summarized his findings and concluded that brain-damaged children suffered from "cognitive disturbances," while Myklebust, Bannochie, and Killen (1971) wrote of integrative-neurosensory learning.

It is quite obvious that the study of patterns of cognition is necessary to understand better the mechanisms of the brain and to improve both the definition of minimal brain dysfunctions and the assessment procedures. It would seem natural to inquire into the differential effects of circumscribed, delimited, neurocognitive disorders on the constructs of learning, intellective skills, and achievement. If this is possible, then the concept of minimal brain dysfunctions need not be approached either skeptically or defensively.

Rationale

The purpose of this chapter is to explore the effects of subclinical neural defect on learning, intellective functions, and achievement. To understand properly the subtle relationships between neural substrata, stimulation, and behavior, it might be well to consider a neurocognitive orientation. There is little doubt that the brain, serving to store, trigger, and rearrange verbal and perceptual memories, requires a most ambitious training period. As the young infant experiences auditory and visual impressions through the sensory receptors, the cortex stores, arranges, and discharges impulses. The ability to absorb and assimilate experiences at the cortical level appears to depend upon the quality and quantity of brain cells, as well as on the efficiency and interaction of the components of the central nervous system, for example reticular and neurotransmitter functions. Engrams, or neural paths, are established enabling the individual to repeat, evaluate, and predict events validly and reliably. These human functions, manifested through language and motor skills, provide the definitional base for the measurement of the constructs of learning, intelligence, and achievement.

Measures of intelligence presumably tap neural efficiencies and complexities. Lashley (1963), in discussing intelligence, wrote,

> That this is primarily a function of the activity of nervous tissue and that its nature is thus finally to be stated in terms of the mechanisms of the brain seem certain.

More specifically he argued that the mechanisms of integration (intelligence) lie in the dynamic relations among parts of the nervous system rather than in structure. It would appear that disorganization at the neural level would logically affect intellectual functioning. If discontinuity or disruption in the dynamic relationship among neural mechanisms can come to define the construct of minimal brain dysfunction, then integrative intellectual skills are necessarily affected. Clearly Lashley referred to the construct of intelligence as a general, integrative function, the essence of which may be tapped by the better tests of intelligence. Yet tests of intelligence are impure measures of integration since much of the variance is dependent upon interactions between brain processes and psychological processes. In 1960 Pribram distinguished between brain processes and psychological processes viewing the latter as representative of a different and more complex level of discourse. This distinction, suggestive of an intangible human quality, is yet another factor in studies of human behavior.

In an attempt to explain the relationship between feeling states and neural interactions, Nicolis and Benrubi (1975) used a multidisciplinary approach in describing the effects of interpersonal communication on the biological rhythms in the individual. This complex model, supported by mathematical arguments, proposes that neuropsychological vigilance precipitated by a cognitive failure (interpersonal conflict) has three main effects. First, the neurotransmitters overload the postsynaptic receptors causing confusion at this hierarchical level. Secondly, highly aroused reticular activities lead to catecholamine depletion in the cortex and hypothalamus which delimits cortical spatial activities. Thirdly, the thalamic-cortical pace-making mechanisms, in conflict with the reticular activities, are severely disrupted. This model effectively demonstrated the contingent nature of cortical-psychologic interactions.

Nicolis and Benrubi argued that anxiety states are the end result of desynchronized hierarchical levels of the nervous system, not the precipitant. From this one could gather that it is the ambiguity (either cortical or environmental) and confusion which increases vigilance and/or anxiety, not the anxiety which distorts the messages.

If interaction between a physical state and a stimulus is as critical as Nicolis and Benrubi attest, the demise of the child with inherently disorganized biologic rhythms is imaginable. Typical interpersonal interactions, positive or negative, may not effectively penetrate the hierarchical levels of the nervous system potentially leading to disorganized efferent feedback which may be misread by observers as bad behavior and further complicate the child's world.

Etiological Considerations

It might be said that a child with a neural defect may be less able to process normal experiences than the normal child. The extent of desynchronization between the defective neural mechanism and its stimulus is likely to be dependent on the degree and type of neural deficit, the nature of the experience, and the protective psychologic mechanisms operating at the time.

Causative conditions may be genetic, congenital, or acquired. Genetic determinants include genetic anomalies as well as innate predisposition towards weakness at one or more neural levels. Congenital determinants include alterations of those inborn traits during the prenatal and/or perinatal periods due to some insult to the organism. Acquired neural defects are obviously those incurred after birth, such as disease or injury. Included in the acquired group is the failure to develop adequate neural mechanisms because of impoverished or aversive experience during the early years of language development.

The manifestation of neural defect may lie in the structure of neural tissue as in the case of a lesion. However Lashley (1963) had argued that the locality and size of a lesion seem not to be as important as the interactions of the parts of the neural system in the organization of a response. Nonetheless the location and size of the lesion would have an effect on the nature and extent of disintegration.

Lashley also asserted that parts fail not so much because of impaired tissue but because transmission from one set of neurons to another and from one hierarchical level to another does not occur smoothly or efficiently. Wender (1973) attempted to operationalize this observation by hypothesizing that the problems of children with learning disabilities rested with amine irregularities. Clearly this may be the case with many children. However the neurotransmitter behavior is responsive to psychologic state, confounding the directness of the relationship between the arousal level and learning.

Another manifestation of neural defect lies at the sensory level or with neural activities below the brain stem. These involve the process of deciphering the sensory impression validly and then of transmitting that impression through regular channels. It is questionable as to whether these should be identified as neuro-cognitive defects since the defect does not lie in the cortex.

Historical Thrust

The concept of minimal brain dysfunction developed from the observation that some children, for no very obvious reason, deviated academically and/or behaviorally both quantitatively and qualitatively from normative patterns. Of average intelligence, they resisted typical and conservative remedial efforts and the problem of underachievement persisted over the years (Menkes, Rowe, and Menkes, 1967; Koppitz, 1971; Eaves and Critchton, 1974–1975). Given the poor motor control, poor impulse control, poor perceptual skills, and possibly emotional problems of these children, it was speculated that the discrepancies between potential and actual skill development in combination with one or more of the above characteristics might be due to a mild neurological dysfunction (Clements, 1966). The notion of minimal brain dysfunction spread among child-care specialists and the informed public and broader classifications such as learning disability and hyperkinesis were used interchangeably to designate some inborn quality. Based on observations, often unreliable and difficult to quantify, the following criteria become the sine qua non of an MBD diagnosis: underachievement, faulty perceptual and motor skills, and hyperactivity. Uncritically and to the discomfort of some professionals, the MBD syndrome came to be accepted as a viable and explanatory construct by many psychologists, educators, physicians, and parents. While the effects of intervention techniques generally are not known, children identified as neurologically handicapped on the basis of the above criteria are subjected to special classes, tutors, opthalmologists, motor training, auditory training, visual training, and so on. In the absence of clearly delineated cause and effect models, the transition from an identification of a cluster of behaviors to a neurocortical etiology and educational intervention (based on correlational and reporting techniques) has led to a confused, circular, and uncomfortable account of childhood behavior.

Diagnostic Issues

Attempts to diagnose MBD in children have failed to reveal homogeneity or agreement among diagnosticians. Most instruments tap behaviors that are not specifically attributable to the degree of neurological integration, and the classical evaluation of neurological signs is too gross to identify subtle problems. The presence of neurological signs is only a potential indicator in those children in whom a lesion is present since there is no evidence that children with neurotransmitter problems have concomitant motor symptomatologies. Some diagnosticians have attempted to isolate neurological soft signs, which are presumed to be associated with MBD. However there is little good evidence to support a diagnosis of MBD based on neurological soft signs exclusively (Wender, 1971; Rutter, 1977).

Through a factor analysis Rie, et al., (1978) isolated three factors which characterized types of neurocognitive patterns. The first was a general intelligence factor, the second, a perceptual-motor-integrative factor, and the third, a language-symbolic integrative factor. Several soft signs were associated with each of these factors. They were characteristically complex motor-integrative tasks such as right-left discrimination tasks, skipping, and so on. Most of the remaining soft signs were associated with age. What was apparent from this study was the close association among reading skill, general intelligence, and perception. That is, despite reports to the contrary, children with presumed neural defect tend to have a lower IQ than the general population. This relationship has been demonstrated in populations of hyperactive children (Palkes and Stewart, 1972; Miller, Palkes, and Stewart, 1973; Stewart, et. al., 1974). Mark Stewart (1966) long argued that lowered achievement among hyperactive children was due to lower intelligence. Should this be the reality, one can then proceed to analyze the relationship between cognition and neural defect with the hope that data regarding information processing might provide greater insight into the cognitive deficits prevalent among children with presumed MBD.

Hyperactivity and MBD

Though constitutional factors are thought to be the determinants of hyperactivity by many experts, there is no evidential link between activity level and brain integrity, perhaps with the exception of those children with demonstrable brain damage who sometime display "organic driveness" (Kahn and Cohen, 1934).

It is possible that the behavioral characteristics of the hyperactive child may reflect a learned pattern of behavior. They may be expressions of defensive coping and of anticipatory behaviors designed to allay anxiety or frustrations. Under these circumstances, rational and cognitive responses are less likely to occur rendering the child less effective academically. As a result an association between achievement and hyperactivity can be demonstrated empirically. However these children may comprise, in part, a disturbed population who fail to learn because of their psychologic state.

Unfortunately these psychologic characteristics, for example distractibility, disruptiveness, and high activity level, have come to define the MBD syndrome. Yet even when measured reliably it is unlikely that they are a sufficient basis for assuming MBD. To demonstrate the relative independence of manifest behavior and perceptual and motor skill, Simensen (1974) correlated several motor tasks with a behavior rating scale. He concluded that the measures tended to be mutually exclusive.

This is not to suggest that children with presumed neurocognitive dysfunctions are not hyperactive as a group. However the behavioral correlates most likely reflect secondary psychologic symptoms. They appear to be high risk for maladaptive patterns. In the normal course of events they do not develop the information processing skills necessary to replace the more infantile modes of interaction as rapidly or consistently as the average child. They are frustrating to their parents in that they fail to meet academic expectations particularly when they enter school. Rutter, Graham, and Yule (1970) point to the close association between psychiatric disorder and neural dysfunction.

Distinction among the Three Constructs

Constructs of learning, intelligence, and achievement tend to be viewed as parallel, correlative phenomena. It may be interesting to speculate regarding the developmental sequence of each construct particularly as they relate to MBD. Certainly a child is not born with intellective functions, such as language, symbolism, and thought, which emerge spontaneously and distinctly from caretaking. He is however born with the ability to hear, see, remember, and copy. What he remembers and how well he remembers depends on the nature of the stimulus as well as on constitutional factors. Fagan (1973, 1974) demonstrated that infants on tests of recognition devote more visual fixation to novel stimuli than to previously exposed stimuli, suggesting a remarkable ability to recall previous exposure. Meyers (1972) found that infant language is enhanced by repeated exposure to a limited set of words to a greater extent than by limited exposure to many words. In addition predictable, nonthreatening, and supportive interactions between the baby and his caretakers appear to be positive reinforcers as well as vigilance reducers. The infant accumulates memories and begins to organize these memories for future reference. The accumulation of memories and/or data and the use to which they are put are basic to the construct of learning. Learning is thus defined as the product of foundational, basic, and primitive mental functions dealing with sensory and primary information processing. Mentally retarded children fail at this level. Children with learning disabilities or MBD may have difficulties at this level but without generalized effect as found in retarded children.

Grouping, regrouping, retrieval of stored data, hypothesis testing, and arriving at solutions are behaviors of a higher order and closer to the integrative function Lashley (1963) describes. Obviously in the absence of learning, such intellective functions would not develop. It is quite evident that children with learning problems have one or more problems at this level, but not necessarily. Some are able to function more or less adequately in this way but are inhibited in skill development because of primary learning problems. Intellective skills are behaviors of a higher order of complexity than learning.

The ability to put to use and produce creative, constructive evaluations of perceived, stored, and retrievable data and to be able to communicate and translate this information into viable conceptualizations, the highest level of human functions, is defined as achievement. The relationships among learning, intellective functions, and achievement are both hierarchical and contingent, and their establishment, as Russell (1959) claimed, is dependent both on reliable and complex experience and on reliable and complex neural propensities.

LEARNING

In discussing the nature of learning in children with presumed neural defect many experts, especially those involved in educational management, speak of auditory and visual discrimination skills. Poor auditory and visual perception all too often are considered symptomatic of minimal brain dysfunction and offered as underlying causes of poor academic performance. Intervention of a direct nature, that is perceptual training, is common though little evidence exists to support the hypothesis that such training has a generalizing effect on academic skills. However more importantly, it is difficult to trace out and differentiate between those perceptual problems which are neurologically determined from those which are environmentally caused. For example attentional problems, potentially the result of anxiety, would affect a child's performance on a test of perception as well as on his performance in the classroom. Habits, oppositionalism, impoverished experience, each affect minimally the performance of perceptual tasks. Consequently many children with functional perceptual problems are categorized as MBD forming heterogeneous rather than homogeneous populations. In our studies we found that 36 children with presumed MBD obtained Bender deviation scores of −3.55 while a matched group of disturbed children deviated by −1.9. The extent of deviation is obviously greater in the MBD group yet the overlap is apparent.

What is of greater concern is the precise relationship between perception and learning. This relationship remains largely unexplored despite continual efforts to remediate learning disabilities through perceptual training. Myklebust, Bannockie, and Killen (1971) postulated that learning varies by type and level. They spoke of three types of learning: intraneurosensory (unimodal), interneurosensory (multi-modal), and integrative-neurosensory (integrative learning). The level of complexity within each type of learning can range from perception to imagery, to symbolism, and to conception. The authors argued that a learning disability should be defined and evaluated according to this model. Perception plays a simple role in this framework and is most likely one of the less important components of learning.

Dykman and Ackerman (1976) stressed attention as the "sine qua non" of learning failure in children with MBD. They reasoned that "attention implies all the neurophysiological mechanisms which determine our conscious awareness at a given point." The authors offer an information processing model organized around memory, attention, and central processing. Problems in any area may cause learning disabilities, however the authors believe that defective central processing, the "strategies for relevant stimulus selection and chunking," account for most learning problems. They concluded that MBD children are able to match the performance of controls on simple tasks but perform less well on more complex concept attainment tasks.

If attention were the basic underlying symptom, the effects of stimulants would indeed be remarkable inasmuch as stimulants enhance attention in many children (Rie, et al., 1976). Yet there is very little evidence, other than reported observations of better performance by teachers and parents, to indicate that the attention sustained artificially physiologically increases the level of information processing or of cognition (Rie, et al., 1976).

Vandevoort, Senf, and Burton (1972) compared retarded and normal readers in matching tasks: visual-visual, auditory-auditory, and auditory-visual. They found that the retarded readers performed less well than controls on all combinations concluding that the problems had more to do with the encoding process than with the crossing of modalities.

Signoret and Lhermitte (1976) addressed themselves to the encoding and translation of verbal and visual stimuli. They found that subjects with frontal vascular lesions were unable to learn six concrete word pairs. From the hypothesis that frontal lobes are instrumental in the choice and initiation of strategies, the authors cleverly introduced "associative mediators" for each pair of words finding that performance was much improved under this condition. Both visual and verbal mediators improved performance. The subjects ultimately learned how to create their own mediators if provided with a model. This example of basic research in learning has practical implications as well as scientific merit and is suggestive of the need for help from the neuropsychologists.

It is not unlikely that visual and auditory perception, in the absence of extenuating circumstances, are functions or symptomatic of substantive neural defect. Greater attention however must be given to purer forms of learning in children with academic problems as well as to those neural functions which determine the nature of learning.

With the exception of studies of adult humans with demonstrable brain damage and studies of the effect of stimulant medication on hyperactivity and learning disability, the search for empirical data regarding the relationship between classical learning and MBD in children has been very disappointing. In a conference sponsored by the Section of Biological and Medical Science of the New York Academy of Sciences titled, "Minimal Brain Dysfunction," mention of learning experiments was not to be found. The absence of classical experimental studies in learning in children with presumed cerebral dysfunction is unfortunate in that important, serious questions cannot be answered comprehensively.

One conclusion reached by many investigators of learning in children with learning problems is that high level mental functions are implicated in the differentiation between learning disabled and control groups. As the solution of the task requires greater complexity the need for the operation of multiple and simultaneous neural cue systems increases. It is at this level that children with neural defect appear to fail. The parts do not function in a unified manner to form a facile and reliable network of communication.

INTELLIGENCE

It has long been understood that the construct of general intelligence describes some attributes of behavior. Measures of intelligence, reflecting both innate predispositions and the training of the individual, give modest but loose estimates of potential. The argument that individual differences on intelligence tests are due to predisposing, genetically determined structures is clearly an overstatement. Nonetheless how do brains differ in people of varying abilities? What are the causative conditions leading to these differences?

As far back as 1929 Lashley addressed the issue arguing for a "general factor of intelligence." Lashey (1963) held the view that complex mental functions were dependent on the quantity of cortical tissue and that global responses of the brain as well as specialized, localized responses operated in problem solving behaviors. He spoke of "some dynamic function of the cortex which is not differentiated with respect to single capacities but is generally effective for a number to which identical neural elements cannot be ascribed." In the middle of the century, Russell (1959) spoke of training the brain via simple conditioning methods. He argued for stimulus repetition, appropriate rewards, and elicitation of concomitant positive emotional arousal. According to Russell as practice and varied experiences lead to the excitation and elaboration of neural pathways, memory, novel associations, and complex reasoning develop. These two views, each reflecting on the dynamic forces in the reasoning process, suggest that intelligence is an expression of multiple, complex, and hierarchical contingencies.

In testing for "g" or for complex reasoning, hypothetical problems are posed for resolution. The intelligence test was designed to ferret out qualitatively and quantitatively the capacity for complex reasoning. Performance on this measure however is confounded by extraneural conditions, such as motivation, psychologic state, and experience, resulting in a comprehensive measure of functioning rather than in a pure ability factor. Consequently conditions other than neural operations appear to be the basic structures upon which complex reasoning is dependent.

While tests of intelligence do not directly measure the components of neural operations, they certainly tap memory and motor performance and sensory and information processing. In this sense they can be sensitive to a defect in the neural structure. A neural defect may affect the reliability and validity of perceptions, profoundly altering the course of the reasoning process as well as the end result. Clearly children with presumed brain dysfunction tend to fall into the low average range of intelligence (Menkes, Rowl, and Menkes, 1967; Paine, Werry, and Quay, 1968; Palkes and Stewart, 1972; Rie and Rie, 1977). Generally it might be said that intellectual behaviors reflect a comprehensive reasoning ability associated with neural operations, psychologic state, and experience.

Level of WISC Performance

Table 12-1 gives a sampling of reported IQs on several subtypes of children, all of whom have a form of learning disability. It is to be noted that in each instance of demonstrable brain damage the IQ falls below average. IQs of populations suspected of some neural defect are almost always lower than controls with the exception of the Francis-Williams study (1976). Her criterion for inclusion in the neurological category was risk in the newborn period. Most investigators use present behavior for that determination. Children classified simply as disabled readers consistently score lower than matched counterparts.

When children are selected on the basis of overt behavior and classified as hyperactive there appears to be less differnece in IQ between them and controls. From our data we found that 42 learning disabled children rated as hyperactive by parent and teacher scored 103.5 on the Verbal, 104.4 on the Performance and 104.2 on the Full Scale. In correlating hyperactive ratings of 80 children with independent neurocognitive ratings, we found a zero order correlation; yet when correlating neurocognitive ratings with Full Scale IQ, the r was .5, significant at the .001 level. A third correlation, IQ and hyperactivity, yielded a zero order correlation.

In a population of hyperkinetic children, Knobel, Wolman, and Mason (1959) reported a Full Scale IQ of 102.8 on the WISC. Palkes and Stewart (1972) found that hyperkinetic children scored 100.3 on the WISC while Dykeman, Peters, and Ackerman (1973) using Clement's definition of minimal brain dysfunction, reported a Full Scale IQ of 105.5. It is suspected that as the delineation for neurological dysfunction is drawn from nonbehavioral but cognitive criteria the IQ tends to drop (Menkes, Rowl, and Menkes, 1967; Paine, Werry, and Quay, 1968; Rie and Rie, 1977). This may be the case for two reasons. The rating of behavioral characteristics tends to be subjective and imprecise, reflecting maladaptive behavior patterns rather than intrinsic neural defect. Secondly, it is likely that populations of hyperactives include many children with primary psychogenic problems rendering these groups considerably more heterogeneous than assumed. Even when the behavior is predictive of a more basic dysfunction it is possibly secondary to the neural defect and not an effect of it. Birch (1964) stated that,

> We never see an individual whose disturbed behavior is a direct consequence of his brain damage. Instead, we see individuals with damage to the nervous system, which may have resulted in some primary disorganization, who have developed patterns of behavior in the course of atypical relations with the developmental environment, including its interpersonal, objective, and social features.

As the accuracy of selection of children with neural defect increases with the elimination of reflexive motor patterns (Rie, et al., 1978), and as the reliability of intelligence tests improves with the elimination of motor items (Bloom, 1964), it is likely that the accuracy of selection of children with neural defect might be enhanced further by eliminating psychogenic behavioral indices.

Rutter, Graham, and Yule (1970) reported that intelligence in epileptic children and in children with lesions below the brain stem is roughly normal (102 and 107 respectively). Yet children with cerebral palsy and other brain disorders scored in the 70's on the WISC. When the damage is manifest and above the brain stem there is a clear effect on intellectual performance.

Effects of noncortical neurologic dysfunction on intelligence appear to be negli-

Table 12-1. Representative Sample of IQs of Children with Learning Disorders

Study	N	Diagnosis	Approx. mean age	Diagnostic method	Reported IQ		Test used
Davids, Goldenberg, and Laufer (1957)	15	Cerebral Palsy	10–6	Medical evaluation		98	WISC
	29	Psychiatric	10–6	Medical and psychiatric evaluations		93	WISC
	24	Normals	10–6	No history of organic impairments		97	California Test of Mental Maturity
Knobel, Wolman, and Mason (1959)	23	Hyperkinetic (with organicity assumed)	10–10	Neurological, psychologic, and psychiatric evaluations	FS VS PS	102.8 104.8 100.3	WISC
	8	Mixed disturbances	10–10		FS VS PS	102.2 107.0 96.2	WISC
	9	Hypokinetic	13–6		FS VS PS	103.9 107.6 99.1	WISC
Birch and Belmont (1964)	149	Retarded readers	10	Scores within lowest 10% on several reading tests		96.7	WISC
	49	Normal readers	10	Not in lowest 10%		110.8	WISC
Belmont and Birch (1965)	29	Reading retarded	9–10	Lowest 10% of readers and failed R-L discrimination items	FS VS PS	90 90 91	WISC
	121	Reading retarded	9–10	Lowest 10% of readers and passed R-L discrimination items	FS VS PS	92 92 94	WISC
	50	Normal readers	9–9	Not in lowest 10% of readers	FS	104.9	WISC
Reed, Reitan, and Klove (1965)	50	Brain damage	12–6	Neurological and medical evaluation		84	WISC
	50	Matched controls	12–6			106	WISC

Study	N	Group	Age (grade level)	Criteria	IQ	Test
Schiffman and Clemmens (1966)	240	Clinically retarded readers	6.1 (grade level)	Identification of reading retardation with word recognition problems	FS 96.0 / VS 91 / PS 101	WISC
Menkes, Rowe, and Menkes (1967)	18	Hyperkinesis with MBD	8	Specific nonbehavioral diagnostic criteria (e.g., clumsiness of fine movements, V-M deficits, delayed or impaired speech)	93	Stanford-Binet
Hughes and Park (1968)	56	Reading retardation with abnormal EEG	11	Neurologist's assessment of EEG results	FS 103.3 / VS 102.5 / PS 103.9	WISC
	101	Reading retardation with normal EEG	10–8	Neurologist's assessment of EEG results	FS 102.9 / VS 100.5 / PS 103.7	WISC
Paine, Werry, and Quay (1968)	83	Suspicion of minimal cerebral dysfunction	8–5	Abnormal neurological signs, abnormal EEG, psychological findings similar to organic encephalopathics	96.3	WISC for older children, Stanford-Binet for younger children
Fuller and Hawkins (1969)	83	Retarded and brain damage	14–6	Medical evidence, social case history, psychological test findings	68.8	Peabody Picture Vocabulary Test
	86	Retarded and non brain damaged	15–2		71	
Rutter, Graham, and Yule (1970)	58	Epileptic	10	Medical evaluation	102	WISC (shortened and scores pro-rated)
	33	Cerebral palsy	11		78	
	20	Other brain disorders	10		74	
	17	Lesions below brain stem	11		107	

Table 12-1. Cont'd Representative Sample of IQs of Children wit Learning Disorders

Study	N	Diagnosis	Approx. mean age	Diagnostic method	Reported IQ		Test used
Wikler, Dixon, and Parker (1970)	24	Experimentals: scholastic and/or behavioral problems (brain dysfunction assumed)	5–15	Identified by teachers, parents, or physicians (neurological evaluations)	FS VS PS	110 112.6 105.6	WISC
	24	Matched controls		Matched for age, sex, race, IQ, social class	FS VS PS	111 113.2 107	WISC
	11	Experimentals with hyperactivity		Checklist re: behaviors at home, school, and with other children	FS VS PS	105.7 108 102.4	WISC
	8	Nonhyperactive experimentals		Checklist re: behaviors at home, school, and with other children	FS VS PS	115 117.5 109.2	WISC
Koppitz (1971)	173	LD (with suspicion of MBD)	8–11	Presence of learning disabilities and belief that child could profit from special class placement as determined by multidisciplinary staff	92		WISC or Stanford-Binet
Myklebust, Bannochie, and Killen (1971)	116	Moderate learning disability (LQs 89–85)	3rd & 4th graders	Learning Quotient technique	FS VS PS	101.5 100.9 102.1	WISC
	116	Matched controls	3rd & 4th graders		FS VS PS	107.6 108 106.6	
	112	Severe learning disability (LQs ≤ 84)	3rd & 4th graders	Learning Quotient technique	FS VS PS	101 100.2 102.1	
	112	Matched controls	3rd & 4th graders		FS VS PS	107.5 107.1 107	

Study	N	Group	Selection criteria	Age	IQ	Test
Ayres (1972)	148	LD	Identified academically by school personnel	7–6	96.5	not reported
Palkes and Stewart (1972)	32	Hyperactive child syndrome	Behavioral criteria applied by MD using Stewart et al. (1966) description	NR	FS 100.3 / VS 101 / PS 99.8	WISC
	34	Matched controls	Matched for age, sex, grade, race, and socio-economic class		FS 111.3 / VS 109 / PS 111.6	WISC
Dykman, Peters, and Ackerman (1973)	82	LD with MBD	Identified by a child guidance team using Clement's diagnostic criteria. Parent/teacher reports used; also presence of developmental delays	8–12	FS 105.5 / VS 103.4 / PS 106.9	WISC
	34	Controls	Identified by teachers		FS 110.1 / VS 112.3 / PS 105.5	WISC
Reitan and Davidson (1974)	29	Unequivocal evidence of cerebral damage (lesions)	Medical diagnosis following detailed physical and neurological evaluation	7–1	FS 78.7 / VS 82.1 / PS 79	WISC
	29	Normal, matched controls	Matched in pairs for sex and age	7–1	FS 104.7 / VS 103.5 / PS 105.3	WISC
Francis-Williams (1976)	31	Neurologically damaged	Neurological damage occurring in the newborn period	8–9	FS 109.2 / VS 110.4 / PS 112.3	WISC
	43	Matched controls	Normal birth history		FS 113.8 / VS 118.1 / PS 115.3	

Table 12-1. Cont'd Representative Sample of IQs of Children wit Learning Disorders

Study	N	Diagnosis	Approx. mean age	Diagnostic method	Reported IQ		Test used
Beaumont (1976)	14	MBD as main diagnosis or principal secondary diagnosis	7-1	Several specialists examining each child over a period of several days	FS VS PS	87 87 90	WISC
	14	Matched controls	7-2	Matched for age, sex, and IQ (within 10 points)	FS VS PS	95 91 98	WISC (shortened form)
Trites and Fiedorowicz (1976)	27	Specific reading disability	11-7	Lag in reading, family history of reading disability, no evidence of gross or focal brain damage	FS VS PS	106 101 110 106	WISC Peabody Picture Vocabulary Test
	10	Reading disability secondary to neurological disease	11-6	Reading lag and medical evidence of neurological damage	FS VS PS	92 90 96 90	WISC Peabody Picture Vocabulary Test
Rie and Rie (1977)	80[1]	Learning disability underachieving children	8	Objective achievement measures	FS VS PS	104.1 103.1 104.6	WISC
		MBD (36)		Neurological and neuro-cognitive scale	FS VS PS	98.6 98.1 99.2	
		Non-MBD (44)		Neurological and neuro-cognitive scale	FS VS PS	108.8 107.2 109	
		Hyperactive (42)		Parent-teacher behavior rating scale	FS VS PS	104.2 103.5 104.4	

Nonhyperactive (38)	Parent-teacher behavior rating scale	FS	104.2
		VS	102.7
		PS	104.7
Hyperactive/MBD (20)	Combination of above methods	FS	98.3
		VS	98.2
		PS	98.9
Nonhyperactive/MBD (16)	Combination of above methods	FS	98.9
		VS	99.8
		PS	99.5
Non-MBD/hyperactive (22)	Combination of above methods	FS	109.6
		VS	108.4
		PS	109.4
Non-MBD/nonhyperactive (22)	Combination of above methods	FS	104.1
		VS	103.1
		PS	104.6

[1]Sample of 80 subdivided into MBD, non-MBD, hyperactive, nonhyperactive groups.

gible. Epilepsy is an exception. As did Rutter, Graham, and Yule, (1970), Hughes and Park (1968) reported no difference in IQ between children with abnormal and normal EEG's.

Arguments that "some children with undoubted brain disorder are of superior intelligence" (Rutter, Graham, and Yule, 1970) logically can only be true of children with lesions below the brain stem or with cortical lesions such as uncomplicated epilepsy which may be under the control of the autonomic nervous system. In six years of research with children from a large metropolitan area having suspected MBD, the highest measured IQ we obtained was in the bright normal, low superior range on the WISC. In assessing children with known lesions, Reitan (1974) found very few children in the average range on the WISC. Loney (1974) found a similar pattern in LD boys. There is evidence to suggest that high IQ and minimal brain dysfunction are incompatible and contradictory conditions; the suspicion of psychogenic determinants of bright children with learning and/or behavioral disabilities must be entertained. Beck and Lam (1955) in a similar statement argue that the lower the IQ, the greater the organicity. Rutter, Graham, and Yule (1970) conclude that "Brain damage can and frequently does, cause a global reduction in intelligence level." However they find that IQ itself is a poor indicator of brain dysfunction.

To summarize Table 12–1, it could be said that disabled children tend to score lower on intelligence tests than controls. When neural defect is associated with neurocognitive problems, IQ is clearly affected . This relationship is less clear in populations of learning-disabled children and in populations of hyperactive children. There is little doubt that these latter two groups do not constitute populations with common etiological factors. The continued use of the category of hyperactivity to infer or to designate MBD is not justified by research, observation, or theoretical formulations. Consequently investigations into the relationship between IQ and brain pathology cannot be found in samples of children characterized solely on the basis of activity level, behavioral indices, or achievement levels.

When children with suspected neural defect are selected on the basis of performance which is more likely to be determined by neural operations than by past experience, intelligence appears to be affected indirectly. Memory, generalization skills, multifaceted thought, ideational stability, reliable conscious retrieval of information are but several possible, somewhat automatic-like, brain functions which may be less affected by past experience than by neural operations. These cortical reflexive activities are basic to the development of intellectual skills. They provide the mechanisms by which experience and information can be stored, utilized, and reorganized. Within the group of children with suspected neural defect, intelligence can range from very low to moderate levels depending on the nature of the defect and/or type of neural dysfunction. The evidence suggests that intellectual functioning is affected adversely.

Pattern of WISC Performance

In our own studies we separated children with learning disabilities into suspected organic and nonorganic groups on the basis of independent judgments of neurocognitive skills (Rie, et al., 1976). Unwilling to utilize behavioral or neurologic indices as designates of minimal brain dysfunction, a rating scale for neurocognitive disorders was derived. The scale was based on the assumption that the brain, processing and recording sensory experience, acts to integrate, connect, and to establish relationships among incoming information as well as retrieving stored data in the act of responding. This complementarity of neural interplay was the essence of a conception of level of neurocognitive skills. The following dimensions were adopted as indicators of neurocognitive dysfunctions: integrative-synthesizing skills, perseverative or impulse control behaviors, conceptualizations, word retrieval, accuracy of retrieval, abstraction, and a compensatory global rating.

Thirty-six of 80 learning-disabled children (behind by an average of 2.1 grade equivalent years in reading) were suspected as having mild but significant neurocognitive dysfunctions. The 36 children identified as having neurocognitive problems differed significantly from the rest on Full Scale IQ (98.6 to 108.8). The two groups did not differ in age, sex ratio, birth order, or grade level. Consistent with the findings of Hopkins (1964), who challenged the argument that Performance IQ is more greatly affected than Verbal IQ among organics, we did not find an imbalance between the means of the two scales for the impaired group. However there was a small tendency for the Performance Score to exceed the Verbal Score in both the neurologically intact and neurologically inferior groups. In the neurologically intact group, Arithmetic was the lowest subtest while Similarities was the highest; in the neurologically impaired group, Information was the lowest and Picture Arrangement the highest. The neurologically impaired differed from the neurologically intact in the direction of lower means on the following subtests: Information, Similarities, Vocabulary, and Block Design. Although no differences were found on the majority of WISC subtests, the impaired children did not function on a higher level than the nonimpaired in any instance. Perhaps it is important to mention that the ratings of neurocognitive dysfunction were made in the absence of data on intelligence. Granted that selection of this population might have been confounded and contaminated by impressions of intelligence, nonetheless there was a sufficient number of children designated as nonimpaired whose IQs fell below 100 as well as a number of impaired children functioning above 100. Psychometric performance and neural operations do not appear to be separate entities, the former being a partial function of the latter. This relationship is reflected by subtle differences in psychometric performance between neurologically impaired and neurologically intact children as well as by low positive correlations between neurocognitive functions and intelligence.

WISC Variation

In the absence of a firm standard of what constitutes a significant variation among WISC subtests, it is unlikely that scatter can be a factor in the identification of neural defect. This is especially true of children with whom the standard error of measurement of the individual subtests is sufficiently large to account for a large range of scores obtainable by chance. Speaking of the WAIS, Wechsler (1958) proposed that a deviation of two or more scaled scores from the mean of the scale is a convenient cutoff point in the determination of an abnormal variation. By averaging the scaled scores of the Verbal and Performance subtests separately, we found that the average mean deviation of a sample of 30 children with learning disabilities was 1.8 on the Verbal Scale and about 1.5 on the Performance. When the children were grouped according to neurocognitive status, some difference in size of deviation was noted between intact and impaired children. The intact group had an average mean deviation of 1.42 for the Full Scale while the impaired group deviation was 1.74. The impaired group had higher deviations than the intact group on both Verbal and Performance Scales. It appears that children with presumed neural defect may differ from other pathological groups in regard to variability of performance on intelligence tests. Rowley (1961) found otherwise.

Myklebust, Bannochie, and Killen (1971) reported that controls had more significant intercorrelations among WISC subtests than the learning disabled. They concluded that the "g" factor was less intact in the disabled group than in the controls and that the "structure of intellect" was different. They found that IQ did not correlate with achievement in the disabled group as well as it did with the controls.

Dykman and Ackerman (1976) remarked that Digit Span is consistently depressed in children with learning disabilities. While not addressing themselves directly to the issue of intelligence, they comment that children with MBD have great difficulty with complex, concept attainment tasks. They summarized by saying that children with learning problems have a basic informational processing deficiency.

Intelligence and Sensory Processing

It is important to distinguish between behaviors which are essentially derived from sensory processing and those derived from higher level comprehensive cortical functions. The somewhat spontaneous developmental switch from dependence on sensory memories to dependence on complex cortical processes in the management of experiences has been a subject of recent interest to clinical child psychologists. The question of what types of environmental interactions lead to or facilitate the development of reliance on the cortex in problem solving in lieu of sensory processes is fundamental. If children continue beyond early elementary years to rely heavily on sensory impressions for one reason or another, then thought, problem solving, generalizing, and so on, become tedious and impossible tasks. The children may appear to suffer from the "minimal brain damage syndrome," but in reality are habituated to a sensory-motor level of functioning. This hypothetical population would not look too different from those children who indeed are neurologically handicapped and who must rely on sensory skills to survive. Conversely some children for whatever reason, for example those with damage below the brain stem, may have grave problems with sensory processing, rendering them highly vulnerable to stress and frustration. These children nonetheless are able to function conceptually at the cortical level when messages do get through. Are these children part of the MBD complex?

Intelligence and the Cortex

In 1942 Hebb argued that brain injury had a more diffuse effect on intelligence in children than in adults. Piercy (1964), in an excellent review, stated that "neurological evidence suggests functional and anatomical differentiation of intellect with maturation and experience." Considering that the proportion of undifferentiated intellectual ability in children is larger than in adults, it is not surprising to find the effects different. Both Cattell (1943) and Hebb (1949) conceived of intelligence as a two phased phenomenon. Hebb distinguished between innate intelligence and the level of development of brain functions, the latter being an effect of experience as well as innate dispositions. Cattell made a distinction between fluid and crystallized intelligence, the former representing an undifferentiated intellectual power (potential energy) while the latter represented the actual ability developed from this energy source.

Studies of the effects of hemispherectomy on intellectual functioning suggest that intellectual performance does not deteriorate as a result of this procedure and sometimes increases (McFie, 1961; Griffith and Davidson, 1966). This finding, which has been corroborated (Piercy, 1964), has led some specialists to conclude that brain damage does not always result in intellectual impairments.

However this conclusion is not entirely justified since premorbid measures, that is measures of intellective functions prior to the damage which led to the removal of the hemisphere, are not usually available. The argument that intelligence increases after surgery because the remaining intact hemisphere is no longer fed extraneous data from the damaged one, and can operate with greater efficiency, is intriguing. The cortex appears to offer a variety of programs or methods for problem solving and when one fails, another assumes the responsibility. Because the multifaceted cortex offers the individual alternative paths, the relationship between cortical functions and intellective skills is indeed a complex one. Some investigators envision future methods of measuring intelligence through electrodermal devices on the basis of small but reliable positive correlation between electrical activities in the cortex and psychometric measures of intelligence (Giannitrapani, 1969).

Special Considerations

The question of the effects of MBD on intelligence is complicated because descriptions of neural operations overlap with descriptions of intelligence. By definition the relationship would be axiomatic, that is measures of intelligence most certainly reflect neural efficiencies. Since pure measures of neural efficiencies and pure measures of potential do not exist, overlap is to be expected.

The analysis of patterns on intelligence tests does not appear to be a fruitful approach simply because cortical activities are both specific and global; interrelating and hierarchical; cross-functional (flexible) and rigid. Intra and inter cortical variances are so great as to preclude the predictability of patterns as well as direct relationships between a set of behaviors and cortical activities.

The incongruous finding that children with minimal brain dysfunction have normal intelligence but fail academically attests to the lack of predictability of IQ for achievement in this population of children. Mark Stewart (1966) nonetheless finding that children with minimal brain dysfunction have lower intelligence than control groups, argues that their corresponding low achievement is commensurate with IQ.

In children aged between 7–9, standardized intelligence tests do not require many integrative-conceptual responses. Items tend to be concrete, cues are often present, specificity, with the exception of several items, is not important. Able to utilize low level sensory imagery and limited cortical memories, children with fairly significant neurological dysfunction may perform reasonably well. When the task loses its general, multimodal flavor and is replaced by one requiring complex memory functions, retrieval, specificity and novelty, the child with neurological dysfunctions fails miserably.

In general it would appear both empirically and theoretically that MBD's are accompanied by both an alteration in problem solving and a reduction in efficiency. That is children with suspected neurological dysfunctions find cortical substitutions for the inoperative cortical function, thus approaching problem solving in circuitous fashion and thereby reducing the efficiency as well as the quality of the mental operation. The establishment and permanence of engrams is affected, rendering the child less able to absorb symbols and memories through repetition and training.

In the last analysis there are many potential alterations of neural operations; there are many forms of MBD; homogeneous effect on an intelligence test should be expected only when subtypes are identified.

ACHIEVEMENT

The principal concern of the parents and teacher of LD children is that of skill mastery. Underachievement and learning are the most frequent initial problems cited to the specialists (Clements, 1966). Even in the more select population of children with presumed MBD the principal complaint is underachievement (Gross and Wilson, 1974). Rutter Graham, and Yule (1970) stated, "Whatever its cause, reading retardation in children with neuro-epileptic disorders constituted one of the most important of their handicaps." Rutter, Graham, and Yule, reported a high rate of reading retardation in children with all kinds of neuroepileptic disorders, however they were most marked in children of low intelligence, a theme commonly repeated in the literature.

Despite the principal complaint of underachievement, little data are available to demonstrate the degree of underachievement or its nature. Attention has been directed to other, less critical symptoms losing sight of the logic that underachievement is, too, a symptom rather than an entity to be explored circuitously.

When a child is observed to have certain difficulties attaining basic skills and when these difficulties persist over time he might be characterized as having learning disabilities. This classification merely describes the child's performance in the classroom and suggests that it is something more than a temporary lag. Though LD carries implications for etiology in some circles, most would agree that the term is descriptive and that the children thus described constitute a heterogeneous population.

Within this group of children with learning problems are subtypes falling into two general causal classes, those with primary psychological problems and those with primary neurological problems. A third type, the child with environmental problems adds to the complexity, however his nature is to be discussed elsewhere. Though all LD children by definition lag academically, not all suffer from primary neurological anomalies. Of those who do, failure to perform academically at an appropriate level is often the first, clear symptom of a major problem. Parents, under gentle probing, often reconstruct retrospectively their observations of early lags in language or in motor development. This is not always the case, yet many children identified as having neurocognitive dysfunctions had subtle but persistent symptoms from early infancy often obvious by nursery school age. Variability in the development of language skills in the general population and the lack of predictability of motor performance for learning disability (Rie, et al., 1978) render early diagnoses difficult and lead to many false positives and negatives.

Failure to read is the first concrete and serious symptom of MBD sometimes occurring in the absence of other telltale signs, but offten suggested by other lags identified in a carefully obtained history. Yet little is actually known about the relationship between school failure and neurologic dysfunction. We have still to demonstrate how level of sensory processing, language processing, memory, and reasoning are related to reading acquisition and to math concepts. Or we have still to demonstrate which neurologic symptoms are associated with which school failures. Our most predictive instrument, though replete with theoretical and statistical problems, remains the intelligence test. This instrument best predicts school failure even within the neurologic population (Rutter, Graham, and Yule 1970).

Review of Pertinent Literature

Myklebust, Bannochie, and Killen, (1971) compared LD and controls on 21 measures of educational achievement. The LD group scored consistently lower on all measures. Those LD children with severe disabilities, as determined by a learning quotient, were the most disparate. To determine which measures were the best discriminators, the authors subjected their data to a discriminant analysis. Surprisingly a syllabication task of matching nonsense words to their auditory equivalents was the most discriminant factor. The authors inspected the most discriminant tasks for common elements to discover that a prominent feature of these tasks was "facility to gain general meaning." It made little difference whether the task was verbal or nonverbal.

Koppitz (1971) reported that 42 LD pupils, achieving at the beginning of the third grade level at age 9, were approximately 6 months retarded in the skill area. Those children with the best initial intellectual, integrative, and academic functioning had the shortest stay in the LD program. The brighter, less disabled children appeared to make the quickest progress.

Rie and Rie (1978) determined that reading retardation was greater in children with neurocognitive disorders when Performance IQ exceeded Verbal IQ by approximately 10 points than when the reverse or no disparity was obtained. The pattern of WISC performance was more closely related to severity of failure than the Full Scale IQ. Curiously the Full Scale IQ had to drop to 92 before reading failure of 6 months or more could be found when the Verbal IQ exceeded the Performance IQ by more than 10 points. Dysfunction in the motor-visual integrative areas appeared to be of less significance in the acquisition of reading than verbal-auditory integration areas.

In another study Rie and Rie (1977) separated 80 LD children according to etiology. Those with presumptive neurocognitive dysfunctions performed less well on each of the tests on the IOWA Test of Basic Skills. In addition the classroom teachers rated the children with neurocognitive dysfunction on a global measure of achievement lower than those LD children who appeared to be intact in this regard. The composite mean grade equivalent for the N-C group was 1.04 (N-35) while the composite score for the intact group was 1.7 (N-43). Their respective ages were 7.89 and 7.94 years. The most discriminant factor was spelling, however the deficit in the N-C group in reading comprehension was approximately 1.5 years while the intact group was behind by 1 year. The N-C group, it should be noted, was less bright, scoring 98.59 on the WISC while the intact group scored 109.02. Though it can be argued that the difference in deficit is due to the difference in IQ, it is also possible that underlying neurologic dysfunction have depressed both kinds of performance. Other investigators have found parallel relationships between IQ and degree of deficit (Hughes and Park, 1968; Ayres, 1972; Palkes and Stewart, 1972)

An interesting incidental finding from these data was that intertest variability was greater for the intact group than for the N-C group. The average deviation from the composite score was .19 (in grade equivalents) for the N-C group while it was .40 for the intact group. This pattern was also true of the pattern of variability on the WISC.

Generally it appears that level of achievement in children with presumptive neurocognitive dysfunctions is less than expected from age and grade levels, is a significant complaint by teachers and parents, is related to intellectual level and to severity of dysfunction. Much research into specific relationships between neuro-cognitive functions and achievement is needed; there are limited available data.

OVERVIEW

Clearly the foundations of learning, intellective functions, and achievement lie in hierarchical neural interactions. A potential effect of disrupted or altered neural interactions is a distortion of perception and thought. Just how perception and thought are affected depends on the age at which the dysfunction occurs as well as on the nature, magnitude, and site of the problem. In one way or another neural dysfunctions almost certainly affect the ability to learn and to achieve in children. Their subtle effect on general intelligence though less dramatic is nonetheless apparent.

It appears that the difficulties of MBD children may not lie exclusively in specific, circumscribed, sensory processing, but also in less tangible, broader, intracortical, extrapsychic information processing. Synthesizing skills, generalizing skills, organizational systems, recording and retrieval of language, and engram stabilization are but a few relevant issues worthy of future exploration.

In general the MBD child is less able to profit from his experiences than the normal child. His poor neural strategy for remembering and for interpreting preclude the development of independent thoughts, unique to him, and available to him for immediate reference. As Kinsbourne (1972) suggested, the MBD child lags developmentally. Unfortunately it is not a question of time, an issue of "catch-up." It is more often an issue of the development of compensatory functions or an issue of circumvention in the method of teaching. It is at last an issue of providing the external connection or structure to enable the child to speak, write, and read sufficiently well to bring gratification to others and to be comfortable with himself.

REFERENCES

Ayres, A. J. "Types of sensory integrative dysfunction among disabled learners." *The American Journal of Occupational Therapy,* 26 (11), 13–18, (1972).

Beaumont, J. G. "The cerebral laterality of 'minimal brain damage' children." *Cortex,* 12, 373–382, (1976).

Beck, H., and R. L. Lam, "The use of the WISC in predicting organicity." *Journal of Clinical Psychology*, 11, 154–158, (1955).

Belmont, L., and H. G. Birch. "Lateral dominance, lateral awareness, and reading disability." *Child Development*, 36, 57–71, (1965).

Birch, H. G. "The problem of 'brain damage' in children," in H. G. Birch, ed., *Brain Damage in Children: The Biological and Social Aspects*, pp. 3–12, Baltimore: Williams & Wilkins, 1964.

Birch, H. G., and L. Belmont. "Auditory-visual integration in normal and retarded readers." *American Journal of Orthopsychiatry*, 34, 852–861, (1964).

Bloom, B. *Stability and Change in Human Characteristics*. New York: Wiley, 1964.

Cattell, R. B. "The measurement of adult intelligence." *Psychological Bulletin*, 40 (3), 153–193, (1943).

Clements, S. D. *Minimal Brain Dysfunction in Children*. NINDB, Monograph No. 3. Washington, D. C. 1966.

Davids, A., L. Goldenberg, and M. Laufer. "The relation of the Archimedes spiral aftereffect and the trail making test to brain damage in children." *Journal of Consulting Psychology*, 21, 429–433, (1957).

Dykman, R. A. and P. T. Ackerman. "The MBD problem: Attention, intention, and information processing," in R. P. Anderson and C. G. Holcomb, eds., *Learning Disability/Minimal Brain Dysfunction Syndrome Research Perspectives and Applications*, 27–93. Springfield, Ill.: Thomas, 1976.

Dykman, R. A., J. E. Peters, and P. T. Ackerman. "Experimental approaches to the study of minimal brain dysfunction: A follow-up study." *Annals of New York Academy of Science*, 205, 93–108, (1973).

Eaves, L. C., and J. U. Crichton. "A five-year follow-up of children with minimal brain dysfunction." *Academic Therapy*, 10 (2), 173–180, (1974–1975).

Fagan, III, J. F. "Infant's delayed recognition memory and forgetting." *Journal of Experimental Child Psychology*, 16, 424–450, (1973).

———"Infant recognition memory: The effects of length of familiarization and type of discrimination task." *Child Development*, 45, 351–356, (1974).

Francis-Williams, J. "Early identification of children likely to have specific learning difficulties: Report of a follow-up." *Developmental Medicine and Child Neurology*, 18, 71–77, (1976).

Giannitrapani, D. "EEG frequency and intelligence." *Electroencephalography and Clinical Neurophysiology*, 27, 480–486 (1969).

Griffith, H., and M. Davidson. "Long-term changes in intellect and behavior after hemispherectomy." *Journal of Neurological Psychiatry*, 29, 571–576, (1966).

Gross, M. B., and W. C. Wilson. *Minimal Brain Dysfunction, A Clinical Study of Incidence, Diagnosis and Treatment in Over 1,000 Children*. New York: Brunner/Mazel, 1974.

Hebb, D. O. "The effect of early and late brain injury upon test scores and the nature of normal adult intelligence." *Proceedings of the American Philosophical Society*, 85, 275–292, (1942).

———*The Organization of Behavior: A Neuropsychological Theory*. New York: Wiley, Inc., 1949.

Hopkins, K. D. "An empirical analysis of the efficacy of the WISC in the diagnosis of organicity in children of normal intelligence." *The Journal of Genetic Psychology*, 105, 163–172, (1964).

Hughes, J. R., and G. E. Park. "The EEG in dyslexia," in P. Kellaway and I. Petersen, eds., *Clinical Electroencephalography of Children*. New York: Grune & Stratton, 1968.

Hunt, J. McV. *The Challenge of Incompetence and Poverty.* New York: Ronald Press, 1961.

Kahn, E., and L. H. Cohen. "Organic driveness: A brain stem syndrome and experience." *New England Journal of Medicine,* 210, 748–756, (1934).

Kinsbourne, M. "School problems, diagnosis and treatment." *Pediatrics,* 52 (5), 596–609, (1973).

Knobel, M., M. B. Wolman, and E. Mason. "Hyperkinesis and organicity in children." *Archives of General Psychiatry,* 1, 310–321, (1959).

Koppitz, E. M. *Children with Learning Disabilities: A Five-Year Follow-Up Study.* New York: Grune & Stratton, 1971.

Lashley, K. S. *Brain Mechanisms and Intelligence.* Chicago: University of Chicago Press, 1929.

———*Brain Mechanisms and Intelligence—A Quantitative Study of Injuries to the Brain.* New York: Dover, 1963.

Loney, J. "The intellectual functioning of hyperactive elementary school boys: A cross-sectional investigation." *American Journal of Orthopsychiatry,* 44, 754–762, (1974).

Luria, A. R. "An objective approach to the study of the abnormal child." *American Journal of Orthopsychiatry,* 31, 1–17, (1961).

———*Higher Cortical Functions in Man.* New York: Basic Books, 1966.

McFie, J. "The effects of hemispherectomy on intellectual functioning in cases of infantile hemiplegia." *Journal of Neurology, Neurosurgery and Psychiatry,* 24, 240–249, (1961).

Menkes, M. M., J. S. Rowe, and J. H. Menkes. "A twenty-five year follow-up study on the hyperkinetic child with minimal brain dysfunction." *Pediatrics,* 39, 393–399, (1967).

Meyers, B. "Early language development as a function of active response and stimulus redundancy" (Ph.D. diss., The Ohio State University, 1972.)

Miller, Jr., R. G., H. S. Palkes, and M. A. Stewart. "Hyperactive children in suburban elementary schools." *Child Psychiatry and Human Development,* 4, (2), 121–127, (1973).

Myklebust, H. R., M. N. Bannochie, and J. R. Killen. "Learning disability and cognitive processes," in H. R. Myklebust, ed., *Progress in Learning Disabilities.* New York: Grune & Stratton, 1971.

Nicolis, J. S. and M. Benrubi. "Inadequate communications between self-organizing systems and desynchronization of physiological rhythms." *Technical Report CSB—2.* Patras, Greece: University of Patras, 1975.

Paine, R. S., J. S. Werry, and H. C. Quay. "A study of minimal cerebral dysfunction." *Developmental Medicine and Child Neurology,* 10, 505–520, (1968).

Palkes, H., and M. Stewart. "Intellectual ability and performance of hyperactive children." *American Journal of Orthopsychiatry,* 42, 35–39, (1972).

Piercy, M. "The effects of cerebral lesions on intellectual function: A review of current research trends." *British Journal of Psychiatry,* 110, 310–322, (1964).

Pribram, K. H. "A review of theory in physiological psychology," in P. R. Farnsworth, ed., *Annual Review of Psychology,* 11, 1–40, Palo—Alto: Annual Review, 1960.

Reed, H. B. C., R. M. Reitan, and H. Kløve. "Influence of cerebral lesions of psychological test performances of older children." *Journal of Consulting Psychology,* 29 (3), 247–251, (1965).

Reitan, R. M. "Psychological effects of cerebral lesions in children of early school age," in R. M. Reitan and L. A. Davison, eds., *Clinical Neuropsychology: Current Status and Applications,* pp. 53–88, Washington, D. C.: Winston & Sons, 1974.

Rie, E. D., and H. E. Rie. "Characteristics of children with learning disabilities." (Paper presented at the 85th Annual Convention of the American Psychological Association, San Francisco, August, 1977.)

———"Reading deficits, intellectual patterns, and hemispheric functions." [1979] forthcoming.

Rie, E. D., H. E. Rie, S. Stewart, and S. Rettemnier. "An analysis of neurological soft signs in children with learning problems." *Brain and Language*, 6, 32–46, (1978).

Rie, H. E., E. D. Rie, S. Stewart, and J. P. Ambuel. "Effects of methylphenidate on underachieving children." *Journal of Consulting Psychology*, 44, 250–260, (1976).

Rosenzweig, M. R. "Conference summary," in M. R. Rosenzweig and E. L. Bennett, eds., *Neural Mechanisms of Learning and Memory*, pp. 593–599. Cambridge: MIT Press, 1976.

Rowley, V. N. "Analysis of the WISC performance of brain damaged and emotionally disturbed children." *Journal of Consulting Psychology*, 25 (6), 553, (1961).

Russell, W. R. *Brain-Memory Learning, A Neurologist's View*. Oxford, England: Clarendon, 1959.

Rutter, M. "Brain damage syndromes in childhood. concepts and findings." *Journal of Child Psychology and Psychiatry*, 18, 1–21, (1977).

Rutter, M., P. Graham, and W. Yule. "A neuropsychiatric study in childhood." *Clinics in Developmental Medicine*, Nos. 35/36, Philadelphia: Lippincott, 1970.

Schiffman, G., and R. L. Clemens. "Observations on children with severe reading problems," in J. Hellmuth, ed., *Learning Disorders*, V.II, pp. 297–310. Seattle, Wash.: Special Child Publications, 1966.

Signoret, J. L. and F. Lhermitte. "The amnesic syndromes and the encoding process," in M. R. Rosenzweig and E. L. Bennett, eds., *Neural Mechanisms of Learning and Memory*. Cambridge: MIT Press, 1976.

Simensen, R. J. "Correlations among Bender-Gestalt, WISC block design, memory-for-designs, and the pupil rating scale." *Perceptual and Motor Skills*, 38, 1249–1250, (1974).

Stewart, M. "The hyperactive child syndrome." *American Journal of Orthopsychiatry*, 36, 861–867, (1966).

Stewart, M., H. Palkes, R. Miller, C. Young, and Z. Welner. "Intellectual ability and school achievement of hyperactive children, their classmates, and their siblings," in D. Ricks, A. Thomas, and M. Roff, eds., *Life History Research in Psychopathology*, vol. 3. Minneapolis: University of Minnesota Press, 1974.

Trites, R. L., and C. Fiedorowicz. "Follow-up study of children with specific (or primary) reading disability," in R. M. Knights and D. J. Bakker, eds., *The Neuropsychology of Learning Disorders: Theoretical Approaches*. Baltimore: University Park Press, 1976.

Vandevoort, L., G. M. Senf, and A. L. Burton. "Development of audio-visual integration in normal and retarded readers." *Child Development*, 43, 1260–1272, (1972).

Wechsler, D. *The Measurement and Appraisal of Adult Intelligence*. Baltimore: Williams & Wilkins, 1958.

Wender, P. H. *Minimal Brain Dysfunction in Children*. New York: Wiley, 1971.

———"Some speculations concerning a possible biochemical basis of minimal brain dysfunction," in F. F. de la Cruz, B. H. Fox, and R. H. Roberts, eds., *Minimal Brain Dysfunction*, 205, pp. 18–28. New York: New York Academy of Sciences, 1973.

Wilker, A., J. F. Dixon, and J. B. Parker. "Brain function in problem children and controls: Psychometric, neurological, and electroencephalographic comparisons." *American Journal of Psychiatry*, 127 (5), 634–645, (1970).

CHAPTER 13

Developmental Language Disorders

Paul S. Weiner

INTRODUCTION

Most children come to speak their native tongues in the expected way and at the expected time. At worst they suffer a relatively transient difficulty in pronunciation. Of those children who do not develop language normally, most show defective sensory, motor, intellectual, or emotional functioning. A small group however does not measure up to expected standards in language development despite adequacy or near adequacy in these areas. They may begin to talk late or, having started to speak, do not expand their comprehension or use of language in the same fashion as does the usual child. It is this group that is usually intended when the language problems of children with minimal brain dysfunction are discussed. In some children the difficulties are evident from the time that language is normally expected to appear. In yet others the difficulties apparently come to notice only some years later when the children begin to have problems with school learning.

There is little information available on the prevalence of these language difficulties. The existing studies all seem to be of British origin, and applicability of their results to other settings is unknown. The most recent and best conceived study (Stevenson and Richman, 1976) involved a one-in-four sample of the entire population of three-year-old children in a London suburb. "Specific language delays," that is, ones not associated with general mental retardation, appeared in 5.7 out of 1000 children. This is considerably higher than the findings of other studies such as those reviewed by MacKeith and Rutter (1972). However the results of these other studies were either obtained from a survey of professionals or else involved older children.

Many terms have been applied to the phenomenon of inadequate language development. Among them have been childhood aphasia, audimutism, congenital auditory imperception, language disorder, linguistic deviance, and delayed language development. Probably the most common designations have involved the use of the term aphasia. This has resulted in seemingly endless and ofttimes acrimonious debate. Objections have centered about such issues as the use of the same term both for the loss of developed language and for failure to acquire language normally, the implication of cerebral dysfunction as the source of the difficulty when the issue is in question, and the further implication of permanence of the language disorder when prediction remains very uncertain. A two-fold classification system, involving a receptive and an expressive category, has ordinarily been used in relation to the term. This too has been subjected to consider-

298

able criticism. The major objection stems from the broadness of the classes. Useful with extreme cases, these classes lose much of their cogency when children with milder problems are involved. Neither aspect of language functioning, understanding or use, stands out as the major focus of difficulty, and a large receptive-expressive group results.

In the face of these criticisms, other designations and classificatory schemes have been proposed. For example T. T. S. Ingram (1972) has proposed the term "developmental speech disorder syndrome" and a scheme which places the children's speech and language problems on a continuum of severity. The designation of "mild" is applied to children who have difficulty acquiring speech sounds but whose language is normal (traditionally termed dyslalia). The "moderate" are those who have a more severe pronunciation or speech articulation problem and are slow to acquire spoken language, while their comprehension of language is normal (expressive dysphasia). The "severe" group is characterized by even greater difficulties with speech articulation and spoken language and in addition by problems with the comprehension of language (receptive dysphasia). The children in the "very severe" group show not only defective comprehension of language, but also of the meaning of other sounds as well (auditory imperception or central deafness). There is inevitably a gross failure in spoken language among these last children.

In the present chapter the terms developmental language disorder (or language disorder) and language delay will be used and will occur interchangeably. No implication regarding the nature of the language acquisition process or prognosis of the language difficulty will be intended. It should be noted that even these terms have been used with some variability. At times language disorder has been used to indicate that the problem is likely to be of long duration. At others it has carried the implication of deviance rather than slowness in language acquisition. For the most part however it seems to be treated as a neutral term, as is language delay. It is this usage which will be followed.

Over the past century investigators interested in the study of language-delayed children have borrowed both their theoretical models and their methods from other fields. In the earliest days, the available medical model of the case study and the methods of examination devised for adult aphasics were used. Later on available neurological and psychological tools were used. Most recently the theories and analytical techniques of the psycholinguists have been applied to the problems of this area. It seems likely that this will continue to be the pattern. While interest in the problems of language-delayed children has increased enormously, the phenomenon still remains peripheral to the interest of all but a small number of investigators.

Many questions must be answered before language disorders can be understood. In broad outline these questions relate to the nature of the language problem, its causes, and its consequences. This presentation will describe existing data and will attempt to indicate the nature of some of the questions needing exploration.

THE NATURE OF LANGUAGE DISORDERS

The language difficulties of concern in this chapter have to some extent been described above. In the presentation of T. T. S. Ingram's (1972) classification scheme, the major areas of language which are explored in a clinical situation were noted. The child's ability to pronounce speech sounds, to express himself in words, and to understand what is said to him are all of concern. The descriptions of a child's language in the earlier case studies tended to be limited to impressionistic statements about these areas with perhaps a few examples of the child's productions included. The children had extreme difficulties so that a limited description seemed reasonably adequate to characterize the nature of the child's language. In addition interest of the investigators both in these case studies and in later group studies was directed toward the child's functioning in other areas, toward what might be called "language related behaviors" (Weiner, 1972a). These behaviors consisted largely of the perceptual and motor functioning of the child. This limitation of interest came in part from the dependence on studies of adult aphasics for a theoretical model and in part from the lack of an appropriate method of analyzing language. The effect of this last factor can be seen also in the research of the same period relating to the development of normal-child language. Studies tended to be atheoretical and to consist of tabulations of the increase in various structures, for example the number of words in sentences, the proportion of complete and incomplete sentences, the complexity of sentences (McCarthy, 1946, 1954). This situation changed only when linguists presented a theory of language structure which seemed to offer the promise of providing greater understanding of language development. This, of course, did not take place until Chomsky presented his theory of generative transformational grammar (1957, 1965). The enormous increase in studies of the language of normal children has been accompanied by at least some attention to that of the language disordered.

Structural Deficits (Delay or Deviance)

The earliest study using Chomsky's transformational theory was made by Menyuk (1964). Using an early version of that theory, she compared the utterances of children with "infantile speech" with those of normal children of the same age, intelligence level, and socioeconomic background. Her findings indicated that the language-disordered group produced more ungrammatical forms and used fewer transformations than did the normal group. Few of the differences were statistically significant. However on the basis of these findings and of a comparison of a language-disordered three-year-old and a two-year-old normal child, she concluded that there was a qualitative difference between the language systems of the two groups. This conclusion has been challenged by Morehead and Ingram (1973). These investigators matched their groups according to a linguistic criterion (mean morphemes per utterance) rather than to the age variable that Menyuk used. The major difference between the two groups was found to be in the "onset and acquisition time necessary for learning base syntax and the use of aspects of that system, once acquired, for producing major lexical items in a variety of utterances" (Morehead and Ingram, 1973, p. 340). The linguistic systems did not differ essentially. However the deviant children were not able to make as effective use of the systems they had acquired as did the normal children. While more complex structures were present, they were less used by the deviant children at each level of linguistic development. Also Morehead and Ingram, in common with Menyuk (1969), concluded that "the utterances produced by deviant children are on the whole less well formed than those of normal children" (1973, p. 343). They essentially opt for a quantitative rather than a qualitative difference. Support for this conclusion is derived from other grammatical studies as well. Ingram (1974) found that the same group of language-disordered children acquired the forms of the verbal auxiliary and the copula in the same order as did the normal control subjects and at the same levels of linguistic development. However they used the forms less frequently. Johnston and Schery (1976) compared the order of acquisition of eight grammatical morphemes by a large group of language-disordered children who varied widely in age with that of three normal children studied longitudinally by Brown (1973). They found that the order of acquisition was much the same, but occurred at later levels of language development.

Two studies have asked the same question about development of semantic relations, that is, the meanings expressed by relationships between words (Freedman and Carpenter, 1976; Leonard, Bolders, and Miller, 1976). The results are those to be expected on the basis of the studies already noted. When the normal and language-disordered children are matched according to level of linguistic development, the semantic relations systems revealed by their utterances do not differ in any essential way.

The question posed by these various studies, that of delay or deviance, has become the central issue in discussions on the nature of the language functioning of these children. To this point the evidence from formal studies would seem to support the hypothesis of delay in acquiring a language system. Only Menyuk's early study (1964), which did not equate groups on the basis of specifically linguistic criteria, lends support to the deviance hypothesis. This is an important issue not only theoretically, but also clinically. It is generally accepted among clinicians (Bangs, 1968; Ingram, 1972) that their charges can be divided into two groups, those whose acquisition of language is simply delayed and those whose language is deviant. There is a very practical referent to this question. If there are indeed children who form deviant language systems, they are the ones most in need of help. Those who can be expected to fashion an adequate system in time may need less intensive help or a different form of help. In fact, if we could make adequate predictions of the future course of their language development, some children might be safely left to their own devices.

The Unity of Language Disorders

Traditionally problems of speech articulation have been treated separately from those involving syntax or semantics. Far more common in occurrence, they have been regarded as less serious. In the speech pathology literature, they have been treated essentially as mechanical problems of sound production, linked primarily to perceptual and motor problems, particularly to the former. In contrast problems of syntax and semantics have been related to knowledge and use of the language system. Increasingly however evidence has accumulated to show that articulation problems too may relate to knowledge and use of an aspect of language, the phonological system (Lorentz, 1976; Compton, 1976). The children's perceptual and motor inadequacies may not be the essential factors (Rees, 1973), as has been assumed. In addition there is increasing evidence that children with articulation problems are likely to show difficulties with syntax as well. The approaches have varied but the results have been consistent. Children who were selected on the basis of their poor articulation have tended also to have difficulties in the use of syntax (Vandemark and Mann, 1965; Shriner, Holloway, and Daniloff, 1969; Whitacre, Luper, and Pollio, 1970) and in its comprehension as well (Marquardt and Saxman, 1972). Groups of children chosen as being language disordered (Menyuk and Looney, 1972a, 1972b; Weiner, 1969c, 1972b) proved to have articulation problems also. In one study (Menyuk and Looney, 1972b), accuracy of the children's repetitions of sounds was found to be related to the meaningfulness of the material used. This at least suggests that problems in all three aspects of the language system—phonology, syntax, and semantics—are interrelated. However it should not be concluded that problems in one of these areas inevitably implicate other areas as well. Crookes and Greene (1963) found that their subjects with articulation difficulties could be divided into two groups, one with syntactical problems and one without. Nonetheless there is some tendency towards such linkages. The child with difficulties in one aspect of language has an increased likelihood of having difficulties in others. In fact it seems possible that a deficit in one area may cause a deficit in another. For example a child with severe articulation problems may restrict the complexity of the grammar he uses as he seeks to avoid exposing his inadequacies (Shriner, Holloway, and Daniloff, 1969).

The Classification of Language Disorders

Despite any limitations, the traditional characterizations of language disorders have offered useful descriptions of the phenomena involved. Many children do seem to fall readily into the broad expressive or receptive categories, and approaches to remediation can be given a general direction by this classification. Explorations of the language behavior associated with each of the categories have provided some potentially useful delineations of language disorders. An example is the observations made on children with expressive problems by Johnson and Myklebust (1967). They have divided such children into three subgroups. The children in one are essentially apraxic, having difficulties with motor patterning of the speech articulators. Those in the second group have problems in retrieving specific words in a needed context. The final group consists of youngsters who have difficulties in formulating grammatically acceptable utterances. This scheme is of course reminiscent of those derived from the study of adult aphasics. The most important point in the present context however is that it stresses the children's difficulties with the production of language, that is with the use of the language system rather than with its acquisition as a system of knowledge.

A comparable scheme for children with receptive problems might well stress the degree to which sound has meaning for a child. Some children do understand language but only to a limited degree. Others find significance only in nonverbal sound, while still others obtain no meaning at all from sound despite adequate auditory acuity. A major question here would be the extent to which a child's problem is essentially one of symbolic formulation, of learning a language system, or one of the ability to transmit sound patterns to a central integrative mechanism so they can be interpreted (Wepman, et al., 1960).

It may be well to conclude with some comments on the frequency and severity of the types of problems in the various categories. Articulation problems are the most common followed by problems in the use of grammatical structure. Least common are problems of language comprehension (Rutter, Graham, and Yule,

1970). This order of frequency is the same as T. T. S. Ingram's (1972) order of severity. Support for that order is provided by McGrady's study of the psychological functioning of expressive and receptive aphasics (1968). The former were more intact in their psychological functioning than were the latter.

Duration

Another issue of importance is the duration of the structural problems of language disordered children. The clinical impression is that most children who begin to talk late eventually do so normally (Rutter, 1972). However some of them do continue to have oral language problems even into adolescence and adulthood. Recent studies have detailed the remaining structural language difficulties of an adolescent (Weiner, 1974) and of a young adult (Kerschensteiner and Huber, 1975). Whether it is only late-speaking children who show disorders in oral language subsequently is not clear. Language disorders have recently been documented in school-age and adolescent learning-disabled children. Vogel (1974, 1975) found that seven- and eight-year-old dyslexic children were inferior to normal children in their use of morphology and syntax in speaking. Wiig and her associates (Wiig and Semel, 1973, 1974; Wiig and Roach, 1975; Semel and Wiig, 1975; Wiig, 1976) established that somewhat older grade-school children and adolescents with learning disabilities had greater difficulty in the production and comprehension of various linguistic concepts than did normal controls. However the age at which the children in these studies began to talk is not noted. It is at least possible that their language problems are ones of slow acquisition not preceded by late onset. Prediction of future development in language delayed children has received attention in only one study (Petrie, 1975). The results suggest that the least affected children are likely to improve the most.

Deficits of Function

The analysis of linguistic adequacy need not be restricted to the study of structure. It is also possible to observe the effectiveness with which a child uses language as a tool in gaining his own ends. Language can serve many purposes in the life of the child. The most important of these are generally considered to be communication and thought. Both are possible without language but each is enhanced by its use. Thus while nonverbal means of communication precede language and continue to be vital throughout life, language soon becomes the major means of initiating and maintaining social contact. Once a child has learned to speak, he is increasingly likely to make his needs, demands, ideas, and feelings known primarily by means of words. Gesturing and crying are but limited substitutes. In turn, if he is to understand fully what his parents are trying to transmit to him, he must be able to respond appropriately to their verbal as well as to their nonverbal messages. The role of language in thought is of course the subject of much discussion and controversy. Contrasting theories abound. Piaget (1963), at one extreme, accords it only a secondary role. Vygotsky (1962), on the other hand, tends to equate language with thought. In the immediate context, concern might well be limited to the children's ability to use language in the solution of cognitive problems, a concern which finds concrete expression in school language arts curricula and in many intelligence tests.

Both of these broad functions, communication and thought, might well be expected to suffer in the language-disordered child. It seems reasonable to expect that as language becomes the major means of communication for children, a youngster with a poorly developed language system would have difficulties in this area. Similarly to the extent that language is important in the development of thought, a language-disordered child would be expected to show deficiencies in that realm.

Studies of how well language-disordered children communicate with others seem to be lacking. Clinical observations indicate that the range is broad indeed. Some of these youngsters develop great skill in nonverbal communication while others seem poverty-stricken. One child may be able to describe a fireworks display without words so vividly that the explosions seem to be occurring in the room. Yet another may be limited to pulling and pointing. The same seems true of various children's use of their limited language systems. One may use a limited stock of words and grammatical structures imaginatively and to great effect while another can only present the most limited of ideas. Such differences my be related to the children's cognitive abilities which have also received only limited exploration.

The study of deficits in the ability to use words in the solution of intellectual problems could potentially take a number of forms. For example the verbal mediation paradigm, involving the covert use of words in problem-solving tasks, has been much employed with both normal and retarded children (Jensen, 1971; Borkowski and Wanschura, 1974). A major hypothesis proposed to account for the intellectual problems of the retarded child is that he lacks the ability to use verbal responses as mediators (or regulators) of voluntary behavior. These mediators are internal verbal responses that a child could use to regulate what he does overtly. Unfortunately the paradigm seems not to have been used with the language disordered. Information on deficits in the use of language in the solution of intellectual problems appears to be restricted to studies of verbal-nonverbal differences in intelligence test results. The studies have not been directed to children who have problems in the comprehension or use of linguistic structure. Much of the interest has arisen rather from a search for the bases of difficulties in learning to read. The Wechsler Intelligence Scale for Children (WISC) has been by far the most favored instrument in this endeavor. The general trend has been for poor readers to show lower functioning on the Verbal subtests than on the Performance subtests (Sattler, 1974). (The latter are not truly nonverbal for they do involve verbal directions. They do not however require a verbal response.) This pattern clearly is not universally true of retarded readers. For example Lyle and Goyen (1969) found greater verbal-nonverbal variations in both directions in a group of retarded readers than in a group of normal readers.

Perhaps most pertinent to the immediate concern of this paper are the studies of correlates of verbal deficits. These are defined as particularly large discrepancies between the results on the two scales of the WISC with the deficiency being in verbal functioning. Speech articulation and reading difficulties were found in all the groups studied. One group with a 20 point verbal deficit (Owen, et al., 1971) showed a significantly greater number of medical and neurological findings than did the control subjects. However another group with a 25 point deficit (Holroyd, 1968) did not reveal increased medical diagnoses of brain damage or of psychiatric disorders. The third group with a 15 point deficit on a short form of the WISC (Weiner, 1969a), did not approach this problem but did find an inferiority in the control group subjects in both auditory perceptual and auditory conceptual tasks.

It is of interest to note that approximately 20% of the language deficient group in the last study were described by their mothers as having been delayed in language development. This was true of none of the control group children. (It should be mentioned that it did not prove possible to interview all the mothers in either group.) The relationship between late onset of speech and verbal deficits has also been approached from the opposite perspective. As part of a longitudinal study of seven late-speaking, dysphasic children (Weiner, 1972b), the WISC was administered at six years of age. The unpublished results revealed that six of the seven children had Verbal Scale deficits. These ranged from 7 to 25 IQ points, with the median deficit being 17 points. Thus, to the extent that these small samples of children are typical of their groups, it may be expected that a minority of children who show verbal deficits on an intelligence test will have been delayed in early language acquisition. Of children who start to speak late and still show difficulties with language structure at five or six years of age, most are likely to show deficits in the use of language in solving intellectual problems. The difficulty may well be a long-lasting one. In the study of language deficient children, the same pattern of verbal deficit was found in most of the children a year later, while in the study of the dysphasics it still existed in most of them two to three years later.

THE CAUSES OF LANGUAGE DISORDERS

Biological Factors

In view of the purpose of this volume, the possible causes of developmental language disorders are of particular interest. Studies in this area have taken a number of directions. One has been the search for evidence of a physical cause. This has been presumed in some definitions of the condition, particularly when the designation of aphasia has been used. For example the definition of aphasia in children used at a major educational and investigative center, the Central Institute for the Deaf, includes the statement that "it is the result of some defect in the central nervous system" (McGinnis, Kleffner, and Goldstein, 1956). In fact several studies of children at the same institution do provide evidence of brain dysfunction in at least some language-disordered youngsters. In one study (Goldstein, Landau, and Kleffner, 1958), neurologic observations on aphasic and deaf children were compared. The aphasic children had severe language disorders; half of them had hearing losses. The groups showed a considerable difference only on "significant defect of motor function," 23.2% of the aphasic group and 3.5% of the deaf group revealing such difficulties. Statistical significance was not noted. Probable etiologies differed between the two groups, with the aphasic children showing a predominance of such problems as "Rh, complications of birth and labor, convulsive disorder, congenital brain abnormality, family history of speech or neurological disorder" (p. 764). Other measures did not reveal differences. In another study by the same group (Landau, Goldstein, and Kleffner, 1960), the autopsy findings on a child with congenital aphasia were reported. "Bilateral old infarctions in the sylvian regions and severe retrograde degeneration in the medical geniculate nuclei" were noted (p. 921). Additional evidence for a biological origin is the occurrence of aphasic or aphasoid language disorders in some children caused by kernicterus, jaundice affecting various cranial nuclear masses (Cohen, 1956; Hannigan, 1956). Finally a recent study of dichotic listening performance of language-disordered children (Sommers and Taylor, 1972) might be considered to provide evidence supporting the thesis of cerebral dysfunction. In this paradigm contrasting auditory stimuli are presented simultaneously to the right and left ear of the subject who is asked to report what he hears. The expected response, that found in the normal control group, was more frequent reports of words and digits heard in the right ear. The language disordered group, in contrast, indicated more frequent left-ear responses. The defective children in this study had had serious speech delays and poor ability to comprehend spoken language. Also virtually all had some soft neurological signs.

Several aspects of the findings of these studies should be noted. First, the subjects were very largely children with severe comprehension problems. Without further study, any implication of brain damage or dysfunction cannot reasonably be extended to children with different kinds or severity of language problems. But even within this group, not all of the children showed signs of brain dysfunction. In the Goldstein, Landau and Kleffner study (1958), 32% of the aphasic children demonstrated abnormalities in none of the neurologic studies done. Yet their auditory and language functioning did not differ from those on whom positive findings were made, nor did their school progress. The existing evidence for cerebral dysfunction as the cause of language disorders in general is not extremely convincing.

Other possible causes have also been implicated. Genetic transmission has been a much favored hypothesis, particularly among European trained investigators, to account for such disorders as greatly delayed onset of speech, long-lasting speech articulation difficulties, and severe problems in learning to read. In fact investigators such as Luchsinger (1959) and Arnold (1961) have proposed a "congenital language disability" involving these and other speech and language disturbances. They have proposed a developmental sequence in which a young child progresses from delayed speech development to an articulation disorder with frequently accompanying "dysgrammatism." Once school age is reached, the child manifests a "specific reading and writing disability." During the succeeding years, the child also has difficulties with various forms of "tachyphemia," such as a tendency toward rapid, precipitate, and cluttered speech. The frequency with which this entire syndrome appears is not noted (Luchsinger and Arnold, 1965). Lenneberg (1967) in his review of the literature on "inherited language potential" describes the familial occurrence of this syndrome as "well documented" (p. 249).

Relevant to the genetic hypothesis is that of a maturational lag (Luchsinger and Arnold, 1965; Eisenson, 1972). The capacities which are important in linguistic development may develop more slowly than usual in language-disordered children whose problems are familial in origin. The result would be a delay in the acquisition of language. This hypothesis does provide a possible biological explanation of developmental language disorders in instances where evidence of brain damage or dysfunction is lacking. To this point however the hypothesis remains simply a theoretical possibility.

Environmental Factors

Environmental factors have had little currency as an hypothesized cause of language disorders. However a number of studies suggest that such factors should be considered. In an early series of studies, Goldfarb (1945) found that stimulus deprivation, such as that endured by children in orphanages, is linked to language delays. Physical restraint in the early months of life has also been related to language delays and speech articulation problems (Sibinga and Friedman, 1971). Further, observations of language development in normal children (Nelson, 1973) have indicated that mothers' acceptance or rejection of their toddlers' utterances is related to the rate at which the children develop language. Whether the negative reactions of one group of mothers to their language-delayed children (Wulbert, et al., 1975) were cause or effect of the language disorder is unknown. However Nelson's findings would suggest that such reactions may further inhibit language development. Finally an experimental study of interaction between a mother and her language-delayed child (Whitehurst, Novak, and Zorn, 1972) provides additional support for the hypothesis of environmental influence. The rate of acquisition of new words was increased by rather small increments in the level of the mother's conversation with and imitative prompts to her child. In all this appears to be a promising area which deserves additional attention.

Perceptual Factors

The greatest amount of attention in the search for causes of language disorders has gone to behavioral or psychological functions, such as perception and memory. "Cause" may not be an entirely appropriate term to use in the context of these studies. The search has been for behavioral deficits which accompany language-learning difficulties and which seem to be logically related to language functioning. The assumption has been that such deficits are basic to the language problem.

For children whose major difficulty has seemed to be in language expression (Ley, 1929), a dyspraxic element has been emphasized as the basic problem. These children have been characterized as being generally clumsy with the awkwardness increasing as the complexity of the act increases. However this has not been universally accepted as a sole underlying deficit even for aphasic subjects whose comprehension seemed normal or near normal. Launay and Soulé (1952) presented cases whch indicated a diversity of underlying defects. Ajuriaguerra and his co-workers (1958) divided their subjects into a dyspraxic group whose members showed a "profound incapacity to organize movements in space and in time" (p. 58) and a group with "prevailing difficulties in temporal organization" (p. 23). Basically they interpret language disorders as involving "a disorder of gestalt formation" (Ajuriaguerra, et al., 1963, p. 134).

These ideas have received greatest currency in the European continental literature. In contrast English and American investigators have favored auditory deficits as the basic problem. Historically the trend seems to have had two sources. The first (and probably original) source was Worster-Drought and Allen's studies of a case of congenital auditory imperception (1929a, 1929b, 1930), in which they emphasized the agnosic aspect of the child's difficulty, his inability to interpret the meaning of sound. The second was Orton's (1937) suggestion that the root of aphasic children's language inadequacies is a difficulty with temporal ordering. This hypothesis has probably received more attention from investigators of developmental language disorders than has any other. The results of the studies have been mixed with reference to visual as well as auditory stimuli. Some investigators (Lowe and Campbell, 1965; Stark, 1966, 1967; Stark, Poppen, and May, 1967;

Monsees, 1968; and Poppen, et al., 1969) interpreted their results as suggesting a deficiency in "temporal ordering" (Poppen, et al., 1969, p. 288). However other investigators (Olson, 1961; Furth, 1964; Furth and Pufall, 1966; Weiner, 1969c, 1972b) interpreted their results as contradicting the hypothesis. The only consistent finding in these varying results is that language disordered children have more difficulty than do deaf or normal children in reproducing nonverbal sequences. In the studies using auditory stimuli (which are more closely related to the language problem being investigated), the results have been mixed. Most of these studies, specifically the ones utilizing vocal responses, may be criticized on the basis of the interpretations made of the findings. These have been based on the nature of the stimuli used and not on the nature of the children's responses. All errors in reproducing stimuli which are sequentially ordered have been treated as though they were equivalent. Errors of omission, substitution, and order have been treated essentially as though they were all errors in reproducing the stimuli in the correct sequence. There seems to be little doubt that language-disordered children have difficulties in reproducing sequentially ordered auditory stimuli such as sentences, series of numbers, or series of sounds. The more relevant question would seem to be whether they reproduce these stimuli in an incorrect order, whether they do indeed have a "difficulty in sequence building" (Orton, 1937, p. 148). Using such a criterion, Weiner (1969c, 1972b) did not find a sequencing problem in his dysphasic subjects. The errors made by them seldom involved order. Further errors of sequence occurred no more frequently among the experimental subjects than among the control subjects. It may be concluded that most of the existing studies do not respond to the essential question. The directly relevant evidence is negative.

Other criticisms of these studies of sequencing problems have been offered (Rees, 1973). For one, they involve the apparent assumption of a Markov, left-to-right view of sentence construction, a theory which receives little support at the present time. Further the research deals for the most part with the ordering of individual sounds or phonemes. However there is evidence indicating that speech sounds succeed each other much too rapidly to be analyzed separately in connected speech.

Several attempts have also been made to determine whether auditory discrimination, the ability to distinguish between sounds, might be deficient in language disordered children (Wilson, Doehring, and Hirsh, 1960; McReynolds, 1966). In each instance the aphasic children did have difficulties with the tasks presented. However in neither study did the investigators conclude that auditory discrimination was the major problem. Instead they suggested that other factors had interfered with the children's responses to the experimental tasks.

The most recent attempt to establish a perceptual basis for language disorders has centered about the rate at which aphasic children can process auditory signals. In a series of studies, Tallal and Piercy (1973a, 1973b, 1974, 1975) tested their dysphasic (or aphasic) subjects' ability to identify and to discriminate binary sequences of stimuli, both in the auditory and in the visual modalities. The auditory testing involved both nonverbal and simulated verbal stimuli (vowels and consonants). The experimental group did not differ from the control group on the visual tests. The major finding in the auditory modality was that the dysphasic children could not process auditory stimuli at a normal rate. On the basis of these studies and those of other investigators, Talla and Piercy (1975) concluded that adequacy in rate of auditory processing is related to adequacy of language functioning. Since the verbal or nonverbal character of the stimuli has proven not to be important, they also concluded that "the language defect of these children is not specifically linguistic but is secondary to an impaired rate of processing auditory information" (1975, p. 73).

Hearing

Before the discussion of perceptual adequacy is closed, the problem of the hearing-related behavior of language disordered children must be touched on at least briefly. The "receptive aphasic" has been described as frequently ignoring "not only speech, but sounds in general," and as being "typically erratic in auditory behavior" (Myklebust, 1954, p. 149). In a study of this characteristic, Reichstein (1964) found that his aphasic subjects varied in the consistency of their auditory behavior. Some were as consistent in their responses to an auditory threshold test as were nonaphasic children with hearing losses or children with normal hearing and language. But another, larger group of aphasic subjects was very inconsistent. This inevitably complicates the determination of the hearing sensitivity of such children. Since some kinds of hearing losses can easily be confused with a developmental language disorder (Ewing, 1930), the question is an important one. Also children with major comprehension problems may show hearing losses (Davis and Silverman, 1960). The losses may not be severe enough to account for the extent of their linguistic deficits but they do complicate the children's language-learning problems.

Cognitive Factors

Contrasting with the perceptual causation hypotheses are those which link developmental language disorders to cognitive deficiencies. One hypothesis (Menyuk, 1969) proposes that language disordered children are deficient in short-term memory. Since they are unable to retain sentences of any length, their analysis of the language they hear is both basic and generalized. This proposal derives from Menyuk's study (1964) of the spontaneous productions and sentence repetitions of the group of children whose speech had been called infantile by speech pathologists. As noted already she concluded that their language was deviant rather than simply delayed or infantile. But she also found, in the repetition task, that there was a significant relationship (r -.53) between length of sentence and failure to repeat correctly. In contrast this relationship was nonsignificant for the normal children in whose failures sentence structure seemed more important than did length. However further study of this issue (Menyuk and Looney, 1972a) indicated that structure was more determinative than length in the repetitions of language disordered children as well. Nonetheless Menyuk continues to support the hypothesis of a short-term memory deficit as basic to these children's language problems.

Recent studies of normal language acquisition have emphasized the necessary cognitive prerequisites (Bloom, 1970; Brown, 1973; Cromer, 1976; Ervin-Tripp, 1971; Sinclair-de-Zwart; 1969). In its broadest form, this hypothesis holds that a child cannot learn language until he has acquired certain cognitive operations. According to Piagetian theory sensory-motor intelligence, the ability to cope effectively with the immediate, concrete environment, is a necessary but not sufficient base. Normally this kind of intelligence develops within the first two years of life. It is only when the child becomes capable of forming symbolic representations, of making something stand for something else which is not present, that he is able to learn language. Indeed it is a deficit in this very ability which has been suggested as the basis for developmental language disorders (Cromer, 1976; Inhelder, 1963; Morehead and Ingram, 1973). To date there apparently have been no attempts to study the question in language disordered children who are just beginning to talk. Published studies involve older subjects. Inhelder (1963) found that the language difficulties of the dysphasic children studied by Ajuriaguerra and his group (1963) were "often accompanied by deficiencies in figurative symbolism" (p. 143). That is, these children had difficulty in forming internal spatial images or representations which would help them solve the problems presented by the investigator. Similarly Lovell, Hoyle, and Siddall (1968) found a "significant relationship between the mean number of morphemes per utterance and the amount of time spent in symbolic play" (p. 50). The relationship, however, held only for the four-year-olds, not the three-year-olds in the study. As the authors recognized neither of these studies can be regarded as establishing the Piagetian hypothesis. In fact Lovell, Hoyle and Siddall raised the opposite question of whether delayed language might not affect intellectual growth. Of course direction of influence is always a problem in essentially correlational studies.

Much of the research on normal children's language acquisition has concerned itself with specific concepts as they are related to specific linguistic structures. For example Cromer (1976) has studied the relationship of the acquisition of time concepts to the expression of these concepts in language. Nothing of this sort has been done with language disordered children. It would certainly be of interest to know whether the lack of a specific linguistic structure (for example tense) is based on an inadequacy in the relevant cognitive operation or is a specifically linguistic lack. This would have a bearing both on the understanding of the nature of language disorders and also on the nature of adequate remediation.

A final cognitive deficit hypothesis should be noted despite the lack of relevant investigation with language disordered children. In order to account for the difference between the brief utterances of young, normal children and the more complex meanings which seem to underlie them, Bloom (1970) proposed a reduction transformation. This is essentially a deletion of some element or elements that seem to be present in the underlying meaning (the deep structure) of an utterance so that it does not appear in the spoken form (the surface structure). Bloom presents an example in a series of sentences spoken by a young child: "raisins; buy more grocery store; grocery store; raisin ə grocery store" (1970, p.138). The intent seems to involve the buying of more raisins at a grocery store. However no one utterance contains all elements of this underlying message. Bloom suggested "that some sort of cognitive limitation in handling structural complexity . . . *underlies* the constraint on length of children's utterances—that the constraint on sentence length reflects an inherent limitation in linguistic operations" (p.165). The question being raised is whether this or a similar hypothesis might be helpful in seeking to understand the linguistic functioning of children with essentially expressive problems. There are young children whose understanding of spoken language seems fully normal but whose utterances show markedly inadequate grammar. While articulation is likely to be very poor at first, the basic problem is clearly not apraxia. Even when the child is understandable, the grammatical structure of his utterances continues to be inadequate for his age over a considerable period. One three-year-old observed by the author was able to pass a grammar comprehension test at the level expected of his age and to obtain a superior score on the Stanford-Binet Intelligence Scale. He did as well on the verbal as on the nonverbal items. However he did not begin to combine words until two weeks before his third birthday. The workings of his superior intelligence were obvious; the phonological and grammatical inadequacies of his spoken utterances were equally obvious. Was he operating under some production span limitation which required him to make reduction transformations to fit his intentions into his limited production means? Further evidence of the need for such a hypothesis comes from the already noted study of an apparently similar group of children by Lovell, Hoyle, and Siddall (1968). As part of their research, they used the ICP (Imitation, Comprehension, Production) test of Fraser, Bellugi and Brown (1963). In this test the same grammatical structures are studied through comprehension, imitation, and production tasks. Among normal children imitation proved to be the easiest, while comprehension and production followed in that order. In contrast the language-disordered children comprehended the various grammatical structures in the test better than they could either repeat or produce them spontaneously. Once again a production deficiency of some kind would seem to be implicated.

CONSEQUENCES OF DEVELOPMENTAL LANGUAGE DISORDERS

The use of the term consequences in relation to developmental language disorders can be misleading. It is difficult to establish that any particular phenomenon is truly a result of a language disorder. Apparently consequent behavior may be linked to a language disorder because both derive from the same source, not because one is the cause of the other. At other times it may be difficult to establish the direction of causality, that is, whether an accompanying phenomenon is indeed the result of the language problem or whether it is one of its causes. Finally behaviors which seem to be consequently related to the language problem may be epiphenomena, neither causal nor consequent. In any event behaviors which seem to be meaningfully attendant upon developmental language disorders will be described in this section. The areas to be explored include thought, reading, and social-emotional adjustment.

Language Disorders and Thought

There is considerable evidence to indicate that language has at best a limited effect upon the thought of the preschool child. This evidence derives particularly from the experiments on verbal mediation. In this paradigm attempts are made to determine whether subjects use verbalizations in working on problems that otherwise would be much more difficult or impossible to solve. Studies of young children have indicated that children below the age of five to seven years fail to use words in the solution of problems. They do so neither spontaneously nor when the words are supplied by the experimenter (Flavell, 1970; Kendler, 1972). Further their preference for visual information when there is a choice would tend to indicate that the preschooler finds rather little use for language in many, perhaps most, problem-solving situations (Blank, 1974). If this thesis is correct, the young language-delayed child should not suffer intellectually provided that he is capable of normal nonverbal learning. However a quite opposed view also seems tenable. In an excellent discussion Blank (1974) presents evidence to indicate that language may indeed be useful in the preschooler's cognitive development. He acknowledges that visual information and gestural communication are preferred by young children when there is a choice between the visual or gestural and the verbal. However a child's gestures are useful communicative tools only when situations include visual cues. When a situation does not permit the meaningful use of gesture, the child must be able to utilize language if he is to communicate or solve problems. Also certain less concrete concepts, such as "how" and "why" or ones with a temporal referent, seem attainable only through language. Other concepts may remain fuzzy and inadequate if the child cannot reveal the nature of his current misconceptions and thereby elicit corrective information. This notion does not involve a negation of the Piagetian contention that certain nonverbal cognitive skills are prerequisite to the grasp of the meaning of their related verbal concepts. Blank's suggestion is rather that these nonverbal skills "remain undeveloped until called upon in situations using higher level language formulations" (1974, p. 242).

To the extent that Blank's thesis is correct, young language-disordered children's cognitive development can be expected to show limitations. Since less doubt tends to be expressed about the role of language in the development of thought in normal school-age children, there would be an even greater expectancy of negative effects of language disorders at this age level. Unfortunately no information is available for either group; only the possibility and the need for relevant research can be noted.

Language Disorders and Reading

Clinicians have long recognized the existence of a link between language disorders and difficulties in learning to read. The most noted observation has been that language delays tend to be succeeded by reading problems when the children reach school age. While retrospective data supporting this hypothesis are available (Ingram, 1963), prospective studies seem to be lacking. Neither the frequency with which this relationship occurs nor the mechanism by which it takes place has been studied. Indeed the opposite tack has been taken. Existing investigations have been directed toward the language deficiencies of dyslexic children. Some studies have sought to determine their knowledge of linguistic structure (Vogel, 1975; Wiig and Semel, 1974; Wiig, 1976). Others have explored the question of whether they have a verbal deficiency. This deficiency has taken a number of forms including dysnomia, difficulty in naming objects or pictures (Denckla, 1972; Jansky and de Hirsch, 1972); a mediational deficiency (Blank, Weider, and Bridger, 1968); and a low verbal IQ (Rabinovitch, 1959). Each of these language deficiencies has been found to exist in some groups of children with reading problems. Despite such findings, the literature on reading difficulties has continued to emphasize perceptual deficits as basic to the problem (Hallahan and Cruickshank, 1973). As a consequence the lack of information on the relationship between language disorders and reading problems persists. Existing studies simply substantiate the existence of the link.

In view of this situation, it seems appropriate to review briefly current thinking on the role of language in reading. Such a review may help to suggest ways in which language disorders may lead to reading retardation.

The importance of language in reading has increasingly been recognized (Kavanagh and Mattingly, 1972). As a result recent theoretical models of reading have included a linguistic aspect in one form or another. A popular current view of the process of reading is that the reader samples the text, predicting what is to come from what he has perceived (Gibson and Levin, 1975). Further sampling permits him to verify his expectations and to make corrections if necessary. In major part his predictions are based on his knowledge of the structure of the language he is reading. This view of reading as a king of "psycholinguistic guessing game" (Goodman, 1967) has been applied to adults (Levin, et al., 1972) and in some measure even to children at the earliest stages of learning the skill (Weber, 1970). A more traditional and contrary view of the process is that the reader proceeds through the text in a letter by letter fashion. Guessing occurs only when the reader does not readily decode the material. But even in this view linguistic knowledge may be seen as entering at a rather early stage. In a recent version of this theoretical model (Gough, 1972), the reader is seen as mapping the printed characters "onto a string of systematic phonemes" (p. 515). Other linguistic levels come into play in later stages of the model.

Thus it would seem that regardless of the nature of the model of reading, the readers' implicit knowledge of language structure is regarded as essential. If this is so, inadequate linguistic knowledge should have negative effects on the process of learning to read. Investigation of the specific effects of the linguistic problems of language-disordered children on their reading is thus very much in order. The results should provide material of considerable interest both in furthering the understanding of the consequences of language disorders and in the verification of various theoretical models of reading.

Language Disorders and Social-Emotional Adjustment

The final area of potential consequence to be discussed is the social and emotional adjustment of language-delayed children. It has occasioned a fair amount of comment, but little in the way of formal study. The most intensive attempt to deal with the area is undoubtedly the study of dysphasic children undertaken by Ajuriaguerra and his colleagues (1963, 1965). Using anamnestic data, school reports, and a direct examination of the children, they concluded that only 27.5% of the children showed completely satisfactory adjustment. The others revealed evidence of major or minor difficulties. A number of factors seemed related to the children's adjustment. The best adjusted group began to talk earlier than did the less well adjusted. Also the desire for communication was greatest for the children in the most normal group and least for the most disturbed. This was true both for verbal and for nonverbal communication. Interestingly there was no relationship between the severity of the language difficulty and adequacy of emotional organization. However such a relationship did exist with the children's style of verbal communication. Most of the well adjusted children used a form of organization which the authors called "verbally restrained" while most of the severely maladjusted children were "verbally unrestrained." The former is characterized by simple sentences and narratives, which largely involve enumeration and description. The latter involves the intermittent use of complex sentences and narratives, which are more complex but largely incoherent. Approximately two years later, it was found that almost all the children reexamined had not changed significantly in emotional organization.

Contrasting with this conclusion that most dysphasic children show at least minor emotional difficulties is that of Rutter (1972). He states that "most children with language difficulties do *not* show abnormalities in social and emotional development" (p. 184). The occurrence of such difficulties may be more frequent than in children in general, but it is still a minority that is affected. While Rutter finds that emotional problems are more frequent in children with the greatest language difficulties, the relationship is not very strong. This conclusion contrasts with that of the Ajuriaguerra group. However both agree that language delays do not lead directly to adjustment problems. Rutter explores various ways in which such delays can lead indirectly to adjustment difficulties: "through educational failure, through the effects of communication difficulties in social relationships, through lack of social integration, through the effects of teasing and rejection by other children and through associated brain dysfunction" (p. 185).

In the discussion Rutter notes the importance of the child's self-image and the effect on it of the parents' bewilderment and anxiety. The child, sensing his parents' feelings, begins to see himself in a negative light and to act in accordance with this view of himself. More directly, if the parents are over-protective, the child does not learn to fend for himself. Some evidence for this description appears in the finding of another study (Weiner, 1969b) that virtually all mothers of a group of language delayed children who were enrolled in a clinic were anxious or guilty about their children's handicap. Also these mothers tended to describe their children as quiet and overly close to them. This seemed to be in agreement with clinical observations of the same children who tended to be quiet and rather inhibited. Rutter's proposal suggests a link between the mothers' reactions and those of the children. Clinical observations would also suggest that as the mothers' level of anxiety and guilt is reduced, the children become less inhibited and more able to benefit from the clinic program.

The behavior of the children at the extreme of the continuum of language disorders (Ingram, 1972), that of severe language comprehension difficulties, requires some special comment. It is generally agreed that the most deviant behavior is likely to occur in these children. At times the withdrawal is sufficient to warrant being called autistic in nature (Myklebust, 1954; Churchill, 1972). This extreme behavior is not a constant concomitant of auditory comprehension problems, even when they are severe. Some children do not withdraw from social contact; others seem to react negatively only when faced with situations involving verbal demands; still others are noted to show social isolation in the preschool years but to improve as they get older. On the other hand, some show serious withdrawal which does not lessen without special intervention. Theories of the basis for the autistic behavior range widely, from one which treats the withdrawal as a response to parental disturbance over the child's language difficulties (Sahlmann, 1969), to one which regards the language difficulty as primary (Rutter, 1972). The latter is the currently most favored theory, especially by those who are engaged in the study of infantile autism. Rutter (1972) stresses the importance of an impairment in "inner language," the difficulty in dealing with symbols in any form. However he proposes that other factors have an influence as well. Other defects in the child, such as low intelligence, and the reactions of others to his difficulties influence his social adjustment, reinforcing or counteracting the effects of the language problem. This theory, it might be noted, has been used to account for the behavior of both autistic and schizophrenic children (Churchill, 1972). The difference between the psychotic children and those considered to have only a central language disorder is laid to the severity of the language problem. Language in this context is considered to include all forms of communication.

DISCUSSION

Despite more than a century of interest and study, rather little is known about developmental language disorders. Generally accepted facts are few, perhaps limited to the existence of language problems in children, the variability of their manifestations from child to child, and their strong tendency to occur in boys. Nonetheless sufficient studies have been made to provide a base for organized investigative efforts and to occasion a number of theoretical conflicts. In this final section some of the more important issues will be discussed and some of the major research needs in the area will be noted.

A basic issue in the study of language disorders is that of definition. A major point in question is the nature of the phenomena that should be included. Regardless of the term used to designate the general area, some definitions are broader than others in their reference. Most investigators (Johnson and Myklebust, 1967; Luchsinger and Arnold, 1965; and T. T. S. Ingram, 1972) include a broad range of phenomena. Their definitions encompass not only problems of comprehension, but also problems of expression which are not accompanied by difficulties in understanding. In contrast Eisenson (1972) would restrict the designation of developmental aphasia to auditory comprehension disorders. When expressive problems are unaccompanied by such auditory difficulties, he considers that oral apaxia is more likely to be involved. The problem would thus be considered as one of motor patterning rather than one entailing a language disorder. The difference could be a vital one. A sample chosen according to Eisenson's definition would be much more restricted than one selected to fit Ingram's "developmental speech disorder syndrome." The results of studies of any aspect of language disorders might differ accordingly. At this point the heuristic value of any definition is unknown. Only careful study could determine whether Eisenson's elimination of expressive problems or Johnson and Myklebust's inclusion and elaboration is the more meaningful or useful. Similarly exploration of the value of the various systems of classification of language problems would seem warranted. T. T. S. Ingram's ordering of the problems according to their severity seems particularly promising.

Another important issue is the relationship of developmental language disorders to minimal brain dysfunction. The usual definition of the later concept includes two aspects, one relating to causation of the condition and the other to its consequences. Thus Clements (1966) describes the affected children as being "of near average, average, or above average general intelligence with certain learning or behavioral disabilities. . . . which are associated with deviations of function of the central nervous system" (p. 9). There is little question that developmental language disorders fit the first part of this definition. However there is considerable uncertainty over the question of causation. The existing information suggests that cerebral dysfunction may be the determining factor in some instances. However the relevant data are derived essentially from children with major comprehension problems. Moreover this source of the problem is only variably in evidence even in this restricted group. The studies which suggest that environmental factors may influence language development do not necessarily contradict this explanation, but do add further complexity to the situation. For the present it seems best to reserve judgment on the extent to which developmental language disorders may be considered a consequence of minimal brain dysfunction. Additional explorations of biological causation using recent methodological advances, more sophisticated designs, and an expanded population base seems very much in order. The need for further study of possible environmental etiologies is evident also. Their role as primary or secondary determinants needs clarification.

The perceptual deficit hypothesis has been the major source of studies seeking a psychological or behavioral cause of language disorders. Eisenson (1968) has even made it the central element in his theory of developmental (auditory) aphasia. However this theory is far from unassailable. Even if the deficiencies of individual studies are set aside, major criticisms can be levied against the entire enterprise of seeking an auditory perceptual explanation for language disorders. As Rees (1973) has pointed out in her highly useful discussion of this hypothesis, the finding of auditory sequencing or of auditory memory deficiencies does not necessarily establish an auditory processing problem as cause. Rather it may simply reflect the fact that the subjects are language disordered. The apparent deficit would in this view be an aspect of the language problem rather than a cause of it. In actuality few attempts have been made to establish specific perceptual deficiencies as the basis of specific aspects of language malfunctioning. While the existing studies (Menyuk, 1969; Tallal, Stark and Curtiss, 1976) have indicated a link between the two phenomena, they have not established a specific causal relationship. In her discussion Rees concludes that the search for auditory factors to account for language disorders seems futile (1973, p. 312). Whether this criticism is exaggerated or not remains to be seen. Studies which are fully adequate to the question are yet to be done.

The recent attention given to cognitive prerequisites of normal language development has brought with it some discussion of intellectual deficit as a possible basis of language disorders. The two published investigations of the Piagetian hypothesis of a prerequisite general representational ability using language disordered samples (Inhelder, 1963; Lovell, Hoyle, and Siddall, 1968) suggest a relationship between this ability and language functioning. Once again however the direction of influence is uncertain. As is true in so many areas, further research is indicated.

Work on the nature of disordered language has centered around the question of the deviance of the children's language. The available evidence would seem to support the thesis that the children's language systems are delayed rather than deviant in form. However some questions must be raised concerning the nature of the samples used. First of all the populations sampled in the different studies may not be the same. The children in the Morehead and Ingram investigation (1973) were obtained in Eisenson's Institute for Childhood Aphasia and therefore undoubtedly had auditory comprehension difficulties. Menyuk's (1964) sample in all probability did not. The differences in the results could relate to this factor as well as to differences in methodology. Another question concerns possible bias in study samples. In studies of language disorders, the investigator is almost inevitably limited to the subjects who happen to be available to him. Since he is not able to make a random selection from the affected population, the sample may well be biased. It is most often small in size so that deviant children (assuming their existence) could be missed. Even if they are included, they may occur so infrequently that their contribution to the data would be lost in group trends. Specific comparisons of individual grammars of a large number of children may be necessary.

The area of potential consequences has not received sufficient study for major conflicting positions to have arisen. The only conflict of any note is over the question of the emotional adjustment of language disordered children. However the discrepant findings (Ajuriaguerra, et al., 1963, 1965; Rutter, 1972) might simply relate to the definitions used. Terms are difficult to define in this area and might easily differ from study to study. Careful delineation of terms and the use of appropriate control groups may resolve the issue without further difficulty. In any event, additional information would be most welcome.

Other research needs in the area of consequences relate to the development of thought and to the learning of reading, as noted in the body of the paper. Studies of the use of language in solving problems, such as those involving the mediational paradigm, would be helpful. Even a simple prospective study of the prevalence of reading difficulties following delay in the development of language would be useful in filling a gap in our knowledge.

This review of the existing knowledge of developmental language disorders leads readily to the conclusion that an adequate data base does not exist. This is true in each of the areas covered, even though in varying degrees. The major consequence of this situation is that adequate theoretical formulations are not yet possible. Much additional research will be necessary before a viable theory of developmental language disorders can be constructed. Fortunately interest in relevant problems has been increasing over the past several decades. Particularly promising are the spread of interest to new fields, such as psycholinguistics and the use of more sophisticated designs. Morehead and Ingram's (1973) study of the grammar of language-disordered children and Talla and her colleagues' studies of their perceptual functioning (1973a, 1973b, 1974, 1975, 1976) are particular cases in point.

An adequate theory of developmental language disorders will undoubtedly prove to be complex. The multifaceted nature of the phenomena involved and the considerable differences among the affected individuals would seem to require such complexity. A single cause is unlikely just as are invariable consequences. It is more likely that developmental language disorders will be found to result from the interaction of a number of causes operating at various levels and differing from individual to individual. Consequences are likely to vary according to the specific cause and nature of a child's language difficulties and his experiences in living with the disorder. At the present time investigations disregard individual variations and are directed toward single factors of cause and of consequence. As additional data accumulate, a more differentiated and complex view of the problem may be expected.

The author would like to thank Mrs. Jessie White and Mrs. Betsy Hill of Trade Winds Rehabilitation Center, Gary, Indiana, for their very helpful critical comments.

REFERENCES

Ajuriaguerra, J. de, S. Borel-Maisonny, R. Diatkine, S. Narlian, and M. Stambak. "La groupe des audimutités." *La Psychiatrie de l'Enfant*, 1, 7–62, (1958).

Ajuriaguerra, J. de, F. Guignard, A. Jaeggi, F. Kocher, M. Maquard, A. Paunier, D. Quinodoz, and E. Siotis. "Organisation psychologique et troubles du développement du langage: Etude d'un group d'enfants dysphasiques," in J. de Ajuriaguerra, F. Bresson, P. Fraisse, B. Inhelder, P. Oléron, and J. Piaget, eds., *Problèmes de Psycho-Linguistique*, pp. 109–142. Paris: Presses Universitaires de France, 1963.

Ajuriaguerra, J. de, A. Jaeggi, F. Guignard, F. Kocher, M. Maquard, S. Roth, and E. Schmid. "Évolution et pronostic de la dysphasie chez l'enfant." *La Psychiatrie de l'Enfant*, 8, 391–452, (1965).

Arnold, G. E. "The genetic background of developmental language disorders." *Folia Phoniatrica*, 13, 246–254, (1961).

Bangs, T. E. *Language and Learning Disorders of the Pre-Academic Child*. New York: Appleton-Century-Crofts, 1968.

Blank, M. "Cognitive functions of language in the preschool years." *Developmental Psychology*, 10, 229–245, (1974).

Blank, M., S. Weider, and W. H. Bridger. "Verbal deficiencies in abstract thinking in early reading retardation." *American Journal of Orthopsychiatry*, 38, 823–834, (1968).

Bloom, L. *Language Development: Form and Function in Emerging Grammars*. Cambridge: MIT Press, 1970.

Borkowski, J. G., and P. B. Wanschura. "Mediational processes in the retarded," in N. R. Ellis, ed., *International Review of Research in Mental Retardation*, vol. 7, pp. 1–54. New York: Academic, 1974.

Brown, R. *A First Language*. Cambridge: Harvard University Press, 1973.

Chomsky, N. *Syntactic Structures*. The Hague, The Netherlands: Mouton, 1957

———*Aspects of the Theory of Syntax*. Cambridge: MIT Press, 1965.

Churchill, D. W. "The relation of infantile autism and early childhood schizophrenia to developmental language disorders of childhood." *Journal of Autism and Childhood Schizophrenia*, 2, 182–197, (1972).

Clements, S. D. "Minimal brain dysfunction in children: Terminology and identification." *Public Health Service Publication No. 1415*. Washington, D.C.: U.S. Department of Health, Education, and Welfare, 1966.

Cohen, P. "Rh Child: Deaf or 'aphasic'? 2. 'Aphasia' in kernicterus." *Journal of Speech and Hearing Disorders*, 21, 411–412, (1956).

Compton, A. J. "Generative studies of children's phonological disorders: Clinical ramifications," in D. M. Morehead and A. E. Morehead, eds., *Normal and Deficient Child Language*, pp. 61–96. Baltimore: University Park Press, 1976.

Cromer, R. F. "The cognitive hypothesis of language acquisition and its implications for child language deficiency," in D. M. Morehead and A. E. Morehead, eds., *Normal and Deficient Child Language*, pp. 283–333. Baltimore: University Park Press, 1976.

Crookes, T. G., and M. C. L. Greene. "Some characteristics of children with two types of speech disorder." *British Journal of Educational Psychology*, 33, 31–40, (1963).

Davis, H., and S. R. Silverman, eds., *Hearing and Deafness*. New York: Holt, Rinehart & Winston, 1960.

Denckla, M. B. "Color-naming defects in dyslexic boys." *Cortex*, 8, 164–176, (1972).

Eisenson, J. "Developmental aphasia: A speculative view with therapeutic implications." *Journal of Speech and Hearing Disorders*, 33, 3–13, (1968).

———*Aphasia in Children*. New York: Harper, 1972.

Ervin-Tripp, S. "An overview of theories of grammatical development," in D. I. Slobin, *The Ontogenesis of Grammar: A Theoretical Symposium*, pp. 189–212. New York: Academic, 1971.

Ewing, A. W. G. *Aphasia in Children*. London: Oxford University Press, 1930.

Flavell, J. H. "Developmental studies of mediated memory," in H. W. Reese and Lewis P. Lipsitt, eds., *Advances in Child Development and Behavior*, vol. 5, pp. 181–211. New York: Academic, 1970.

Fraser, C., U. Bellugi, and R. Brown. "Control of grammar in imitation, comprehension, and production." *Journal of Verbal Learning and Verbal Behavior*, 2, 121–135, (1963).

Freedman, P. P., and R. L. Carpenter. "Semantic relations used by normal and language-impaired children at Stage I." *Journal of Speech and Hearing Research*, 19, 784–795, (1976).

Furth, H. G. "Sequence learning in aphasic and deaf children." *Journal of Speech and Hearing Disorders*, 29, 171–177, (1964).

Furth, H. G., and P. B. Pufall. "Visual and auditory sequence learning in hearing-impaired children." *Journal of Speech and Hearing Research*, 9, 441–449, (1966).

Gibson, E. J., and H. Levin. *The Psychology of Reading*. Cambridge: MIT. Press, 1975.

Goldfarb, W. "Effects of psychological deprivation in infancy and subsequent stimulation." *American Journal of Psychiatry*, 102, 18–33, (1945).

Goldstein, R., W. M. Landau, and F. R. Kleffner. "Neurologic assessment of some deaf and aphasic children." *Annals of Otology, Rhinology and Laryngology*, 67, 468–479, (1958).

———"Neurologic observations on a population of deaf and aphasic children." *Annals of Otology, Rhinology and Laryngology*, 69, 756–767, (1960).

Goodman, K. S. "Reading: A psycholinguistic guessing game." *Journal of the Reading Specialist*, 6, 126–135, (1967).

Gough, P. B. "One second of reading," in J. F. Kavanagh and I. G. Mattingly, eds., *Language by Ear and by Eye: The Relationships between Speech and Reading*, pp. 331–358. Cambridge: MIT Press, 1972.

Hallahan, D. P., and W. M. Cruickshank. *Psychoeducational Foundations of Learning Disabilities*. Englewood Cliffs, N. J.: Prentice-Hall, 1973.

Hannigan, H. "Rh Child: Deaf or 'aphasic'? 3. Language and behavior problems of the Rh 'aphasic' child." *Journal of Speech and Hearing Disorders*, 21, 413–417, (1956).

Holroyd, J. "When WISC verbal IQ is low." *Journal of Clinical Psychology*, 24, 457, (1968).

Ingram, D. "The acquisition of the English verbal auxiliary and copula in normal and linguistically deviant children," in L. V. McReynolds, ed., *Developing Systematic Procedures for Training Children's Language*, pp. 5–14. ASHA Monograph No. 18. Washington, D.C.: American Speech and Hearing Association, 1974.

Ingram, T. T. S. "The classification of speech and language disorders in young children," in M. Rutter and J. A. M. Martin, eds., *The Child with Delayed Speech*, pp. 13–32. Clinics in Developmental Medicine No. 43. Philadelphia: Lippincott, 1972.

———"Delayed development of speech with special reference to dyslexia." *Proceedings of the Royal Society of Medicine*, 56, 199–203, (1963).

Inhelder, B. "Observations sur les aspects operatifs et figuratifs de la pensée chez des enfants dysphasiques," in J. de Ajuriaguerra, F. Bresson, et al., eds., *Problèmes de Psycho-Linguistique*, pp. 143–152. Paris: Presses Universitaires de France, 1963.

Jansky, J., and K. de Hirsch. *Preventing Reading Failure: Prediction, Diagnosis, Intervention*. New York: Harper & Row, 1972.

Jensen, A. R. "The role of verbal mediation in mental development." *Journal of Genetic Psychology*, 118, 39–70, (1971).

Johnson, D. J., and H. R. Myklebust. *Learning Disabilities: Educational Principles and Practices.* New York: Grune & Stratton, 1967.

Johnston, J. R., and T. K. Schery. "The use of grammatical morphemes by children with communication disorders," in D. M. Morehead and A. E. Morehead, eds., *Normal and Deficient Child Language,* pp. 239–258. Baltimore: University Park Press, 1976.

Kavanagh, J. F. and I. G. Mattingly, eds., *Language by ear and by eye: The relationships between speech and reading.* Cambridge,: MIT Press, 1972.

Kendler, T. S. "An ontogeny of mediational deficiency." *Child Development,* 43, 1–17, (1972).

Kerschensteiner, M., and W. Huber. "Grammatical impairment in developmental aphasia." *Cortex,* 11, 264–282, (1975).

Landau, W. M., R. Goldstein, and F. R. Kleffner. "Congenital aphasia." *Neurology,* 10, 915–921, (1960).

Launay, C., and M. Soulé. "Trois cas d'audimutité." *Archives Francaises de Pédiatrie,* 9, 754–759, (1952).

Lenneberg, E. H. *Biological Foundations of Language.* New York: Wiley, 1967.

Leonard, L. B., J. G. Bolders, and J. A. Miller. "An examination of the semantic relations reflected in the language usage of normal and language-disordered children." *Journal of Speech and Hearing Research,* 19, 371–392, (1976).

Levin, H., J. Grossman, E. Kaplan, and R. Yang. "Constraints and the eye-voice span in right and left embedded sentences." *Language and Speech,* 15, 30–39, (1972).

Ley, J. "Un cas d'audi-mutité idiopathique (aphasie congénitale) chez des jumeaux monozygotiques." *L'Encéphale,* 24, 121–165, (1929).

Lorentz, J. P. "An analysis of some deviant phonological rules of English," in D. M. Morehead and A. E. Morehead, eds., *Normal and Deficient Child Language,* pp. 29–59. Baltimore: University Park Press, 1976.

Lovell, K., H. W. Hoyle, and M. Q. Siddall. "A study of some aspects of the play and language of young children with delayed speech." *Journal of Child Psychology and Psychiatry,* 9, 41–50, (1968).

Lowe, A. D., and R. A. Campbell. "Temporal discrimination in aphasoid and normal children." *Journal of Speech and Hearing Research,* 8, 313–314, (1965).

Luchsinger, R. "Die vererbung von sprach-und stimmstörungen." *Folia Phoniatrica,* 11, 7–64, (1959).

Luchsinger, R., and G. Arnold. *Voice-Speech-Language.* Belmont, Cal.: Wadsworth, 1965.

Lyle, J. G., and J. Goyen. "Performance of retarted readers on the WISC and educational tests." *Journal of Abnormal Psychology,* 74, 105–112, (1969).

Mac Keith, R. C., and M. Rutter. "A note on the prevalence of language disorders in young children," in M. Rutter and J. A. M. Martin, eds., *The Child with Delayed Speech,* pp. 48–51. Clinics in Developmental Medicine, No. 43. Philadelphia: Lippincott, 1972.

McCarthy, D. "Language development in children," in L. Carmichael, ed., *Manual of Child Psychology,* pp. 476–581. New York: Wiley, 1946.

———"Language development in children," in L. Carmichael, ed., *Manual of Child Psychology,* 2 ed., pp. 492–630. New York: Wiley, 1954.

McGinnis, M. A., F. R. Kleffner, and R. Goldstein. "Teaching aphasic children." *Volta Review,* 58, 239–244, (1956).

McGrady, H. J. "Language pathology and learning disabilities," in H. R. Myklebust, ed., *Progress in Learning Disabilities,* vol. 1, pp. 199–233. New York: Grune & Stratton, 1968.

McReynolds, L. V. "Operant conditioning for investigating speech sound discrimination in aphasic children." *Journal of Speech and Hearing Research,* 9, 519–528, (1966).

Marquardt, T. P., and J. H. Saxman. "Language comprehension and auditory discrimination in articulation deficient kindergarten children." *Journal of Speech and Hearing Research,* 15, 382–389, (1972).

Menyuk, P. "Comparison of grammar of children with functionally deviant and normal speech." *Journal of Speech and Hearing Research,* 7, 109–121, (1964).

——*Sentences Children Use.* Cambridge: MIT Press, 1969.

Menyuk, P., and P. L. Looney. "A problem of language disorder: Length versus structure." *Journal of Speech and Hearing Research,* 15, 264–279, (1972a).

——"Relationships among components of the grammar in language disorder." *Journal of Speech and Hearing Research,* 15, 395–406, (1972b).

Monsees, E. K. "Temporal sequence and expressive language disorders." *Exceptional Children,* 35, 141–147, (1968).

Morehead, D. M., and D. Ingram. "The development of base syntax in normal and linguistically deviant children." *Journal of Speech and Hearing Research,* 16, 330–352, (1973).

Myklebust, H. R. *Auditory Disorders in Children.* New York: Grune & Stratton, 1954.

Nelson, K. "Structure and strategy in learning to talk." *Monographs of the Society for Research in Child Development,* 38, Serial No. 149, 1973.

Olson, J. L. "Deaf and sensory aphasic children." *Exceptional Children,* 27, 422–424, (1961).

Orton, S. T. *Reading, Writing and Speech Problems in Children.* New York: Norton, 1937.

Owen, F. W., P. A. Adams, T. Forrest, L. M. Stolz, and S. Fisher. "Learning disorders in children: Sibling studies." *Monographs of the Society for Research in Child Development,* 36, Serial No. 144, 1971.

Petrie, I. "Characteristics and progress of a group of language-disordered children with severe receptive difficulties." *British Journal of Disorders of Communication,* 10, 123–133, (1975).

Piaget, J. "Le langage et les opérations intellectuelles," in J. de Ajuriaguerra, F. Bresson, et al., eds., *Problèmes de psycho-linguistique,* pp. 51–61, Paris: Presses Universitaires de France, 1963.

Poppen, R., J. Stark, J. Eisenson, T. Forrest, and G. Wertheim. "Visual sequencing performance of aphasic children." *Journal of Speech and Hearing Research,* 12, 288–300, (1969).

Rabinovitch, R. D. "Reading and learning disabilities," in S. Arieti, ed., *American Handbook of Psychiatry,* vol. 1, pp. 857–869, New York: Basic Books, 1959.

Rees, N. S. "Auditory processing factors in language disorders: The view from Procrustes' bed." *Journal of Speech and Hearing Disorders,* 38, 304–315 (1973).

Reichstein, J. "Auditory threshold consistency in differential diagnosis of aphasia in children." *Journal of Speech and Hearing Disorders,* 29, 147–155, (1964).

Rutter, M. "The effects of language delay on development," in M. Rutter and J. A. M. Martin, eds., *The Child with Delayed Speech,* pp. 176–188, Clinics in Developmental Medicine No. 43, Philadelphia: Lippincott, 1972

Rutter, M., P. Graham, and W. Yule. *A Neuropsychiatric Study in Childhood.* Clinics in Developmental Medicine Nos. 35/36. Philadelphia: Lippincott, 1970.

Sahlmann, L. "Autism or aphasia?" *Developmental Medicine and Child Neurology,* 11, 443 –448 (1969).

Sattler, J. M. *Assessment of Children's Intelligence.* Philadelphia: Saunders, 1974.

Semel, E. M. and E. H. Wiig. "Comprehension of syntactic structures and critical verbal elements by children with learning disabilities." *Journal of Learning Disabilities,* 8, 53 –58, (1975).

Shriner, T. H., M. S. Holloway, and R. G. Daniloff. "The relationship between articulatory deficits and syntax in speech defective children.'' *Journal of Speech and Hearing Research*, 12, 319–325, (1969).

Sibinga, M. S., and C. J. Friedman. "Restraint and speech." *Pediatrics*. 48, 116–122, (1971).

Sinclair-de-Zwart, H. "Developmental psycholinguistics," in D. Elkind and J. H. Flavell, eds., *Studies in Cognitive Development*, pp. 315–336, New York: Oxford University Press, 1969.

Sommers, R. K., and M. L. Taylor. "Cerebral speech dominance in language-disordered and normal children." *Cortex*, 8, 224–232, (1972).

Stark, J. "Performance of aphasic children on the ITPA." *Exceptional Children*, 33, 153–158, (1966).

———"A comparison of the performance of aphasic children on three sequencing tests." *Journal of Communication Disorders*, 1, 31–34, (1967).

Stark, J., R. Poppen, and M. Z. May. "Effects of alterations of prosodic features on the sequencing performance of aphasic children." *Journal of Speech and Hearing Research*, 10, 849–855, (1967).

Stevenson, J., and N. Richman. "The prevalence of language delay in a population of three-year-old children and its association with general retardation." *Developmental Medicine and Child Neurology*, 18, 431–441, (1976).

Tallal, P., and M. Piercy. "Defects of non-verbal auditory perception in children with developmental aphasia." *Nature*, 241, 468–469, (1973*a*).

———"Developmental aphasia: Impaired rate of non-verbal processing as a function of sensory modality." *Neuropsychologia*, 11, 389–398, (1973*b*).

———"Developmental aphasia: Rate of auditory processing and selective impairment of consonant perception." *Neuropsychologia*, 12, 83–93, (1974).

———"Developmental aphasia: The perception of brief vowels and extended stop consonants." *Neuropsychologia*, 13, 69–74, (1975).

Tallal, P., R. E. Stark, and B. Curtiss. "Relation between speech perception and speech production impairment in children with developmental dysphasia." *Brain and Language*, 3, 305–317, (1976).

Vandemark, A. A., and M. B. Mann. "Oral language skills of children with defective articulation." *Journal of Speech and Hearing Research*, 8, 409–414, (1965).

Vogel, S. A. "Syntactic abilities in normal and dyslexic children." *Journal of Learning Disabilities*, 7, 47–53, (1974).

———*Syntactic abilities in normal and dyslexic children.* Baltimore: University Park Press, 1975.

Vygotsky, L. S. *Thought and Language.* Cambridge: MIT Press, 1962.

Weber, R. M.,"First graders' use of grammatical context in reading," in H. Levin and J. P. Williams, eds., *Basic Studies on Reading*, pp. 147–163, New York: Basic Books, 1970.

Weiner, P. S. "The cognitive functioning of language-deficient children." *Journal of Speech and Hearing Research*, 12, 53–64, (1969*a*).

———"Mothers' reactions to delayed language development in their children." *Exceptional Child*, 36, 227–279, (1969*b*).

———"Perceptual level functioning of dysphasic children." *Cortex*, 5, 440–457, (1969*c*).

———"The language-related behavior of dysphasic children," in R. L. Schiefelbusch, ed., *Language of the Mentally Retarded*, pp. 188–207. Baltimore: University Park Press, 1972*a*.

———"The perceptual level functioning of dysphasic children: A follow-up study." *Journal of Speech and Hearing Research*, 15, 423–438, (1972*b*).

————"A language-delayed child at adolescence." *Journal of Speech and Hearing Research*, 39, 202–212, (1974).

Wepman, J. M., L. V. Jones, R. D. Bock, and D. Van Pelt. "Studies in aphasia: Background and theoretical formulations." *Journal of Speech and Hearing Disorders*, 25, 323–332, (1960).

Whitacre, J. D., H. L. Luper, and H. R. Pollio. "General language deficits in children with articulation problems." *Language and Speech*, 13, 231–239, (1970).

Whitehurst, G. J., G. Novak, and G. A. Zorn. "Delayed speech studied in the home." *Developmental Psychology*, 7, 169–177, (1972).

Wiig, E. H. "Language disabilities of adolescents: Implications for diagnosis and remediation." *British Journal of Disorders of Communication*, 11, 3–17, (1976).

Wiig, E. H., and M. A. Roach. "Immediate recall of semantically varied 'sentences' by learning-disabled adolescents." *Perceptual and Motor Skills*, 40, 119–125, (1975).

Wiig, E. H., and E. M. Semel. "Comprehension of linguistic concepts requiring logical operations by learning-disabled children." *Journal of Speech and Hearing Research*, 16, 627–636, (1973).

————"Logico-grammatical sentence comprehension by adolescents with learning disabilities." *Perceptual and Motor Skills*, 38, 1331–1334, (1974).

Wilson, L. F., D. G. Doehring, and I. J. Hirsh. "Auditory discrimination learning by aphasic and nonaphasic children." *Journal of Speech and Hearing Research*, 3, 130–137, (1960).

Worster-Drought, C., and I. M. Allen. "Congenital auditory imperception (congenital word-deafness): With report of a case." *Journal of Neurology and Psychopathology*, 9, 193–208, (1929A).

————"Congenital auditory imperception (congenital word-deafness): Investigation of a case by Head's method." *Journal of Neurology and Psychopathology*, 9, 289–319, (1929b).

————"Congenital auditory imperception (congenital word-deafness): And its relation to indioglossia and other speech defects." *Journal of Neurology and Psychopathology*, 10, 193–236, (1930).

Wulbert, M., S. Inglis, E. Kriegsmann, and B. Mills. "Language delay and associated mother-child interactions." *Developmental Psychology*, 11, 61–70, (1975).

CHAPTER 14

Personality and Behavior

Kenneth Berry and Valerie J. Cook

The effect of unequivocal brain injury upon behavior and personality has been repeatedly studied and discussed during the last 80 years. In 1903 Bailey investigated several children who had experienced cerebral injury and reported that they became irritable, aggressive, boisterous, and engaged in behavior indicative of emotional lability. In their classic work Strauss and Lehtinen (1947) found and reported that brain-injured children exhibited erratic, uncontrolled, and uninhibited behavior, indicative of extreme lability. They described these children as being, among other things, impatient, fearful, flighty, erratic, excitable, unreliable, and impulsive—in general difficult children with whom to deal and to educate.

Early in the century, from the work of researchers such as Kasanin (1929), Bailey (1903), and Ford (1926) the picture of the child who had experienced injury to the brain was that of extreme lability, aggressiveness, disobedience, instability, and antisocial behavior. In the period from 1920 until about 1940, the notion of the so-called post-encephalitic syndrome was quite popular. These children displayed behavior much like that of children who had experienced frank injury to the central nervous system. They were reported to exhibit antisocial tendencies, emotional lability, moodiness, hostility, aggression, and frequently increased activity levels.

A related concept which enjoyed a good deal of popularity in the early 1900s and until about 1940 was that of the so-called "epileptoid personality" (Kanner, 1966). During that period a good deal was written about the personality makeup of individuals with epilepsy. Many writers and clinicians accepted as fact (Kanner, 1966; Guerant, et al., 1962) that children with epilepsy exhibited definite personality characteristics. These were typically described as emotional instability, impulsiveness, pugnacity, egocentricity, selfishness, circumstantiality in speech and actions, and some writers included religiousness and self-righteousness. Others felt that cruelty was a common personality characteristic. The idea of the epileptic personality was disseminated between 1914 and 1933 by Clark (1914) and Kanner (1966). In 1953 Sullivan and Gahagan in a study of 103 epileptic children found high correlations between home situations and the described personality characteristics. Lennox in 1941 effectively repudiated the notion of an epileptoid personality by his failure to find any common characteristic; however this term can still be found today in the *Diagnostic and Statistical Manual of Mental Disorders* (DSM II) published by the American Psychiatric Association (1968).

There has not been as great a fervor to develop a concept of the minimal brain dysfunction personality. However a number of characteristics have been advanced as "typical or diagnostic signs indicative of minimal brain dysfunction." Mendelson, Johnson, and Stewart (1971) cited the following behaviors: overactiv-

324

ity, distractibility, impulsiveness, excitability, aggressiveness, poor school performance, and socially "constantly in trouble." Clements and Peters (1962) classified many of these characteristics under the term of "lability of emotions." Wender (1972) put forth the concept of "primary functional deficits" as opposed to "secondary characteristics." He viewed the primary functional deficits as an abnormality in arousal (activity level, concentration, impulse control, and so on) and a diminished capacity for positive and negative affect (lessened responsiveness to pain and pleasure and imperviousness to positive and negative reinforcement). As secondary characteristics he cited impulsiveness, disobedience, increased sensation and pleasure seeking, increased attention demanding, paradox performance, increased anxiety and guilt, and decreased self-esteem. Huessy, Marshall, and Gendron (1973) listed the following characteristics: emotional overactivity, temper tantrums, group difficulty, language deficits, coordination and learning problems. Katz, et al., (1975) cited poor frustration tolerance, immaturity, and aggressiveness as common characteristics of the child with minimal brain dysfunction. In 1975 Wender added to the list the following: delinquency, extroversion, resistiveness to social demands, and altered reactivity. Becker (1974) perhaps should be credited with the longest list of characteristics of the child diagnosed as having MBD. Becker listed over 50 characteristics. Among these he included anxiety, anger, a tendency toward unprovoked temper tantrums, aggressiveness, poor tolerance for dissonance and frustration, difficulties with concentration, obstinateness, negativism, obstreperousness, boisterousness, arbitrariness, oppositionalism, unhappiness. He also reports that the MBD child is temperamental, "highstrung," sensitive, arrogant, has a defiant facade, is provocative, depressed, confused, has low self-esteem, and an "inordinate need for unconditional acceptance" (page 94). In addition he reported that the MBD child is flighty, aimless, indiscriminately destructive, and dissocial. He stated that parents tend to view their MBD child as being defiant, impulsive, narcissistic, egocentric, manipulative, uneven, demanding, irrational, and often inappropriate and inconsistent. In contrast Becker reported that some MBD children are likely to be withdrawn, quiet, hypokinetic, inaccessible, unresponsive, shy, self-effacing, mute, and lacking in outgoing aggressive impulses; however at times these children unpredictably will become "driven, impulse ridden, labile, explosive, or hyperkinetic" (page 94).

There are a number of problems in attempting to develop a coherent review of personality variables related to the syndrome of minimal brain dysfunction. Basic of course is the fact that there is little agreement on what the term personality means. Exploration and investigation of personality characteristics and development is difficult in children who have been labeled as having minimal brain dysfunction for several reasons. There has been no definitive structure of child personality achieved in normal children, much less in the case of the child with any psychological disability. There has been little actual research into the personality variables of the child labeled as having MBD; the research with few exceptions has been highly equivocal. Even more basic—nowhere is there a clear definition of the MBD syndrome to allow for correlation of data from one study to another (Twitchell, 1971). Much has been written, but the bulk of this is based upon opinion and clinical data and there is very little actual research into behaviors commonly called personality characteristics. With this in mind a survey of the literature was done and the most frequently appearing characteristics attributed to the MBD child (not necessarily consistently defined) were selected. This review is an attempt to bring some degree of organization to a chaotic area. The following characteristics will be discussed:

1. Emotionality-stability.
2. Self-control (reflection-impulsivity and distractibility).
3. Social behavior (aggression-inhibition, extroversion-introversion).
4. Miscellaneous (anxiety, need-achievement).

EMOTIONAL STABILITY

Emotional stability or lability has been one of the features most commonly mentioned in discussions of characteristics of the child with MBD. Most have written that the mood of the child is highly labile, that he/she is irritable, moves rapidly from laughter to tears, and may tend to become panicked by what would appear to be minimally stressful situations. Gross and Wilson (1974) in a statistical comparison of 817 MBD patients with 239 non-MBD patients found temper outbursts, frequent crying, insecurity, and depression in a high percentage of patients. Temper outbursts occurred in 19.2% of their sample; moodiness, depression, and frequent crying were present in 9.7%. These characteristics were statistically significant when compared with their non-MBD sample. In the administration of the Peterson Quay Questionnaire they found that the following characteristics related to emotional instability were greater in the MBD patients: crying over minor annoyances or hurts, temper tantrums, irresponsibility, and undependability. Weiss and Minde (1974) in a follow-up study of children diagnosed as having MBD found that excitability decreased over the five-year period of the study; however when compared with matched normal controls, the adolescent subjects scored significantly higher on excitability than did the controls. Menkes, Rowe, and Menkes (1967) in reporting on 14 children seen in an outpatient psychiatric clinic found that emotional lability (which they subsumed under the term hyperactivity) was a significant factor affecting the children's function.

Clements (1973) in a review and an attempt at refining the diagnosis of MBD children reported that they often exhibit frequent rage reactions and tantrums and that they experience excessive variations in mood and responses from day to day and from hour to hour, along with poor adjustment to environmental changes. He found that emotional lability was the third most frequent characteristic reported by authors. Quinn and Rapaport (1974) in a study of 6- to 12-year-old boys in the Hyperactivity Clinic at Georgetown University Hospital, found that 53 out of 81 of the boys were classified as exhibiting labile behavior and 13 of the youngsters demonstrated outbursts of anger. Wender (1975) states that increased lability and dysphoria is a common behavioral alteration. He further reported that mood fluctuations from day to day and hour to hour were frequently reported by parents, and he describes MBD children as having a "short fuse" and "low boiling point" with frequent temper tantrums. However he does not report any specific data. Stevens, et al., (1968), in a study of reaction time, impulsivity, and autonomic lability found that MBD children were more autonomically labile than their normal controls in heart rate and skin resistance; however the differences were not significant.

In contrast with other writers, Routh and Roberts (1972) found no good evidence that emotional lability distinguished between MBD children and non-MBD children. Routh and Roberts defined emotional lability,

as behavior associated with internal conflict which is a specialized diagnostic term applied to the behavior of children who show certain signs of conflicting feelings and attitudes toward themselves. The signs of this type of disturbance may be of the following four general types: inhibition of activity, social withdrawal, anxiety, or schizoid reaction. [P. 309]

Routh and Roberts derived 112 intercorrelations of a number of variables, including emotional lability, in 89 children. Emotional lability was not correlated with any of 16 measures utilized. They concluded that their failure to find much clustering among the measures was somewhat damaging to the basic idea of an MBD syndrome.

Langhorne, et al., (1976) did a factor analysis (using a varimax rotation) of Routh and Roberts' data. In spite of the fact that few of the correlations were significant, they found six factors, the fourth of which accounted for 8.2% of the variance, and included three variables, emotional lability, hyperactivity, and hearing impairment. These variables were not significantly intercorrelated. Langhorne's data yielded three primary factors accounting for 44.6% of the variance. It appears that the correlations of these three variables can be explained by the method of assessment. Langhorne and his co-workers believe that the three factors were the following: psychoeducational testing, teacher factors, and pediatrician factors. It appears that the general factor analytic studies of MBD symptoms produce many small factors which are independent of each other and which, as in Routh and Roberts' data, correspond to the source of information (Langhorne, et al., 1976).

Langhorne and his colleagues further examined what they called the core of primary symptoms of MBD children, only one of which would roughly correspond to emotional lability, namely the symptom of excitability. They examined a clinic sample of 135 boys with the mean age of 8.2 years and mean IQ of 99.5. They selected 11 variables which seemed to agree with their core behavioral symptoms. They gained much of their information from four sources: parents, teachers, psychiatrists, and medical chart raters. They used the Conners Teacher Rating Scale and the Conners Parent Rating Scale. They found four factors, the second of which accounted for 14.2% of the variance and consisted of the teachers' characterization of the child as being restless, overactive, and excitable. All of their factors had small intercorrelations and they concluded that limiting their analysis to a few primary behavioral symptoms did not reduce the impression of heterogeneity. The work was like that of previous analyses in that a large number of small factors were found which were not significantly related to one another. Crinella (1973) reported similar findings.

SELF-CONTROL

Reflection-Impulsivity

One characteristic which has a relatively good research base relevant to MBD is that of reflection-impulsivity. This has been described as the tendency to reflect on the validity or solution of a problem when several possible alternatives are present and there is uncertainty about which is the most appropriate (Messer, 1976). Tasks used to measure this characteristic usually present the subject with an array of possible alternatives of which only one is correct. The children who respond quickly (high on impulsivity) make more errors; those who reflect on the alternatives (high on reflectivity) are more often correct. The task most often used to measure this trait is Kagan's (MFFT) Matching Familiar Figures Test (Kagan, et al., 1964), which provides different forms dependent on the age of the child or adult being examined. Essentially this task involves a presentation of certain figures with four, six, or eight other highly similar figures which differ in only a few details. The subject is then asked to select the figure which exactly matches the standard figure. Response time and number of errors are measured. The child who is below the median on response time, but is above the median point in error measurements, is termed impulsive; whereas the reflective child is the one who is above the median point on response time and below the median point on errors. The reliability of this test is variable, but tends to be relatively high, .34 on error reliabilities to as high as .96 on response time reliabilities (Adams, 1972; Duckworth, et al., 1974; Hall and Russell, 1974). There is some degree of variability and stability over ages. In children under six years of age errors are moderately stable, but response time is not. Whereas in children beyond six response time is stable over time, but errors are not stable.

The general findings in normal populations indicate that children become more reflective with age. Test scores and intelligence are only slightly to moderately correlated, depending upon the level of verbal skills required by the particular intelligence test, in that nonverbal skills are more highly correlated with MFFT scores. Kagan (1965) reported a relationship between impulsivity and later reading skills in first grade children. Several studies have reported that MFFT scores predictive of impulsivity are related to diagnosis of MBD (specifically hyperactivity). Campbell, Douglas, and Morgenstern (1971) reported that children diagnosed as hyperactive had high impulsivity scores on the MFFT which decreased following the administration of methylphenidate. Campbell (1973) found that hyperactive children differed from normal reflectives, but obtained scores which were comparable to the scores of normal impulsives, that is children who are found to be impulsive but with no symptoms of hyperactivity or MBD.

In normal populations impulsivity as measured by the MFFT appears to be modifiable (Messer, 1976). However there has been little discussion about directly modifying impulsivity in MBD subjects, with the exception of Meichenbaum's work (1977).

Related to reflectivity and impulsivity is another variable, namely that of field dependence-independence. This has typically been measured in two major ways, the Embedded Figures Test (EFT) and the classic rod-and-frame test (Witkin, et al., 1962). In general it has been found that reflectives are significantly more field independent than are impulsives (Campbell and Douglas, 1972). Campbell and Douglas also reported that hyperactive and impulsive subjects did not differ in degree of field independence-dependence and that both tended toward being more field dependent than did reflective children.

Distractibility

A review of the literature indicates that distractibility is one of the more frequently reported symptoms of MBD. Various characteristics described as attentional disorders and short attention span were included in this category, in that such terms have been used interchangeably by most authors. The MBD child is commonly described as distractible, unable to pay attention, prone to focus on irrelevant aspects of the learning situation (Rourke, 1975), and to daydream (Conners, 1969), as having poor concentration (Gross and Wilson, 1974), and as unable to focus attention (Wender, 1972). References to distractibility as a characteristic of MBD children are overwhelmingly based on clinical observations and have a small data base (Clements, 1973).

Lievens (1974) attempted to quantify such clinical observations by analyzing the presenting problems of 22 children (10 girls, 12 boys) ages 7 to 12 who were being seen at a clinic in Brussels. The children had been referred for learning and/or behavioral problems referrable to perinatal cerebral origins. Of the 22 cases studied, 14 had indicated weaknesses in attention or concentration and 13 of these were referred primarily for dysfunction of attention. While such data are descriptive of this small group of children, no comparison was made with a group of comparable "normal" children. Gross and Wilson (1974) recognized the necessity of comparison groups when analyzing the complaints of parents bringing their children to the psychiatric clinic. Parents completed the Peterson-Quay Questionnaire identifying areas of concern. Gross and Wilson examined the data on a total of 1056 children ages 2 to 18 of which 817 were MBD and 239 were non-MBD. Five factors were identified as accounting for 64% of the complaints concerning MBD children, while eight factors accounted for 74% of the total complaints about the non-MBD children. Three of these factors were common to both groups: (1) underachievement, (2) aggressiveness, and (3) temper outbursts. Those factors unique to MBD children were restlessness and distractibility, whereas the non-MBD children were described as depressed, insecure-anxious, rebellious, having temper out-bursts, having psychosomatic complaints, and acting out in the form of running away, truancy, and so on. Gross and Wilson thus identified distractibility as a symptom unique to the MBD subgroup of a psychiatric population.

Conners (1969) used a four point rating scale completed by teachers in a pre- and posttreatment design examining the effects of dextroamphetamine on the behavior of 103 children (82 boys, 21 girls) who were described as having behavior disorders, hyperactivity, poor attention spans, and IQs over 80. Diagnosed psychotic and grossly brain-damaged children were omitted from the study. In validating the teacher behavior rating scale, a factor analysis was completed. Five factors were identified:

1. Defiance or aggressive conduct
2. Daydreaming-inattentive
3. Anxious-fearful
4. Hyperactivity
5. Health

The items which clustered to form the second factor of distractibility included those describing poor coordination, inattentiveness, difficulty in concentrating, daydreaming, appearing to be easily led, and appearing to lack leadership. Another group of researchers (Rie, et al., 1976) used teacher and parent behavior rating scales in a pre- posttreatment design to evaluate the effects of methylphenidate (Ritalin) on underachieving children. It was found that the drug increased attention and decreased distractibility, especially in brighter, less organic children. Weiss, et al., (1971), using a rating scale completed by both mothers and teachers in a five-year follow-up study of the hyperactive child, found distractibility to be the chief problem. On the follow-up portion of the study, 56% of the mothers reported distractibility as a continuing problem. A special problem in such studies using rating scales relates to the original diagnosis of MBD in making the diagnosis. If these MBD subjects had been diagnosed partly on the basis of the complaint of distractibility, the findings on follow-up simply confirm the persistence of MBD, but do not identify distractibility as inherent in MBD. Other than the clinical statements and the remarks of teachers and parents, there are few experimental studies which clearly show an attentional deficit in such children.

Rather than start with a defined group of MBD children, Conners (1973) chose to start with a large group, to give tests, then categorize by subgroup patterns. All of his subjects, ages 6 to 12, were referred to the hospital clinic for evaluation of learning and/or behavior disorders. All had IQs of 80 or above, good physical health, and no gross organic, visual, or auditory defects. Each child received a complete evaluation including traditional psychometric assessment, a continuous performance test, a paired-associates learning test, motor tests, EEG, and tests of auditory and visual perception. A factor analysis of the data revealed five factors:

1. General intelligence
2. Achievement
3. Rote learning
4. Attentiveness
5. Impulse control

Six groups of children were identified based on their performance patterns on the five factors:

1. Low IQ, together with poor rote-learning, but good impulse control.
2. Low achievers and poor learners who are somewhat inattentive.
3. Very poor impulse control, poor rote-learning, and moderate inattentiveness.
4. Bright, high achievers, good impulse control, slightly inattentive.
5. Average in most areas ("normals").
6. Low IQs, poor impulse control but good rote-learning.

Conners argued against the conglomerate label MBD and advocated descriptors of functioning. Conners furthered his hypothesis by examining the groups' differential responses to drug therapy. He designed a double-blind, placebo-controlled study examining the effects of three stimulants: dextroamphetamine (Dexedrine), methylphenidate (Ritalin), and magnesium pemoline (Cylert). Using a pre- posttreatment design with measures on teacher- and parent-symptom lists, Conners found that general behavior was significantly improved by drugs as compared with placebo. However, in his one, two, and three groups, drugs had little effect on inattentiveness.

Some researchers are beginning to question whether distractibility and inattentiveness are interchangeable. Dykman and Ackerman (1976) suggested two kinds of distractions: (1) distraction as the interfering effect of specific irrelevant stimuli and (2) distraction as a state of being dazed, scatterbrained, or daydreaming—that which William James discussed as the opposite of attentiveness. The concepts of attention and distraction require closer scrutiny. Is inattention the result of being distracted by the irrelevant? While researchers have not addressed those concerns directly, some specific work has been completed in the areas of attention and distraction.

Sykes (1971) examined attention of hyperactive children by using performance measures on the Continuous Performance Test requiring the subject to monitor a screen on which letters appear at regular intervals and to respond to previously specified stimuli. The performance of 40 hyperactive children, 5 to 12 years of age, IQs not less than 80, was compared with the performance of the normal control children, matched for age and IQ. The hyperactives made significantly fewer correct responses than the normals, however they did not differ in respect to the overall number of errors. Half of the hyperactive children then received active drug (Ritalin) and half placebo, under double-blind conditions. The performance of the drug group was similar to normal children on the attention task. Sykes concluded that the hyperactive children do have a deficit in the ability to maintain attention to a task.

Rourke (1975) reviewed his previous studies examining attention of children by using reaction times to stimuli. In investigations with Czudner (1970, 1972), he had found that younger brain-damaged children exhibited a deficit in visual reaction time relative to young normal children, older brain-damaged children, and older normal children, while performance of older brain-damaged children did not vary significantly from normals.

These results were upheld in a later study (1972) by auditory reaction time as well. Thus the slower reaction time of the younger brain-damaged children was not found to be modality specific but to be a more general, perhaps attentional deficit. Douglas (1974) presented a general report of a series of her studies examining reaction time and accuracy of responses in children, comparing the performance of normal and hyperkinetic children. She concluded that the hyperactive child had little trouble making a correct response so long as he was warned shortly before the stimuli occurred. The hyperactive child's performance deteriorated more rapidly than did the normal child's. She suggests that the performance difference is due to poor attention or careless-impulsive responding behavior. To investigate the relationship of attention and distraction, she designed a vigilance task during which distracting-competing stimuli occurred. Performance on this task did *not* discriminate between hyperactive and normal children. Douglas cautions clinicians and researchers against considering impaired attention and distractibility as identical problems.

On the other hand if the inability to attend were due to the distractibility of the MBD child, it would make sense to eliminate potential distractions to increase attentiveness, that is to create a sterile environment. This is a general description of the educational intervention suggested by Cruickshank and others (Cruickshank, et al., 1961). They further hypothesize that if attention should improve, so should academic progress. Meyer (1968) criticized the studies of Cruickshank, et al., used to support their recommendation. Only 7 of 64 statistical tests were significant in terms of differential improvement between control and experimental groups, and 1 of these 7 indicated a *loss* for the experimental group. Gains on the remaining 6 appear to be mostly related to improved performance on the Bender-

Gestalt, which may have been due to instructional methods rather than environment. Rost and Charles (1967) designed a sterile environment in the form of individual study cubicles to eliminate environmental distractors. All subjects were diagnosed brain-injured or hyperactive, half received the experimental condition of individual cubicles, half served as controls. Though the experimental group spent 1 1/2 to 2 hours of each 5-hour school day in cubicles, no significant gains were made. Somervill, Warnberg, and Bost (1973) designed a more elaborate study of the same question. Forty-eight boys were chosen from a population of 113 first graders from four elementary schools. Their inclusion was based on teacher ratings which identified 24 distractible and 24 nondistractible boys. The two groups were matched on a measure of intelligence and on age. Subjects were assigned to one of these treatment conditions, each having an equal number of distractible and nondistractible children:

1. Normal stimulation, testing four subjects at a time in a room.
2. Reduced stimulation, testing four subjects at a time in individual cubicles.
3. Increased stimulation, testing four subjects at a time in a room given additional auditory (tape of noises) and visual (moving objects) stimulation.

The subjects were tested on 10 tasks, 1 per day, which were primarily perceptual-motor in nature. The results were intriguing in that the overall task time for distractible subjects was significantly longer than that for the nondistractible and *no* significant differences were found for any of the three treatment conditions. Unfortunately the experiment had some weaknesses in control of task instructions and difficulty. Furthermore a relationship between task performance and intelligence was demonstrated. The authors also hypothesized differential performance by race, which was not controlled. However it remains an interesting study of distractibility and more studies of this nature are recommended.

In a study comparing 70 brain-injured children with normal preschoolers (Graham, et al., 1963), the stereotyped behavior pattern of hyperactivity, distractibility, and impulsivity was not found among the majority of the children based on results of a standardized battery of cognitive, perceptual-motor, and personality tests. Wolff and Hurwitz (1973), being dissatisfied with both the term MBD and the research, designed a study starting with a group of 1300 normal children, ages 10 to 12. These children were screened for a neurological indicator associated with MBD, choreiform movements. The investigators identified 103 boys and 25 girls with unequivocal choreiform movements (CM+) and compared them with their normal peers; however attention span did *not* discriminate between normal and CM+ boys. The research reviewed tends to support the clinical observation that the MBD child has some kind of disorder in the area of attention and/or distraction.

However the research discussed here must be weighed in relation to the pervasive problems of subject description (brain damaged, brain injured, hyperactive, distractible) and concept definition (attentional problems versus distractibility) and their interrelationship. More research is needed in examining the attentional problem versus the distractibility issue.

In general it appears from the research that has been done that the responses to distracting stimuli do not clearly distinguish MBD children from normal controls.

It also appears that decreasing distraction in the classroom does not seem to benefit the MBD child (Safer and Allen, 1976).

SOCIAL BEHAVIOR

Aggression

"Aggressive" is a recurrent descriptor of the MBD child and adolescent. Aggressiveness as a symptom has been based on clinical observations and reports of destructiveness, roughness in play, lacking sense of fair play, lying, stealing, rudeness, fighting, and boisterousness. Frequently mothers describe their children as not being intentionally mean but appearing mean.

When validating a teacher rating scale for use in drug studies with children, Conners (1969) identified one of five major behavior factors as that of defiance or aggressive conduct. Items indicating an aggressive nature which loaded on this factor dealt with destructiveness, lying, stealing, lack of fair play, destructiveness, stubbornness, and disturbing others. Weiss, et al., (1971) in their follow-up studies of hyperactive children indicated that aggressive behavior persisted in most. Teachers' and mothers' ratings indicated that aggressiveness had decreased, but not reached the lower levels of normal control children.

Conners (1970) later used parent ratings of symptoms to compare the psychiatric clinic population (neurotics and hyperkinetics) with a sample of normal children. The 316 clinic patients were nonpsychotic, nondelinquent, without signs of organic brain damage, and having IQs above 80 on the WISC. The patients were classified as neurotic or hyperkinetic based on their history. The 365 normals were children of parents attending PTA meetings in four Baltimore schools, two middle class, two lower class, one each all white, one each all black. While the clinic population as a whole was more aggressive than the normals, an interesting contrast occurred within the clinic population. The hyperkinetic children were identified as having significantly more severe aggressive conduct disorders than the neurotics. Conners found a relationship between severity and social class, with children from low socioeconomic status groups showing more severe problems. Paternite, Loney, and Langhorne (1976) further investigated and confirmed the relationship finding it to be more fully explained by parenting variables. Conners (1970) also found that the specific items from the Peterson-Quay Questionnaire that differentiated the MBD from the non-MBD child were boisterousness, attention-seeking, destructiveness, and fighting, among others.

An observational study was designed to examine the level of aggressive behavior of hyperactive children compared with that of normal children (Schleifer, et al., 1975). The observers used Beller's Nursery School Rating Criteria to quantify the behavior of 28 hyperactive children with 26 matched control children. Aggressive behaviors were those defined as attacking others physically by throwing things or by teasing, striking, kicking, biting, and so on. The hyperactives were found to be significantly more aggressive than their normal counterparts.

On the basis of the research reviewed here, "aggressive" would be an appropriate adjective describing hyperactive and MBD children, but one can only speculate about the cause of such behavior. Aggressive behavior might be explained by the MBD child's lack of impulse control as described earlier. This might be relabeled as the MBD child's lack of aggression-inhibition. A second possible explanation for aggressive behavior is that of poor social-perception, discussed later in this chapter.

Antisocial Behavior

MBD children are frequently said to have classroom behavior problems. The child reportedly does not respond well to discipline, is negativistic, uncooperative, has poor peer relations, and is occasionally charged with juvenile delinquency. Research in this area is lacking; most studies are tangential to the issue.

Touliatos and Lindholm (1975) examined the need affiliation of 16 MBD and 16 normal children matched for age, sex, birth order, and father's education. Measures used were projective devices including the Thematic Apperception Test (TAT) and other like instruments. No differences or relationships were found on the measure of affiliation motive between MBD and normal children or their parents. It is suggested then that MBD children desire to be socially accepted, though their behavior often interferes.

Peer Relations

Bryan (1974) administered a sociometric technique to 63 classrooms of third, fourth, and fifth graders in which there was at least one learning disabled (LD) child. Scores of social attraction and rejection were computed. Each LD child was matched with a normal child of the same classroom for purposes of comparison. LD children, particularly white and female, were significantly less attractive and more rejected than achieving children. More specifically, white LD children received the greatest number of rejection ratings, while controls the fewest; the least number of acceptance votes went to white LD children, the most to the white controls. The relationship to achievement was examined and while correlations were significant, they do not explain why black children were not more rejected than whites since their achievement scores were much lower. Bryan suggests that acceptance-rejection might be related to peer expectations. Girls are expected to do better, therefore are more rejected if they do not do well; black children are not expected to do as well, therefore are not as rejected if they fail to do well. If this is the case, the black LD youngster is not under as much pressure to achieve and is not as socially outcast for underachieving.

Bryan (1976) replicated her study with a subsample of the same subjects one year later. This added another dimension. Even though there was a greater than 75% change in classroom composition, LD children did not enhance their social attractiveness with a fresh start in a new school year. This is consistent with Conners' (1970) finding that the psychiatric clinic population had significantly more difficulty making and keeping friends and had problems with their siblings. Within the clinic population there were no differences in ability to make friends between neurotic and hyperkinetic patients; however the hyperkinetic children had significantly more difficulty maintaining friendships.

Negativism-Uncooperativeness

The MBD child is frequently labeled negativistic, defiant and uncooperative, yet very little research is offered to support the attributions of these negative characteristics. Conners (1969) identified a factor called "defiance or aggressive conduct" in his factor analysis of a teacher rating scale used in drug studies with children. Some of the items which appear to account for the defiance portion are: sullen, quarrelsome, stubborn, and impudent behavior and acting "smart." Uncooperativeness was also identified by Wolff and Hurwitz (1973) in their assessment of CM+ children. These children, both boys and girls, were found to have more signs of classroom behavior problems and were less cooperative than the normal controls. Research is very much needed in this area to achieve better definition of the behavior, clarify its prevalence in both MBD and normal children, and to develop intervention strategies for dealing with such behavior problems.

Extroversion-Introversion

Many authors refer to the MBD child's tendency to be extroverted and relate it to general antisocial and aggressive behaviors. Lerner (1974) has been alone in addressing the extroversion-introversion range in children having minimal brain dysfunction. Thirty children, ages 6 to 10, were selected from special education classes for the brain injured. All had been diagnosed as MBD with specific learning disabilities. These 30 had been chosen due to identification as hyperactive (n = 15) or hypoactive (n =15) based on Bucks Behavior Rating. Two measures were used to assess extroversion-introversion: the Child-Audit Research Form of the Pittsburgh Scales of Social Extroversion and Bucks Behavior Rating Scale. Significant differences were identified. The hyperactives scored high on extroversion whereas the hypoactives were markedly introverted.

Based on these results and supporting data from other segments of his study, Lerner refutes the stereotyped personality characteristics associated with MBD. He suggests two types, related to the conditions of hyperactivity and hypoactivity. The hyperactive child is described as having a high activity level, showing greater incidence of destructive behavior, becoming easily frustrated and reacting motorically, responding rapidly to stimulation, demanding the teacher's attention, and readily involving himself in classroom activities. He is perceived by his teachers as assertive, outgoing, and gregarious. The hypoactive child is perceived by his teachers as slow-moving and lethargic, nondisruptive, inattentive and daydreamy in response to frustration, nondemanding of attention, seemingly bored and disinterested. He is described as shy, withdrawn, passive, and closed-off from teachers.

Lerner's work is a beginning in this area. Much more research needs to be conducted. Even a replication of Lerner's study with a larger number of subjects and perhaps a normal control group comparison would be helpful.

Social Perception

Various rationale have been offered to explain the reputedly poor social relationships of MBD children. Two basic hypotheses have been suggested: (1) a primary deficit in the MBD child's ability to perceive the emotions and needs of others, and/or (2) a deficit in the ability to perceive his own emotions.

Johnson and Mykelbust (1967) state that children and adolescents with learning disabilities have been described as having reduced ability to interpret the significance of nonverbal aspects of communication which would indicate the attitudes, feelings, and intentions of others. They discussed this low social perception in relation to visual processing problems, but did not substantiate their discussion with research. Wiig and Harris (1975) designed a study to address this issue. They compared the perceptions and interpretations of a young female's videotaped, nonverbal expressions of anger, embarrassment, fear, frustration, joy, and love made by 17 learning-disabled and 17 achieving adolescents, matched for age, IQ, sex, ethnic, and socioeconomic backgrounds. Learning-disabled adolescents misinterpreted the emotions significantly more frequently than achieving controls. Furthermore the number of correct interpretations of emotions correlated significantly and positively with scaled scores on the Block Design and Object Assembly subtests of the WISC and WAIS and converted scores on the Design subtest of the Detroit Tests of Learning Aptitudes. Social perception was *not* significantly related to performance on the Picture Arrangement subtest of the WISC or WAIS, as is so often clinically suggested. Wiig and Harris demonstrated a relationship between the LD adolescent's ability to recognize nonverbal affective cues and general visual-motor-organizational ability. Sulzbacher (1975), discussing related patterns, found it necessary to teach LD children to listen to each other's stories. He observed that LD children fail to notice when others become angry with them.

Sulzbacher further described the LD child's inability to perceive himself as irritated or frustrated and the fact that he generally has difficulty communicating his feelings, except inappropriately. Several authors hypothesize a generalized deficit in the MBD child to anticipate and experience pleasure (rewards), and displeasure (punishment) (Klein and Gittelman-Klein, 1975; Virkkunen and Nuutila, 1976; Wender, 1972). Should this inability exist, it might be related to the child's reported resistance to discipline and corrective measures. None of the descriptions of this deficit in self-perception of emotions have been based on research data.

The entire area of the social perceptions of MBD children and adolescents is in need of research. If this afiility, or lack thereof, is related to the child's social relations as has been hypothesized, definitive research may be the key to development of effective intervention strategies.

OTHER CHARACTERISTICS

Need-Achievement

Low motivation or need-achievement has been one of the descriptors associated with the MBD child. While several authors have named this characteristic or symptom, only one designed a study specifically to examine the achievement and affiliative needs of brain-injured children and two addressed the issue tangentially. Wolff and Hurwitz (1973) in their previously described study of children having unequivocal choreiform movements noted the CM+ boys were significantly less motivated than the normal boys though no differences were noted for girls. In the five-year follow-up study by Weiss, et al., (1971) lack of ambition was identified as one of the continuing characteristics reported by teachers and mothers of hyperactive children.

Touliatos and Lindholm (1975) directly addressed need achievement and need affiliation in MBD children as compared to normal children and their parents. The 16 MBD and 16 normal children, ages 8 to 13, were matched on age, birth order, father's education, and sex (12 boys and four girls in each group). The TAT and like projective techniques were administered to the children and their parents. MBD children and their mothers were found to have significantly lower achievement motive than the normals and their mothers. Results for fathers were in the same direction but were not significant. No differences were indicated of affiliation motive. Touliatos and Lindholm demonstrate a lower need achievement for MBD children but can only hypothesize reasons for the difference. They raise two possibilities: (1) the lower need achievement is due to repeated failure in school or (2) the lower need achievement is reflective of lower expectations because of the handicap. The implications for intervention are opposite: if hypothesis (1), demand less; if hypothesis (2), demand more.

Anxiousness-Fearfulness

The MBD child has been described as anxious and fearful, however very little has been done to substantiate these descriptors. Lievens (1974) in his statistical description of children having problems perinatal-cerebral in origin, identified psychosomatic manifestations of anxiety (nightmares, problem sleeping, sleepwalking) in 12 of 22 children. These symptoms did not persist beyond age 6 or 7; however a marked general anxiety, including fear of new experiences, was pervasive (18 of 22 subjects). Conners (1969) identified an anxious-fearful factor as one of five factors resulting from a teacher rating form. His experiment was described earlier. The items that clustered on the anxious-fearful factor included: falls apart under stress, oversensitive, overly serious or sad, excessive demands for teacher attention, and overly anxious to please. Both the Lievens (1974) and the Conners (1969) studies share the problem of not having a comparison group. In a later study Conners (1970) compared the parent ratings of symptoms of psychiatric clinic patients (hyperkinetic and neurotic) with those of the normal population. While the clinic group as a whole were rated significantly higher on anxiety behaviors, such as sleeping problems, fears, and worries, than the normal controls, the neurotics were rated significantly higher than the hyperkinetics. It would seem then that the hyperkinetic child is somewhere between the normal and the neurotic child on a factor of anxiousness and fearfulness.

Poor Self-Concept

Professionals who work with MBD children identify the child's poor self-concept as a problem which affects the child's learning and social relationships. However most references to poor self-concepts in MBD children are based on clinical observations. Lievens (1974) and Paternite, Loney, and Langhorne (1976), in describing their MBD clinic populations, identified unsatisfactory self-esteem as a pervasive problem. The MBD child was described as insecure, having a weak sense of reality and difficulty in identification. MBD children from lower socioeconomic groups had significantly lower self-esteem. Furthermore self-esteem deficits were found to be related to specific parenting variables. In two studies which followed hyperactive children over a period of time (Mendelson, Johnson, and Stewart, 1971; Weiss, et al., 1971), low self-esteem was one of the characteristics which continued over the years. These studies, none of which focused on the self-concept of the MBD child, had significant flaws. Comparison groups were needed in all, most reported results in a general descriptive manner with little detail of methodology and statistical analysis.

DISCUSSION

The major conclusion that can be drawn from the literature is that we can say nothing definitive in regard to personality characteristics peculiar to children diagnosed as having minimal brain dysfunction. The research findings to date are highly equivocal. There are a number of problems in attempting to study personality and behavioral characteristics of children labeled as having MBD. Perhaps the most evident one is that of the circularity involved when subjects are selected because of certain characteristics which are then examined in the subject group, thus insuring that the characteristic will be found. In much of the literature surveyed, this kind of approach had been taken. Personality characteristics used to describe the child having MBD have been derived primarily from clinical impressions, yet when these have been put to the test by such investigators as Routh and Roberts (1972), Crinella (1973) and Langhorne, et al., (1976), even the commonly attributed characteristic of emotional lability finds little support. Therefore no unequivocal, definitive statements can be made about the personality characteristics of a child purported to have minimal brain dysfunction.

It seems likely that there are a number of alternative hypotheses that can be developed to account for the unsupported clinical impressions of certain characteristics in children diagnosed as having minimal brain dysfunction.

Some light can be shed on this area from examination of the work of Thomas, Chess, and Birch (1968), and Thomas and Chess (1977). They developed nine categories of temperament:

1. Activity level
2. Rhythmicity
3. Approach-withdrawal
4. Adaptability
5. Threshold of responsiveness
6. Intensity of reaction
7. Quality of mood
8. Distractibility
9. Attention span and persistence

From these characteristics they developed three constellations of temperament: the easy child, the slow-to-warm up child, and the difficult child. Their description of the difficult child (Thomas and Chess, 1977, p. 23) is highly similar to what has been described in the clinical literature as the child with MBD. They found that the difficult child constituted 10% of the 141 subjects they followed in the New York Longitudinal Study (NYLS).

Temperament appears to be established by three months of age. Thus prenatal, genetic, and very early postnatal factors probably determine whether a child is a difficult child or an easy child. Presence or absence of brain injury is seemingly not related to the category of temperament. Only one of the three impaired children in this sample fell into the category of difficult-child temperament and this child was also rated high on "inconsistent and contradictory parental attitudes and practices" (Thomas and Chess, 1975). Admittedly their sample was small. However in their rubella sample (n = 243), they came to similar conclusions and reported that in general, presence or absence of difficult-child characteristics did not distinguish among their rubella group, their retarded group, and their earlier data from NYLS (1977). Similarly they reported a lack of correlation between temperament and perinatal brain damage, which they point out flies in the face of Wender's (1971) postulation that the traits of activity, distractibility, intensity, and approach-withdrawal are "relevant to the minimal brain dysfunction syndrome."

Their work to date has indicated that the categories and constellations are also not clearly related to parental care practices. However genetic variables appear to have some influence over the development of temperamental traits. From their own small twin sample and the larger twin sample of Torgerson (53 same-sex twin pairs, 34 of which were monozygotic) Thomas and Chess present data strongly suggesting that genetic variables are contributory but not sole determinants of temperamental characteristics.

Parental and perinatal factors exert some influence upon the development of a difficult-child temperament, but the relationship is not entirely clear. Carey, Lipton, and Myers (1974) in a study of temperament in adoptive and foster babies, examined the effects of maternal pregnancy anxiety. They found that the more anxious mother did *not* produce difficult babies. They reported no significant differences between their control group and the group of adoptive and foster children in regard to the difficult-child personality. Cadoret, et al., (1975) found that male children of disturbed mothers manifested a number of difficult-child traits, even though they were separated from their mothers at birth.

In their more recent work, Thomas and Chess (1977) concluded that parental attitudes and functioning at the very most have only a slight etiological influence on temperament type. However this conclusion is based largely on unpublished data and thus the studies cannot be thoroughly evaluated. The general conclusion was that, regardless of the role of environmental influences on the development of temperament, these influences do accentuate, modify, and in some cases even change temperamental traits of the developing child.

Although taking a different approach, Wender (1971) hypothesized that the MBD child presents three primary reactions and theorized that all other personality characteristics stem from the three primary symptoms or reactions. These reactions are:

1. Decreased experience of pleasure and pain.
2. Generally high and poorly modulated levels of activation.
3. Extroversion.

He believed that other characteristics were derived from these. However he presented no hard data in support of these hypotheses nor are there any firm data to be found in the present literature.

From the examination of research literature it seems highly probable that personality traits and behaviors which appear to be clinically present in children who are experiencing brain dysfunction are a result of an interaction between a mildly nonintact child and environmental variables. It seems plausible that so-called MBD children like any other group of children with handicaps, are more highly susceptible to adverse variables within their environment.

Some of the apparent disparity between clinical impressions and research findings may be the consequence of inadequately refined methods of measurement. The necessarily subtle problems of children believed to have minimal brain dysfunctions may become apparent after fairly extensive observation of a child undertaking a great variety of tasks in a typical clinical encounter. Yet the ostensibly more objective research measures of personality characteristics may be too delimited in their focus to tap these subtle problems, may elicit them inconsistently, and are unlikely to offer opportunities for observation of informal behavior.

Among the personality and behavioral characteristics attributed to children with MBD a few are supported by the literature. Attentional problems and/or distractibility seem to occur with some frequency in children designated as having MBD, although this may be due partly to the fact that these are among the characteristics used for selection of such children. Aggressive behavior has been observed in some children said to have MBD and there appear to be problems with need achievement in some. Finally anxiety and/or fearfulness has characterized some research samples although less so than neurotic children with whom the MBD subjects were compared.

Inevitably one must conclude that minimal brain dysfunctions cannot now be reliably diagnosed or consistently described by means of personality characteristics, even when personality is used to designate a broad array of behavioral phenomena. A major obstacle (not simply to deriving less equivocal conclusions from the available literature, but to undertaking definitive research) lies in the definitions of the personality and behavioral characteristics on the one hand and of MBD on the other hand. For the present MBD clearly refers to a rather heterogeneous group of children. There would appear to be no reason, under this circumstance, to expect to find an MBD personality and the failure to do so is far less remarkable than the persistence of the belief that a significant set of common personality characteristics exists.

REFERENCES

Adams, D. Z. "Strategy differences between reflective and impulsive children." *Child Development*, 43, 1076–1080, (1972).

American Psychiatric Association, Diagnostic and Statistical Manual of Mental Disorders, p. 42. Washington, D.C.: American Psychiatric Association, 1968.

Bailey, P. "Fracture at the base of the skull: Neurological and medicolegal considerations." *Medical News*, 82, 918–926, (1903).

Becker, R. D. "Child psychiatry—The continuing controversy." *The Israel Annals of Psychiatry and Related Disciplines*, 12, 87–106, (1974).

Bryan, T. H. "Peer popularity of learning disabled children." *Journal of Learning Disabilities*, 10, 621–625, (1974).

————"Peer popularity of learning-disabled children: A replication." *Journal of Learning Disabilities*, 9, 307–311, (1976).

Cadoret, R. J., L. Cunningham, R. Loftus, and J. Edwards. "Studies of adoptees from psychiatrically disturbed biologic parents." *Journal of Pediatrics*, 87, 301–306, (1975).

Campbell, S. B. "Cognitive styles in reflective, impulsive and hyperactive boys and their mothers." *Perceptual and Motor Skills*, 36, 747–752, (1973).

Campbell, S. B., B. Douglas, and G. Morgenstern. "Cognitive styles in hyperactive children and the effect of methylphenidate." *Journal of Child Psychology and Psychiatry*, 12, 55–67, (1971).

Campbell, S. G., and V. I. Douglas. "Cognitive styles and responses to the threat of frustration." *Canadian Journal of Behavioral Science*, 4, 30–42, (1972).

Carey, W. B., W. L. Lipton, and R. A. Meyers. "Temperament in adopted and foster babies." *Child Welfare*,53, 352–359, (1974).

Clark, L. P. "Psychology of essential epilepsy." *Journal of Nervous and Mental Disease*, 63, 575–585, (1926).

Clements, S. D. "Minimal brain dysfunction in children," in S. G. Sapir and A. C. Nitzburg, eds., *Children with Learning Problems: Readings in a Developmental-Interactions Approach*, pp. 159–172. New York: Brunner/Mazel, 1973.

Clements, S. D., and J. E. Peters. "Minimal brain dysfunction in the school age child." *Archives of General Psychiatry*, 6, 17–29, (1962).

Conners, C. K. "A teacher rating scale for use in drug studies with children." *American Journal of Psychiatry*, 126, 884–888, (1969).

———"Symptom patterns in hyperkinetic, neurotic, and normal children." *Child Development*, 41, 667–682, (1970).

———"Psychological assessment of children with minimal brain dysfunction." *Annals of the New York Academy of Sciences*, 205, 283–302, (1973).

Crinella, F. M. "Identification of brain dysfunction syndrome in children through profile analysis: Patterns associated with so-called, 'minimal brain dysfunction.'" *Journal of Abnormal Psychology*, 82, 33–45, (1973).

Cruickshank, W. M., F. A. Bentzen, F. H. Ratzeburg, and M. T. Tannhauser. *A Teaching Method of Brain-Injured and Hyperactive Children*. Syracuse N.Y.: Syracuse University Press, 1961.

Czudner, G., and B. P. Rourke. "Simple reaction time in 'brain-damaged' and normal children under regular and irregular preparatory interval conditions." *Perceptual and Motor Skills*, 31, 767–773, (1970).

Czudner, G., and B. P. Rourke. "Age differences in visual reaction time of 'brain-damaged' and normal children under regular and irregular preparatory interval conditions." *Journal of Experimental Child Psychology*, 13, 516–526, (1972).

Douglas, V. "Differences between normal and hyperkinetic children," in C. K. Conners, *Clinical Use of Stimulant Drugs in Children*, pp. 12–23. New York: American Elsevier, 1974.

Duckworth, S., G. D. Ragland, R. E. Sommerfeld, and M. D. Wyne. "Modification of conceptual impulsivity in retarded children." *American Journal of Mental Deficiency*, 79, 59–63, (1974).

Dykman, R. A., and P. T. Ackerman. "The MBD problem: Attention, intention, and information processing," in R. P. Anderson and C. G. Holcomb, *Learning Disability/ Minimal Brain Dysfunction Syndrome: Research Perspectives and Applications*. Springfield, Ill.: Thomas, 1976.

Ford, F. R. "Cerebral birth injuries and their results." *Medicine*, 5, 121–194, (1926).

Graham, F. K., C. B. Ernhart, M. Craft, and P. Berman. "Brain injury in the preschool child: Some developmental considerations." *Psychology Monograph*, 77, 1–16, (1963).

Gross, M. D., and W. C. Wilson. *Minimal Brain Dysfunction*, pp. 23–51. New York: Brunner/Mazel, 1974.

Guerrant, J., W. Anderson, A. Fischer, M. R. Weinstein, R. M. Jaros, and A. Deskins. *Personality in Epilepsy*. Springfield, Ill.: Thomas, 1962.

Hall, Z., and W. Russell. "Multitrait-multimethod analysis of conceptual tempo." *Journal of Educational Psychology*, 66, 923–939, (1974).

Huessy, H. R., C. D. Marshall, and R. A. Gendron. "Five-hundred children followed from grade two through grade five for the prevalence of behavior disorder." *Acta Paedopsychiatrica*, 39, 301, (1973).

Johnson, D. J., and H. R. Myklebust. *Learning Disabilities: Educational Principles and Practices.* New York: Grune & Stratton, 1967.

Kagan, J. "Reflection-impulsivity and reading ability in primary grade children." *Child Development*, 36, 609–628, (1965).

Kagan, J., B. L. Rosman, D. Day, J. Albert, and W. Phillips. "Information processing in the child: Significance of analytic and reflective attitudes." *Psychological Monographs*, 78 (1964).

Kanner, L. *Child Psychiatry*, 3rd ed. pp. 314–344. Springfield, Ill.: Thomas, 1966.

Kasanin, J. "Personality changes in children following cerebral trauma." *Journal of Nervous and Mental Disease*, 69, 385–408, (1929).

Katz, S. K., R. Saraf, D. S. Gittelman-Klein. "Clinical pharmacological management of hyperactive children." *International Journal of Mental Health*, 4, 157–181, (1975).

Klein, D. F., and R. Gittleman-Klein. "Diagnosis of minimal brain dysfunction and hyperkinetic syndrome," in C. K. Conners, ed., *Clinical Use of Stimulant Drugs in Children*, pp. 1–11. New York: American Elsevier, 1974.

Langhorne, J. E., Jr., J. Loney, C. E. Paternite, and H. P. Bechtoldt. "Childhood hyperkinesis: A return to the source." *Journal of Abnormal Psychology*, 85, 201–209, (1976).

Lennox, W. C. *Science and Seizures.* New York: Harper, 1941.

Lerner, H. D. "Hypoactivity and hyperactivity in minimal brain dysfunction children: A comparative study of psycholinguistics abilities, visual-perceptual processes and social extroversion-introversion" (Ph.D. diss., Rutgers University, 1974).

Lievens, P. "The organic psychosyndrome of early childhood and its effects on learning." *Journal of Learning Disabilities*, 7, 626–631, (1974).

Meichenbaum, D. *Cognitive-Behavior Modification: An Integrative Approach.* New York: Plenum, 1977.

Mendelson, W., N. Johnson, and M. A. Stewart. "Hyperactive children as teenagers: A follow-up study." *Journal of Nervous and Mental Disease*, 153, 273–279, (1971).

Menkes, M. M., J. S. Rowe, and J. H. Menkes. "A twenty-five year follow-up study on the hyperkinetic child with minimal brain dysfunction." *Pediatrics*, 39, 393–399, (1967).

Messer, S. B. "Reflection-impulsivity: A review." *Psychological Bulletin*, 83, 1026–1052, (1976).

Meyer, W. J. "Cerebral dysfunction," in G. O. Johnson and D. Blank, eds., *Exceptional Children Research Review*, pp. 181–209. Washington, D.C.: The Council for Exceptional Children, 1968.

Paternite, C. E., J. L. Loney, J. E. Langhorne, Jr. "Relationships between symptomatology and SES-related factors in hyperkinetic/MBD boys." *American Journal of Orthopsychiatry*, 46, 291–301, (1976).

Quin, P. O., and J. L. Rapaport. "Minor physical anomalies and neurologic status in hyperactive boys." *Pediatrics*, 53, 742–747, (1974).

Rie, H. E., E. D. Rie, S. Stewart, and J. P. Ambuel. "Effects of methylphenidate on underachieving children." *Journal of Counseling and Clinical Psychology*, 44, 250–260, (1976).

Rost, L. J., and D. C. Charles. "Academic achievement of brain-injured and hyperactive children in isolation." *Exceptional Children*, 33, 459–467, (1967).

Rourke, B. P. "Brain-behavior relationships in children with learning disabilities: A research program." *American Psychologist,* September, 911–920, (1975).

Routh, D. K., and R. D. Roberts. "Minimal brain dysfunction in children: Failure to find evidence for behavioral syndromes." *Psychological Reports,* 31, 307–314, (1972).

Safer, D. J., and R. P. Allen. *Hyperactive Children,* p. 25. Baltimore: University Park Press, 1976.

Schleifer, M., G. Weiss, N. Cohen, M. Elman, H. Cvejic, and E. Kruger. "Hyperactivity in preschoolers and the effect of methylphenidate." *American Journal of Orthopsychiatry,* 45, 38–50, (1975).

Somervill, J. W., L. S. Warnberg, and D. E. Bost. "Effects of cubicles versus increased stimulation on task performance by first-grade males perceived as distractible and nondistractible." *Journal of Special Education,* 7, 169–185, (1973).

Stevens, D., A. Ackerman, and R. A. Dykman. "Reaction time, impulsivity, and autonomic lability in children with minimal dysfunction," *in Proceedings of the Seventy-Sixth Annual Convention of the American Psychological Association,* 367–368, (1968).

Strauss, A. A., and L. E. Lehtinen. *Psychopathology and Education of the Brain-Injured Child.* New York: Grune & Stratton, 75–97, 1947.

Sullivan, E. B., and L. Gahagan. "On intelligence of epileptic children." *Genetic Psychology Monograph,* 17, 309–376, (1935).

Sulzbacher, S. I. "The learning-disabled or hyperactive child: Diagnosis and treatment." *Journal of the American Medical Association,* 234, 841–938, (1975).

Sykes, D. H., V. I. Douglas, G. Weiss, and K. K. Minde. "Attention in hyperactive children and the effect of methylphenidate (Ritalin)." *Journal of Child Psychology and Psychiatry,* 12, 129–139, (1971).

Thomas, A., and S. Chess. "A longitudinal study of three brain-damaged children." *Archives of General Psychiatry,* 32, 4557–465 (1975).

Thomas, A., and S. Chess. *Temperament and Development.* New York: Brunner/Mazel, 1977.

Thomas, A., S. Chess, and H. G. Birch. *Temperament and Behavior Disorders in Children.* New York: New York University Press, 1968.

Touliatos, J., and B. W. Lindholm. "TAT need achievement and need affiliation in minimally brain-injured and normal children and their parents." *Journal of Psychiatry,* 89, 49–54, (1975).

Twitchell, T. E. "A behavioral syndrome," a Review of *Minimal Brain Dysfunction in Children* by P. H. Wender, *Science,* 174, 135–136, (1971).

Virkkunen, M., and A. Nuutila. "Specific reading retardation, hyperactive child syndrome, and juvenile delinquency." *Acta Psychiatrica Scandinavica,* 54, 25–28, (1976).

Weiss, G., and K. K. Minde. "Follow-up studies of children who present with symptoms of hyperactivity," in C. K. Conners, ed., *Clinical Use of Stimulant Drugs in Children,* pp. 67–78. New York: American Elsevier, 1974.

Weiss, G., K. K. Minde, J. S. Werry, V. Douglas, and E. Nemeth. "Studies on the hyperactive child: Five-year follow-up." *Archives of General Psychiatry,* 24, 409–414, (1971).

Wender, P. H. *Minimal Brain Dysfunction in Children.* New York: Wiley, 1971.

——"The minimal brain dysfunction syndrome in children." *The Journal of Nervous and Mental Disease,* 155, 55–71, (1972).

——"The minimal brain dysfunction syndrome." *Annual Review of Medicine,* 26, 45–62, (1975).

Wiig, E. H., and S. P. Harris. "Perception and interpretation of nonverbally expressed emotions by adolescents with learning disabilities." *Perceptual and Motor Skills*, 38, 239–245, (1974).

Witkin, H. A., R. B. Dyk, H. S. Saterson, D. R. Goodenough, and S. A. Karp. *Psychological Differentiation*. New York: Wiley, 1962.

Wolff, P. H., and I. Hurwitz. "Functional implications of the minimal brain-damage syndrome." *Seminars in Psychiatry*, 5, 105–115 (1973).

CHAPTER 15

MBD: Critical Diagnostic Issues

Gabrielle Weiss

INTRODUCTION: HAVE WE BEEN "COUNTING JARS OF RASPBERRY JAM?"

I hope Dr. Robert Sprague (1976) will forgive me for plagiarizing his title "Counting Jars of Raspberry Jam," which was the colourful and provocative title he once gave to a talk on Minimal Brain Dysfunction (MBD).

The jars of raspberry jam refer to an incident that took place during the Napoleonic Wars in 1812. A British cavalry regiment fighting in Spain had considerably upset the Foreign Office in Britain because it was unable to account for all the jars of raspberry jam that had been consumed. The Duke of Wellington responded in a historical letter to the Foreign Office that he could either "train an army of uniformed British clerks in Spain for the benefit of the accountant and copy boys in London or perchance, see to it that the forces of Napoleon were driven out of Spain," but he could not do both.

How does this story apply to the problems of diagnosis of MBD? When we look at the historical aspects of the diagnosis of MBD (which will be briefly covered later) it becomes apparent that a great deal of highly skilled professional time has been spent on finding new names for old problems and then clarifying, defining, and redefining the newer terminology. For example Minimal Brain Damage was superceded by the term Minimal Brain Dysfunction. Under the latter rubric, several subcategories of children were included, for example children with specific learning disabilities, with hyperkinetic impulsive disorders, children who showed soft signs on a neurological examination, clumsy children, those with cognitive or motor developmental lags, and possibly those who fell below the median of a normal distribution curve for the various cognitive and motor developmental tasks. These subcategories are not too clearly defined themselves, sometimes distinct and sometimes overlapping.

Has the time and effort been worth while? Have the children involved and their families benefited by having better and more readily available services? Was MBD a heuristic concept for research?

In contributing yet another chapter on problems of the diagnosis of MBD, am I continuing to "count the jars?" This will certainly be the case unless my long clinical and research experience with children who would be diagnosed MBD by others but called hyperactive by me, will enable me to view the problems of diagnosis of MBD in a somewhat different light. My experience with these children and their families has in fact influenced me towards a more holistic frame of reference for looking at the age-old dichotomy of mind-body as it applies to this heterogeneous group of children.

HISTORICAL ASPECTS:
A SERIES OF ILLOGICAL CONCLUSIONS

As far back as the early Greeks connections have been made between organic factors (for example the body humours) and personality and behavior.

In the nineteenth century the medical literature contained many detailed case histories of personality changes following accidents that resulted in brain damage. Following the First World War, an epidemic of encephalitis lethargica was noted to result in post-encephalitic behavior disorders in some of its child victims (Hohman, 1922; Ebaugh, 1923; Kahn and Cohen, 1934). The children were described as suffering from hyperactivity, impulsivity, antisocial behavior and emotional lability and were referred to by Kahn and Cohen as "organically driven." Even then it was recognised that the children's behavior could be improved in a residential treatment center, but that their behavior deteriorated when they were returned to parents who themselves were maladjusted (Bond and Smith, 1935). Bradley, working at the Bradley Home in Rhode Island (a residential treatment center for disturbed children), found that the stimulant drugs benzedrine and dexedrine when given to disturbed children of mixed etiology and diagnosis had certain beneficial effects on the majority of them. He described a paradoxical quietening effect on the hyperactive children and an improvement of mood and school performance in most of the children thus treated (Bradley, 1937).

The discovery of the paradoxical quietening effect and the marked improvement of hyperactive children when treated with stimulants may well have influenced the selection of the term MBD many years later. For example Paul Wender writes, "...one of the additional common properties of this heterogeneous group of children (MBD) is the dramatic response of many of them to treatment with stimulant and antidepressant drugs" (1973a). Bradley's original finding (1937) that children with *diverse psychopathology* responded favorably to stimulants has remained largely forgotten.

Laufer and Denhoff gave an excellent behavioral description of children who had what they termed "hyperkinetic impulse disorders" (1957). Their classical description is still the one used to describe MBD children, although many clinicians will also include children who display only some of the symptoms of the hyperkinetic impulse disorder. They even include those children who have no behavior problems at all, but have one or more specific learning disabilities; or those who are clumsy and have soft signs on a neurological examination, the latter indicating an immature sensimotor apparatus.

Historically the designation Minimal Brain Damage syndrome preceded Minimal Brain Dysfunction syndrome. The former terminology seems to have originated from the work of Strauss and Werner which began in the 30s. These workers differentiated a group of brain-damaged and nonbrain-damaged retarded children and described the former as having difficulties in perception, concept formation, language and emotion, and behavior. Strauss suggested in Volumes 1 and 2 of *Psychopathology and Education of the Brain Injured Child* (Strauss and Kephart, 1948, 1955 respectively) that if children with known brain damage (as detected in his studies by a neurological examination and/or history suggestive of brain damage) showed specific behavioral and cognitive problems, then children exhibiting these same behavioral difficulties but without any evidence of brain damage, probably suffered from brain damage. However the latter could not be diagnosed because "the common neurological examination is known not to be infallible"

(Strauss and Kephart, 1955). The authors were fully aware of the circularity of their reasoning but felt justified in their assumption. The prefix Minimal in Minimal Brain Damage probably testifies that the Damage is so small as to be missed by the neurological examination. According to Benton however the adjective minimal betrayed doubt that real brain disease could be detected solely in the form of behavioral deviation without classical neurological evidence of disease (1973). He pointed out that,

> Radical excision of an entire hemisphere (with occasional sparing of one or another area such as the occipital lobe or hippocampus) rarely harms the child.

He suggests that cerebral lesions in children must either be quite extensive or have specific disorganising functional properties in order to produce important behavioral abnormalities. Benton states that,

> If the behavioral deviations defining MBD are to be ascribed to brain damage or dysfunctions, then that damage or dysfunction can hardly be 'minimal' in character. [1973, p. 30]

However the terminology of Minimal Brain Damage as the cause of a specific behavioral syndrome came into widespread use in spite of the fuzzy thinking behind it. This popularity probably resulted from Strauss' emphasis (1948, 1955) on the importance of recognition of the syndrome he had described, so that the affected children could be identified and placed into special educational settings where their ability to learn would be enhanced. In fact most states in the United States, largely as a result of this work, passed legislation to provide special educational programs (special classes) for the minimally brain damaged. While these special classes are now used for children with specific learning difficulties and/or hyperactivity and distractibility, as late as 1972 Clemmens and Kenny pointed out that in some school systems it is the practice to require a neurological examination, medical diagnosis, and even an EEG prior to placement of learning-disabled or hyperactive children into special classes. This is so in spite of the fact that it is known that children with learning disabilities and/or hyperactive impulse disorders may not have abnormal neurological or EEG findings, and even if they had (aside from the rare treatable neurological conditions, such as brain tumors or frank epilepsy) the findings would make no difference whatever to their educational and psychological rehabilitation or their total management.

Clements and Peters were the first workers to use the term "MBD" (1962). They broadened the term Minimal Brain Damage to include also constitutional factors and temperament. These authors were reacting to the then prevalent purely psychogenic causes of behavior disorders and wrote:

> It is necessary to take into account the full spectrum of causality from the unique genetic combination that each individual is, to his gestation and birth experiences, to his interaction with significant persons and finally to the stresses and emotional traumata of later life, after his basic reaction patterns have been laid down.

Clements and Peters felt it was not uncommon in child guidance clinics to blame good parents for their children's problems suggesting to them that there was "some magical subtle aberration in their attitudes and behavior" (1962, p. 195).

There is no doubt in my mind that some psychiatrists and other professionals have in fact blamed parents and have thus increased feelings of guilt, thereby practicing incompetently. There is also no doubt that such a holistic approach as suggested by Clements and Peters is essential both for good diagnosis and treatment, but the errors made in the past by incompetent mental health workers who erroneously blamed parents or did not take constitution and heredity into account do not provide logical evidence to coin a new syndrome.

Soon after Clements and Peters' classical paper, "Minimal brain dysfunction in the school-age child" (1962), an international study group was convened at Oxford in 1962 to examine further the concept of MBD. In his introductory remarks to the proceedings of this conference, Ronald MacKeith writes,

> The main achievement of the conference was in fact the negative one of deciding that the concept of 'minimal brain damage' should be discarded....there are reasons for using (in its place) the convenient but possibly illogical term 'Minimal Brain Dysfunction' (1963).

In 1963 the U.S. Public Health Service and the National Easter Seal Society for Crippled Children and Adults sponsored a conference in Washington. As a result of this conference two task forces were established. Task Force I was to prepare working papers on terminology and identification of MBD and Task Force II was to prepare working papers on the diagnosis of MBD.

Task Force I, adopting the terminology MBD, listed almost 100 signs and symptoms (described in the literature) exhibited by children falling under this diagnosis (Clements, 1966). A formal definition of MBD was given in their report:

> The term MBD refers to children of near average, average or above average general intelligence with certain learning and/or behavioral difficulties ranging from mild to severe, which are associated with deviations of the CNS. These deviations may manifest themselves by various combinations of impairments in perception, conceptualization, language, memory and control of attention, impulse or motor function. These aberrations may arise from genetic variation, biochemical irregularities, perinatal brain insults or other illnesses or injuries sustained during the years which are critical for the development and maturation of the CNS or from unknown causes. (Pp. 9–10]

Task Force II reflected the different interests and concerns of: (1) physicians who, working on a medical model, were concerned with medical diagnosis and management and (2) educators and psychologists who were concerned with the assessment of learning disabilities and techniques of remediation.

Noteworthy is the fact that both the Oxford Conference (1962) and the Task Forces (1963) considered that the children included under the diagnosis of MBD are a heterogeneous group and that efforts should be made to subclassify them into more homogeneous subgroups. It is obvious that neither follow-up studies of MBD, nor evaluation of treatment efficacy of any treatment modality for MBD children, nor biochemical research on MBD (for example brain catecholamine studies) can produce valid results unless MBD is subclassified into more homogeneous subgroups of children and the children in these more homogeneous subgroups become the subjects of the research. In fact given the present state of knowledge (or lack of it) of the etiology, pathophysiology, or phenomenology of MBD, it is impossible to conceive of a treatment for such a heterogeneous group of children. Rather each child will require unique combinations of therapies and/or remediation depending on his individual profile of cognitive skills and behavior patterns. This raises doubt about the value to practicing clinicians of an entity as vague as that of MBD.

While interest in MBD began to wane in the late 60s, it was revived by Paul Wender's book, "*Minimal Brain Dysfunction in Children,*" which appeared in 1971. Wender's book was stimulating in that he postulated some primary psychological defects in MBD children in an analogous way to Bleuler's primary defects in schizophrenia (for example disorder of association). These primary defects Wender suggests are present in all MBD children no matter how diverse their symptomatology. There are two primary defects: (1) an apparent increase in arousal and (2) a diminished capacity for positive and negative affect, resulting in diminished sensitivity to positive and negative reinforcement. He further postulates that these primary defects result from a disorder of monoamine metabolism, which may occur on a genetic basis. Wender subdivides children with MBD into phenotypic subgroups, including the classical hyperactive, the neurotic, psychopathic, psychotic, and the child with specific learning disorders.

It was pointed out by Klein and Gittleman-Klein that Bleuler's work led to a rapid proliferation of the diagnosis of schizophrenia, particularly in the United States (1974). These authors wrote, "The diagnosis came to include patients whose thinking did not exactly match their psychiatrist's (whose associative processes were adjudged to be an impeccable standard)." In fact Wender's hypothesis and his enthusiasm with stimulant therapy probably led to an increase in both the diagnosis of MBD and to the use of stimulant drug therapy. Wender himself states that MBD probably constitutes the single most common cause of chronic behavioral problems in the pediatric age group (Wender, 1973b). Unfortunately a very large proportion of disturbed children could be fitted into Wender's description of MBD and the primary defects which he describes are hard to specify. Just when is a child said to be "unresponsive to reinforcement?" What is the average level of responsiveness and to what reinforcement? So far I know of no work that has clearly supported the validity of the presence of Wender's primary defects of increased arousal and decreased positive and negative effects (or reduced sensitivity to positive and negative reinforcement) in MBD children. This is a heuristic area for research.

The renewed popularity of the term MBD following Wender's book seems to follow the same path as the popularity of the earlier term Minimal Brain Damage. Both Strauss and Wender counteracted therapeutic nihilism and provided discouraged parents and professionals with the optimistic view that "something could be done." For children with minimal brain damage it was placement into special educational classes and for many children with MBD it was the excellent behavioral response to stimulant medication. It is this writer's point of view that neither special classes nor medication are the answer for this diverse group of children, although either or both may be most valuable for some children. Both special classes and stimulant medication have their unique drawbacks, even though for some children they may be essential and for others valuable for limited periods of time.

PROBLEMS OF DIAGNOSIS

Conceptual Problems

Factor Analytic Studies

Is MBD a syndrome or are there different syndromes within the MBD category? Clements used the term "MBD syndrome" and listed 99 symptoms which he found when he perused the available literature (1966). In the same article he listed the 10 most widely cited symptoms:

- Hyperactivity
- Perceptuomotor impairments
- Emotional lability
- General coordination deficits
- Disorders of attention
- Impulsivity
- Disorder of memory and thinking
- Specific learning disabilities
- Disorders of speech and equivocal neurological signs
- EEG irregularities

A syndrome is a cluster of signs and symptoms which occur together more frequently than by chance. A few studies have attempted to use statistical techniques in order to assess the evidence of a behavioral syndrome or syndromes within the MBD category. Rodin took a group of 72 children referred by school authorities for behavior or academic problems and performed factor analyses on their various signs and symptoms (Rodin, Lucas, and Simson, 1964). The analyses revealed a disappointing lack of relationship among history of brain damage, neurological findings, EEG, intellectual deficits and behavior. It was concluded that the clinical picture observed in a child was most probably the result of a unique combination of innate, traumatic psychological and social causes. There was little evidence that MBD was a single homogeneous syndrome or that it was caused by a single etiology.

In a study of 103 chronically hyperactive children Werry (1968) confirmed the findings of Rodin, both in terms of factor structure and in the lack of relationship among behavioral problems, the history, the EEG, intellectual assessment, and neurological examination. Schulman, Kaspar, and Throne (1965) using the technique of cluster analysis concluded that there was no such thing as the brain-damage syndrome. Paine, Werry, and Quay (1968) reported on 83 children with a diagnosis of MBD on whom correlational and factor analytic studies were performed. It was concluded that MBD is not a homogeneous diagnostic entity, but rather a way of describing a variety of unrelated minor dysfunctions—some neurological, some behavioral, some cognitive—which may put a child in difficulties with his social and familial environment. They suggested that "professionals should be circumspect in hypothesizing about cerebral status in individual cases and concentrate on adequate psychosocial and educational assessment and rehabilitation programs" (p. 516).

Finally in a paper by Routh and Roberts (1972) 16 measures were obtained for a sample of 89 children including most of the 10 variables described by Clements. Few instances of significant relationships were found especially when age and IQ were statistically controlled. Results indicated a failure to find evidence of a behavioral syndrome in a group of MBD children.

We can conclude that the studies which have used covariate or factor analytic techniques have without exception failed to find a syndrome (or different syndromes) within the category of MBD children. From a statistical point of view most of the studies criticized some of their own shortcomings, nevertheless the weight of all studies together is strong evidence against the existence of an MBD syndrome.

In addition there is no evidence at the present time that children referred to as having MBD have in common certain formal qualities of dysfunctions, such as conceptual difficulties, concreteness, perseveration problems with laterality, and so on. If no syndrome can be shown to exist either with respect to behavioral problems or formal cognitive dysfunctions and if there is no single dysfunction which is common to a group of children designated as having MBD, then it seems to the author that in the light of present-day knowledge there is no justification in regarding individual dysfunctions as pathognomonic of a clinical entity such as MBD. Also we cannot term various *different* combinations of these dysfunctions a syndrome.

Problems Associated with the Etiology of MBD

If an etiological factor common to MBD children could be demonstrated, it would support the concept that MBD is indeed a disease entity even if its symptoms do not form a unitary cluster. However no one such etiological factor has been demonstrated. Various diverse etiologies have received varying degrees of empirical support, but none has been demonstrated to be etiological for all MBD children.

One of the earliest etiologies described is brain damage caused by such factors as foetal malnutrition, birth injury, perinatal anoxia, head injuries, encephalitis, lead poisoning, and so on. More recently cerebral allergies have received attention as another possible cause (Crook, 1975). Evidence is also accumulating that food additives may be etiological for a few hyperkinetic children (Conners, et al., 1976; Williams and Cran, 1977).

Disorders of brain catecholamine metabolism in hyperkinetic children have been studied (Shaywitz, Cohen, and Bowers, 1977) following Wender's (1973a) speculations that these may form the common physiopathology of MBD.

A genetic causation was suggested by the work of Cantwell (1972), Goodwin, et al., (1975), and Morrison and Stewart (1971), while the work of Werry, et al., (1972) suggested that the condition may be simply a biological variation made manifest by universal compulsory education. Maturational lags have also been described as etiological.

Environmental factors, such as neglect, lack of emotional and intellectual stimulation at home and at school, a chaotic disorganized home, or certain child rearing practices have been implicated. While it is difficult to prove or disprove the environmental theory of etiology, it is evident that environmental factors can influence both behavioral and cognitive problems of MBD children, while not necessarily being the cause of them.

One must conclude that the etiology of MBD is presently unknown and likely to be multifactorial and heterogeneous, and that no single etiology is sufficient to explain causation in MBD children. In addition etiology may well be multiple in any one child assessed.

At the present time the heterogeneity of the etiological factors studied does not support the view that we are dealing with a single disease entity. It seems rather that we are dealing with a group of different disorders with different etiologies.

Problems of Definition of Individual Symptoms

How poor must concentration or hyperactivity be before a child is referred for these problems and diagnosed as having MBD on the basis of these symptoms? Probably none of these behavioral traits can be quantified because they contain a dimension over and beyond the quantitative. For example it would be of little practical value if attention were quantitatively measured by giving each child a Continuous Performance Test and coming out with an "error of omission and commission score!" What we really need to know is whether the child's inattentiveness affects his various school subjects and if so, whether he is more attentive in some subjects than in others, and why? In a similar way when hyperactivity was measured mechanically in some hyperactive children, it was found that they were not necessarily more active (in the quantitative sense) than other children. It seems that what is referred to as hyperactivity is activity that is aimless and that has an annoying quality to others. However adults (parents and teachers) have varying tolerance to being annoyed, a child may be called normal in one setting in the presence of more tolerant adults and hyperactive in another setting with less tolerant adults. Hence these symptoms are difficult to quantify and are usually socially and not mechanically or quantitatively defined.

In addition each symptom has a dimension of intensity and frequency. Thus a child could be extremely inattentive occasionally, or moderately inattentive most of the time. Also it is not uncommon to find that a child shows the behavioral problems only in some situations, for example in the school or in the home, but not in all situations. These are inherent difficulties of diagnosis when we are dealing with the behavioral sciences and, in my opinion, the problem is not resolved by substituting a more reliable and quantifiable laboratory task in place of the life situation. The laboratory task, for example the Matching Familiar Figures Test, as a task of reflectivity may be reliable and quantifiable but how well does it correlate with a child's reflectivity in a classroom where the whole social situation is different?

While quantification of symptoms can be carried out in any setting (at home, at school, and in the laboratory) the correlation between these different sources of information is sometimes poor, which suggests that a child's symptomatology has a strong relationship to the setting in which it is expressed and thus represents an interaction among factors within the child and the specific qualities of the environment in which the child finds himself.

There is no perfect solution to the difficulty of defining these symptoms. The most accurate information is obtained by multifaceted approaches, such as observation of the child in the natural setting, obtaining a description of the problems (or symptoms) from teachers and parents, as well as assessing the child's performance on laboratory tasks. It is also an aid to both understanding and helping the child to know in what specific situations his behavioral problems are most prominent. Most hyperkinetic children are situational to some degree, in the sense that their behavior problems are more prominent in some settings than in others.

Problems Arising from Professionals from Different Disciplines Diagnosing and Treating MBD Children

There is a tendency for the more behaviorally disturbed MBD children to be referred for assessment and treatment to a psychiatrist or psychologist, for the learning-disabled child to be referred for assessment and remediation to an educator, and for the neurologically handicapped child to be referred to a neurologist or pediatrician. Ideally for the patient each professional should be equally able to evaluate the child as described in the following section. In practice, since this is rarely the case, children usually require multidisciplinary evaluation. Because the latter is not always available and is expensive, one suspects that children with suspected MBD may receive different kinds of evaluation and subsequent treatment depending on who first sees them. Thus the psychiatrist may concentrate on family counseling (with or without the use of medication), the psychologist may concentrate on behavior modification, the educator on remedial educational programs, and the neurologist and pediatrician on medical management (medication). There is no hard evidence that this bias operates frequently, but when it does it is detrimental for the child and his family. Not infrequently one hears a distraught parent report that every person who evaluated his child observed a different problem and suggested a different solution. (Intervention and coordination are discussed in a subsequent section of this book.)

CONCLUSIONS:
THE APPLICATION OF A BIOPSYCHOSOCIAL MODEL FOR UNDERSTANDING MBD CHILDREN

It is in my opinion preferable to classify children by the older descriptive terms which refer to more homogeneous subgroups of children (for example those with specific learning disabilities, those who have hyperkinetic impulse disorders and, of course, those children who have both). The older descriptive terminology has the advantage that it does not imply any etiology, whereas the term MBD implies biochemical or physiological aberration in the brain, which has not been demonstrated to exist. Shaywitz, Cohen, and Bowers (1977) have demonstrated a possible abnormality in brain dopamine in six hyperkinetic children, but the evidence for this is not yet convincing. Even if a biochemical abnormality is later demonstrated to occur in some hyperkinetic children, there would be no simple direct relationship between this and the deviant behavior. The latter will occur in its specific forms as a result of interaction between the biochemical aberration, the child's personality, and the child's environment. The concept that a biochemical abnormality is directly responsible for behavior is to me an oversimplified and reductionist point of view.

In this connection George Engel's article "The need for a new medical model: A challenge for biomedicine" (1977) is most timely. Engel states that the dominant model of disease today is biomedical with molecular biology its basic scientific discipline. This model requires that disease be dealt with as an entity independent of psychological or social factors. It also requires that behavioral deviations be explained on the basis of disordered biochemical or physiological processes in the brain. Engel points out that such a model has two main disadvantages. It embraces a mind-body dualism (a dichotomy that has long plagued medicine) and furthermore the model is reductionist because it implies that complex behaviors are ultimately attributable to a single primary determinent. Engel recognizes that the biomedical model with its firm base in the biological sciences together with modern technology has a record of astonishing achievement. He feels however that the model is no longer adequate for the scientific tasks and social responsibilities of either medicine or psychiatry today.

Children with various symptoms that have been subsumed without adequate support under the heading of MBD require a comprehensive diagnostic assessment using the broad frame of reference discussed above. It must be kept in mind that the etiology in any one child may be multiple: organic and environmental. Thus the following evaluation of each child is important:

1. A careful *history* of organic and environmental factors during pregnancy, delivery, and throughout the child's development from infancy on.

2. Assessment of the child's *behavioral aberrations*—the specific symptoms present, their severity, frequency, the degree to which symptomatology is situational, and the duration of the problems.

3. An *educational assessment* to determine if learning disabilities are present and, if so, their nature. Current functioning of the child in written and oral language, reading, arithmetic, and handwriting must also be evaluated.

4. Assessment of the *intrapsychic processes* of the child; how he views himself, his family, his peers, his school, and so on; evaluations of his personality strengths and weaknesses; during this assessment (at which the diagnostician should be alone with the child) a positive therapeutic relationship is established which becomes of great value if the diagnostician is also the person responsible for the rehabilitation program and continues to work with the child.

5. *Interactions* of the immediate family of the child require assessment. These interactions may be highly supportive and constructive to the child or may be exacerbating and in some cases perhaps causing some of the child's symptomatology. Even healthy families may get into unhappy vicious cycles with difficult children, and not infrequently difficult children produce strains on the marriage of the parents and feelings of resentment in the siblings.

6. *Assessment of the child's school.* Is he in a school environment that is conducive to his learning? Can a specific remedial program be incorporated into his regular school curriculum? Placement of children into special classes has some built-in disadvantages, a discussion of which is beyond the scope of this chapter.

7. Assessment of the child's *neurological status.* I feel this is only necessary if a treatable neurological condition is suspected (epilepsy, brain tumors, or encephalopathies, and so on). In that case a neurological examination, EEG and, if necessary, other techniques need to be carried out. There is no good evidence that children who have soft signs on a neurological examination or who have abnormalities of EEG (such as slow diffuse dysrythmia) have a better therapeutic response to stimulants than do chil-

dren in whom these signs are absent. Hence neurological evaluation is not required for a decision regarding the question of medication; the latter decision must be made on the basis of the behavioral assessment. This is confirmed by the study of Kenny, et al., of 100 children referred for hyperactivity, from which the authors concluded that

The poor correlation of the neurological examination and the electroencephalogram with the final diagnosis indicates that these procedures are of limited utility in assessing hyperactivity in childhood. [1971]

I have chosen two clinical vignettes which I think illustrate the application of the biopsychosocial model to the group of children under discussion. The first is an example of how an emotionally traumatic event worsened temporarily all the classical symptoms of a hyperkinetic 9-year-old boy, whose primary etiology was probably brain damage. The second illustration is a short summary of the progress of a hyperkinetic boy whom I followed between the ages of 5 and 22 years.

John was a hyperkinetic boy of nine years, who had weighed two pounds at birth. He was first treated with methylphenidate which reduced his behavioral difficulties, but not sufficiently to stay in a regular classroom. He had average intelligence and no specific learning disabilities although he had severe gross and fine motor problems and his handwriting was sometimes illegible. Behavior modification was initiated both in his home and in his class. This together with medication enabled John to remain in a regular class and learn at an average rate. The episode to be described occurred at the end of grade three at a time when his behavior had been stable all year. John was wrongly accused by a teacher of taking money from her desk. (Only later was the real culprit identified.) Following this, some children in his class teased him about stealing and the problem came to a climax during John's ninth birthday party to which he had invited some of his friends. One child lost something at the party and accused John of taking it. John's mother appeared on the scene too late because the children had their coats on and wanted to go home and John began to cry. Following this episode John began to talk about "no one liking him" and did not wish to return to school. The parents insisted that he go to school. His behavior deteriorated and the parents stated that the medication was not working any more and the behavior modification programs "had become useless," as John had relapsed into his original unacceptable behavior patterns both at home and at school. Increasing John's medication was tried but found not to be helpful. Finally six weeks later at a time when the teacher once more wanted John out of the class, I had an opportunity to talk with John alone. I saw him three consecutive times. I convinced him of the relationship between his worsened behavior and his perceived social failure, that is his problems with his friends. I helped him work out a way to win his friends back. At the same time the teacher talked to the whole class about teasing and how much it could hurt any one of them. Immediately after this twofold intervention John's behavior returned to its previous fairly stable level and John in fact won back his friends.

My second clinical vignette concerns Peter whom I first met 17 years ago when he was 5 years old. At that time a comprehensive evaluation, as outlined above (of which only some highlights will be described) indicated that Peter was a hyperkinetic child with severe aimlessness, restlessness, poor concentration, short attention span and gross motor clumsiness. He was the younger of two boys born prematurely to an upper middle class family. His father, a university teacher, was an ambitious person, well known and respected in his field. Peter's mother was a highly strung, very conscientious woman whose life had become almost totally devoted to Peter. At the time of being seen she said, "I am at the end of my rope" and was suffering from acute anxiety. She felt she could at no time let Peter out of her sight as he was unaware of danger and did not learn from experience (such as almost being hit by a car at age 3 years). She did not allow him to play outside as he still had a habit of darting impulsively into the street. The adolescent boy in the family, Jeffrey, indicated that Peter was the family pet and said that both parents were constantly involved with him. Jeffrey had developed some antisocial behaviors within the past year. The parents on their part felt that their disagreements as to how to handle Peter were causing marital stress. Peter's father considered his wife too soft with Peter, and she indicated that her husband did not accept the child and was too demanding.

Peter's IQ on the Stanford-Binet was 79, and a diagnostic educational assessment indicated that he had gross motor and perceptuomotor problems. A remedial program was initiated in Peter's kindergarten. In addition his father (who did not believe the results of the Stanford-Binet as accurately reflecting his son's intelligence) spent much time with Peter over homework he constructed for him each evening, some of which sessions ended with Peter in tears. An electroencephalogram indicated that Peter had slow diffuse dysrhythmia.

Family therapy was initiated with the aim of ameliorating some of the difficult family interactions. The therapist attempted to:

1. Help the adolescent boy communicate his needs for more parental attention.

2. Help the mother feel more sure of herself in limit setting and to become less protective of Peter (father's common sense helped mother in this respect).

3. Help father better accept Peter with his handicaps (mother particularly wished to facilitate this).

4. Decrease the differences in approach to Peter between his two parents and thus decrease resulting marital tension.

These goals were only partially achieved. When Peter was nine years old his father asked if the intellectual evaluation could be repeated. This time Peter was given a Wechsler Intelligence Scale for Children and the results were: full scale IQ, 85; verbal, 86; performance 86, with little subtest scatter. Father was naturally disappointed in the results and again felt that they did not reflect Peter's ability as he was now doing close to average work in most subjects in grade two, whilst receiving tutoring at home (father) and remedial education at school. Psychiatric evaluation of Peter at this time showed a deterioration. He was somewhat less restless and distractible, but he now showed a degree of withdrawal not noticed previously and had become afraid of playing with other children, saying they were too rough. His mother still took him to and from school and he still rarely played outside, preferring solitary activities. Because of this deterioration and because of the stress this child caused the family, a boarding school for children with learning disorders was recommended. Peter did well at this school and no longer required medication. At age fifteen he was able to transfer to a regular boarding school where he remained another four years.

At the present time Peter is an immaculately dressed, very polite young man in his early twenties. His parents are proud of him and he is presently completing a third year at a university. He tends to be silent in the presence of his parents, but opens up when seen alone. He complains of severe self-consciousness and does not feel he can relate to people. He says he has never felt accepted by others and works hard to be liked. He is hoping to be accepted into graduate school in an out-of-town university since he is aware of being emotionally dependent on his parents and sees living away from them as a difficult challenge.

He has learned to compensate for some continued problems of the hyperkinetic impulse disorder and is fully aware of this. He is no longer overly restless although he feels restless. He counteracts poor concentration by great effort and will power and divides his various assignments into smaller units to be done at one time. He deals with low frustration tolerance by going off to listen to music when he becomes acutely frustrated with a situation. He tries to deal with poor social skills by carefully controlled politeness which works better with adults than with peers. He has not yet succeeded in making a friend although he now has a relationship with an older student which is helpful to him and he feels he will soon make other friends. He has never had a girlfriend as yet, but is attracted to girls.

This case was cited because it seems to me that Peter's final outcome as a young adult was determined by: possible brain damage (prematurity), unique family interactions, excellent schools, including the financial means to make the educational facilities possible, and lastly, Peter's own personality (with high motivation and no antisocial traits). Peter's continued low self-esteem is seen as secondary to his earlier hyperkinetic behavior disorder and learning difficulties which resulted in specific interactional problems with his parents, teachers, and peers. I suggest that the prognosis of any other child with Peter's identical handicaps and Peter's identical brain damage (or dysfunction), but living in a different family, going to different schools, having a different genetic background and personality, and different financial resources, would be entirely different.

At The Montreal Children's Hospital we have carried out prospective 10-to 15-year follow-up studies on 75 hyperactive adults aged 18–24 years and 45 matched normal controls (Weiss, et al., 1978). The findings indicate that there is indeed great variability in outcome which is best explained on the biopsychosocial model of etiology. Only a small minority of the hyperactive adults became chronic offenders of the law, none was psychotic, and two were diagnosed as borderline personalities. Immature and impulsive traits persisted in many of the hyperactive adults. An interesting finding was that their work records (measured by employer's ratings and Hollingshead Job Status) were as good as those of normal controls, whereas their school records (as measured during their last year at school by teachers' behavioral ratings and school achievement) were significantly worse than those of controls. This indicates the situational aspects of the behavioral problem and is not a surprising finding within the framework of the broader medical model for understanding this condition.

The biopsychosocial model is also valuable in understanding the difference in incidence of hyperkinesis in the various studies which range from 1/2000 (Rutter, Graham, and Yule, 1970) to 5% (Miller, Palkes, and Stewart, 1973). This difference is partially explained by different criteria for making the diagnosis, but it is very likely that there is a different incidence of the condition in a more stable and cohesive community like that of the Isle of Wight than, for example a city slum.

My conclusions are that there is insufficient evidence at the present time for the existence of a syndrome or a disease entitled "Minimal Brain Dysfunction." Children generally classified under this rubric are a diverse group of children who should be classified into more homogeneous subgroups. While many children in these subgroups have an organic or constitutional etiology, the various biological, psychological, and social factors invariably interact to produce the specific symptomatology and the final adult outcome.

REFERENCES

Benton, A. L. "Minimal brain dysfunction from a neuropsychological point of view." *Annals of the New York Academy of Science*, 205, 29–37, (1973).

Bond, E., and L. H. Smith. "Post encephalitic behavior disorders—A 10-year review of the Franklin School." *American Journal of Psychiatry*, 92, 17–33, (1935).

Bradley, C. "The behavior of children receiving benzedrine." *American Journal of Psychiatry*, 94, 577–585, (1937).

Cantwell, D. "Psychiatric illness in the families of hyperactive children." *Archives of General Psychiatry*, 27, 414–417, (1972).

Clements, S. D., and J. E. Peters. "Minimal brain dysfunctions in the school-age child." *Archives of General Psychiatry*, 6, 185–197, (1962).

Clements, S. D. *Minimal Brain Dysfunction in Children*. NINDB, Monograph No. 3. Washington, D.C.: 1966.

Clemmens, R. L., and T. J. Kenny. "Clinical correlates of learning disabilities, minimal brain dysfunction and hyperactivity." *Clinical Pediatrics*, 11, 311–313, (1972).

Conners, C. K., C. M. Goyette, D. A. Southwick, J. M. Lees, and P. A. Andrulonis. "Food additives and hyperkinesis: A controlled double-blind experiment." *Pediatrics*, 58(2), 154–165 (1976).

Crook, W. G. "Food allergy—The great masquerador." *Pediatric Clinics of North America*, 22(1), 227–238, (1975).

Ebaugh, F. G. "Neuropsychiatric sequelae of acute epidemic encephalitis in children." *American Journal of Diseases of Children*, 25, 89–97, (1923).

Engel, G. C. "The need for a new medical model: A challenge for biomedicine." *Science*, 196 (4286), 129–136, (1977).

Goodwin, D., F. Schulsinger, L. Hermansen, J. Guze, and G. Winokur. "Alcoholism and the hyperactive child syndrome." *Journal of Nervous and Mental Diseases*, 160, 349–353, (1975).

Hohman, L. B. "Post-encephalitic behavior disorders in children." *Johns Hopkins Hospital Bulletin*, 33, 372–375, (1922).

Kahn, E., and L. H. Cohen. "Organic driveness: A brain stem syndrome and an experience." *New England Journal of Medicine*, 210, 748–756, (1934).

Kenny, T. J., R. L. Clemmens, B. W. Hudson, G. A. Lentz, R. Cicci, and P. Nair. "Characteristics of children referred because of hyperactivity." *The Journal of Pediatrics*, 79, 618–622, (1971).

Klein, D. F. and, R. Gittelman-Klein. "Problems in the diagnosis of minimal brain dysfunction and the hyperkinetic syndrome." *International Journal of Mental Health*, 4, 45–60, (1974).

Laufer, M. W., and E. Denhoff. "Hyperkinetic behavior syndrome in children." *Journal of Pediatrics*, 50(4), 463–474, (1957).

MacKeith, R. "Foreword: Minimal brain damage—A concept discarded." *Proceedings of the International Study Group on MBD.* Little Club Clinics in Developmental Medicine, No. 10. London: Heinemann, 1963.

Miller R., H. Palkes, and M. Stewart. "Hyperactive children in suburban elementary schools." *Child Psychiatry and Human Development,* 4, 121–127, (1973).

Paine, R. S., J. S. Werry, and H. C. Quay. "A study of minimal cerebral dysfunction." *Developmental Medicine and Child Neurology,* 10, 505–520, (1968).

Rodin, E., A. Lucas and C. Simpson. "A study of behavior disorders in children by means of general purpose computers," in *Data Acquisition and Processing in Biology and Medicine,* vol. 3, pp. 115–124. Proceedings of the 1963 Rochester Conference, New York: Pergamon, 1964.

Routh, D. K., and R. D. Roberts. "Minimal brain dysfunction in children: Failure to find evidence of a behavioral syndrome." *Psychological Reports,* 31, 307–314, (1972).

Rutter, M., P. Graham, and W. Yule. *A Neuropsychiatric Study in Childhood.* Spastics International Medical Publications. London: Heinemann, 1970.

Schulman, J. L., J. C. Kaspar, and F. M. Throne. *Brain Damage and Behavior: A Clinical Experimental Study.* Springfield, Ill.: Thomas, 1965.

Shaywitz, B. A., D. J. Cohen, and M. B. Bowers. "CSF monoamine metabolites in children with minimal brain dysfunction: Evidence for alteration of brain dopamine." *Journal of Pediatrics,* 90, 67–71, (1977).

Sprague, R. L. "Counting Jars of Raspberry Jam," in R. T. Anderson and C. G. Halcomb, ed., *Learning Disability/Minimal Brain Dysfunction Syndrome.* pp. 94–125. Springfield, Ill.: Thomas, 1976.

Strauss, A. A. and N. C. Kephart. *Psychopathology and Education of the Brain Injured Child,* vol. 1. New York: Grune & Stratton, 1948.

Strauss, A. A. and N. C. Kephart. *Psychopathology and Education of the Brain Injured Child,* vol. 2. New York: Grune & Stratton, 1955.

Weiss, G., L. Hechtman, T. Perlman, J. Hopkins, and A. Wener. "Hyperactives as young adults: A controlled prospective 10 year follow-up of the psychiatric status of 75 hyperactive children." *Archives of General Psychiatry,* 1978, in press.

Wender, P. H. *Minimal Brain Dysfunction in Children.* New York: Wiley, 1971.

———"Some speculations concerning a possible biochemical basis of minimal brain dysfunction." *Annals of the New York Academy of Science,* 205, 18–28, (1973a).

———"Minimal brain dysfunction in children: Diagnosis and management." *Pediatric Clinics of North America,* 20, 187–202 (1973b).

Werry, J. S. "Studies on the hyperactive child, IV: An empirical analysis of the minimal brain dysfunction syndrome." *Archives of General Psychiatry,* 19, 9–16, (1968).

Werry, J. S., K. Minde, A. Guzman, G. Weiss, K. Dogan, and E. Hoy. "Studies on the hyperactive child, VII: Neurological status compared with neurotic and normal children." *American Journal of Orthopsychiatry,* 42, 441–451, (1972).

Williams, I. J., and D. M. Cran. "Testing the Feingold diet for the management of hyperkinesis." (Paper presented at the Annual Meeting of the Canadian Psychiatric Association, Saskatoon, September 1977.)

CHAPTER 16

Psychological and Psychoeducational Assessment Techniques

Theodore H. Wohl

The editors have allowed an apparent redundancy to stand in the chapter title which the writer is pleased to exploit. In recent years there has been little reason to differentiate the terms psychological and psychoeducational when applied to children with minimal brain dysfunction. The latter has come to convey a broad spectrum of interrelated approach strategies utilized in diagnostic conceptualization and in programmatic remediation and therapy. No longer may academicians and experimentalists work in splendid isolation; they are, in a real sense, being induced to bring forth discoveries in psychophysiology, perception, memory, and cognition appealing directly to the professional or applied worker. They are generally aware of the literature relating to MBD and evidence much more interdisciplinary awareness of relevant discoveries and opinions. This contrasts sharply with the parallel research lines in medicine, psychology, and education stemming from the latter part of the nineteenth century. The present chapter is concerned with psychoeducational assessment as a major approach to diagnostic conceptualization. As already noted the term itself is a dynamic appellation applied to the whole child. It addresses itself not only to the identification and description of perceptual, integrative, and expressive functions, but also to etiology and ongoing flexible prognoses and treatment. It follows that those professionals implementing psychoeducational approaches are more likely to consider a wide variety of contributory data and to be more flexible in modifying remedial goals and techniques in view of the child's needs. This contrasts sharply with the doctrinaire approach of a few investigators and their lay followers who view deviations from certain implicit assumptions as a sin before the deity. More specifically this chapter will be concerned with a variety of techniques. They include assessment interviewing, intellectual and personality measurement, language and perceptual-motor testing, classroom adjustment surveys, behavioral or operant diagnosis-task analysis and orientation, and projective and psychodynamic evaluation.

Chapter 18, "Other Assessment Techniques," is isolated from the psychoeducation approaches with considerable presumption. It includes assessment approaches more classifiable under what Bateman (1966-1967) has termed an etiologic diagnostic approach based on more narrowly focused investigations and which purport to identify causal factors underlying minimal brain dysfunction. Language, visual, and auditory assessments frequently *do* lead towards more precise treatment or teaching. They are however most often accomplished outside of the context of the educational establishment by professionals and scientists

362

who are not intimately involved in the day-to-day diagnosis and teaching of the MBD child. To the extent that these approaches are integrated within a special or general education program, they become part of the psychoeducational strategy. The current field contains a number of models or approaches which may provide a general framework permitting the reader to integrate better the divergent views besetting him. The writer has frequently utilized either the three approaches of Bateman (1966-1967), that is etiologic, diagnostic-remedial, and task analysis, or Hewett's (1968) psychodynamic-interpersonal, sensory-neurological, and behavioral modification strategies. A more recent model has been advanced by Johnson and Morasky (1977) oriented toward what seems to them "basis emphases in theories and approaches." This illustrates the shifts of emphases among current writers from theoretical and etiologic concerns to utilitarian problems of diagnosis, remediation, and the delivery of adequate services. Each approach or technique discussed in this chapter may be viewed as dimensional continuum along which one can locate interacting nodal points representing the MBD child and his problems.

DIAGNOSTIC CONSIDERATIONS

Educators, behavioral clinicians, and the full array of nonmedical therapists often make the wistful observation that their medical colleagues are blessed with a diagnostic system in which given causes have regular and predictable effects. Clinical medical procedures have evolved over the last few centuries which allow unique classification of the patient on the basis of symptom patterns usually coexistent with a specific microorganism, structural or functional defect, or chromosomal aberration. This would lead easily to a more or less predictable sequence of prognosis and treatment. Such an approach however cannot be applied effectively to the problems of minimal brain dysfunction.

We are bereft of known test patterns; questionnaires; rating scales; or physiologic, psychologic, and social measures which can be said to be *certainly* diagnostic of *any* given underlying condition. Even when the source of lesion underlying MBD is known, one cannot surely predict its manifestation in thinking and behavior. Children with grossly similar patterns of learning deficit may develop strikingly dissimilar life- and task-coping strategies. The medical-etiologic approach is probably a feasible way of organizing and integrating disparate data available about MBD, but may obscure the fact that genetic, physical, and psychological components exist not in isolation, but in constant interaction with one another. Most children classified as MBD *cannot* be assigned to any particular symptom category. The syndrome identification or arrival at a diagnostic label should not be regarded as the main goal concerning the MBD individual. In the psychoeducational realm, in particular, a system is greatly needed which will permit the orderly description of each child on a large number of different dimensions: perceptual, intellectual, motivational, interpersonal, and so on. The beginnings of such a system may be embodied in the current American Association of Mental Deficiencies classification scheme (Heber, 1959, 1961) which stresses current functional impairment, the rating and complete description of seven major subcategories of development, and places relatively less emphasis on etiologic factors. It is still a matter of some disagreement among researchers and clinicians whether to study each individual in his own terms (idiographic philosophy) or whether the greatest value lies in discovering generalized laws which are applied to all human behavior (nomothetic philosophy). The latter approach does form a recognizable basis for psychoeducational assessment since it attempts to identify and describe the individual's perceptual, integrative, and expressive functioning eventuating in a diagnostic label. The classification may suggest that a particular deficit is indeed causing the manifest problems of the child. The identification of a cause in one person leads to the fallacious assumption that the identical deficit may be the causal factor in another individual. This may result in a disregard of other important data about the individual and his diagnosis.

The above observations suggest caution. Yet there is a pressing need for psychoeducational assessment and potentially constructive applications to the MBD problem. Bateman (1966-1967) notes the relationship of assessment data to the how and what of teaching. The teacher is committed to the synthesis of the test data and active interaction with the child. Kessler (1971) has noted that psychoeducational assessment provides an opportunity for interaction and utilization of clinical experience and intuition in discovering what a child is thinking or feeling. Kessler further alludes to a "descriptive phenomenology." She emphasizes the difficulty in obtaining necessary data from which concepts and principles can be induced for logical classification. She argues compellingly for more behavioral analysis and observational data to be integrated and related to plans helpful to the professional.

Currently investigators and professionals alike are preoccupied with questions of validity and reliability relating to all assessment instruments and measures. The measurer and measuring instrument are difficult to separate. An interpretation of results is often predicated on the manner in which original standardized instructions are followed, on knowledge of scoring criteria, on general interpretation of the infinite varieties of specific test behaviors, on the solicitation of top motivation, and on adequate attention to the qualitative as well as quantitative aspects of a child's response (Wohl, 1978). All psychoeducational approaches are designed to reduce the tremendous burden on the interviewer or examiner as a recording or evaluating instrument. The success of these approaches may very well depend on the adequacy of standardization of both materials and methods yielding:

1. Satisfactory criteria of adequacy.

2. Assessment of the representativeness or typical aspect of test behavior.

3. Care in selecting the normative populations so that the child's behavior can be compared to a representative sampling of his peers.

The validity of an assessment is limited to the decision that must be made. Great caution must be used in generalizing the results of certain measures to questions and populations lying outside the primary purview of the test.

Comprehensive subsequent interventions and prognoses should be built on a foundation of thorough and extensive evaluation of the MBD child. Kessler (1971) has argued for a "working diagnosis" which may be modified frequently in view of the child's status. The development of proper criteria (that is improvement in areas such as reading, writing, and speaking) can only help the professional to focus his efforts. All of this does not denigrate the view of the child as a complex totality rather than as a collection of discrete and isolated functions.

EDUCATION AND SPECIAL EDUCATION

Despite the awareness that only a multidisciplinary approach will allow adequate measurement of the varying parameters of MBD as manifest in the individual child, the applications lie primarily within the educational arena. The child manifests a learning deficit and all types of professional efforts seem directed toward the more optimal achievement of educationally related goals. The special educator in particular provides the interface between the MBD child and the broad array of interdisciplinary conceptualizers. On the firing line, so to speak, the special educator is the principal trainer of specialists within the field. By his efforts he produces a continuous data pool which probably should be more effectively utilized. Currently educators are much more interested in function than structure. It is probably correct to state that most educators would proceed with a diagnosis and remediation plan, frequently without the input of more etiologic diagnostic statements from medicine or psychology. Johnson and Morasky (1977) have postulated discriminatively different facets of the learning-disability problem. These are developmental status, basic processes, deficit behaviors, assessment, and management. The involved professionals, preoccupied with educational relevance, stress principally the assessment and management emphases.

Clinical Methodology

From the early child biographers of the last century through the inception and influence of early child guidance clinic movements at the beginning of this century, clinical method and judgment has pervaded work with the individual child and his family. Lerner (1971) observes that a teaching plan results from a sequence of four prior steps of the diagnostic process:

1) determine whether the child has a learning disability, 2) measure the child's present achievement, 3) analyze how the child learns, explore why he is not learning, and 4) collate and interpret data and formulate a diagnostic hypothesis.

Implicit is the assumption that any teaching plan is modifiable in view of the continuous accumulation of data. Truax and Carkhuff's (1967) well-known compilation and analysis of counseling and psychotherapy cite the three basic ingredients for the successful therapist. These are accurate empathy, nonpossessive warmth, and genuineness. It is likely that these are essential for the successful interviewer as well. Despite the universality of the interview, it seems to have lost ground in recent years before the plethora of scales and tests. It is still the most flexible and perhaps indispensable means of developing a case or educational history replete with information and clues about a child's physical, social, and educational background. The astute interviewer will modify his style in deference to the characteristics of the interviewee. He will strive to obtain correct identifying data and a clear statement of the problems of the child: as the child perceives it, as the family perceives it, and even as the interviewer himself perceives it. A careful description of each of the child's maladaptive behaviors must be obtained: when they were first noticed, whether they are persistent or sporadic, their severity, the circumstances that influence each behavior for better or worse, and their effect on the child's life and on significant others of his environment. What are the specific and general environmental circumstances in which maladaptive behaviors evolve? What is the child's concept of himself, his attitudes towards his educational problems and any possible secondary gain? Does the child have any sense of needing help? The child's history may contain information about early genetic, familial, economic, and social influences impinging on the child throughout his life. The child after all is born in a milieu which will provide the peculiar cultural, sociological, and familial value systems through which he interprets the world and his educational tasks. It is therefore important to have a detailed picture of the parents and siblings with whom the child lives. The personal history of the child is really a developmental analogue of his maturation and the interviewer must be thoroughly familiar with the range of typical behavior displayed by children of various ages, intelligence, and socioeconomic levels in interview settings.

Behavioral observation helps the evaluator to obtain a cross-section view of the child as he appears to the evaluator, the parents, and other significant people in his environment. An extensive description might include general appearance, manner and attitude, associations and thought processes, affect and mood, thought content, sensorium, and cognitive functions. The noneducator will probably utilize one or another variety of mental status exams. The educator and the school psychologist may have at their disposal a number of brief, nonstandardized approaches, such as the guidelines for information techniques offered by Smith and Neisworth (1969), and various pupil rating scales, for example the Northwestern University research project (Myklebust and Boshes, 1969), classroom studies from Bryan and Wheeler (1972), Shedd's (1967) collation of behavioral characteristics of dyslexic children, and Royal's (1973) listing of performance and criterion reference objectives developed for young preschoolers in the area of reading.

Despite the central importance of interviewing in the diagnostic approach, there has been relatively little research on reliability or validity of the interview or other informal means of behavioral description. Representative studies such as Beck, et al. (1962) indicates that diagnostic classifications made from psychiatric interviews usually are not reliable. A series of more systematic studies reported by Rutter and Graham (1968) found that gross agreement relating to the question of psychiatric versus no psychiatric abnormality could be obtained between raters but there is much lower agreement for specific items on the rating scale. They noticed that overall reliability appeared to be highest when normal children were interviewed but reliability decreased in direct proportion to the degree of disturbance in the children.

Formal Standardized Methods

Inevitably the individual general intelligence test is a major part of any psycho-educational assessment. The Wechsler Intelligence Scale for Children (WISC) revised edition and the Stanford-Binet Intelligence Scale are two commonly used global tests. Both may be considered examples of Spearman's "g" factor theory, that is, the various tests and subtests contain varying amounts of a basic intelligence factor. However both tests can also be conceptualized as measuring different kinds of intelligence and being broad enough to tap a multiplicity of variables related to thinking and learning. Although these tests have been reduced by mathematical means to a few basic elements, they do not fulfill the need of the practitioner to break these elements down to specific perceptual and cognitive abilities which bear a direct relationship to learning and classroom achievement.

A major approach to meet this need has been the Illinois Test of Psycholinguistic Abilities (ITPA) in both its original experimental and revised form (Kirk, McCarthy, and Kirk, 1968). The test is based on a model for language-communication behaviors largely developed by Osgood (1953, 1957), which postulates two progressively complex levels of language behavior—the automatic and representational; three major processes—decoding, encoding, and association of symbolic material; and three different channels—visual, auditory, and haptic. The scale includes twelve subtests sampling behavior representing all of the interactions on all of the previously mentioned dimensions. The test has suffered severe criticism about its use of the term psycholinguistic (Carrol 1972). It does not after all yield detailed information pertinent to the way in which individuals acquire and use language systems, and over half of the subtests do not seem concerned with language at all. Earlier criticisms (Weiner, Barritt, and Semmel, 1967) relating to low reliability and intercorrelations of the subscales of the experimental test edition have given way to more serious concern regarding the restrictive normative sampling and doubtful validity of the tests or subscales when used with lower socioeconomic groups. Despite a large number of attempts, only a few relevant factor analytic studies have been completed with only minimum support for the validity of the ITPA model. Probably the ultimate validity will be proven by use. Evidently the test constitutes a major line of assessment in the armamentarium of the educator who assists in the delineation of deficit areas and it is being included in programs of remediation (Wiseman, 1970). However before one can draw direct inferences from the criterion behaviors on the test to appropriate specific remedial techniques, considerably more data will have to be accumulated.

Another major criticism of the ITPA as an approach to MBD is that it is limited to predominantly language-type behaviors. By the same token, the Developmental Test of Visual Perception (DTVP) is an assessment model purporting to deal predominantly with visual perception (Frostig and Horn 1964; Frostig, 1963, 1966a, 1966b). An outgrowth of the founding and operation of the Mary Ann Frostig Center for Educational Therapy in Los Angeles, it purports to measure five areas which are predominantly visual-perceptual:

1. Eye-motor coordination
2. Figure ground
3. Form constancy
4. Position and space
5. Spatial relations

These areas were probably selected because pragmatically they are early and frequent areas of deficit behavior in MBD children. The DTVP yields both a perceptual quotient (PQ) and a perceptual age (PA) that is an estimate of the developmental level which may be compared to chronological age for interpretation. It also makes a close transition to an instructional-remedial program (the Frostig-Horn), but there is a lack of data as to whether this results in specific translation to remedial activity and whether gain in some exterior criterion measures, such as reading, can be attributed specifically to the remedial program. Various factor-analytic studies (Silverstein, 1965; Ward, 1970) have shown a lack of independence among the subtests of the DTVP standardized on a predominantly middle class population. The monograph for the test does not contain adequate information on validity or for prediction of school achievement on older children. Mann (1972) notes in summary that the DTVP does not appear to be able to assess specific areas of perception differentially, but it is noted that the amalgam of subtests as represented by the PQ has a reasonable reliability and predictive powers for subsequent achievement. Both Kephart (1971) and Mann (1972) caution against uncritical use of this test in assessing preacademic basic learning skills which are presumed to determine later learning and academic achievement. Kephart notes the danger of uncritical use of Frostig materials by inadequately trained personnel. He opines that such fractionalization of the program is manifestly contrary to the author's intent. Indeed Mann and Phillips (1967) made an early attempt to highlight the inappropriate attention directed toward the dysfunctions themselves, frequently disregarding the child as a complex interacting organism. Some 13 years later the authors' warnings that tests with limited empirical substantiation are determining the type of remediation employed and even leading to professional and faculty training have a remarkably contemporary ring. Underachievers are still being trained to manage their bodies, to discriminate words more efficiently, and to perceive embedded figures more accurately, even though they do not make significant *reading* progress. Thus the original diagnosis and training give rise to the problem. Both the ITPA and the DTVP have been criticized as not measuring what they purport to measure and as really yielding only measures of poorly delineated cognitive functions similar to those measured by the Binet or WISC (Carroll, 1972; Mann, 1972). Yet these tests and others continue to be enthusiastically employed, yielding copious data which are probably underutilized for accountability purposes.

The (PPMS) Purdue Perceptual-Motor Survey (Roach and Kephart, 1962) follows in the tradition of a series of tests presented by Kephart (1971) in *The Slow Learner in the Classroom.* The test enables the examiner to identify children who lack the preceptual-motor readiness skills necessary for academic progress. It is unclear what attainment levels of the scale are normally achieved by certain age groupings. The subtests are inherently interesting; seem to have face validity; and measure a range of abilities, some of which seem to tap simple sensory motor processes and other more cognitive functions. Despite the ease of administration, the survey cannot insure that interexaminer differences and occasional ambiguity in directions will not seriously decrease the reliability of the survey. The manual of the test gives little information; certainly the examiner (usually the classroom teacher) has no way of appreciating the wealth of clinical observation and rich theorizing that forms the foundation of the survey. Kephart states that every normal child establishes an adequate orientation to the basic realities of the universe, space, and time. But in a significant percentage of children accidents occur during the developmental period and the effect of these accidents is to interfere with the establishment of a stable perceptual-motor world. These theories draw from such sources as Sherrington, Gesell, Piaget, Hebb, and Strauss and lead the serious reader to the study of the principles of development in general as well as the principles of the development of motor skills and motor patterns. They show how a cognitive awareness of the surrounding world emerges from the data obtained by a well-developed motor exploratory system, concepts of sensory and organ development, the perceptual-motor "match," the development of the visual world duplicating motor world, and the fusion of all this with the time dimension. Kephart made the point that the MBD child's orientation to the surrounding physical universe is atypical. He asked for greater attention to a child's *methods* in dealing with his world rather than simply consideration of whether or not a task is performed successfully. The PPMS, at its present stage of development, probably can assist the teacher in identifying both skill deficits and the faulty generalization of these skills to other situations. However more effort is needed to establish norms once test directions have been clarified to render the survey method more consistent with Kephart's theorizing.

Robert Valett's (1967) Developmental Survey of Basic Learning Abilities and his psychoeducational resource programs are best described as an overall programmatic or systems approach to psychoeducational growth. The developmental survey presents operational definitions of gross-motor development, sensory-motor integration, perceptual-motor skills, language development, conceptual skills, and social skills. These six areas are further subdivided into 53 separate tasks. A broad rationale as well as a justification for the selection of items and any subsequent inferences are provided the psychologist, educator, and teacher. The author devises some of the items on the basis of past experience but prominently borrows from such sources as Terman, Wechsler, Gesell, and Kephart. Not infrequently some items selected from reputable test batteries such as the Stanford–Binet are arbitrarily used and interpreted out of context. Valett (1967) offers little or no information on validity or reliability and little explanation of the appropriateness of item placement by age level. In fact his survey has been criticized as being in violation of the standards for educational psychological tests and manuals of the American Psychological Association (Rutte, 1972). Valett has ambitiously provided a tempting package for psychologists and kindergarten and elementary school teachers. He provides a format for establishing operationally defined goals and devising relevant educational programming techniques utilizing attractive workbooks and materials. He even considers nuts-and-bolts factors, such as classroom organization and scheduling needs. All of this may be an excellent example of the current American merchandising ideal. Indefatigably he presents normative and clinical data and step-by-step planning for use in education and grouping. This approach has worked well in industry and seems widely employed in general education in this country today. It is not surprising that Valett's work has been classified as fitting the management paradigm of psychoeducational assessment practices.

The reader should briefly consider several more typical formal standardized methods of psychoeducational assessment. This is not an extensive review, but it should nonetheless convey the current flavor of diagnostic efforts.

The Predictive Index (Hirsch, Jansky, and Langford, 1966) consists of a large battery of tests administered to kindergarten children. Best predictive measures of children in the second grade experiencing academic problems were further expanded by Trimble (1970) and published as a revised predictive index. It is viewed as a useful screening device for predicting reading problems of children completing the first grade.

The Pupil Rating Scale (Myklebust, 1969) consists of screening techniques presumably linked to learning disabilities developed as part of the comprehensive study which attempted to determine both medical and psychological correelates of learning disability. Subsequent studies of validity and factor structure have supported the validity and reliability of this scale in detecting learning problems.

The Peabody Picture Vocabulary Test (PPVT) can be individually or group administered (Dunn, 1959). Designed initially for use with handicapped children who might have difficulty with verbal responses to test items, it is quick and easy to score despite relatively high correlations with the WISC and Stanford-Binet, it almost certainly does not measure similar kinds of intellectual functioning. Primarily it seems to be a measure of verbal comprehension of single words.

The Bender Visual-Motor Gestalt Test (1938) is a brief test originally developed to assess brain injury in adults, but it is now used in a wide variety of clinical and educational assessments of children. Koppitz (1964) has provided procedures and normative information for use of the test with children between ages of 5 and 11. She has presented data correlating children's scores on the test with performance on other intelligence, reading, and achievement tests. Although the test correlates positively with certain psychopathologic classifications of children, the high frequency of false positives and false negatives should restrain the professional from attempting to make uncritical inferences from this kind of data.

The Developmental Test of Visual-Motor Integration (Beery and Buktenica 1967) is another brief test consisting of 24 geometric forms presented in ascending difficulty suitable for children ages 2 through 15. The child is required to copy each from within the provided test booklet space. Specific format directions allow more precise and reliable scoring.

Auditory Discrimination Tests (Wepman 1958) were designed to measure the ability of children five to eight years of age to discriminate between pairs of spoken words. There are norms, but the child must be able to understand the concepts of "same" or "not the same." It is quickly administered and scored but may not be sensitive to cultural differences nor can it differentiate between an auditory perceptual and discriminative deficit by itself.

The Northwestern Syntax Screening Test (Lee 1970) is a narrow spectrum test which assesses essentially a single language area: syntax. Usually administered to children who manifest delayed syntactical skills, it measures both the receptive and expressive use of language. Sampling is inadequate and unrepresentative.

The Wide Range Achievement Test, revised edition (Jastac and Jastac 1965) is a widely used screening achievement test that provides scores in three subtests: reading (word recognition), spelling, and arithmetic. It seems useful in diagnosing disabilities in these areas and in estimating intelligence. This is probably attributable to the sensitivity and experience of the examiner rather than the properties of the test. Merwin (1972) has noted a paucity of information about the sample and sampling procedures and questions are raised concerning test reliability and validity.

The Peabody Individual Achievement Test (PIAT) assesses achievement in reading recognition, reading comprehension, spelling, general information, and mathematics (Dunn and Markwardt, 1970). Applicable to individuals from preschool to adulthood, it is quickly administered, easily scored, and has been widely standardized. The manual is specific in providing the consumer with precise information relating to reliability and validity. It is primarily useful as a rough estimate of educational achievement and points to where more intensive assessment might be needed.

Various reading tests are widely used in general and special education with reference to all forms of achievement, underachievement, and learning problems. They may be conceptualized generally as survey or diagnostic. The latter attempts to analyze the processes by which children read and leads directly to remedial planning. The former generally yields only the level at which a child reads and may indicate his position within his group. A few of the many published tests in this area are: the Gates-MacGinitie Reading Tests (1965), the Gates-McKillop Reading Diagnostic Tests (1962), the Gray Oral Reading Test (1962), the Stanford-Binet Achievement Test: Reading (1965), the Metropolitan Achievement Test: Reading Test (1971), the SRA Achievement Scales: Reading (1963), the Durrell Analysis of Reading Difficulty (1955), the Roswell-Chall Diagnostic Reading Test of Word Analysis Skills (1964). These tests vary somewhat in length, clarity of instructions, utility of scores, relevance of measurement areas, and in coverage in the manual of information regarding sampling, reliability, and validity. Apparently they have been found diagnostically useful and are widely adopted.

Illustrative Findings

Accurate and enlightened assessment should have much to do with educational policy and the future of special education programs. Methods of evaluation help in making decisions on administrative priorities and the allocation of funds for the identification of remediation goals, teaching approaches, programmatic variables, and matters having to do with the effectiveness of a total program for the MBD child. It is a matter of some disappointment that parents, lawmakers, and educators alike seem to be satisfied with placebo programs which apparently totally ignore the research evidence relating to them. Several interesting but unintegrated studies are cited as representative of the flood of research occurring during the seventies. Silberberg (1969) has cynically observed that,

Rather than serving as a basis on which carefully conceived educational programs are constructed, such research often functions as a rationalization invented after the fact for educational programs popular with teachers and administrators.

Silver and Hagan (1968) culminated a long series of neurologic, perceptual, and educational evaluations with the observation that a deficit in any modality influences overall effectiveness of mental function. They addressed teaching effort to specific deficit areas revealed by perceptual profiles.

A recent program evaluation report by Proger (1975) provided the results of new Stanford Achievement Test administrations in four Pennsylvania programs for physically handicapped, emotionally disturbed, minimally brain injured, and learning-disabled children. The study attempted to establish realistic expectancy levels of performance for children at various abilities and levels within each program. Results are reported showing patterns of gain ranging from less than half a year to somewhat less than a full year for each year of instruction. Reiss (1975) provided an evaluation report of a special education program in New York City designed to improve the reading and arithmetic skills of brain-injured children in mainstream classes, grades 1 through 8. He studied the extent to which the actual program coincided with the proposed program and found that children in grades 1 to 4 achieved statistically significant improvement in both reading and mathematics. A combination of careful assessments and observations indicated that the program operated essentially as described in the proposal. Badian (1975) screened 300 kindergarten children with a battery of tests (including the Draw-A-Man Test, Metropolitan Readiness Test, and Primary Mental Abilities Test) to identify high-risk children. He selected children according to the general principle of discrepancy between achievement and potential. At the *beginning* of grade one, they were tested with the Wechsler Adult Intelligence abilities. At the *end* of grade one, these high-risk children scored within *the average range* on the Metropolitan Achievement Test indicating that selection criteria in kindergarten were woefully inadequate. Whitehead (1973) attempted to determine the effectiveness of a method of screening children early in their school careers, to identify potential learning disabled students. The experimental index was designed to accomplish this and attempted to quantify all observations and judgments of kindergarten teachers concerning each pupil. Two hypotheses were made: (1) that certain behaviors of subjects of kindergarten level, recorded by their teachers on a cumulative record and quantified on the experimental index, will discriminate between the learning-disabled group and a normally achieving group, and (2) that there will be an inverse relationship between the kindergarten experimental index and the composite Stanford Achievement Test scores obtained at the end of the fifth grade. The obtained results demonstrated that, utilizing teacher observations, learning-disabled students can be identified at the kindergarten level and that kindergarten experimental index scores do discriminate between learning-disabled and normally achieving students as measured by their composite Stanford Achievement Test scores at the end of the fifth grade.

PSYCHOEDUCATIONAL ASSESSMENT CONTRIBUTIONS OF ACADEME

Current work in psychophysiology, perception, memory, and cognition might well provide the basis for the ultimate understanding and effective remediation of the multifaceted problems of the MBD child. These findings stem from narrowly focused investigations couched in the formidable terminology and frequent statistical complexity of science. Many findings would be of great help in psychoeducational assessment as utilized within psychology and education. Basic research in neurophysiology and neuropsychology has recently advanced more carefully delineated patterns of brain and behavior relationships that typify the MBD child. This will be discussed in a later chapter. Use of mathematical approaches, experimental methodology applied to the reading process, and experimentation with isomorphic brain and perceptual functions typify current academic research efforts of immediate use to the applied scientist. De Ruiter (1974) studied a group of psychometric instruments which were selected to measure a set of component disabilities described as "highly diagnostic" for MBD. These instruments were used with two matched groups consisting of 25 MBD children and 25 normal achievers. The efficiency and effectiveness of all identification procedures based on tests were studied through a comparison of Bayesian techniques and discriminate analysis. Both approaches were equally effective for identification of MBD, but Bayesian procedures were easier to compute and permitted the use of a varied number or set of tests within a given comparison. Both types of analysis correctly classified from 88 to 100% of the samples correctly using sets of 2 to 17 variables. It would seem that this type of investigation would assist greatly in specific identification procedures which might be useful for cross-validation studies and in school conferences for making decisions about placement in learning disability classrooms.

The work and conceptualizations of Gibson (1966; Gibson and Shepela 1968;

Gibson, et. al., 1963) seem most exemplary in translating the data of the scientific laboratory to the applied classroom setting. Referring to a 1959 research project grant to Cornell University by HEW, she empirically fashioned an "experimental psychology of learning to read." This simple but classic work traced the young child's evolving ability to differentiate graphic symbols and to decode gross patterns into the processing of higher order units, spelling, and morphological patterns of language. All this is described in great detail. Gibson propounded the conviction that good teaching is based only on a deep understanding of the subject to be taught and the nature of the learning process involved. When one analyzes the discriminating, decoding, semantic, and syntactical aspects of the reading task together with the thorough analysis of the learning process, he is in a much better position to know what must be learned and how it must be learned—only then can formal instruction be devised. Gibson and Levin (1975) culminated a series of theoretically based reading research studies by proposing a coordinated theory of how one learns to read. It is an attempt to overcome 40 years of experimental psychological indifference to the area of reading by painstakingly developing concepts best indicated from the book's chapter headings:

- A Theory of Perceptual Learning and Its Relevance for Understanding Reading.
- The Development of Cognitive Strategies.
- Linguistic Concepts Necessary to Study Reading. Language Development. Writing Systems.
- An Application of Basic Concepts Relating to Word Perceptions.

The reader is led by the hand, so to speak, along the bothersome terrain of the study of reading. He is tutored in the development of prereading skills and led into an experimental phenomenology of the beginning-to-read process, and then on to the transition to skilled reading, learning from reading, and models of the reading process in the mature reader. The authors demonstrate the value of theory-based research on how a child learns to read. Nearly always there is dependence on laboratory experimentation. Representative of the rich data contained in this book is the information regarding trends in perceptual development. Learned material includes distinctive features of things as well as coded symbolic material in various relations to events and structure (both superordinate and subordinate), which may also be thought of as higher order relations and rules. Processes involved include: ignoring irrelevant information, adaptive use of peripheral sense-organ adjustments, and perhaps reinforcement by discovery of structure and reduction of uncertainty. Relying on empirical investigation, the authors do not forgo generalizations. It is clear that reading is above all an adaptive process. It is a flexible processing combination of strategies that continually change to meet the demands of the text and the purpose of the reader. A second major principle is the tendency toward increased economy in the adult reader. According to Gibson and Levin (1975) economic processing of textual material is accomplished in four ways:

1. By selecting relevant information.
2. By ignoring irrelevant information.
3. By processing the largest units that are appropriate for the task.
4. By processing the least amount of information compatible with the task.

It is important to reemphasize the fact that recent years have witnessed an increased rapprochement between basic and applied scientists regarding reading research and an overall view of perceptual and cognitive learning development. Kershner (1970) iterated an isomorphism between cognitive functioning and central brain processes requiring a multidisciplinary theory. He felt that the pioneering work of Piaget deserved special mention, pointing to the fact that the central processes characterizing reading are best conceptualized as active, problem solving, and integrative. Utilizing a complex apparatus consisting of figures, tracks, and mirrors, he created four field configurations, each of which was presented to a child. The value of this approach as psychoeducational assessment lies in its emphasis on the primacy of central processes rather than on the importance of figurative or absolute spatial dimensions. It was noted that the visual-imagery strategy was not significantly influenced by verbal knowledge of direction or motor participation, but that certain laterality effects were obtained. The author interpreted this finding as consistent with recent neurophysiological evidence attesting to the asymmetrical functioning of the cerebral hemispheres with regard to the kinds of information each stores and processes. In her systematic attempt to devise an experimental psychology of reading, Gibson (1975) utilized and devised many and varied instruments and techniques which possess psychoeducational usefulness. By employing a standard laboratory memory drum, Gibson, et al. (1963) used a matching-judgments method involving letters with four-year-old children. A visual discrimination task was later employed by Gibson, Shapiro, and Yonas (1968). Two letters were simultaneously exposed by projection on a small screen. An index and error count was obtained as was a measure of latency to indicate the sameness or differences of the projected figures.

Methods of identifying and measuring processes by which the child selects or differentiates distinctive features from the omnipresent surrounding stimuli are extensively treated by Gibson. She cites Lehman's (1972) experiment in which kindergarten and second- and fourth-grade children, were asked to match objects differing in at least two properties from a standard. He was able to show a developmental trend in the children's search strategies, in their being able to extract and notice a distinguishing variable and to ignore irrelevant cures. Dichotic listening techniques were utilized by Maccoby (1967) with kindergarten and second- and fourth-grade students. A child is required to listen to a man's and a woman's voice, each of whom speaks a different word at the same time. The subject is then asked to report the word spoken by only one of the voices. Gibson (1975) reports an improvement with age in the ability to report correctly the word spoken by the asked-for voice and a progressive decline in the number of intrusion errors, that is reporting the word spoken by the voice that was to be ignored. Gibson (1975) states that in the case of graphic shapes (or letters) differing from one another only slightly, "an increase in specificity of correspondence between discrimination and stimulus information is critical for the development of reading skill." Gibson, et al. (1962) developed a set of graphic forms similar to Roman capital letters and possessing the kinds of transformations that were considered to give children either minimal or maximal problems. Some transformations (for example, straight into curve, open into closed) are considered critical for distinguishing letters. The forms were put on small cards and the subjects were asked to compare a standard form with each of its transformations and to select only exact copies of the standard. The subjects matched for 12 different standards, each with all 12 transformations. It is noted that the children were progressively increasing the specificity of their discrimination in accordance with changes in the stimulus. Analysis of errors was accomplished and curves by age group were computed for at least four classes of transformations. The present author is convinced that the experimental techniques and instrumentation presented in this section are potentially useful and relevant psychoeducational assessment methods that can be related to school achievement and remedial approaches in a highly relevant and specific manner. Further they constitute tangible evidence that the scientific method can facilitate a true collaboration between basic and applied science.

PROJECTIVE AND PSYCHODYNAMIC ASSESSMENT

This section deals with subject matter classifiable under the diagnostic remedial approach of Bateman (1966-1967). The goal of projective testing and psychodynamic diagnosis is to provide information that will lead to specific and appropriate treatment. It is of increasing concern that diagnostic procedures of this sort should so frequently go beyond totally objective gathering of data. When contrasted with previous methodology, which seemed preoccupied with measurement and quantification (for example a child might be located in a particular developmental sequence or scale), the current approach places much more emphasis on the individual child.

This approach received impetus from the early emphases by anatomists and pediatricians on the broad implications of configurations rather than narrowing attention to absolute norms. By direct measurement of bodily contours, angles, and proportions, they came to the conclusion that children of the same chronological age differed in bodily dimensions and capacity for physical performance. These findings tended to fuse with the early twentieth-century influence of child guidance clinics, wherein for the first time physicians, psychologists, and social workers began to be concerned with *individuals* who could not meet the expectations of society or their parents. They propounded the notion that an individual was truly unique and had a unique history with important implications for diagnosis. They wielded the clinical method as a mighty weapon, insisting that all techniques and approaches are relative, and they then insisted that the use of all instruments, norms, and techniques be ordered in the idiosyncratic frame of reference of the individual. Needless to say this approach is roundly criticized today as introducing an element of uncontrolled subjective judgment. It is said that the helping professional often cannot adequately describe how he arrived at a diagnosis and that the weights assigned to certain clinical findings may be arbitrary. On the other hand these assessments were often *highly controlled* and often a product of many years of experience and heightened sensitivity. After all a neurosurgeon or an orchestra conductor cannot with certainty describe all of the intricate movements of fingers or baton which may achieve a complex effect. Professionals began to appreciate that their precise measurements are always subject to modification in the light of case history and clinical interview material. The psychodynamically oriented clinician attempts to deal with the MBD child as an active, grappling, and aggressively coping organism, rather than as a passive recipient of environmental stimuli or a carrier of certain traits and characteristics. The personality is viewed as an open system in a state of internal flux, but in direct homeostatic interaction with the external world. This is suggestive of Lennenberg's (1951) earlier opinion that it is extremely difficult to suppress language development and that maturation gives language a self-propelling quality.

Hewett (1968) stressed the

> high priority . . . to understanding psychological causal factors and the development of a positive trusting relationship between adult and child and formal educational training.

Certainly psychodynamic theory has influenced special education approaches to the MBD child. Teachers have been directing more than passing attention to the why of a reading problem, consideration of feeling states, and interpersonal relationships both at school and at home. However there has probably been more of an attempt to help teachers cope with a disturbed child six hours a day, thereby establishing a more optimal climate for learning. The intensive training and quasi-therapist role required for this emphasis has "not produced a truly translatable strategy for the typical classroom" (Hewett, 1968). Thus the contribution to assessment and amelioration of MBD is provided more in the forms of publications, interprofessional meetings, and probably most pertinently through direct consultation among school psychology, clinical psychology, and psychiatry. The consultant may lessen the reliance on tests and measurements. Kessler (1966) has already indicated the tremendous advantages of testing as an opportunity for verbal interaction and noted that clinical experience and intuition may be the optimal means of finding out what a child is thinking or feeling. She even suggests simply asking or guessing. Berlin (1975) describes the development of mental health consultation as a direct method based on the development of a collegial relationship between the consultant and the educator, which introduces new sources of data and helps the educator change as the student develops. The effect of the consultation process is almost to compel one to collect data from many sources and to stress pertinent observation as a means of ascertaining the context of a specific behavioral problem. This is followed by the phase of hypothesis generation where various empirical hypotheses followed by interventions are scrutinized and continually revised. As a means of psychoeducational assessment, the consultation paradigm may enhance the educator's involvement in the nonjudgmental evaluation process, focus attention on the more relevant aspects of the educational day, and stress the poorly understood and very important role of the affective aspects of education, that is emotional expression in every aspect of learning. The reciprocal relationship between family setting and child-school functioning as well as the interaction between psychological and somatic factors demonstrate an increasing role for the consultant who can couch his diagnostic observation in a manner that will fit the use of specific remedial and modification techniques. Parents and teachers who realistically understand the role of maturational factors, of family disturbance, the meaning of poor self-concept, and the depressing and disruptive effect of constant failure, are better able to cope with their children's special problems as well as their own lives.

Certain conceptions and assumptions have influenced the diagnostic posture of the dynamically oriented consultant. The professional recognizes that: (1) there is a classification of school problems whose deficit patterns result from organic brain dysfunction and that (2) there is another major category in which family interactions and individual emotional reactions have produced neurotic processes as well as attitudinal and motivational problems relating to the various aspects of the learning process. This conceptualization has progressed beyond the early analytic speculation that there was a symbolic relationship between a learning problem and type of symptomatology (Hawke, 1966). Poor reading for example was attributed to a child's repressing and inhibiting visual "looking behavior" in response to anxiety aroused by having witnessed parental sexual activity. Current concepts seem to center more on the fact that in his inability or refusal to learn at school, a child is defending himself against the potential results of expression of his own impulse life. The conflicts then inhibit or may block the various aspects of learning and interfere with growing up. A displacement of anger and anxiety to the school-learning situation may generally enable children to function without disruptive anxiety. Constant failure may serve both as moderate punishment to the child and as a form of hostile reproach to his parents. Gardner and Sperry (1974), in a recent review of learning disabilities and school phobias, report an early study by Liss (1943) who discriminated two basic types of children with learning problems: (1) those who had a primary acquisition problem manifested by inability to acquire basic school skills in reading, spelling, and arithmetic and (2) those who showed more of an expressive problem despite fairly intact skills. Clinically both groups were viewed as dealing with depressive affect arising both from traumatic life experiences and their (perceived) devalued role in the family.

Wender and Eisenberg (1974), separately and together, prominently represent a significant group of physicians who believe it is important to diagnose and treat a child with a *demonstrable* CNS lesion differently from the child with MBD. Both investigators define the term "minimal" as indicating that the symptom does not fit an otherwise recognized pattern and is associated with soft signs and presumptive evidence of brain disorder. They chide other psychiatrists for being too preoccupied with psychogenesis and failing to consider that a behavior disorder may be secondary to brain dysfunction. Naturalistic observations of the child's behavior and a structured format for obtaining history of the problem are the major diagnostic tools. They recommend open-ended questions and the use of multiple informants and multidisciplinary observation. Unlike other physicians, psychiatrists, and psychologists, they put little reliance on the utility of the clinical interview, pointing to the real possibility that the child will not manifest his typical or representative functioning and mislead the interviewer. Projective testing is eschewed in favor of diagnostic educational testing that reflects specific perceptual cognitive difficulties that will require remedial special education.

Projective techniques and projective tests as utilized by dynamically oriented consultants are apparently in frequent use within the psychoeducational approach. English and English (1958) define a projective technique as

> a procedure for discovering a person's characteristic modes of behavior by observing his behavior in response to a situation that does not elicit or compel a particular response. . . . [A projective test is defined as] a relatively unstructured yet standard situation in which a testee is asked to respond but with as few restrictions as possible upon the mode of response.

A projective test then is an unstructured but essentially standardized event. It is interesting to consider that the variance in responses to specific questions and tasks of the Wechsler Intelligence Scale for Children may in fact constitute a projective response, e.g., that a projection apparently has occurred the examiner might gain valuable insight as to how a child's affect and anxiety are influencing his intellectual functioning. One may note that the receptive attitudes manifested by the child are both specific reaction tendencies towards incoming experience as well as an individualized way of interpreting the environment. Similarly on presentation of a projective stimulus, we see an expressive set or disposition to respond in a consistent manner. The individual's style of responding will be somewhat representative of his manner outside of the test situation. Since *style* of response is peripheral to the assigned task, it is perhaps least susceptible to manipulation or distortion by the child.

Gallagher (1966) devised a psychoeducational definition of the brain-injured child by approaching the problem from the point of view that certain combinations of developmental imbalances led to typical shades of characteristics by which the brain injury could be identified. Rappaport (1964) conceptualized the matter from breadth rather than from the perspective of education alone as did Gallagher. Almost all psychoeducational dynamicists concur with his statement that

> children erect response patterns aimed at protecting them from awareness of their deficiencies and which interfere further with their academic and interpersonal growth.

He admits the frequent presence of central nervous system lesions, but feels that an inclusive definition of the brain-injured child cannot overlook the highly personalized, uniquely dynamic nature of the ego deficit. The Rappaport definition seems to indicate that educators must expand beyond their traditional areas of responsibility and encompass the ego factors of the MBD child into daily school programming. Indeed Rappaport concluded that behavior and learning disturbances are *not* due solely to pathologic brain tissue per se and are therefore not necessary irreversible. More importantly these disturbances are due greatly to the alterations which central nervous systems damage causes in the epigenesis of the ego. Deviant ego maturation fosters a disturbed parent-child relationship, which in turn further interferes with proper ego development.

The concept of ego development and function constitutes a nodal point of confluence for the disparate threads of dynamic assessment. Hartman (1939) postulated that primary ego functions included such important skills as motility, perception, concept formation, and language. Deficits in primary ego functions in turn distort the response pattern of mother to child. For example the perinatally brain-injured child may present an altered stimulus to the mother so that she responds differently than she would to an normal offspring who would be viewed as an extension of herself. Her altered response pattern may manifest itself in not stimulating the child adequately and in rejecting or overprotecting him, thereby robbing him of his opportunity for growth. Secondary functions are also developed; these include defense mechanisms such as repression, reaction formation, and so on. Without functional intactness of both primary and secondary functions, the ego has difficulty in maintaining its autonomy or adaptive balance in regard to instinctual drives from within and stimuli from the world around it. To varying degrees all MBD children find difficulty in achieving mastery over themselves and in successfully coping with the external environment. The result is often a strong and pervasive sense of inadequacy and contributes greatly to the nonadaptive behavior responses so characteristic of the MBD child.

BEHAVIORISM AND TASK ANALYSIS

Behavioristic psychology has contributed strongly to current assessment practices employed with the MBD child. Behaviorists are conceptualizing problems and utilizing techniques generally classified under the rubric of the operant methodology of B. F. Skinner (1938) and the behavioral therapies of Eysenck (1960) and Wolpe (1964). Educational settings today are replete with various behavioral approaches to learning, including behavioral methods of observing and recording data, contingency management, token economies, social modeling, programmed learning, reinforcement, and aversive methodology.

Essential to any behavior approach is the collection and analysis of clinical data, that is, a behavioral analysis consisting of an objective and most often quantitative description of maladaptive responses that constitute the child's problem. Kanfer and Phillips (1970) have summarized what may be regarded as a general behavioral approach

To select specific symptoms or behaviors as targets for change, employ concrete planned interventions, manipulate these behaviors and monitor progress continuously and quantitatively.

It is evident that the behavioral analysis generates a series of clinical hypotheses about what is controlling and maintaining the patient's problematic behaviors. Browning and Stover (1971) view behavioral assessment as an experimental-clinical method using experimental designs in routine clinical practice. These authors criticize usual psychometric instruments as yielding data which are "too distant from critical referral problems." They advocate the obtaining of in vivo data regarding a child's behaviors towards teachers, peer group, and family. In vivo data are readily obtainable from classrooms and residential facilities. Narrative charts and rating scales that focus on clinically important behaviors and that allow reliable quantitative measurement on a large number of behaviors or traits are commonly utilized. Measurement devices of all kinds must meet rigorous standards of reliability and validity. They should also be eminently practical as an indication of the real-life behavior of an individual child.

An MBD child with typical problems in underachievement in school and disordered behavior at home presents a problem in the screening out of the central problem from a large array of negative behaviors. It is possible that a careful shaping of more mature adaptive behaviors that are largely *absent* may be the best approach to use. Lovitt (1967) suggested a four point diagnostic procedure based on methodologic assessment including:

1. Baseline assessment.
2. Assessment of behavioral components.
3. Assessment based on referral.
4. Generalization of assessment.

To obtain needed data for this kind of approach the therapist must utilize research notes; critical incident techniques, that is emergence of a type of behavior within a given situation; and all types of behavioral charting and counting. Behavioral charting allows the monitoring of a variety of behaviors and may adequately reflect the impact of different treatment approaches. More precise electromechanical systems to supplement behavioral chartings have also been used (Ferster and Skinner, 1957), particularly behavioral coding systems and recorder-timers which can measure the appearance and duration of selected antecedent stimulation and contingent reinforcing conditions maintaining behavior. Behavioristic approaches cannot ignore both etiologic and diagnostic-remedial factors. There is a need to collate and integrate data in such a manner that it can be incorporated into specific treatment paradigms for changing specific behavior. It is important to consider that within the more traditional assessment frameworks, the nature of the situation in which a child is functioning is of less interest than are underlying dynamics or structural components. In contrast the behavioral approach would assume that a person's behavior in a sample or experimental situation is directly representative of behavior in an analogous nontest situation. Goldfried (1976) while stressing the use of naturalist observation, also supports a wide variety of behavioral assessment methods: situation testing, role playing, self-report, and intake evaluation. Situation tests remedy the lack of examiner control over the situation to which the child is responding. The MBD child could be closely observed within situations likely to elicit the types of overactive behavior towards which an assessment is specifically directed.

It is possible on some occasions to obtain relevant and subjective measures of anxiety. The behavioral avoidance test (BAT) was used by Bernstein and Nietzel (1973) as a means of evaluating the strengths of fears and phobias. Role playing allows a child to work through in fantasy or react as if an event were occurring to him in real life. A face-to-face role playing interaction could be utilized with a teacher and an MBD child by constructing a situation in which the teacher confronts the child with challenging seat-work in the 10 minutes before morning recess. Self-report procedures focus on subjective experience of emotional response and perceptions of environmental settings. Wolpe and Lazarus (1966) have devised a widely used questionnaire measuring assertiveness in different situations. Fear survey schedules have been used as quick and easily administered screening devices. The S-R inventory of anxiousness (Endler, Hunt, and Rosenstein 1962) and Zuckerman and Lubin's (1965) Multiple Affect Adjective Checklist have had value in allowing persons to reflect their feelings in anxiety producing situations and describe themselves by checking off a series of descriptive statements. A relatively recent attempt to understand the nature of a particular social environment of the MBD child by Insel and Moos (1974) has been described as social ecology. Questionnaires were used to assess the impact made by varying environmental settings (home and school) on the child's behavior and his perception of various aspects of his total social environment. Behavior modifiers and behavior therapists alike have the general problem of defining general problems in operational terms. Goldfried (1976) has focused on obtaining a detailed account of a specific situation which would make an individual anxious or, more specifically, of situational antecedents of behavior. An MBD child frequently manifests consistent patterns of unadaptive behavior in response to anxiety (defined in terms of autonomic response patterns). According to Goldfried (1976), it is likely that early in life the child developed a cognitive set in regard to his surrounding world which in distorted form is mediating various maladaptive responses and emotional reactions. The child might then be behaviorally analyzed in his response to areas of excessively learned fearfulness and the generalization of this fearfulness to benign situations.

A major objective of behavioral therapies, which in the frame of reference of this chapter could be viewed as further assessment, is to replace the anxiety responses with more adaptive emotional responses. Wolpe and Lazarus's (1966) experimental desensitization procedures consist of stimuli that evoke maladaptive responses. These are repeatedly presented at low intensities and thus do not provoke the full-blown response. Then the stimulus intensity is systematically increased until even high intensity no longer provokes maladaptive responses. A child may be assisted in devising anxiety hierarchies with subsequent training and relaxation techniques in which he is asked to imagine scenes ranging (initially) from least threatening to most threatening.

Phillips and Mordock (1970) have stressed the use of operant procedures and assertiveness training in helping children who are withdrawn or who appear to be experiencing anxiety in social situations. Drawing freely from the work of Wolpe and Lazarus (1966), these authors stress much work with parents and helping the child in the home and school evnironments. The behavioral analysis typically extends over several sessions with the focus upon detailed descriptions of a child's behavior, parental handling of the child's behavior, parent-child interaction, child peer relations, school functioning, and so on. Several objective instruments, such as Phillips's (1969) Reinforcement Survey Schedule for Children (RSSC) and the Fear Survey Schedule of Wolpe (1969) are used frequently. The writings of Bandura (1969; Bandura, Blanchard, and Ritter, 1969) are representative of the social learning theorists who continue in the forefront of innovative concern with children's home and classroom-coping problems. He stresses behavioral analysis with subsequent desensitization approaches based on modeling techniques that employ the actually feared stimuli rather than a child's mental representations of them.

Task analysis may be considered a behavioristic distillation of all conditions that alter or maintain behavior. It is based on direct observation and objective specification. This writer recalls several consultative visits to self-contained MBD classrooms where he was asked by the teacher, "How do you teach reading to an MBD child?" The inappropriateness or prematurity of the question was underscored by the fact that the child was not in his seat long enough to be taught by any method. Teachers seem to need a means of obtaining and collating data; task analysis can provide the means to explore the nature of the reading process by considering the specific behavior required for successful performance. Johnson and Morasky (1977) state that task analysis has very little to do with instructional methodology; Johnson (1967) emphasizes that "task analysis will shift the teacher's orientation from subject matter in the curriculum to processes." Bateman (1966–1967) simply asks, "What specific behavior does the child need to be taught?"

Hewett's (1968) model of the engineered classroom represents a largely successful attempt to integrate developmental theory, behavior modification technology, and the requirements of special education. He posits developmental stages in the context of diagnostic and treatment efforts. These stages are attending, response, order, exploratory, social, mastery, and achievement. Reinforcements are carefully defined and assessed. This writer (Wohl, 1974; 1978) has previously described behavioristic psychology as a bridge between data classification and the utilization of this information for instructional purposes. Hewett's project is a reification of such a view and constitutes a viable educational program for children with learning disorders.

SUMMARY

Psychoeducational assessment has been examined and discussed as a dynamic process concerned with the whole child and addressing itself not only to the identification and description of perceptual, integrative, and expressive functions, but also to etiology and ongoing flexible prognoses and treatment. The helping professional or educator is quickly confronted with important diagnostic considerations. Etiologic preoccupations must give way to an approach which will permit the orderly description of a child from a large number of different dimensions. Unwise labeling is currently eschewed in favor of psychoeducational processes that provide an opportunity for interaction and the utilization of clinical experiences in order to make inferences regarding cognitive and emotional experiences. The validity of any assessment is limited to the decision that must be made. It follows that great care must be taken relating to scale and test construction, standardization, sampling, and so on. Consistent with the educator's interests in a here-and-now description of function, there continues to be a wide reliance on all forms of cross-sectional evaluation. A wide variety of approaches are in use: interviews; scaling; life history; and both standardized and unstandardized means of assessing intellectual, cognitive, perceptual-structure, and perceptual-motor abilities. Many of these approaches have violated current professional and scientific guidelines for test construction. They seem to be an outgrowth of the clinical method wherein any methodology, intuition, or even hunch is allowable if it leads to the amelioration of the problems of the individual child and his family. Professionals have utilized some of these tests uncritically and made inferences deviating from the theories and practice of the test originators.

Academicians and experimental investigators are bringing forth discoveries in psychophysiology, perception, memory, and cognition couched in understandly pertinent terminology. Gibson (1975) is representative of a growing cadre of workers fashioning an experimental psychology of reading. These investigators utilize rigorous methodology in attempting to provide the basis for ultimate understanding and effective remediation of reading problems.

Psychodynamically oriented consultants are making significant contributions within educational settings. Current dynamic concepts seem to be centered on the fact that because of either a manifest inability or a refusal to learn at school, a child may be defending himself against the potential results of any expression of his own impulse life. Conflicts are then viewed as inhibitory and as blocking various aspects of learning. Naturalistic observations of the child's behavior and a structured format for obtaining history of the problem are the major diagnostic tools. Projective tests and questioning are useful in helping to analyze the process of perception and often give valuable insight as to how a child's affect influences his intellectual functioning. Rappaport (1964) has advised educators to progress beyond their traditional areas of responsibility and consider the ego factors of the MBD child. Deviant ego maturation may foster disturbed parent-child relationships which in turn will further interfere with proper ego development.

Behaviorism and task analysis constitute the final major emphasis of this chapter. Investigators in this field are conceptualizing and utilizing techniques generally classified under the rubric of the operant methodology of B. F. Skinner (1938) and the behavioral therapies of Eysenck (1960) and Wolpe (1964). They emphasize collection and analysis of clinical data, that is an objective and most often quantitative description of maladaptive responses that are conceived to constitute the child's problem. Behavioral analysis then generate a series of clinical hypotheses about what is controlling and maintaining problem behaviors. Psychometric instruments are often criticized as too distant from critical referral problems. In vivo data concerning a child's behaviors towards teachers, peer group, and family are recommended instead.

Most investigators are increasingly aware that psychoeducational analysis can be undertaken only within the context of the development and growth of the whole child. Hewett (1968) has provided a model based on a developmental sequence of educationally relevant skills with an incorporated behaivor modification paradigm which is used in defining and assessing reinforcements for the students. The psychodynamic workers bring empathy, flexibility, and sensitivity to the study of the MBD child. Behaviorists bring task analysis and orientation, pragmatism, goal directedness, and empiricism, without which current diagnostic and training efforts would surely founder. This writer is convinced that the MBD child requires and deserves detailed and intensive assessment. It should not be forgotten that diagnoses and classification are also tools. It is not likely that diagnosis and subsequent remediation or treatment can be truly separated. Observational data, developmental profiles, test scores, and the resultant diagnostic labeling should be integrated into planning which will help the child and promote better family adjustment and happiness.

REFERENCES

Badian, N. "The identification of high risk children: A retrospective look at selection criteria." *Journal of Learning Disabilities,* 8(5), 283–287, (1975).

Bandura, A. *Principles of Behavior Modification,* New York: Holt, 1969.

Bandura, A., E. Blanchard, and B. Ritter. "The relative efficacy of desensitization and modeling approaches for inducing behavioral, affective, and cognitive changes." *Journal of Personality and Social Psychology,* 13, 173–199, (1969).

Bateman, B. "Three approaches to diagnosis and educational planning for children with learning disabilities." *Academic Therapy,* 2, 215–222, (Winter 1966-1967).

Beck, A. T., C. H. Ward, M. Mendelson, J. E. Mock, and J. K. Erbough. "Reliability of psychiatric diagnoses, 2: A study of consistency of clinical judgments and ratings." *American Journal of Psychiatry,* 119, 351–357, (1962).

Beery, K., and N. Buktenica. *Developmental Test of Visual-Motor Integration,* Chicago: Follett, 1967.

Bender, L. *A Visual-Motor Gestalt Test and Its Clinical Use.* American Orthopsychiatry Association Research Monograph No. 3. New York: 1938.

Berlin, I. "Psychiatry and the school," in A. Freedman, H. Kaplan, and B. Sadack, eds., *Comprehensive Textbook of Psychiatry,* vol. 2, 2nd ed. Baltimore: Williams & Wilkins, 2251–2262, 1975.

Bernstein, D., and M. Nietzel. "Procedural variation in behavioral avoidance tests." *Journal of Consulting and Clinical Psychology,* 41, 165–174, (1973).

Browning, R., and D. Stover. *Behavior Modification in Child Treatment,* pp. 1–17. Chicago: Aldine-Atherton, 1971.

Bryan, T., and Wheeler. "Perception of learning-disabled children: The eye of the observer." *Journal of Learning Disabilities,* 5, 484–488, (1972).

Carrol, J., in O.K. Buros, ed., *The Seventh Mental Measurements Yearbook,* vol. 1, pp. 819 –823. Highland Park, N.J.: Gryphon, 1972.

Dale, E., and J. S. Chall. *A Formula for Predicting Readability.* Columbus, Ohio: Ohio State University Bureau of Educational Research, 1948.

Dunn, L. M. *Peabody Picture Vocabulary Test.* Minneapolis: American Guidance Services, 1959.

Dunn, L. M., and F. Markwardt. *Peabody Individual Achievement Test.* Circle Pines, Minn.: American Guidance Services, 1970.

Durrell Analysis of Reading Difficulty. New York: Harcourt Brace Jovanovich, 1955.

Endler, N., J. McV. Hunt, and J. Rosenstein. "An S-R inventory of anxiousness." *Psychological Monographs,* 76, 1–33, (1962).

English, H., and A. English. *A Comprehensive Dictionary of Psychological and Psychoanalytic Terms.* New York: Longmans, Green, 1958.

Eysenck, H. *Behavior Therapy and The Neuroses.* New York: Pergamon, 1960.

Ferster, C., and G. Skinner. *Schedules of Reinforcement.* New York: Appleton-Century-Crofts, 1957.

Frostig, M. "A developmental test of visual perception of evaluating normal and neurologically handicapped children," *Perceptual and Motor Skills,* 12, 383–394 (1963).

Frostig, M. *The Developmental Program in Visual Perception: Intermediate Pictures and Patterns.* Chicago: Follett, 1966*a.*

———*The Developmental Program in Visual Perception: Advanced Pictures and Patterns.* Chicago: Follett, 1966*b.*

Frostig, M., and D., Horn. *The Frostig program for the development of visual perception: Teacher's guide.* Chicago: Follett, 1964.

Gallagher, J. "Children with developmental imbalances," in W. Cruickshank, ed., *The Teacher of Brain-Injured Children,* p. 23. Syracuse, N.Y.: Syracuse University Press, 1966.

Gardener, G., and B. Sperry. "School problems, learning disabilities, and school phobia," in S. Arieti, ed., *American Handbook of Psychiatry,* 2nd ed., vol. 2, pp. 116–130. New York: Basic Books, 1974.

Gates, A., and W. MacGinitie, *Gates-MacGinitie Reading Tests.* New York: Teachers College Press, 1965.

Gates, A., and A. McKillop. *Gates-McKillop Reading Diagnostic Tests, Manual of Directions.* New York: Teachers College Press, 1962.

Gibson, E. "Experimental psychology of learning to read," in J. Money, ed., *The Disabled Reader,* pp. 41–59. Baltimore: Johns Hopkins University Press, 1966.

Gibson, E., and H., Levin, *The Psychology of Reading,* Cambridge, Mass.: MIT Press, 1975.

Gibson, E., and S. Shepela. "Some effects of redundant stimulus information on learning to identify letters," in *The Analysis of Reading Skill: A Program of Basic and Applied Research,* pp. 63–75. Ithaca, N.Y.: Cornell University; Washington, D.C.: U. S. Office of Education, Final Report, Project No. 5–1213, 1968.

Gibson, E., F. Shapiro, and A. Yonas. "Confusion matrices for graphic patterns obtained with a latency measure," in *The Analysis of Reading Skill: A Program of Basic and Applied Research,* pp. 76–96. Ithaca, N.Y.: Cornell University; Washington, D.C.: U. S. Office of Education, Final Report, Project No. 5–1213, 1968.

Gibson, E., J. Gibson, A. Pick, and H. Osser. "A developmental study of the discrimination of letter-like forms." *Journal of Comparative and Physiological Psychology,* 55, 897–906, (1962).

Gibson, E., H. Osser, W. Schiff, and J. Smith. "An analysis of critical features of letters, tested by a confusion matrix," in *Final Report on a Basic Research Program on Reading.* Ithaca, N.Y.: Cornell University Press; Washington, D.C.: U.S. Office of Education, No. 639, 1963.

Goldfried, M. "Behavioral assessment," in I. Weiner, ed., *Clinical Methods in Psychology,* vol. 5, pp. 281–331. New York: Wiley, 1976.

Gray Oral Reading Tests. Indianapolis, Ind.: Bobbs Merrill, 1962.

Hartman, H. *Ego Psychology and The Problem of Adaptation.* New York: International Universities Press, 1939.

Hawke, W. "The psychiatric aspects of learning disabilities." *The Bulletin,* 28, (1966).

Heber, R. "A manual on terminology and classification in mental retardation." *American Journal of Mental Deficiency,* 64 (1959); Monogr. Suppl. (rev. ed.), 1961.

Hewett, F. *The Emotionally Disturbed Child in the Classroom,* pp. 9–20. Boston: Allyn & Bacon, 1968.

Hirsch, K. de, J. Jansky, and O. Langford. *Predicting Reading Failure.* New York: Harper and Row, 1966.

Insel, P., and R. Moos. "Psychological environments: Expanding the scope of human ecology." *American Psychologist,* 29, 179–188, (1974).

Jastak, J., and S. Jastak. *The Wide Range Achievement Test,* rev. ed. Wilmington, Del.: Guidance Associates, 1965.

Johnson, D. "Educational principles for children with learning disabilities." *Rehabilitation Literature,* vol. 28, No. 10, 318, (October, 1967).

Johnson, S., and R. Morasky. *Learning Disabilities,* Chap. 6. Boston: Allyn & Bacon, 1977.

Kanfer, F., and J. Phillips. *Learning Foundations of Behavior Therapy,* pp. 389–390. New York: Wiley, 1970.

Kephart, N., *The Slow Learner in the Classroom,* 2nd. ed. Columbus, Ohio: Merrill, 1971.

Kershner, J. "Psychoeducational diagnosis of learning disorders: A cognitive perspective." (Paper presented at the Annual Meeting of The American Psychological Association, Miami Beach, Florida, September, 1970.)

Kessler, J. "Psychological services to the retarded—after testing what?" Groton, Conn.: Read before Training Institute of the State Department of Health (September 10–17, 1966).

———"Nosology in child psychopathology," in H. Rie, ed., *Perspectives in Child Psychopathology.* New York: Aldine–Atherton, 1971.

Kirk, S., J. McCarthy, and W. Kirk. *Illinois Test of Psycholinguistic Abilities,* rev. ed. Urbana: University of Illinois Press, 1968.

Koppitz, E. M. *The Bender-Gestalt Test for Young Children.* New York: Grune & Stratton, 1964.

Lee, L. "A screening test for syntax development." *Journal of Speech and Hearing Disorders,* 35, 103–112, (1970).

Lehman, E. "Selective strategies in children's attention to task-relevant information." *Child Development,* 43, pp. 197–209, (1972).

Lennenberg, E., *Biological Foundations of Language.* New York: Wiley, 1951.

Lerner, J. *Children with Learning Disabilities,* p. 46. Boston: Houghton Mifflin, 1971.

Liss, E. "Physiology of learning." *American Journal of Orthopsychiatry,* 13, 275. (1943).

Lovitt, T. "Assessment of children with learning disabilities." *Exceptional Children,* 234, (December, 1967).

Maccoby, E. "Selective auditory attention in children," in L. Lipsitt and C. Spiker, eds., *Advances in Child Development and Behavior,* pp. 99–124. vol. 3, New York: Academic Press, 1967.

Mann, L. in O.K. Buros, *The Seventh Mental Measurements Yearbook,* vol. 2, pp. 1274–1276. Highland Park, N.J.: Gryphon, 1972.

————in O.K. Buros, in *The Seventh Mental Measurements Yearbook,* vol. 2, p. 1274. Highland Park, N.J.: Gryphon, 1972.

Mann, L., and W. Phillips. "Fractional processes in special education." *Exceptional Children,* 33, 311–319. (January 1967).

Merwin, J. in O.K. Buros, in *The Seventh Mental Measurements Yearbook,* vol. 1. Highland Park, N.J.: Gryphon, 1972.

Metropolitan Achievement Tests: Reading Tests. New York: Harcourt Brace Jovanovich, 1971.

Myers, P., and D. Hamill. *Methods for Learning Disorders.* New York: Wiley, 1969.

Myklebust, H. *Pupil Rating Scale.* New York: Grune & Stratton, 1969.

Myklebust, H., and B. Boshes. *Minimal Brain Damage in Children.* Final Report U.S. Public Health Service, Contract 108–65–142, U.S. Department of HEW. Evanston, Ill.: Northwestern University, 1969.

Osgood, C. *Method and Theory in Experimental Psychology.* New York: Oxford University Press, 1953.

————"Motivational dynamics of language behavior," in M. Jones, ed., *Nebraska Symposium on Motivation.* Lincoln: University of Nebraska Press, 1957.

Phillips, D. "A reinforcement therapy for children," mimeographed paper, Princeton Center for Behavior Therapy, N.J., 1969.

Phillips, D., and J. Mordock, "Behavior therapy with children: Some general guidelines and specific suggestions." (Paper presented at the Annual Convention of the American Association of Psychiatric Services for Children, Philadelphia, November, 1970.)

Proger, B. "Trends and patterns in achievement test results and baseline expectancy data for future performance." Annual Program Evaluation Report, Montgomery County, Pennsylvania, 1975.

Rappaport, S., *Childhood Aphasia and Brain Damage.* Narberth, Penn.: 1964.

Reiss, P. "Reading and arithmetic for mainstreaming brain-injured children." [Evaluation report.] New York, 1975.

Roach, E., and N. Kephart. *The Purdue Perceptual Motor Survey,* Columbus, Ohio: Merrill, 1962.

Roswell-Chall Diagnostic Reading Test. Planetarium Station, New York (1964).

Royal, M. "Performance objectives and C-R tests: We wrote our own." *The Reading Teacher,* 26, 572–580, (1973).

Ruiter, J. De "A Bayesian approach to the use of test data for the identification of learning disability in school-age children," *Dissertation Abstracts International,* 34(8A), 4919–4920, (February, 1974).

Rutte, R. in O.K. Buros, ed., *The Seventh Mental Measurements Yearbook,* vol. 2, pp. 1192–1194. Highland Park, N.J.: Gryphon, 1972.

Rutter, M., and P. Graham. "The reliability and validity of the psychiatric assessment of the child: Interview with the child," *British Journal of Psychiatry,* 114, 563–579, (1968).

Shedd, C. "Some characteristics of a specific perceptual motor disability: Dyslexia," *Journal of the Medical Association of Alabama,* 37, 150–162, (1967).

Silberberg, N., and E. Silberberg, "Myths in remedial education." *Journal of Learning Disabilities,* 2, 209–217, (1969).

Silver, A., and R. Hagen. "Specific reading disability: An approach to diagnosis and treatment." *Journal of Special Education,* vol. 1, No. 2, (1968).

Silverstein, A. "Variance components in the developmental test of visual perception." *Perceptual and Motor Skills,* 20, 973–976, (January 1965).

Skinner, B. F. *The Behavior of Organisms.* New York: Appleton, 1938.

Smith, R., and J. Neisworth. "Fundamentals of informal educational assessment," in R. Smith, ed., *Teacher Diagnosis of Educational Difficulties.* Columbus, Ohio: Merrill, 1969.

SRA Achievement Scales. Science Research Associates, (1963).

Stanford Achievement Test: Reading Tests. New York: Harcourt Brace Jovanovich, 1965.

Trimble, A. C. "Can remedial be eliminated?" *Academic Therapy Quarterly,* 5, 207–213 (1970).

Truax, C., and R. Carkhuff. *Toward Effective Counseling and Psychotherapy,* p. 2. Chicago: Aldine, 1967.

Valett, R. *The Remediation of Learning Disabilities: A Handbook of Psychoeducational Resource Programs.* Palo Alto, Cal.: Consulting Psychologist, 1967.

Ward, J. "The factor structure of the Frostig Developmental Test of Visual Perception." *British Journal of Educational Psychology,* 40, 65–67, (February 1970).

Wiener, P., C. Barritt, and M. Semmel. "A critical evaluation of the Illinois Test of Psycholinguistic Abilities." *Exceptional Children,* (February 1967).

Wender, P., and L. Eisenberg. "Minimal Brain Dysfunction," in S. Arieti, ed., *American Handbook of Psychiatry,* vol. II, 2nd ed., pp. 130–131. New York: Basic Books, 1974.

Wepman, J., *Test of Auditory Discrimination.* Chicago: Language Research Associates, 1958.

Whitehead, B., "The experimental index: A proposed screening instrument of early identification of learning disabled students." *Dissertation Abstracts International,* 34(3A), 1157–A, (1973).

Wiseman, D. "Remedial education: Global or learning-disability approach," *Academic Therapy,* 5, 165–175, (1970).

Wolpe, J. "Behavior therapy in complex neurotic states." *British Journal of Psychiatry,* 110, 28–34. (1964).

Wolpe, J. *The Practice of Behavior Therapy.* New York: Pergamon, 1969.

Wolpe, J., and A. Lazarus, *Behavior Therapy Techniques.* New York: Pergamon, 1966.

Wohl, T. "Thorough behavioral analysis and description." *Mental Retardation,* 21–23, (August, 1974).

Wohl, T. "Psychologists working with learning-disabled children," in K. Donelly, ed., *Communicative Disorders.* Boston: Little, Brown, [1978] in press.

Zuckerman, M., and B. Lubin. *Manual for the Multiple Affect Checklist.* San Diego, Cal.: Educational and Industrial Testing Service, 1965.

CHAPTER 17

Medical and Neurological Differential Diagnosis

Richard J. Schain

The primary responsibility of the physician dealing with a child who is thought to exhibit minimal brain dysfunction is in thoroughly dealing with the issue of associated medical disorders. This requires consideration of a variety of physical problems that may interfere with a child's behavioral or cognitive development. Recognition of the presence of such disorders will assist in placing total treatment plans in a realistic perspective by more accurately focusing on the origins of the child's difficulties. Conversely, clearly establishing the absence of detectable medical disorders can provide medical closure, thus helping parents and other clinicians to concentrate on the educational and psychological needs of the MBD child.

The medical syndromes to be considered are:

1. Brain damage behavioral syndromes.
2. Seizure disorders.
3. Mental retardation.
4. Cerebral palsy.
5. Ocular, auditory, and speech disorders.
6. Progressive neurologic and metabolic disorders.
7. Childhood psychosis.
8. Developmental hyperactivity.

It should be emphasized that one may not be able definitively to assign the majority of children with symptoms suggestive of MBD to any of these syndromes.

BRAIN-DAMAGE BEHAVIORAL SYNDROMES

The cardinal features of MBD: hyperactivity, distractibility, emotional lability, and impulsivity were originally regarded as sequels to brain damaging events in the life of a child (Strauss and Lehtinen, 1947). The exact causes of behavioral disturbances in children who have suffered earlier brain damage may be difficult to specify with precision, but there can be little doubt that brain damage can interfere with learning abilities of children. It is of value to recognize that the symptoms of MBD may date from a brain-damaging event even though this association may have little in the way of treatment implications. Parents wish to know the origin of the problems of their children and they have a right to have all relevant facts presented to them.

The major method of identifying brain-damage behavioral syndromes is the determination of a careful history oriented to eliciting the occurrence of brain-damaging events and relating such events to subsequent behavioral changes. Causal relationships may be difficult to establish with absolute certainty, but highly probable associations are occasionally discovered. The more important causes of brain damage in childhood are outlined below.

Low Birth Weight

There is substantial evidence that infants who are small at birth are high risks for the development of the brain-damage behavioral syndrome as well as specific neurological deficits (Kawi and Pasamanick, 1958; Drillien, 1964, 1970; Wiener, et al., 1968). This high risk status of low birth-weight infants has persisted in spite of major improvements in nursery care. It may even be that the incidence of neurological deficits associated with low birth weight has increased because of lowered mortality rates. While the conventional definition of prematurity still applies to an infant with birth weight under 2500 grams or 5.5 pounds (World Health Organization), it is the smaller infants under 3.5 pounds at birth who are at the greatest risk for later neurological disorders. Lubchenco and her co-workers (1963) found 25 of 63 children born with a birth weight of 3.5 pounds or under to be slow learners at 10 years of age. It is pertinent that they reported a lack of correlation between intelligence quotients and poor school performance. Drillien (1964) reported a high incidence of hyperactive behavior and frequent difficulties of school adjustment in small prematurely born infants. Of course the association of low birth weight with MBD syndromes does not mean that the environment has no role in the genesis of symptoms.

In fact longitudinal studies (Werner, et al., 1967) have provided evidence that the home and social environment play a major role in determining school performance of children who have had adverse perinatal experiences. It is likely that the role of the environment is more important in determining subsequent behavior in high risk newborns than in infants born under optimal conditions.

Birth Injuries

Unlike low birth weight, birth injuries do not appear to be an important cause of MBD syndromes in spite of frequent assumptions to the contrary. Compared to the clear evidence implicating low birth weight with subsequent learning disorders, the relation between later development and birth difficulties is less clear. Most behavioral differences between stressed and unstressed newborns disappear with increasing age. A follow-up study of 41 infants subjected to profound anoxia at birth revealed that 20% subsequently manifested major retardation syndromes (Benaron, et al., 1960). The remainder of the group were performing equally well in school as a control group. The authors concluded that even the severest forms of anoxia produced deficits in only a small group of affected infants. A well controlled study of infants subjected to perinatal anoxia revealed little impairment of functioning evident by seven years of age (Corah, et al., 1965).

In spite of the difficulty in demonstrating that birth anoxia produces vulnerability for learning disorders by prospective means, retrospective studies have often suggested an increased incidence of perinatal stresses in children with evidence of minimal brain dysfunctions (Kawi and Pasamanick, 1958; Gubbay, et al., 1965; Prechtl and Stemmer, 1962; Brenner, et al., 1967; Paine, Werry, and Quay, 1968). Towbin (1971) has discussed the mechanisms of cerebral hypoxic lesions occurring at birth and has suggested that minimal cerebral lesions occurring at this time are a cause for later minimal brain dysfunction syndromes. However data correlating pathological findings with clinical syndromes of minimal brain dysfunction are not available. Probably environmental factors gradually supervene as the most important determinant of behavior and performance by the time the infant reaches school age.

Postencephalitic and Posttraumatic Syndromes

The concept of a brain-damage behavioral syndrome was first developed in the 1920s when it was noted that children recovering from acute attacks of epidemic encephalitis lethargica (von Economo's encephalitis) often manifested persistent behavioral disturbances. Since that time postencephalitic behavioral syndromes have become less common but still occur.

It is evident that many behavior disorders loosely attributed to encephalitis or head injuries are associated with family disturbances and often antedate the supposed cerebral insult. Blau (1954) in a classic paper reversed his earlier view that many childhood behavior disorders were due to encephalopathies, and he stressed the environmental origins of these disorders. Some studies attributing behavior disorders to encephalitis (Greenbaum and Lurie, 1948; Levy, 1956) are found on detailed scrutiny of published data to provide uncertain evidence for the association.

These remarks should not be interpreted to mean that viral encephalitis may not result in permanent brain damage with subsequent neurological and behavioral sequelae. This has been especially well documented in relation to outbreaks of western encephalitis in California (Finley, et al., 1967). Finley and his collaborators concluded that the extent of brain damage is related to the age at onset of encephalitis; the younger the infant at the time of illness, the more likely the occurrence of permanent sequelae. These are likely to be overt neurological disorders such as hemiplegias, seizures, and mental retardation. Finley (1971) believes that some of these children are left with subtle neurological deficits which may be identified only in the area of learning performance. In general the physician should be cautious in attributing MBD syndromes to poorly documented episodes of encephalitis.

Head injuries have also been widely believed to produce behavior problems in children even when the injury is apparently minor (Bakwin and Bakwin, 1966). However only severe trauma with protracted coma have been clearly implicated in subsequent personality disturbances (Richardson, 1963). Studies by Russell and Smith (1961) on sequelae of closed head injuries have revealed that youth is a favorable factor in assessing prospects for complete recovery. The premorbid personality is also an important factor determining subsequent symptoms.

The occurrence of a definite alteration of previous personality characteristics with irritability or dulling of mental functions following trauma should alert the examiner to the possible presence of a space-occupying lesion, such as a brain tumor, intracranial hematoma, or brain abscess. Under such circumstances signs and symptoms of increased intracranial pressure such as headache, vomiting, or papilledema may be present. In the absence of this type of overt complication, closed-head injuries in children rarely result in prolonged post-traumatic symptoms except where litigation is an issue or preexistent symptoms of behavior disorders are present.

Lead Poisoning

Heavy metal intoxication from lead is a not uncommon cause of acute neurological symptoms in preschool-age children from low income areas. Children may absorb lead by chewing on wall peeling from older homes (pre-World War II), by eating crayons containing lead compounds, or by being exposed to lead fumes from burning auto battery casings. Lead encephalopathy can result in chronic brain damage with behavioral manifestations similar to other types of acquired brain damage, that is hyperkinesis, impulsivity, and perceptual deficits (Thurston, Middleman, and Mason, 1955; White and Fowler, 1960). There is growing suspicion that many children from poorer neighborhoods are exposed to chronic lead intoxication without developing acute symptoms that ordinarily lead to the diagnosis of lead poisoning. Evidence exists that lead exposure in early childhood is associated with later depression of intellectual levels and poor school performance (Zarkowsky, 1976). One important clue in suspecting the possibility that lead poisoning may have occurred undetected at an earlier age is a history of pica, the indiscriminate ingestion of nonedible objects.

If lead poisoning is suspected, elevated lead levels in blood and urine will usually confirm the diagnosis. However if lead is no longer being ingested and only the residual of brain damage remains, it may be difficult to prove the suspicion. Characteristic X-ray changes in the long bones may be helpful in confirming prior exposure to harmful quantities of lead.

Other Causes of Brain Damage

Meningitis, hydrocephalus, cerebrovascular accidents, status epilepticus, and severe intoxications from drug ingestion or poisonous fumes constitute other causes of brain damage. Survivors of bacterial meningitis may exhibit intellectual deficits in the absence of overt neurological syndromes (Sell, et al., 1972). A recent study has indicated that viral forms of meningitis in early life may also result in some degree of permanent cerebral deficits (Sells, Carpenter, and Ray, 1975). These episodes can be readily elicited by a detailed history which is usually obtained in the course of a medical evaluation.

SEIZURE DISORDERS

The hallmark of seizure phenomena is an abrupt alteration of behavior. Psychomotor seizures may manifest themselves as behavioral automatisms, such as complex motor acts, lip smacking, chewing, abrupt disorientations, or agitation. Drowsiness may follow the episodes. Fugue states refer to prolonged periods during which the child may walk about or engage in customary activities in a trance-like manner. On occasion prolonged behavioral disturbances associated with continuous electroencephalographic seizure activity may occur (Goldensohn and Gold, 1960). Children may appear withdrawn or confused during periods of abnormal cerebral discharge. These episodes may last for hours.

Petit mal seizures refer to brief lapses of consciousness lasting for up to 30 seconds. The child may suddenly stare blankly or perhaps blink momentarily. The episode may be so inconspicuous that others in the child's presence are not aware of the event. It is characteristic of this type of seizure that the patient is not aware of its occurrence and that there are no after effects as in the case of other seizure types. Occasional petit mal seizures rarely interfere with normal mental or motor activities. However frequent spells may disturb a child's ability to concentrate and engage in learning activities.

There are paroxysmal symptoms that may be difficult to classify as seizures with certainty. Migraine episodes, syncopal spells, episodic vertigo (dizziness), motor tics, or hysterical pseudoseizures may be seen in individual children with learning problems. In these situations analysis of EEG patterns will be of great value in deciding about the presence of a seizure disorder.

The occurrence of major EEG abnormalities (Figure 17–1), such as polyspike or spike and wave discharges can occasionally be found in children with MBD syndromes in the absence of overt clinical manifestations of seizures (Schain, 1970). Paine (1962) has suggested that this phenomenon represents a borderline form of epilepsy. Paroxysmal subclinical EEG bursts have been shown to result in amnesic episodes (Hutt, Lee, and Ounsted, 1963; Geller and Geller, 1970) or slowing of response time (Tizard and Margerison, 1964), especially if the bursts last more than one second. Mirsky and Van Buren (1965) report that behavioral alterations may precede wave spike discharges. The effect of subclinical EEG bursts upon behavior and learning is one of the most important interfaces of neurology and the problem of minimal brain dysfunction.

Neurologists usually do not feel justified in administering anticonvulsant agents in the absence of clinical seizures even when the EEG reveals epileptiform abnormalities. This attitude is based upon good reasons: the problem of labeling a child

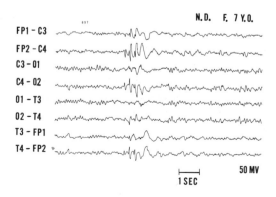

Figure 17–1.   Paroxysmal spike-slow discharge from right-central parietal area. Seven-year-old girl with behavioral and learning problems. No history of seizures.

as epileptic by administration of anticonvulsants, inappropriateness of chronic drug usage without clear indications, and perhaps most important, lack of clear-cut criteria of drug effectiveness.

The resolution of this issue requires appropriate outcome criteria that acknowledge the fact that behavior and learning styles may be slow to change in response to anticonvulsant drug effects on EEG seizure patterns. At the present time the presence of subclinical EEG seizure discharges in children with clear-cut MBD syndromes provides some justification for a therapeutic trial with an anticonvulsant agent. Such a trial should include measures of the effects on the MBD symptoms since, in the absence of such effects, changes in the EEG patterns would be of uncertain consequence. This issue is greatly in need of careful clinical research.

MENTAL RETARDATION

It is important to distinguish children with learning difficulties due to intrinsic limitations in intelligence from those who manifest MBD syndromes. Many parents of children with mild but global retardation syndromes regard their children as having specific learning disabilities. Some retarded children are trained in verbal skills far beyond their actual abilities in judgment and performance.

A careful developmental history of retarded children often reveals evidence of delayed motor and speech development. Any child who was not walking unaided by 18 months of age is suspect for some major deficit in mental or neurologic function. Persistent inability to develop peer relationships is suggestive (but not pathognomonic) of mental retardation. Conversation with a child will often suggest to the physician the presence of dullness of mental faculties.

Whenever the presence of a mental-retardation syndrome is suspected, administration of one of the standard psychometric tests of intelligence is required. This is often one of the Wechsler Intelligence Scales which have the virtue of being divided into verbal and performance sections or the Stanford-Binet. Performance on such scales is best regarded as a measure of a child's achievement in acquisition of cognitive skills; it is clear that many factors affect these abilities besides constitutional ones. In spite of the undeniable influence of cultural and other environmental factors upon intelligence test performance, this measure is a valuable aid to the clinician and often the only available objective measure of mental skills.

The physical examination of children with suspected mental retardation should include careful inspection of the skin for evidence of neurocutaneous syndromes. Multiple cafe au lait spots, subcutaneous nodules, or heavy freckling may suggest neurofibromatosis. Short stature and thickening of the neck folds in a girl should raise the possibility of Turner's syndrome (45 chromosomes, XO karyotype). Buccal smear examination revealing a chromatin-negative pattern establishes this diagnosis in girls. Turner's syndrome is of special interest in the area of learning disorders because it involves specific impairment of spatial abilities and of right-left directional sense in affected children (Garron and Stoep, 1969). It is this space-form deficit that may account for the high incidence of mild mental retardation in children with Turner's syndrome.

Microcephaly as defined by head circumference of more than two standard deviations below the mean is highly correlated with subnormal intelligence (O'Connell, Feldt, and Stickler, 1965). This repeatedly noted observation emphasizes the importance of routine head circumference measurement and use of standard curves of head growth for its interpretation. Head growth in children with metabolic or endocrine growth disturbances is less affected than body growth. However many microcephalic children function in the normal range of intelligence (Martin, 1970) so that this parameter is not to be regarded as pathognomonic of mental retardation.

Other specific medical disorders to be considered in mild mental retardation are hypothyroidism, hypoparathyroidism, phenylketonuria, and other disorders affecting sex chromosomes. These conditions can be identified by appropriate laboratory procedures.

The final diagnosis of mental retardation should be based on judicious consideration of developmental and historical information, data from psychometric testing and the physical examination, together with awareness of environmental factors. If doubt exists, the decision should be postponed pending further observation and studies. The physician should keep in mind the lifelong implications of labeling a child as mentally retarded, even if the diagnosis is reversed at a later date.

CEREBRAL PALSY

Definition and Manifestations

The term cerebral palsy refers to a group of disorders of motor function caused by nonprogressive brain lesions acquired in early life. These lesions may be due to noxious agents affecting the brain during prenatal life, brain damage occurring during a difficult or premature birth, or an illness or injury damaging the brain in early infancy. This general concept has been hammered out by physicians over the course of a long controversy in past years not unlike present discussions about the nature of minimal brain dysfunction (Ingram, 1964).

One of the most important facts about cerebral palsy is that affected children are often multiply handicapped. Approximately one-third of cerebral-palsied children are significantly mentally retarded. Seizures are a common associated neurological problem. Ocular, hearing, and speech problems complicate the life of many children with cerebral palsy. Some of these children manifest a severe hyperactivity syndrome which seriously interferes with classroom adjustment. All of these features are familiar to clinicians interested in minimal brain dysfunction, and in fact an earlier expression commonly used for MBD was minimal cerebral palsy.

In addition to these obvious handicaps, cerebral-palsied children also reveal evidence of perceptual disturbances that interfere with learning processes (Cruickshank, et al., 1965; Holt and Reynell, 1967). Spastics are said to be more prone to perceptual problems than are children with athetoid or ataxic cerebral palsy (Abercrombie, 1964). Birch and Belmont (1965) have suggested, as a result of their demonstration that cerebral-palsied children are deficient in the capacity to perform auditory-visual integrations, that the perceptual disturbance may be due to defective capacity for intersensory integration.

While overt forms of cerebral palsy are readily recognized, borderline forms present greater difficulties in diagnosis. It is important to remember that, even though cerebral palsy is often regarded as a fixed disorder, early signs of cerebral palsy not infrequently disappear during later development (Lubchenco, et al., 1963; Illingworth, 1968). Clinicians with opportunities for longitudinal surveys will find children who as infants may have manifested unmistakable signs of diplegias or movement disorders, but who at school age appear perfectly normal. It is to be expected therefore that borderline manifestations of cerebral palsy will exist. Some of the symptoms that have been thought to indicate minimal cerebral palsy are discussed below.

Clumsiness

Children with MBD syndromes are often noted to be clumsy by examiners. The expression clumsiness generally refers to awkwardness of physical performance (for example running, playing ball, dressing oneself). Walton and his co-workers (Walton, Ellis, and Court, 1962; Gubbay, et al., 1965) have described a group of clumsy children who were excessively awkward in daily activities and manifested signs of constructional apraxia. Dysgraphia and copying difficulties were striking in these children. This constellation of symptoms was regarded as an apraxic-agnosic syndrome due to developmental delay or actual structural damage of undetermined origin.

Clumsiness is particularly prominent in ataxic diplegia or other forms of cerebral palsy in which ataxia is prominent. The plantar responses are almost always extensor in even mild forms of ataxic diplegia. It is important to recognize the presence of ataxia in clumsy children. Ataxia is a disturbance of postural fixation which in children is usually due to cerebellar dysfunction. This can be demonstrated by a number of standard neurological tests of cerebellar function, such as the finger to nose maneuver; performance of alternating movements, such as pronation-supination of the forearm; touching each finger against thumb in sequence; and ability to maintain hands in an outstretched position. Tandem walking and ability to hop on one foot are especially sensitive tests of cerebellar functions. Ataxic children are always clumsy to some extent but many clumsy children manifest no true signs of cerebellar ataxia.

Clumsiness is a highly unspecific symptom, often a manifestation of tension or uncertainty in a child. Many clumsy children are otherwise perfectly normal. It is unwise to attribute clumsiness to a borderline cerebral palsy syndrome unless definite supporting evidence is present such as spasticity, extensor plantar responses, or definite ataxia. One may regard clumsiness as evidence of cerebral dysfunction in children, but this is an assumption impossible to support in the absence of other signs of neurological disturbance. As in the case of language development, there is great variability in acquisition of motor skills in normal children.

Involuntary Movements

Many MBD children are restless and fidgety much of the time. They may manifest involuntary choreic-like (Prechtl and Stemmer, 1962) movements that can be demonstrated by asking the child to extend the arms or place hands on knees for a moment or two. Engaging the child in conversation or the existence of some tension-provoking circumstance may bring out these movements. Sometimes voluntary activity results in overflow phenomena, that is the occurrence of unwanted movements in addition to the desired movements. Mirror movements refer to overflow into the opposite side of the body and may be particularly prominent in hemiparesis with overflow into the normal side (Cohen, et al., 1967).

Involuntary movements or choreoathetosis are a prominent sign of extrapyramidal forms of cerebral palsy. This type of movement disorder is often associated with muscle rigidity of varying degree. However, as in the case of clumsiness, caution must be exercised in attributing minor involuntary movements as an isolated finding to the existence of cerebral palsy. Stereotyped involuntary movements or tics may be of psychogenic origin. Psychogenic tics are often prominent in the facial and ocular muscles. Whatever its cause, there can be little doubt that the fidgety child is an especially difficult problem for classroom teachers.

Gait Disturbances

Observations of gait and posture will uncover mild forms of cerebral palsy when gross abnormalities are not evident. Walking is a complex neuromotor task that involves many reflex integrative functions. The different gait abnormalities found in cerebral-palsy syndromes are described in detail by Paine and Oppe (1966). Observation should be made of walking, running, ability to reverse direction rapidly, and heel to toe (tandem) walking. Head posture, arm swinging, pelvic movements, and foot position should be noted during walking and the condition of the soles of the shoes should be inspected for clues of asymmetrical wear. The different gait abnormalities seen in cerebral palsy are outlined in Table 17–1.

Table 17–1   Gait Disturbances in Cerebral Palsy

Type	Manifestations
Cerebral diplegia	Stiff, shuffling gait with excessive lower extremity aduction (scissors gait). Toe walking with wearing out of tips of soles bilaterally. Crouching if flexion contractures are present in hip and knees.
Hemiparesis	Circumduction of leg affected. Stiff knee and scraping of foot (due to functional elongation of affected leg). Diminished swinging of arm on affected side.
Dyskinesia	Writhing movements during walking; posturing, involuntary jerks. Throwing head backward or sideward.
Ataxia	Wide-based gait. Reeling or staggering. Truncal tremor. Difficulty with tandem walking. Inability to hop on one foot.

Source: Adapted from R. J. Schain, (1977)

Muscular Hypertonia

The examiner should routinely test the responses of large muscle groups, especially the antigravity muscles (arm flexors, leg extensors) to fast and slow stretching. Gross shortening of the heel cords or hip adductors will produce the gait abnormalities mentioned above. Spinal deformities such as lordosis (forward curvature) or scoliosis (lateral curvature) may be present in varying degrees of severity.

There is little difficulty in recognizing frank spasticity. Mild forms may be less evident with manifestations limited to deep tendon hyperreflexia, slight awkwardness during activity, and shortening of the heel cords resulting in a tendency to toe walking or equinovarus deformities. Certain forms of hypertonia may manifest as cogwheel rigidity with resultant clumsiness of motor skills.

OCULAR, AUDITORY, AND SPEECH DISORDERS

Ocular Disorders

It is common for children with MBD to exhibit poor performance on ocular-tracking tasks or to demonstrate endpoint nystagmus (jerking eye movements on lateral gaze). These are some of the principal soft signs used to justify the diagnosis of minimal brain dysfunction.

There is a consensus among ophthalmologists who have studied the relationship of ocular disorders to reading problems that minor disturbances of visual acuity or ocular muscle imbalance do not themselves produce reading problems although they may aggravate an existing situation (Goldberg and Drash, 1968). Many claims have been made relating poor ocular skills, eye-hand coordination problems, or constricted visual fields to learning problems, but there is little evidence that ocular-training programs in themselves are of value in assisting children to learn. Intermittent squints and refractive errors are equally common in children with or without reading problems (Park, 1966). These statements do not mean that squint, eyestrain, and poor visual acuity do not require appropriate treatment. It should not be expected however that these measures will prevent or reverse reading disorder in children except in very rare cases.

Auditory Disorders

Hearing deficits may produce classroom impairment in the absence of gross deafness. These are usually due to high frequency hearing loss, which results in a sloping configuration of the audiogram (Matkin, 1968). High frequency deficits result in loss of consonant recognition, which is functionally more disabling than low frequency losses. Severe high frequency losses are always associated with some degree of speech impairment. Less severe deficits may not affect speech noticeably, but may require the child to concentrate intensively in order to hear. Such children may seem to lose interest in classroom activities or may be accused of uncooperative behavior when in fact they cannot maintain the effort required to hear the teacher.

Screening audiometry should be performed on all children with unexplained learning problems. This is a simple office procedure, which can be performed by a nurse or an assistant. Any evidence of a deficit indicates the need for full-scale audiologic evaluation. Failure to recognize hearing deficits in children with school problems results in misdirected effort that produces little result. The length of time that high frequency hearing deficits in children may go undetected is surprising.

It is common for children with MBD to also exhibit speech disorders. Speech is intimately associated with higher cortical functions representing man's efforts at communicating ideas. It is a purely human activity closely allied to reading. It should not be surprising that children who exhibit difficulties with speech acquisition often have later problems in acquisition of reading and spelling skills.

It is necessary to distinguish between comprehending and expressing spoken language from articulatory motor skills. The former are higher cortical functions residing in language centers of the brain (frontispiece); the latter depend upon upper motor neurone systems, peripheral nerves, and muscular structures of the mouth. Disturbances of speech based upon defective language functions of the brain are termed aphasias, while speech disorders due to faulty motor systems are called dysarthrias. The theoretical difference between these two terms is quite clear, although the distinction may not be apparent in clinical practice.

In general if a child is not speaking by the age of three years, some defect in speech mechanisms is usually present. Milestones in acquisition of ability to speak words, phrases, and sentences have been delineated (Lillywhite, 1958). By six years of age speech should generally be clear, fluent, and syntactical. However there is greater variability in acquisition of speech skills than of motor skills in children, so that the clinician should be cautious in attributing too great a significance to age of appearance of speech skills.

The services of a speech pathologist will often be of assistance in determining the nature of the speech problem as well as considering the possibilities of speech therapy.

PROGRESSIVE NEUROLOGICAL OR METABOLIC DISORDERS

Degenerative Brain Disorders

The onset of a number of degenerative disorders of the brain may be in middle childhood and the early symptoms of these disorders may be most prominent in the areas of mental or coordinative functions. These children often first reveal signs of their disease by inability to function at school. Gradual worsening of symptoms is the hallmark of a degenerative disorder. These disorders are rare, but their recognition is an important responsibility of the consulting physician. Even if a specific therapy is not available, early recognition of these diseases will at least provide the family with definite information regarding the outlook for the affected child and permit them to plan in a realistic manner. Genetic counseling is essential for families of children affected by degenerative brain disorders.

Huntington's Chorea

This hereditary disorder, transmitted by an autosomal dominant gene, may manifest itself by clumsiness, emotional lability, and restlessness for some years before the presence of a progressive disorder is recognized. Onset of symptoms in childhood has now been documented as a common occurrence (Jervis, 1963; Markham and Know, 1965; Byers and Dodge, 1967). The presence of a family history of this disease should be sought if Huntington's chorea is suspected. In the absence of a family history, confirmation of the diagnosis may require prolonged clinical observation because there is no specific means of laboratory diagnosis. Eventually the appearance of hypokinesia, incoordination, chorea, and rigidity will clarify the clinical picture. Seizure or psychotic behavior are not uncommon in this disorder.

Choreiform movement disorders may be seen in association with Sydenham's chorea, lupus erythematosus, and phenothiazine intoxications. These conditions must be distinguished from Huntington's chorea.

Hepatolenticular Degeneration (Wilson's Disease)

This is a rare disorder transmitted as an autosomal recessive trait in which recognition is especially important because of the value of dietary and drug treatment at all stages of the disease. The occurrence of mild intellectual or emotional disturbances may be the first manifestation of the disease. Fantasies of death and other morbid thoughts in affected children have been noted (Denny-Brown, 1964). Muscle rigidity, dysarthria suggestive of pseudobulbar palsy, mask-like facies, and the classic wing-flapping tremor are later manifestations of this disease. Evidence of liver disease may precede the neurological symptoms. A greenish brown pericorneal ring may or may not be seen on visual inspection, but it is invariably noted in slit-lamp examination performed by an ophthalmologist. The diagnosis is based upon absent or low blood ceruloplasmin levels and high direct reacting copper levels in serum and urine.

Torsional Dystonia (Dystonia Musculorum Deformans)

This basal ganglia disorder is characterized by abnormalities of gait and bizarre involuntary movements. Toe walking, facial grimacing, and torsional spasms of neck and trunk are perplexing symptoms to those not familiar with this disorder. Torsional dystonia is almost invariably regarded as psychological in origin during the early and sometimes even during the later stages of the disease.

The diagnosis is established by recognition of the steady progression of the characteristic dystonic movements affecting a previously well child. The pattern of inheritance is mixed, but a familial form is found in families of eastern European Jewish extraction. Excellent results have been claimed for the surgical treatment of this disorder by placement of lesions in the basal ganglia (Cooper, 1970).

Juvenile Cerebromacular Degeneration (Spielmeyer-Vogt Disease); Juvenile Lipidosis

The characteristic first symptom of juvenile cerebromacular degeneration, an autosomal recessive disorder, is the rapid loss of visual acuity beginning between five and eight years of age. Often an ocular problem is initially suspected as the cause of the visual disturbance. Within several years the appearance of coordination and mental difficulties reveals the presence of a global neurological disorder. A characteristic stuttering speech disorder has been noted as symptoms evolve (Schain and Wiley, 1965). The disease is slowly progressive and results in death by the third decade of life.

Schilder's Disease

Gait disturbance and intellectual impairment are common early symptoms of Schilder's disease, occurring as a result of diffuse degeneration of cerebral white matter. Rapidly progressive blindness of cortical origin (normal optic discs) is commonly present in Schilder's disease. The disease usually results in massive cerebral deterioration within one to two years. It is usually a sporadic disorder although hereditary forms have been described.

Friedreich's Ataxia (Spinocerebellar Degeneration)

This disorder initially involves spinocerebellar tracts and posterior columns of the spinal cord resulting in early symptoms of a slowly progressive gait ataxia. A high arched foot (pes cavus) and back deformity (scoliosis) are usually present. Signs of brain involvement including dysarthria, nystagmus and mental changes make a later appearance. Ultimately the patient with Friedreich's ataxia is severely disabled. The disorder seems usually to be transmitted as an autosomal recessive trait, although some variations have been reported. No treatment is available.

Subacute Sclerosing Panencephalitis (Dawson's Encephalitis)

This is an uncommon disorder of recent interest because of the identification of the etiological agent, measles virus acting as a slow virus. The first symptoms may be mild intellectual impairment and coordination difficulties. After a variable period of time, evident intellectual deterioration and myoclonic seizures are noted. Electroencephalogram (EEG) abnormalities in the form of rhythmic bursts of spike and wave complexes are characteristic. The diagnosis is confirmed by evidence of high levels of measles antibody in blood and cerebrospinal fluid. The disorder is progressive, resulting in severe deterioration or death within one to two years (Freeman, 1969).

Brain Tumors

Brain tumors in children are more common than was believed in years prior to the development of special procedures capable of detecting intracranial masses. The majority of brain tumors in children of primary school age are located in the posterior fossa of the intracranial cavity. Tumors in this location typically result in rapidly developing signs of postural difficulties, cranial nerve paralyses, or increased intracranial pressure. These signs are not likely to be confused with minimal brain dysfunction. However it is often unappreciated that 10 to 15% of brain tumors in young children occur in the cerebral hemispheres (Low, Corell, and Hammill, 1965; Matson, 1968). Tumors in this area may result in relatively subtle signs of impaired cortical functions for many years prior to the appearance of more florid neurological symptoms. Listlessness, indifference, and a tendency to withdraw from activities are characteristic personality alterations. The presence of persistent severe headaches in children with recent personality alterations should alert the examiner to suspect the presence of brain tumor. Sometimes the occurrence of focal seizures is the first definite clue to the presence of a brain lesion. Ultimately focal neurological signs such as hemiparesis, reflex changes, and muscle tone disturbance indicate the presence of a hemispheric lesion. EEGs, skull radiographs, and radioisotope brain scans are procedures that should be performed as soon as brain tumor is suspected.

Hyperthyroidism

Hyperkinetic behavior in an adolescent girl should raise a suspicion of hyperthyroidism, although this disorder can occur at any age or in either sex. Associated findings include tremor, tachycardia, and excessive sweating. An enlarged palpable thyroid may be noted, and exophthalmos may be visible. Graefe's sign (lagging of the upper eyelid as the eye looks down) and Mobius' sign (inability of the eyeballs to converge) may be present. Determination of protein-bound iodide or a similar measure of thyroid function will confirm the diagnosis.

CHILDHOOD PSYCHOSIS

Children with infantile autism manifest early behavioral disturbances characterized by lack of affective interest in caretaker adults, stereotyped behaviors, and varying degrees of speech deficits. These children may manifest continuous activity that superficially resembles the behavior of severely hyperkinetic children, but the conditions are different in that the autistic child lacks the ability to form human relationships. Seizure disorder (Schain and Yannet, 1960; Rutter, Greenfield, and Lockyes, 1967) and epileptiform EEG abnormalities (White, DeMyer, and DeMyer, 1964) are found commonly in autistic children. Wing (1966) suggests that autism should be regarded as a learning disability involving failure of the child to develop abilities in interpersonal relationships. Ornitz and Ritvo (1968) have argued that the symptoms of autistic children indicate the presence of global perceptual dysfunction.

Many autistic children functionally become severely retarded, while others may develop sufficiently to make marginal adjustments in classroom situations. Their odd behavior may perplex teachers and result in referral for suspected minimal brain dysfunction.

The conventional adult type of schizophrenic reaction characterized by paranoid ideology, hallucinations, delusions, and disorientation may be seen in older children with previous patterns of normal personality development. Bizarre, withdrawn, or asocial behavior may be the external manifestations of this condition. A number of organic disorders may produce schizophrenic-like behavior in children. The occurrence of a seizure in a child manifesting psychotic behavior should always be regarded as strong evidence of an organic origin of the psychosis. Medical conditions that may produce psychosis are diffuse collagen disease (especially lupus erythematosus), deep lying brain tumors in the limbic region, subacute encephalitis, and chronic forms of meningitis (tuberculosis, cryptococcosis.

coccidioido mycosis). Psychotic behavior may be part of a progressive degenerative disorder such as Huntington's chorea or Wilson's disease. Juvenile paresis (neurosyphilis) is now a medical rarity, but once was a cause of delusional behavior in children. Of greater importance in terms of present prevalence are observations that chronic drug abuse may precipitate prolonged psychotic reactions in certain individuals.

DEVELOPMENTAL HYPERACTIVITY

The concept that hyperactivity may reflect a constitutional trait was first introduced by Bakwin and Bakwin (1966) and greatly elaborated by Werry (1968). The essential element of this condition is that the hyperactivity, beginning in the first years of life, is present in a child who is otherwise mentally and neurologically intact (Table 17–2). Parents may have regarded the restless, inquisitive, impulsive behavior of their child as signs of a vigorous (usually male) personality, but these traits become a handicap when the child is expected to conform to classroom restrictions. Male preponderance is as high as 90%. Hyperactivity usually diminishes with age, but may be replaced by conduct disorders if the child has failed to enter into the learning process at school because of hyperactive behavior.

Table 17–2   Developmental Hyperactivity

1. Early hyperactivity.
2. No evidence of major CNS damage, mental retardation or psychosis.
3. Distinguished from restlessness of anxiety states or reactive behavior by its chronicity.
4. High male preponderance (90%).
5. Perceptual-motor deficits.
6. Soft neurologic signs.
7. Hyperactivity disappears by adolescence.

Source: R. J. Schain, (1975)

Thomas, Chess, and Birch (1968) have provided evidence that hyperkinesis may be a temperamental trait, constitutional in origin, and evident during the early months of infancy. Such children naturally manifest high activity levels and development of impulse control is delayed. If these personality traits are incompatible with the way in which classroom or home activities are organized, symptoms of adjustment problems arise. The physician may choose not to regard this situation as a medical problem, but its destructive effect on the child's social and academic progress is often profound.

Many such children are regarded as exhibiting minimal brain dysfunction, even though they appear perfectly normal in all other respects. In spite of disclaimers in the literature, this term implies a morbid process in the central nervous system to most parents and nonmedical clinicians. The expression developmental hyperactivity has the merit of avoiding this implication in children whose sole problem appears to be a restless disposition.

SUMMARY

Because of the prevalence in our society of children labeled with the term minimal brain dysfunction, physicians who treat children must develop a point of view toward the syndrome and a working procedure for assisting affected children. An approach to this problem can be divided into two parts: detection of somatic disorders and comprehensive management of school problems. The detection of somatic disorders that may have produced or substantially contributed to the school problem requires conventional medical skills for recognition and treatment. Comprehensive management of school problems requires a broader approach by the physician, including counseling of the parents regarding adverse family interactions, advice about educational resources, and consideration of the question of drug therapy for behavioral disorders. Parents should be able to rely on the physician to act as a scientific source of guidance regarding complex terminology and regarding the merits of the numerous therapies directed toward the child with MBD. The ability to function competently in these areas will enable the physician to provide a service for children and their families that may profoundly affect their lives.

REFERENCES

Abercrombie, M. L. J. *Perceptual and Visuo-Motor Disorders in Cerebral Palsy.* Little Club Clinics in Developmental Medicine, No. 11. London: Heinemann, 1964.

Bakwin, H., and R. M. Bakwin. *Clinical Management of Behavior Disorders in Children,* p. 351–353. Philadelphia: Saunders, 1966.

Benaron, H. B. W., B. E. Tucker, J. P. Andrews, B. Boshes, J. Cohen, E. Fromm, and G. K. Yacorzynski. "Effect of anoxia during labor and immediately after birth on the subsequent development of the child." *American Journal of Obstetrics and Gynecology,* 80, 1129–1142, (1960).

Birch, H. G., and L. Belmont. "Auditory-visual integration in brain-damaged and normal children." *Developmental Medicine and Child Neurology,* 1, 135–144, (1965).

Blau, A. "The psychiatric approach to posttraumatic and postencephalitic syndromes." *Research Publications of the Association for Research in Nervous and Mental Disease,* 34, 404–423, (1954).

Brenner, M. W., S. Gillman, O. L. Zangwill, and M. Farrell. "Visuo-motor disability in school children." *British Medical Journal,* 4, 259–262, (1967).

Byers, R. K. and J. A. Dodge. "Huntington's chorea in children." *Neurology,* 17, 587–596, (1967).

Cohen, H. J., L. T. Taft, M. S. Mahadeviah, and H. G. Birch. "Developmental changes in overflow in normal and aberrantly functioning children." *Journal of Pediatrics,* 71, 39–47, (1967).

Cooper, I. S. "Neurosurgical treatment of dystonia." *Neurology,* 20, 133–148, (1970).

Corah, N. L., E. J. Anthony, P. Painter, J. A. Stern, and D. L. Thurston. "Effects of perinatal anoxia after seven years." *Psychological Monographs: General and Applied,* 79, No. 3, (1965).

Cruickshank, W. M., H. V. Bice, N. E. Wallen, and K. S. Lynch. *Perception and Cerebral Palsy: Studies in Figure-Background Relationship.* Syracuse, N. Y.: Syracuse University Press, 1965.

Denny-Brown, D. "Hepatolenticular degeneration. (Wilson's disease)." *New England Journal of Medicine,* 270, 1149–1156, (1964).

Drillien, C. M. *The Growth and Development of the Prematurely Born Infant,* p. 258. Baltimore: Williams & Wilkins, 1964.

———"Fresh approaches to prospective studies of high risk infants." *Pediatrics,* 45, 7–8, (1970).

Finley, K. H., *Personal communication,* 1971.

Finley, K. H., L. H. Fitzgerald, R. W. Richter, N. Riggs and J. T. Shelton. "Western encephalitis and cerebral ontogenesis. *Archives of Neurology,* 16, 140–164, (1967).

Freeman, J. "The clinical spectrum and early diagnosis of Dawson's encephalitis." *Journal of Pediatrics,* 75, 590–603, (1969).

Garron, D. C., and L. R. V. Stoep. "Personality and intelligence in Turner's syndrome." *Archives of General Psychiatry,* 21, 339, (1969).

Geller, M., and A. Geller. "Brief amnestic effects of spike-wave discharges." *Neurology,* 20, 1089–1095, (1970).

Goldberg, H. K., and P. Drash. "The disabled reader." *Journal of Pediatric Ophthalmology,* 5, 11–24, (1968).

Goldensohn, E. S., and A. P. Gold. "Prolonged behavioral disturbances as ictal phenomena." *Neurology,* 10, 1–9, (1960).

Greenbaum, J. L., and L. A. Lurie. "Encephalitis as a causative factor in behavior disorders of children." *Journal of the American Medical Association,* 136, 923–930, (1948).

Gubbay, S. S., S. Ellis, J. N. Walton, and S. D. M. Court. "Clumsy children. A study of apraxic and agnostic defects in 21 children." *Brain,* 88, 295–312, (1965).

Holt, K. S., and J. K. Reynell. *Assessment of Cerebral Palsy II. Vision, Hearing, Speech, Language, Communication and Psychological Function.* London: Lloyd-Luke, 1967.

Hutt, S. J., D. Lee, and C. Ounsted. "Digit memory and evoked discharges in four light sensitive epileptic children." *Developmental Medicine and Child Neurology,* 5, 559–571, (1963).

Illingworth, R. S. "Delayed motor development." *Pediatric Clinics of North America,* 15, 569–580, (1968).

Ingram, T. T. S. *Pediatric Aspects of Cerebral Palsy.* Edinburgh, Scotland: Livingston, 1964.

Jervis, G. E. "Huntington's chorea in childhood." *Archives of Neurology,* 9, 244–257, (1963).

Kawi, A. A., and B. Pasamanick. "Association of factors of pregnancy with reading disorders in childhood." *Journal of the American Medical Association,* 166, 1420–1423, (1958).

Levy, S. "Postencephalitic behavior disorder — A forgotten entity. Report of 100 cases." *American Journal of Psychiatry,* 115, 1062–1067, (1956).

Lillywhite, H. "Doctor's manual of speech disorders." *Journal of the American Medical Association,* 167, 850–858, (1958).

Low, N. L., J. W. Corell, and J. F. Hammill. "Tumors of cerebral hemispheres in children." *Archives of Neurology,* 13, 547–554, (1965).

Lubchenco, L. O., F. A. Horner, L. H. Reed, I. E. His, D. Metcalf, B. Cohig, H. C. Elliott, and M. Bourg. "Sequelae of premature birth." *American Journal of Diseases of Children,* 106, 101–115, (1963).

Markham, C. H., and J. W. Know. "Observations on Huntington's chorea in childhood." *Journal of Pediatrics,* 67, 46–57, (1965).

Martin, H. P. "Microcephaly and mental retardation." *American Journal of Diseases of Children,* 119, 128–131, (1970).

Matkin, N. D. "The child with a marked high-frequency hearing impairment." *Pediatrics Clinics of North America,* 15, 677–690, (1968).

Matson, D. *Neurosurgery of Infancy and Childhood,* 2nd ed., p. 480–484. Springfield, Ill.: Thomas, 1968.

Mirsky, A. F., and J. M. Van Buren. "On the nature of the absense in centrencephalic epilepsy: A study of some behavioral electroencephalographic and autonomic factors." *Electroencephalography and Clinical Neurophysiology,* 18, 334–348, (1965).

O'Connell, E. J., R. H. Feldt, and G. B. Stickler. "Head circumference, mental retardation, and growth failure." *Pediatrics,* 36, 62–66, (1965).

Ornitz, E. M., and E. R. Ritvo. "Perceptual inconstancy in early infantile autism." *Archives of General Psychiatry,* 18, 76–98, (1968).

Paine, R. S. "Minimal chronic brain syndromes in children." *Developmental Medicine and Child Neurology,* 4, 21–27, (1962).

Paine, R. S., and T. Oppe. *Neurological Evaluation of Children,* p. 142–149. London: Heinemann, 1966.

Paine, R. S., J. S. Werry, and H. C. Quay. "A study of 'minimal brain dysfunction.'" *Developmental Medicine and Child Neurology,* 10, 505–520, (1968).

Park, G. E. "Functional dyslexia (reading failures) vs. normal reading." *Eye, Ear, Nose and Throat Monthly,* 45, 74–80, (1966).

Prechtl, H. F. R., and C. J. Stemmer. "The choreiform syndrome in children." *Developmental Medicine and Child Neurology,* 4, 119–127, (1962).

Richardson, F. "Some effects of severe head injury. A follow-up study of children and adolescents after protracted coma." *Developmental Medicine and Child Neurology,* 5, 471–482, (1963).

Russell, W. R., and A. Smith. "Post-traumatic amnesia in closed head injury." *Archives of Neurology,* 5, 4–17, (1961).

Rutter, M., D. Greenfield, and L. Lockyer. "A five to fifteen year follow-up study of infantile psychosis." *British Journal of Psychiatry,* 113, 1183–1199, (1967).

Schain, R. J. "Neurological evaluation of 40 children with learning disorders." *Neuropediatric,* 3, 307–317 (1970).

Schain, R. J. *Neurology of Childhood Learning Disorders, 2nd ed.* Baltimore: Williams & Wilkins, 1977.

Schain, R. J., and J. Wiley. "Evolution of a characteristic speech disorder in juvenile cerebral lipidosis." *Transcations of the American Neurological Association,* 23, 290–291, (1965).

Schain, R. J., and H. Yannet. "Infantile autism: An analysis of 50 cases and a consideration of certain neurophysiologic concepts." *Journal of Pediatrics,* 57, 560–567, (1960).

Sell, S. H. W., W. W. Webb, S. E. Pate, and E. O. Doyne. "Psychological sequelae to bacterial meningitis: Two controlled studies." *Pediatrics,* 49, 212–217, (1972).

Sells, C. J., R. L. Carpenter, and C. G. Ray. Sequelae of central nervous system enterovirus infections." *New England Journal of Medicine,* 293, 1–4, (1975).

Strauss, A. A., and L. E. Lehtinen. *Psychopathology and Education of the Brain-Injured Child,* New York: Grune & Stratton, 1947.

Thomas, A., S. Chess, and E. G. Birch. *Temperament and Behavior Disorders in Children.* New York: New York University Press, 1968.

Thurston, D. L., J. N. Middlekamp, and E. Mason. "The late effects of lead poisoning." *Journal of Pediatrics,* 47, 413–423, (1955).

Tizard, B., and J. H. Margerison. "Psychological functions during wave-spike discharge." *British Journal of Social and Clinical Psychology,* 3, 6–15, (1964).

Towbin, A. "Organic causes of minimal brain dysfunction. Perinatal origin of minimal cerebral lesions." *Journal of American Medical Association,* 217, 1207–1214, (1971).

Walton, J. N., E. Ellis, and S. Court. "Clumsy children: A study of developmental apraxia and agnosia." *Brain,* 85, 603–612, (1962).

Werner, E., K. Simonian, J. M. Bierman, and F. E. French. "Cumulative effect of perinatal complications and deprived environment on physical, intellectual and social development of preschool children." *Pediatrics,* 39, 490–505, (1967).

Werry, J. S. "Developmental hyperactivity." *Pediatric Clinics of North America,* 14, 581–599, (1968).

White, H. H., and F. D. Fowler. "Chronic lead encephalopathy. A diagnostic consideration in mental retardation." *Pediatrics,* 25, 309–315, (1960).

White, P. T., W. DeMyer, and M. DeMyer. "EEG abnormalities in early childhood schizophrenia: A double blind study of psychiatrically disturbed and normal children during promazine sedation." *American Journal of Psychiatry,* 120, 950–958, (1964).

Wiener, G., R. V. Rider, W. C. Oppel, and P. A. Harper. "Correlates of low birth weight. Psychological status at eight to ten years of age." *Pediatric Research,* 2, 110–118, (1968).

Wing, J. *Early Childhood Autism: Clinical Educational and Social Aspects.* London: Pergamon, 1966.

Zarkowsky, H. S. "The lead problem in children: Dictum and polemic.'" *Current Problems in Pediatrics,* 6, 1–47, (1976).

CHAPTER 18

Other Assessment Techniques

Theodore H. Wohl

The author has noted in Chapter 16 the theoretical areas and assessment techniques—based on relatively narrowly focused investigations—that purport to identify causal factors underlying minimal brain dysfunction. Assessments of brain and behavior relationships, language, visual, visual-motor, auditory, and gross- and fine-motor coordination frequently lead toward more precise teaching or treatment. These assessments often take place outside of the formal educational context and are frequently not integrated with day-to-day diagnostic efforts and teaching of the MBD child. There are certainly no pejorative connotations in the title *Other Assessment Techniques.* However Silver (1975) arbitrarily dissects the field into "acceptable and controversial approaches," listing in the latter category Doman and Delacato's neurophysiological retraining approaches (patterning), optometric therapy, and sensory integrative therapy as described by Ayers. He also discusses orthomolecular medicine, alpha-wave conditioning, and food additives, but strongly urges physicians to become more familiar with these approaches in order to be better resources for parents who seek guidance. Assessment approaches discussed in this chapter are often based on an overriding concern with past factors which may have contributed to the current status of the child in painstaking comparisons with known diagnostic categories. Bateman (1966) and Chalfant and Scheffelin (1969) have cautioned that these kinds of data, of undeniable value in their own right, may not provide clear-cut remedial or therapeutic directions for helping a child. Chalfant and Scheffelin reviewing research literature, succinctly summarized evidence indicating that educators believe additional knowledge of brain dysfunction does *not* tell them what to do:

1. The educator cannot fix the brain.
2. He does not know what he would do differently if he knew that the brain was damaged.
3. Such emphasis may tend to stop intensive remedial work on the assumption that the damage or its behavioral consequences are permanent.

To make matters worse, the multidisciplinary field of human development is continually providing educators with conceptualizations, diagnostic findings, and treatment recommendations couched in varying terminology and of formidable complexity. Wohl (1978) has recently emphasized the need for a human transducer who will collate, translate, and reduce cumulative multidisciplinary scientific findings to manageable form. Simply stated the various disciplines too often fail to keep themselves informed about what is going on in other fields. In defense of such ignorance they often deny that other findings have relevance for their work.

The fact that a theory or assessment methodology may be couched in neurophysiologic terms does not make it less relevant to the educator. Currently such findings probably do *not* have narrower applications, but simply represent unexploited findings of possible value. The assessment approaches and techniques will be discussed in reference to general diagnostic considerations, general brain and behavior relationships, language, sensorimotor integration, and developmental patterning. The MBD child and his problems can be located along the dimensional continua represented by these approaches. There is a major need to utilize these techniques in an integrative manner within the educational establishment and in reference to the whole child.

DIAGNOSTIC CONSIDERATIONS

Behavioral scientists and educators still are attempting unsuccessfully to understand the multiplicity of interacting factors that occur between a specific cause and an MBD child, a child who, in turn, is attempting to cope with learning tasks as well as the people around him. Since a child is much *more* than the result of central nervous system damage or dysfunction, we continue to describe and collate carefully characteristic behaviors in brain-injured children. Even so, adequate findings for purposes of subsequent remediation are often based as much on the professional's sagacity and sophistication as on specific test instruments. The task is further complicated by our awareness of the almost infinitely long list of behavioral abnormalities that may result from damage to the developing human brain. Disordered function may manifest itself in hardly noticeable circumscribed deficits in sensori-motor abilities, or it can pervade every aspect of the child's intellectual and personality functioning, disrupting abilities to cope with everyday problems of living or interfering with congenial interpersonal relationships.

Variance in the nature, site, timing, extent, and source of CNS lesions gives rise to a bewildering variety of symptoms. The interaction between the resourceful human personality and lesion variance is apparent in the example of two MBD children who respond to the competitive pressure of the schoolroom in opposite fashions: one responds with dogged effort to learn; while the other, with precisely the same pattern and level of mental abilities, may respond by refusing to learn at all. A child suffering from a brain dysfunction or injury behaves as a fusion of self and parental perceptions. Intellectual retardation may be manifest as well as variable levels of activity, difficulty in sleeping and deficiencies in inhibitions and attention. Decrease in overall intellectual efficiency may stem from deficits in a few basic factors or diffuse disruption of multiple patterns and functional organization of the brain.

Professionals attempting to assess part functions or relatively discrete reflexes and behavioral responses have long been plagued with the apparent transiency of neurologic reflexes. Even the much elicited Babinski response (stimulations of the sole of the foot followed by dorsiflexion of the big toe) may be here today and gone tomorrow. Although it is usually associated with interruption of pyramidal tract functions, it is commonly present in some cases of established corticospinal lesions in humans. Peculiarities of neuronal and synaptic conductivities with unknown factors of neurosecretory activity further depict the central nervous system as a tenuous field for measurements by relatively gross intrumentation (Truex and Carpenter, 1964). Reitan (1967) early called for data useful for clinical tests. He noted that the first step was to "formulate some kind of statement of an adequate set of psychological measurements," that is a battery of tests to reflect the behavioral correlates of brain functions. Yet the attempt to develop such test batteries and other measures of neurologic function has encountered measurement problems concerning reliability and the representativeness of the manifest behavior. Such questions are often predicated on the assessor's ability: (1) to follow original standardization instructions or skillfully depart from the same instructions and (2) to pay attention adequately to the qualitative as well as quantitative aspects of a child's response. Assessment instructions should be standardized in relation to both material and methods so that satisfactory criteria of adequacy have been met. The assessor is concerned with the question of the child's fundamental capacity and the question of how representative of the child's typical mode of performance are the results obtained. Frequently the results are compared with those obtained from a representative group sample of other children the subject's age. Complex statistical methodology for adequate standardization groups in the interpretation of test and scaling results have been developed. This also serves as a type of post-assessment control and is viewed as preventing undue dependence on the individual examiner's subjectively established norms. It is important to note that a test which helps in making one decision may have no value for another kind of decision. A sophisticated approach to the complex issue surrounding evaluation is encouraged. Rather than the general question, "Is this a valid test?" A more cogent rephrasing might be, "How valid is the test for the decision that is to be made?" Apparently the assessment processes treated in this chapter have at least a validity of use. They are considered by their devisors, proponents, and consumers as possessing a few principal uses for which their validity has been fairly well established.

Lezak (1976), in a recent comprehensive source book on adult neuropsychology, notes that central nervous system damage always includes underlying loss and implies behavioral impairment. The loss or deficit may be frank or subtle, with the latter often unobservable under ordinary conditions but sometimes becoming apparent in complex judgmental tasks or under emotionally charged conditions. This has led to a deficit assessment methodology that permits the identification of patterns of intellectual impairment and that relates directly to subsequent educational and rehabilitation planning.

BRAIN AND BEHAVIORAL RELATIONSHIPS: NEUROPSYCHOLOGICAL PROCEDURES

The purpose of the neuropsychological assessment is to "provide detailed indices of behavior allowing an integrated description, prediction, modification or control of behavior" (Lezak, 1976). At the same time there is often a need to provide data to the physician relating to the underlying condition of the nervous system. The contribution of the evaluation can be understood best within the total context of past and current theories of brain function and dysfunction, problems and techniques of measurement, and consideration of several representative studies concerning the results of neuropsychological assessment.

Brain Function and Dysfunction

Most investigators argue that primary sensory and motor functions are relatively well localized in the central nervous system. However there has been major emphasis on a compromise between extreme and specific localization theories, the higher mental functions viewpoint versus the viewpoint that such functions are equally dependent on all parts of the cerebrum. Serious consideration of animal and human experimentation lead to three major areas of conceptualization regarding brain function and deficit: (1) association or neuronal theory, (2) theory of equipotentiality, and (3) theory of regional equipotentiality or functional equivalence. The latter seems to attract the majority of adherents. Before one is prepared to utilize test results confidently, there must be a certainty that the presence or absence of a psychological function can be ascribed to a particular region of the brain. It is extremely difficult in many instances to delimit accurately the extent of anatomical and physiologic dysfunction produced by a brain lesion. Even laboratory investigations are sometimes frustrated by intracranial pressure, disruption of pathways between brain anatomical centers, contiguous cerebral edema, and functional interruption of normal neural tissue by immediately proximal pathologic tissue, and so on. Based on what has already been explained regarding the effect of various lesion characteristics on behavior, not only can different types of lesions in the same locus produce differing results, but also apparently similar lesions with respect to locus may have dissimilar effects. It is unfortunate that often there is little knowledge of the premorbid levels of certain psychological abilities. It then becomes necessary to compare the performance of the subject with data from a normal control group. Ross (1976) thoroughly discusses this form of assessment citing a study by McIntosh (1973) which strongly suggested that psychological tests do not provide unequivocal indices for brain damage in children. The results indicated that neither clinical judgment nor actuarial norms were able to classify children significantly better than chance. If children with demonstrable lesions are so difficult to classify, the task of classifying the MBD child must constitute a problem of impressive dimensions (Ross, 1976).

Lezak (1976) considers it useful to analyze behavior in terms of three functional systems: (1) intellect, the information processing aspect of behavior; (2) emotionality, concerning feelings and motivation; and (3) control, which alludes to the expression of behavior. Defects in one of these systems has inevitable repercussions within another. The processing capacity of the child lends itself to further subdivision in terms of receptive and expressive functions and within these categories such activities as awareness, recognition, orientation, speech, writing, and gross and fine-motor manipulation. These factors lead to the identification and discussion of various dysphasias and dyspraxias, which together with the general cluster of related dysfunctions known as language disturbance will be discussed later. All are subject to such variables as attention, concentration, personality, and control functions. The latter is viewed as an integral quality of all ongoing behavior. Impulsivity may seriously disrupt behavior no matter how muich intellectual or emotional residue is retained. It is probably correct to emphasize that direct, one-to-one correlations do not currently exist between specific neuroanatomical structures and such factors as overall intellectual retardation; deficiencies in inhibition and attention; unusually high, low, or variable level of activity; and difficulties in sleeping, eating, or toilet training. All may be the concomitance of central nervous system damage, but each also accompanies emotional disturbance, cultural-familial retardation, and even normal development. Overall reduction in a child's mental capacity may result because of lesion-caused deficits in a few specific basic elements, such as the development and use of verbal concepts or the maintenance of attention. Disorganization and idiosyncratic approaches are reflected in the performance of brain-injured and MBD children on tasks involving concept formation, purposive use of language, and perceptual-motor processes. The neuropsychologist today has appropriated Luria's (1966) fundamental hypotheses, if not his specific instrumentation.

If a brain lesion directly causes loss of a factor, then all functional systems which include this factor suffer, while at the same time all functional systems which do not include the disturbed factor are preserved.

Advocating a system of syndrome analysis, Luria (1966) infers physiologic differences between seemingly similar functions as well as physiologic similarities between seemingly different functions.

During the last decade Reitan (1964b) has continued to emphasize the agreement between independent judgment of neuropsychological data and data from the neurological disciplines based on individual patient assessments. Agreement significantly exceeds chance expectancy for the following categories:

1. Diffuse focal, focal and diffuse, or bilaterally focal cerebral damage.
2. Right or left hemisphere involvement.
3. Lobular localization of areas of maximal involvement within each hemisphere.
4. Static, slowly progressive, moderately progressive, or rapidly progressive character of the lesion.
5. Lesion categories including cerebral vascular disease; tumor; degenerative or demyelinating disease; inflammatory, infectious disease; and trauma.

The high positive correlations suggest that the cited study includes relevant independent variables with respect to CNS disease and psychological measurement. However agreement seems based more on the training and perspicacity of the investigators than on the power of tests to accomplish mathematical prediction of certain classification outcomes by utilizing relevant constellations of variables.

The above interpretive efforts would lack effectiveness without the recent findings, results, and implications of hemispheric asymmetry (Milner, 1954; Kimura, 1966; Sperry, 1970; and Gazzaniga, 1970). The study of brain structures reveals three major divisions of hindbrain, midbrain and forebrain, with the functional organization showing a pattern of increasing complexity from lower brain stem levels up through the cerebral cortex of the forebrain. Generally the lower centers mediate basic life-preserving functions, while more complex integrative functions seem to be largely in the province of the cerebral cortex. Through the hindbrain are intertwined nuclei and axonal fibers mediating complex postural reflexes, muscle tone, motor control and coordination, level of consciousness, alertness, stimulus screening, and overall responsivity. The midbrain nuclei seem most concerned with integration of visual and auditory automatic respones. Motor nuclei also play a role in smooth integration of muscle movements and in the patterning of automatic posture. The diencephalic and telencephalic divisions of the forebrain seem to play a major role as way stations continuously transmitting data to the cerebral cortex. They mediate emotional experience through the limbic system, memory functioning through some thalamic nuclei, and autonomic visceral functions and mood states (hypothalamic control). The two cerebral hemispheres show predictable cortical functional organization in regard to homologously positioned sensory, motor, and association areas. Each cerebral hemisphere, with the exception of certain aspects of the visual and auditory systems, mediates the function of the contralateral half of the body. Apparently the two hemispheres differ with respect to the location of perceptual and cognitive functions and in reference to selective processing of certain behaviors. Left hemisphere lesions commonly give rise to verbal and language problems and thus basically interfere with interpersonal communication. Patients with right hemisphere involvement will experience visual spatial deficit and pervasive inability to handle serial or patterned data, which cannot be readily processed by the contralateral (left) hemisphere. Language functions may be localized in homologous areas of the right hemisphere in less than 10% of left-handed persons and fewer than 1% of right-handed persons (Goodglass and Quadfasel, 1954; Penfield and Roberts, 1959). Recently the development of surgical commissurotomy procedures is proving a valuable supplement to observations of behavioral impairments arising from lateralized lesions. These procedures permit the study of differences between hemispheres relating to *how* each processes information at its disposal in addition to what is processed. Sperry (1964) characterized the left hemisphere as the analyzer and the right as the synthesizer. Lezak (1976), analyzing the mediation of spatial relationships, explains how left hemisphere processing analyzes a visual percept into details that can be identified and conceptualized verbally in meaningful qualities. The right hemisphere deals with the same visual stimuli as spatially related wholes. Thus for most people spatial recognition, pattern analyses, and appreciation of differences in the formation of complete impressions from fragmented percepts (the closure function) depends on the intact functioning of the right hemisphere. Diller (1968) and Gainotti (1972) have argued for hemispheric differences in emotional changes that accompany brain injury. Milner (1967) heavily stresses the contribution of premorbid personality predispositions when viewing patients' behavior subsequent to brain lesions.

Functional organization of behavior along the anterior-posterior axes of the brain, while seemingly less emphasized, has important implications and meaning for the interpretation of test behavior. Cortical functional patterning seems to correspond to anterior-posterior locations as well as rough demarcations of lobular divisions. Luria (1965), Benton (1967), and Hecaen (1969) have ascribed a variety of dysgnosias and dysphasias to posterior hemisphere lesions, many in the parie-to-temporo-occipital area. Hecaen and Assal (1970) state that left hemisphere lesions are apt to disrupt the serial planning and activation of neural sequences necessary to achieve a copying task, while right hemisphere constructional dyspraxias result from visuo-spatial defects. Milner (1971) noted that the more posterior left temporal lesions were more likely to produce dyslexia and verbal dysphasias than more anteriorly placed left temporal lesions. Luria (1966), in a careful neuropsychological analysis, attempted to identify different factors underlying different types of writing disturbances. He explained that in order to write accurately in response to dictation, a person must be able to accomplish a clear choice of phonemic signs by means of acoustic analysis and synthesis. He considers this possible only when the posterior section of the left temporal lobe (zone of Wernicke) is intact. Geschwind (1969) termed this disorder "Wernicke's aphasia," attributing a patient's lack of comprehension of human speech to interruption by local lesions of neural fibers connecting Wernicke's with Broca's area.

Measurement Techniques

Neuropsychological assessment usually constitutes an individually tailored approach designed to meet the needs of the patient or subject and addresses both general and specific questions of diagnosis and description. Interest is seldom restricted to the question of the presence or absence of CNS impairment. More often there is a need for delineation of capacities, strengths, limitations, emotional problems, and social and vocational implications. Test batteries of varying length consist of both standardized and unstandardized tests and are often used by those working with the MBD child. A battery of tests should measure simple sense modalities (auditory, visual, and haptic) as well as the effector responses used in communication, that is spoken, written, graphic, and constructional responses. Ideally the battery should be sensitive to varying levels of intellectual function and adequately delineate complex, abstract cognitions as well as purer and simpler sensory-motor acts. The battery and component invidual tests should provide a format for the efficient quantification and collation of data useful in establishing baselines, accomplishing subsequent comparisons, and specifically detailing areas of intellectual functioning. The examiner must flexibly consider motivational factors, low IQ, and the severity of sensory or orthopedic impairment, both in his selection of test instrumentation and in relation to whatever necessary liberties are taken with the standardized test instructions. It is important to emphasize that except for research purposes, test findings alone are seldom used for MBD remediation and diagnosis. Reitan and Davison (1974) suggest the inclusion of a modified clinical neurologic exam, estimates of cerebral dominance and laterality, and even use of projective measures in order to help clarify and support the validity of test findings and diagnostic inferences. For example in the presence of lateralizing neurologic signs, it is unlikely that uniformly low test scores could be attributed solely to deficient intelligence. Clinicopathological correlation is still regarded as the ultimate criterion in judging the validity of test results relating to central nervous system lesions. It is not realistic to consider that children will be available for anatomic exploration of their brains at postmortem. Instead examiners must content themselves with careful descriptions of behavior which are consistent with data obtained from similar children of comparable developmental levels who manifest demonstrable brain lesions as visualized by laboratory procedures, that is cerebral contrast studies, brain scans, electroencephalograms, skull films, and so on. Davison (1974) interestingly portrays American clinical psychology's preoccupation with organic damage as a unitary concept. He explains that Lashley's (1929) early animal experimentation and Goldstein's (1941) clinical theory concerning the mass action of the brain cells deemphasized notions of differential function of the brain substance depending upon topological organization. Their work mediated that brain damage had similar effects in different patients varying only in severity. This seemed to encourage the search for an ideal or single most reliable test which could accurately measure these general effects. Clinical neuropsychology has expanded and redirected this approach with a deficit or localization model which generally prevails in most medical neurologic settings. The major external criterion is lesion localization with or without support of neurologic or neurosurgical findings. Halstead's battery (1947) as modified and applied by Reitan (1955), and Benton's (1963, 1967) studies of language disorders are good examples of psychological test batteries which attempt to delineate behavior resulting from any manner of cerebral lesion. The interactional effect of many factors is acknowledged. These often obscure the meaning of individual scores and literally demand a sophisticated knowledge of diagnostic criteria and the natural history of clinical neurological disease.

Reitan and Davison (1974), while discussing Halstead's battery, note that an experiment was performed with every subject which consisted of

1. An intensive study of the test results (dependent variables) for each individual subject.
2. A written evaluation of these results, a set of predictions of neurological variables based on behavioral measurements.
3. An actual comparison of these predictions with the independently obtained neurological criterion information.

Several individual tests from the adult battery briefly explained are as follows: *Category Test:* Utilizes a projection apparatus for briefing the patient on stimulus material. The patient is required to abstract principles based upon variables such as size, shape, number, position, brightness, and color around which to organize his responses. *Tactual Performance Test:* Time, memory, and localization phases; utilizes a modification of the Seguin-Goddard form board. The blindfolded subject is not permitted to see the form board or blocks at any time. First the blocks are fitted in their proper places with the preferred hand, then the procedure is repeated with the other hand, and finally the task is repeated a third time using both hands. Board and blocks are then removed. The blindfold is taken off and the patient is required to draw a diagram of the board representing blocks in their proper spaces. Scoring is for total time needed to place the blocks on the board under all conditions. Memory component is based on the number of blocks correctly reproduced and drawn on the board, while correct localization of the blocks is also scored. *Speech Sounds, Perception Test:* Sixty spoken nonsense words which are variants of the "e" sound are presented in multiple-choice forms on a tape recorder. The intensity of sound is adjusted to the patient's preference. The patient's task is to select the spoken syllable from the alternatives printed on the test form. The research for development of the Halstead Neuropsychological Battery for Children was accomplished by Reitan from 1951 through 1954 for children 9 through 14 years of age. Directions were modified and various adult component tests were simplified. This evolved into the Reitan-Indiana Neuropsychological Battery for Children (1964b), retaining many of the tests within the Halstead battery, but permitting additional tests which were viewed as holding promise of maintaining the attention and interest of young children (5 through 8). Most neuropsychological test batteries are supplemented and extended by addition of individual tests or even supplementary batteries. These are specialized in content and administered to enhance findings when special populations are studied or certain questions are being asked of the data. The use of clinical neuropsychological test batteries is usually designed to reflect the full range of deficits associated with brain lesions and they are fully integrated and carefully systematized. However there is still a current tradition of psychometric investigation which attempts to set up unique testing situations for each patient in order to detect deviations from average or "normal" functioning in dichotomous fashion. These investigators tend to work and develop professionally in medical settings and have acquired many years of experience with large numbers of children with cerebral difficulties. Dr. Elizabeth Lord (1973) was one such worker who joined the newly organized Neurological Division of Children's Hospital in Boston in 1929 and pioneered in testing children with cerebral palsy. Using then current clinical testing instruments, she taught her collaborators how better to assess children with serious physical impairment and to appreciate the predictive significance of patterns of strengths and weaknesses in the brain-injured child. After Dr. Lord's death in 1943 her position was filled by Edith Taylor whose roots were in German genetic and Swiss Piagetian psychology. Dr. Taylor's (1959) methodological approach appreciated the examiner's personality as an integral part of examination planning. Case history interview with parents; understanding of the patient's medical condition; use of developmental norms; and use of standardized and unstandardized tests of special abilities, attention, learning ability, perceptual skills, motor situation, language facility, and so on, were utilized to the fullest extent. This approach does not differ substantively from that of the behavioral neurologist who may utilize varying conceptual rather than operational definitions of behavior.

The individual case study rather than group statistics is emphasized as a legitimate basis for generalizations. Cohn (1964) stresses the central importance:

in all neurological testing . . . is the experience of the neurologist with essentially normal children without gross problems in language function . . . child must be treated as a biologic system with disturbed function . . . the role of the neurologist is to determine whether the disturbances disclosed are likely to be associated with central nervous system lesions. [He] does not equate minimal neurologic findings with 'minimal brain damage' and that it is most sensible, through precise examination, to delineate relatively normal input systems and thereby indicate the instrumentalities through which language can be developed in the most fruitful way possible for the individual.

Luria (1966) in the context of Russian physiological emphases, armed with little more than a paper and pencil, utilizes a complex methodology, highly individualized according to the neurologic problem of the patient. Lord (1937), Taylor (1959), Luria (1965, 1966), and Cohn (1964) all attempt to elicit conceptually similar behaviors from different patients and different situations. In contrast to the neuropsychologist's emphasis on operational definitions of deficit behaviors and propensities to view behavior on a continuum, the above investigators attempt to separate clearly abnormal from normal behavior.

The administration of assessment test batteries is frequently a time consuming, expensive procedure. A major attempt to apply the law of parsimony is embodied in the employment of discriminate function analysis to obtain the best linear combination of variables in a test battery. The purpose is to predict criterion group membership utilizing various mathematical procedures. Test batteries can be shown to be producing the diagnostic discriminations asked of them (Wheeler,

Burke, and Reitan, 1963; Wheeler and Reitan, 1962). Russell, Neuringer, and Goldstein (1970) have attempted to make the reasoning involved in analyzing the results of Reitan's neuropsychological batteries explicit and objective. The authors, in explicating the decision rules, assess agreement between the classification of patients by these rules as opposed to the neuropsychologist's and clinical neurologist's categorization of patients based on the same protocols. Davison (1974) notes an impressive level of agreement, but states that the work was handicapped by arbitrary values used in place of empirical data which were not available. He argues for a neuropsychological manual which would produce a systematic casebook allowing the collation of many different kinds of knowledge and conditions contained in the literature. Such a manual would facilitate learning and certainly help weave the threads of experimentation during the last decade into a recognizable design.

Representative Studies

Methodological and developmental factors continue to bedevil the serious investigator gingerly picking his way through the welter of studies concerning the MBD child. The perception among certain professionals that brain damage is a unitary concept has already been noted. There is increasing recognition that assessment procedures within the context of brain pathology impose on the assessor the need to become familiar with the full range of cerebral pathologies in order to develop a reasonable understanding of associated psychological deficits. Medical and nonmedical investigators alike, in order to study the test performances of child groups, assign their subjects on the basis of a clinical neurologic examination which may be variable in content from one neurologist to another. It is also not uncommon to note groups divided on the basis of a provisional diagnosis, often stemming from a history of clinical neurologic examination. These are frequently found to be in error when additional information is obtained from laboratory procedures such as angiography, surgical notes, and findings from histological sections of autopsies. McFie (1975) has ruefully noted the tendency of the literature to utilize heterogeneous groups of brain-injured children (defined as having abnormal neurologic findings or abnormal EEGs) who are then tested and the results compared with a group of normal children (or children not characterized by those signs). This procedure, in rare incidences, may be helpful to identify effects which are related to a very pervasive or general factor. However if one accepts the differential effects of cerebral lesions separately located, it would appear that there could very well occur a canceling effect or that other confounding influences on the measurement could arise, resulting from the indiscriminate compounding of possibly relevant factors. Reitan (1974) has reflected that it is probably naive to hope that a single differential score index will reflect consistent findings over a range of variables as broad as that represented by brain damage of varying durations, types, premorbid characteristics, and so on. This again leads back to the previously described advantages of a neuropsychological test battery and Halstead's (1947) pioneer emphasis that only a battery of psychological tests covering a wide range of functions could effectively delineate the effects of brain damage in one patient after another.

The reader may profit from a brief survey of studies in which neuropsychological assessment is basic to clinical and educational management and to the formulation of useful theory relating to minimal brain dysfunction in children.

Clinical

Reed (1968) used the Reitan modification of the Halstead battery to assess school-age children. He proposed that the test battery was convincing "in understanding the unique constellation of problems of the individual subject." He left open the question of whether the social and educational problems suffered and manifested by large groups of school-age children could be effectively studied. He stressed that the obtained data together with rating scales and checklists could provide momentum for the development of a clinical research program relating neuropsychological test data to educational achievement. Reed seems convinced that logical relationships do exist between diagnosis and remediation. He made several suggestions regarding educational technique, behavior modification, and depictive sociograms which could lead to programmatic therapy and remediation of well-documented neuropsychological deficit. Unfortunately the individual case history and neuropsychological evaluation of a ten-year-old girl presented by Dr. Reed does not illustrate the specific application of remedial approaches to the described pattern of deficits: right-sided motor and sensory deficit, consistent evidence that the left cerebral hemisphere was functioning on a less adequate level than the right, mild right hemisphere dysfunction, and low scores on screening achievement measures.

Normative Development

Reitan and Davison (1974) discuss varying attempts and a 15-year history of broad investigations of behavioral disturbances associated with cerebral damage —he prominently quotes his own studies and that of Ernhart, et al., (1963) and Reed (1965). He discusses the utilization of extensive psychological procedures of children in the 5- to 8-year-age range with known cerebral lesions and subsequently compares them with normally functioning children in the same age range. He concludes that it is possible to draw reasonable inferences regarding brain and behavioral relationships in children who have both serious and mild deficits. He notes that behavioral measurements may provide a more sensitive measure of impairment than would clinical neurologic investigation utilizing the interindividual relationships among test results and the comparison of functioning of the two sides of the body. He advocates that neuropsychological data provide the ideal objective supplement to anamnestic and medical sources of information.

Older Children

Boll (1974) provides an excellent review of the literature relevant to children with known cerebral lesions. Three previously cited major articles authored by Ernhart, et al., (1963); Reed, Reitan, and Klove (1965); and Klanoff, Robinson, and Thompson (1969), provided information regarding neurologic issues and documented initial deficits as well as the effect on personality and developmental patterning (including the rate and pattern of overall ability development). Boll utilizing data from Klanoff, et al., (1969) and Reitan (1974), considered 13 categories of variables important in the study of a matched group of 27 brain injured and a control group. Categories were composed as a means of organizing the total number of variables and were arbitrarily grouped as follows:

- Verbal tests of the Wechsler Bellevue scale.
- Performance tests of the Wechsler Bellevue scale.
- Pure motor skill.
- Motor problem-solving.
- Visual motor problem-solving.
- Tactile perception.
- Academic development.
- Auditory perception (verbal and nonverbal).
- Visual motor reaction of temporal estimation.
- Incidental memory and alertness.
- Concept formation.
- Summary intelligence measures.
- Name writing.

After computing all possible inter-test correlations, the data indicated significant differences among correlations for groups of children with and without brain damage on a wide variety of psychological behavioral measures. Boll speculates concerning the possibility that the *same* abilities were *not* being measured in children with and without brain damage.

Theory Formulation

Satz and Sparrow (1970) and Sparrow and Satz (1970) thoroughly review the literature on specific developmental dyslexia with attention to certain patterns of deficit:

- Directional or left-right confusion.
- Calculation difficulties.
- Finger differentiation problems.
- Spontaneous writing and spelling impairments.
- Impairments in formed perception.
- Impairments in verbal intelligence.
- Cross-modal integration.
- Disconnection syndromes.
- Maturational lag hypothesis.
- The concept of hierarchical levels in hemispheric specialization.

Citing educational (de Hirsch, et al., 1966) and genetic factors (Halgren, 1950; Owens, Adams, and Forrest, 1968) and a variety of achievement measures, Satz and Sparrow conclude that the literature suggests that both neurological and psychological organization result from genetic and environmental factors which constitute a maturational lag and that this usually retards the acquisition of reading skills. The authors also attempt to determine how dyslexics differ from normal readers by monitoring the development of laterality across several age levels. Assuming, as did Penfield and Roberts (1959), that verbal skills represent the summit of language differentiation and lateralization in man, Satz and Sparrow note the difficulty of investigating problems in central lateralization. They describe several forms of dichotic auditory stimulation techniques that provide an indirect method for determining the cerebral lateralization of speech (Satz, Achenbach, and Fennell, 1967). In addition some 80 children were examined for possible developmental aspects of laterality and dyslexia, utilizing levels of manual preference, dexterity, strength, controlling eye, ear asymmetry, verbal intelligence, lateral awareness, and finger differentiation tests. Information was obtained regarding family history of left-handedness. The Harris (1957) scale of lateral dominance, electric tappers, Keystone telebinoculars, Piaget's hole-in-mirror technique, and serial questions were among specific techniques used to measure important variables. Satz and Sparrow concluded that there were no differences between older dyslexics (9 to 12) and controls on early lateralized functions, whereas there were substantial differences on those functions hypothesized to lateralize at later ages (9 to 12). Their results are viewed as consistent with a developmental theory of laterality as it relates to dyslexia. Rourke, et al., (1973) utilized the Bellevue Intelligence Scale and a grooved pegboard test with a large number of children referred for assessment of learning problems which were thought to have resulted from cerebral dysfunction. They reported that their results supported the inference of cerebral dysfunction, but mainly for older children. Younger children were viewed as having a different pattern of psychological test performance. Ross (1976) concludes that the study was ambiguous and went considerably beyond the data. However he felt that a possible difference between younger and older learning-disabled children could be explained by developmental hypotheses. Older children have probably received much more cumulative stress, resulting in a disorganized, anxious child who is functionally much more similar to a brain-injured person. Gallagher (1966) and later Ross (1976) suggest that much less emphasis should be put on neurologic etiology and much more emphasis put on descriptive measures that can delineate patterns of academic deficit. Any program based on such assessment procedures must allow for considerable individual attention and tutoring.

LANGUAGE

It is fair to state that theoretical and applied workers in educational fields have not emphasized language factors in understanding or remediating academic performance of MBD children. Experimental psychology and research in clinical medicine have long been aware of the relationship of language development and pathology to intellectual and perceptual functioning, but have not in past years adequately facilitated the translation of laboratory findings to the applied situation. Yet language represents the summit of evolutionary development and is basic to a person's ability to cope and adapt. Horton (1968) has referred to it as the major vehicle through which we organize our world and achieve some degree of order out of the chaos arising from the infinite number of sensory impressions that we take in during a lifetime. An analysis of the behavior of an MBD child cannot escape the pervasive effect of language deficit. There is a growing body of literature, compiled by linguists and psycholinguists, stressing the various components of language as crucial to the acquisition of skill in reading. Vellutino (1977), in a recent systematic review and critique, thoroughly explored several conceptualizations of dyslexia. He proposed that poor readers lack the syntactic, semantic, and chronologic cues that ordinarily alert one to the critical differences in letters and words. This is considered a dysfunction in visual-verbal learning and results in marked perceptual inefficiency. In explaining difficulties in semantic processing, Vellutino explains that poor readers may have difficulty both in linguistic coding of incoming information and in the retrieval of linguistic reference associated with given stimuli. He stresses, as did Gibson (1971), the multitudinous classes of information that must be processed to decode even a single word. Subtle syntactic deficiencies are increasingly recognized as impeding development of reading skills. Goodman (1968) has found that inaccuracies at various stages of reading are typically determined by semantic and syntactic contexts. Vellutino concludes that the influence of a faulty single linquistic system may chronically impair the ability to read. The other major emphasis, from the point of view of assessment, is disordered language or dysphasia resulting from central nervous system dysfunction, either congenital or acquired. Despite the implicit assumption of a central nervous system lesion as the principal significant "cause" of the dysphasic problems of children, most authorities view the dysphasias and dyspraxias as collections of essentially disparate conditions with the sole commonality being a failure or difficulty in the acquisition of language skills. Assessment of this condition requires close examination of symbol-formulation disorders as reflected from behavior in each communicative modality: listening, speaking, reading, writing, and gesturing. Lezak (1976) contrasts aphasia assessment with other kinds of verbal tests,

which measure aspects of verbal function that may be affected by perceptual or response disabilities, by learning and memory disorders . . . when symbol formulation remains essentially intact.

Wepman (1960), Jones and Wepman (1968), Myklebust (1963), and others have provided models suitable for assessment of organically caused language disturbance. They also provide therapeutic and educational guidelines for subsequent remediation and therapy. Most of the assessment techniques are actually test batteries that are modality oriented, sensitive to transfer across modalities, and yield a detailed description of the child's communication problems. Test items and levels of individual tests most often progress from the simple to the complex. Horton (1968) suggests that levels of assessment within any one sense modality should proceed from:

1. Sensation
2. Attention
3. Recognition
4. Retention
5. Discrimination

6. Imagery
7. Recognition of the verbal symbol
8. Retrieval and use of the verbal symbols.

Many writers mention the fact that dysphasic children (very likely all children) learn principally through one major channel modality. It is therefore necessary to identify visile and audile children for purposes of confronting the consistent problem in special education, that is whether to focus remediation efforts on the assets or strengths of the individual. Horton (1968) describes the role of auditory processing as a major contributor to organic language disturbance. It is therefore not accidental that major sections of aphasia batteries are devoted to the measurement of auditory function or that methodologies such as the McGinnis method (1963), originally developed for deaf children, have found welcome and wide application throughout many categories of special education. It is unfortunate that the best standardized, best known, and most discriminative aphasic batteries were standardized principally on adult populations, that is mainly patients having acquired a brain lesion resulting in some kind of communicative disability. At least two of these batteries are briefly discussed here because they can be administered to children, interpreted qualitatively, take into account the developmental level and intelligence of the child, and describe in detail the disordered language functions themselves.

The Porch Index of Communicative Ability (PICA)

Eighteen subtests are administered, four of them requiring a spoken response eight gestural, and six graphic. The tests rely on visual recognition, understanding spoken word functions, and basic reading ability. The same common items are generally used for each subtest and responses must be scored according to a 16-point multidimensional scoring system. No response is scored as 1; an active response after a cue is given is described as "cue" and is scored as 8, and so on. PICA (1967) examiners must undergo a rigorous 40-hour training period. This leads to high score reliability correlation and has been shown to be valid in its applications. A battery takes anywhere from 1 hour to 1/2 hours and has been criticized in terms of its length and to some extent for its emphasis on visual and graphic abilities at the expense of aural areas.

The Minnesota Test for Differential Diagnosis of Aphasia

Schuell (1965) culminated pioneering work in measurement of aphasic disturbance by devising a lengthy test involving 47 subtests requiring on the average from one to three hours for suitable administration. The battery measures different aspects of five factor, analytically derived areas:

- Auditory disturbances.
- Visual and reading disturbances.
- Speech and language disturbances.
- Visuo-motor and writing disturbances.
- Disturbances of numerical relationships and arithmetic processes.

Classifying a patient using Schuell's system involves great familiarity with the data reported in the technical manual. The test does not seem adequately standardized, perhaps due to the number and frequency of revisions (eight). The examination booklet also contains a six-point scale for rating a patient's test-taking behavior or extra-test observations.

Brief screening tests are used frequently to supplement the more careful language evaluation of complete aphasia test batteries. They usually do not require technical knowledge of speech pathology for satisfactory administration or interpretation. The Halstead-Wepman (1949) and the token test of De Renzi and Vignolo (1962) fairly represent the usefulness and flexibility of the screening test. The former has no rigid scoring standards and is oriented around the nature of the language problem once it has been delineated. The token test only requires that a patient comprehend the token names, verbs, prepostitions, and instructions (Lezak, 1976). The tokens come in two shapes, two sizes, and five colors. The examiner gives a series of 62 oral commands in five sections of increasing complexity. The test often unmasks symbolic processing problems that are not readily recognizable and is remarkably sensitive to a wide variety of disruptive linguistic processes. Spreen and Benton (1969) developed a shortened, still more abbreviated modification of the Token test which proved to be an adequate screening form for distinguishing aphasic and nonaphasic patients.

Our interest in language assessment continues to be stimulated by such questions as:

- What is the connection between language and the thinking process? (Lerner, 1971)
- What is the nature of its relationship with social learning processes and perceptual, motor, and conceptual development?
- What are the specific links and how are they developmentally manifest in learning disabilities?
- What is the extent to which dysphasia impairs intellectual functioning? (Valenstein 1976)

Since disorders of symbol processing and language development are not unique to minimal brain dysfunction, it is of crucial importance to explore and describe the reciprocal relationship between developing language and intelligence. Valenstein approaches this problem from the standpoint of the effects of demonstrable localized brain lesions and resultant specific impairments of linguistic function. Individually administered intelligence tests tend to rely heavily on linguistic skills while similar nonlinguistic tests usually rely on categorization or generalization. Congenitally deaf children, prior to language instruction, may do well on the latter performance-oriented tests. Goldstein (1948) postulated that pure aphasia is only a surface manifestation of an underlying impairment of prelinguistic intellectual abilities. If this is true, there is no real difference between impairment in higher-order abstract abilities and language impairment. Valenstein (1976) rather favors the point of view that many aphasics may retain nonverbal intelligence and may be able to learn through alternate means of communication. He explores the recent literature for evidence that language and intellectual abilities are highly correlated, and discusses research evidence relating to gestural communication, understanding of nonlanguage sounds, drawing, tests of categorization (De Renzi, et al., 1966), and tests of generalization (Basso et al., 1973). Valenstein, citing preliminary results, suggests that some patients with poor verbal comprehension do well on verbal matching tasks involving categorizations and generalizations. The general range of conclusions seems to indicate that there are identifiable groups of aphasics who are able to understand nonlinguistic cues and who may be able to learn other means of symbolic communication. These findings, when applied to the MBD child, add particular emphasis to the importance to indentifying residual or remaining abilities, so that appropriate remediation may be accomplished through developing patterns of strengths rather than perseveratively quantifying failures.

SENSORY-MOTOR INTEGRATION AND DEVELOPMENTAL PATTERNING

There is little question that the momentum and thrust of professional concern and treatment of MBD children has centered around sensory-motor and perceptual-motor development. Itard's (1962) inspired attempt to teach the feral child Victor in the locale of Aveyron, through Seguin's (1971) major contributions to the educational experimental literature in France and the United States, culminated in the representative philosophies and investigations of Piaget (1952), Gesell and Ilg (1948), Strauss and Lehtinen (1947), and Hebb (1949). Current investigators and treatment methodologies draw heavily from and have stressed the importance or receptor-effector processing as the focal area for assessment and remediation. The work of Ayres (1972), Doman, et al., (1960), Kephart (1960), and Getman (1965) seem related closely to their specialities, occupational therapy, psychology, language pathology, education, and so on. All emphasize the importance of developmental stages and conclude that adequate thinking and conceptualization can occur only when the various perceptual-motor systems have been fully developed and integrated. Interruption in the development of normal motor learning will affect future learning potential. Heinz Werner's (1948) concepts of the "action qualities of objects" and "action space" may be related to a toddler's understanding of an object and the orientation to its location in space totally dependent on its functional use (action). This illustrates the visual role or movement and manipulation in the development of cognition. Assessment attempts within this context are usually concerned with the presence or absence of a particular behavioral segment, or whether the behavior under study is appropriate for the child's chronologic age. There is a consistent attempt to order the diagnostic findings in a manner which will lead towards future appropriate therapies and remediation. In the case of the MBD child, there is the clear inference that coordinated diagnostic descriptions and appropriate remediation will cause the child to be more amenable to reading and mathematical instruction.

Ayers (1967) proposes that the brain stem and certain other subcortical structures have a facilitating or disruptive effect on higher cortical function. She has adapted a series of hypothetical constructs (much misused and uncritically applied by many) which are designed to enhance cognition. Crediting Luria (1966), Ayers describes the brain as operating on the basis of functional systems involving many levels which are relatively separate but in some ways related to each other. Primary defects may result in the disturbance of several different systems manifested by symptoms which may seem unrelated. In other situations higher functions are simply depressed and are reflected by general weakening of neural processes. The constructs and subsequent treatment philosphy of Ayers also flows naturally from the work of Bobath and Bobath (1964) and from that of Rood (1967). Every muscle spindle and every surface hair activated by small movements will create an afferent sensory stimulus pattern in the brain. Much of body image and mental alertness are dependent on proprioceptive and kinesthetic stimuli. If low threshold myelinated pathways are used first, the same pathways are primed for speedier transmission immediately following stimuli. Thus the Fernald (1943) method of tracing a word several times prepares the neural tracts for what is to follow. Semans (1967) correctly classifies these concepts with the older Jacksonian (1932) view of the hierarchical organization of integrative brain function and with the more recent Denny-Brown (1962) interpretation of the motor and perceptual disorders of patients with regard to lesions at various levels of the neuroaxis. A fundamental principle seems to be the identification of abnormal postural patterns and the facilitation of normal postural reaction. This is described by Semans (1967) as accomplished by simultaneous inhibiting of certain reflex patterns controlled at key points, while active (more adaptive) automatic reactions are introduced. Ayers (1965) completed a factor analytic study in which she identified four major types of dysfunction which she characterized as: (1) deficits in motor planning (praxia, dyspraxia), (2) deficits in postural and bilateral integration, and (3) disorders in form and space perception, and (4) tactile defensiveness (avoidance reaction). Two major diagnostic and treatment principles are: (1) recapitulation of the sequence of perceptual-motor development, and (2) control of sensory input—continuous maturation of the process of organizing tactual and proprioceptive impulses along with visual stimuli into meaningful perception. In assessment one must explore the protective or spinothalamic pathway with its discriminating system which differentiates among various tactile sensations. Interwoven is the posterior column medial-leminiscal system—touch and proprioception utilized more for perceptual processes than for survival functions.

A series of test batteries have been devised by Ayers (1964, 1965-1969, 1966*a*, 1966*b*) and her associates which purport to measure sensory integrative mechanisms. They are the Southern California Kinesthesia and Tactile Perception Test, Southern California Motor Accuracy Test, and the Southern California Perceptual-Motor Test. They are best utilized with children from 4 to 10 years of age. Many of the subtests are normed and the directions standardized. The batteries are easily administered and scored and offer useful information in terms of hypothesized brain mechanisms and providing specific bases for subsequent remediation and therapy. Children are said to enjoy the tests and seem motivated generally by the format. Several reviewers (Gaines, 1972, Kephart, 1972, Landis 1972, and Proger, 1972) have criticized these batteries as variously lacking appropriate test-retest reliability measures, presenting little or no validity data, accomplishing gross and superficial measurement of abilities, and as possessing questionable stability coefficients which decrease with age.

Both Ayers (1965) and Kephart (1960) emphasize assessment as an important means of identifying children who lack the developmental readiness skills necessary for academic progress. Their surveys and batteries seem psychometrically inadequate and are conceptually far short of the stimulating material contained in the writings of both of these investigators.

Optometry has contributed also to the general assessment and treatment of the MBD child. Getman (1965) postulates a hierarchy of skills based on innate response systems and progressing through gross and more specialized motor systems. Development eventuates in eye–hand relationships and perfection of ocular motor systems where matched and precisely balanced movement of both eyes are achieved. When these ocular mechanisms are ready, speech-motor, visualization, and perceptual systems can occur. Perception develops into cognition, which in its highest form is viewed as abstraction, imagination, relativity, and expression. The total constitutes the highest level of intellectual development. Getman and his associates offer planned exercises for developing perception and intelligence. Programs stress practice in general coordination, balance, eye-hand coordination, eye movements, general movement patterns, form recognition, and visual memory (imagery). Flax (1967), and a significant proportion of optometrists concerning themselves with learning problems, tend to down-play the role of visual acuity measurements as clearly differentiating those who are successful in learning to read from those who have reading difficulties. Most believe that the role of vision becomes increasingly dominant as normal development proceeds. Assessment usually proceeds along the lines of thorough description of levels of visual development. These include acuity measurements, refractive error, binocular coordination, accommodative facility, eye movement control, inter-sensory relationships, and the ability to integrate sensory-motor and postural data as a means of structuring signals received through the eyes (Flax, 1967). Learning to read is defined as the ability to match visual configurations to language constructs and ultimately form concepts. Optometric theories have been judged valuable in leading to important specific assessments in methods of treatment. However individual authorities (Silver, 1965; Hagin, 1965) have criticized lack of documentation, unwarranted speculation, reliance on anecdotal evidence, and seeming unwillingness to undertake planned experimental validation studies. More severe criticisms have been leveled by ad hoc committees of several medical specialties with the nominal support of the National Council for Exceptional Children. A few of the objections seem guild oriented, while others correctly emphasize that the teaching and assessment of the MBD child properly belongs in the context of education, and eye care should never be instituted in isolation when a patient has a reading problem.

Still another developmental-perceptual approach brought forth by Doman (1967), Delacato (1963), and associates at the Institutes for the Achievement of Human Potential (IAHP) in Philadelphia is frequently classified as "sensorimotor patterning or neurological organization treatment approach." Stemming from the earlier work and writings of Fay (1948), the fundamental rationale is that central nervous system damage may be treated directly by prescribing activities which will strengthen specified neurologic organizations and thereby prevent and eliminate a wide range of language problems. The basic theory of neurological organizations assumes that the process of individual development recapitulates the process of species development. Humans perceive in predetermined order through the medulla and cord, pons, midbrain, and cortex eventuating in hemispheric dominance. The individual's development of vison, audition, mobility, and language parallels and is functionally related to his anatomical progress (Robbins, 1966). Advocates of the method infer that parents may be able to improve normal development significantly in their children and that this can result in easing world tensions and enhancing the evolutionary process. Assessments and diagnoses seem to center around the "Developmental Profile" (1965). According to McDonald (1968), baseline functional areas consisting of three expressive or motor functions—mobility, language, and manual competence (writing); perceptive or sensory functions and visual competence (reading); auditory competence (understanding man's spoken language); and tactual competence (stereognosis—are plotted on a developmental profile chart. Neurological age which falls below chronological age is indicative of neurologic disorganization. Severity of impairment is equated with the total number of functions involved and the size of the discrepancy between neurological and chronological age. The performance on each of 42 subcriteria are totaled and then converted to a neurological age equivalent. One is then able to determine a child's neurologic organization relative to that of his chronological age peers. The developmental profile seems to have developed from the ongoing cumulative clinical work of the institute. Similar to most developmental scales, a behavior or skill that is either present or absent is matched chronologically with the typical or mean appearance of that behavior in the child's age range. It is a well know fact, by this time, that deviations from normative averages do not necessarily indicate pathology. Use of the profile as justification for putting restrictions on certain age-appropriate activities of which the child is capable and to restrict many typical child rearing practices as damaging to the child's potential, are regarded by many authorities as misuse of diagnostic procedures. This author is unable to discover pertinent data relating to the construction of the profile and attempts to cross validate it against other accepted methods are rare or nonexistent. Since the early sixties, the medical, psychological, and educational literature (Robbins, 1966; Cohen, Birch, and Taft, 1970; Freemen, 1967; and a published joint statement of 10 medical, health, and educational associations) has advanced severe criticism of the Doman-Delacato (1960, 1967) assessment and treatment methodology. Their ire was directed against certain theoretic and practical implications of the theory of neurological organization, the constant promotion of publicity devoted to the technique, insufficient exposures of ideas in scientific journals, seeming lack of documentation, lack of empirical evidence, and regidification of therapeutic procedures which are demeaning and may lead to disruption and neglect within the patient's family. Neman, et al., (1974) evaluated a sensorimotor patterning program with 66 institutionalized mentally retarded children and adolescents. Using adequate experimental groupings and procedures, they found significantly greater improvement in language ability resulting from sensorimotor training than occured with two other control groups. Intellectual functioning was not enhanced by the procedures, nor was validation of the developmental profile attemted.

   The Doman-Delacto treatment approach, while receiving severe criticism for its generally uncritical attitude and generally overoptimistic tone of publicity and communications, does not seem to differ substantially from other approaches discussed in this chapter. The author appreciates and sympathizes with the fact that parents and even therapists under stress, coping with the multitudinous problems of a special child, may reach out to grasp the extended helping hand. It seems foolish to wait until science and basic research produce final answers. All of the methods and approaches discussed in this chapter offer evaluation which constitutes the first step of remediation. Motor readiness, perception, and concept formation remain linked in inevitable stepwise progression. Yet remediation of motor deficits does not necessarily lead to improvement in academic skills. Language development, a central factor in assessing and remediating minimal brain dysfunction, is omitted from consideration within most perceptual-motor theoretical approaches.

SUMMARY

A wide range of assessments often takes place outside of formal educational contexts and frequently is not integrated with day-to-day diagnostic efforts and teaching of the MBD child. This chapter has emphasized principally assessments of brain and behavior relationships, language development, visual-motor, auditory, and gross and fine-motor coordination. It is assumed that the MBD child and his problems can be located along several dimensional continua represented by these approaches.

Various tests and scales have been developed to describe carefully and collate characteristic behaviors in brain-injured children. However subsequent analysis and therapeutic remedial planning are often based more on general professional knowledge than on the test instruments themselves. Disordered central nervous system functioning may manifest itself in hardly noticeable circumscribed deficits of sensorimotor abilities, or can pervade every aspect of a child's intellectual and personality functioning.

Neuropsychological assessment is presented as an individually tailored approach, addressing both general and specific questions, prognosis and description. The individual subtests vary from complex abstractive to simple sensorimotor and usually measure auditory, visual, and haptic sensory modalities. Such batteries are designed to measure the presence and nature of brain impairment in spite of its varying dimensions within different people. This has led to a primary methodology permitting the identification of patterns of intellectual impairment and directly related to subsequent educational or rehabilitative planning. The concomitants of central nervous system damage, such as impulsivity and distractibility, also may seriously disrupt behavior and interfere with learning. Luria's (1966) fundamental maxim continues to provide a major foundation for neuropsychological efforts today:

If a brain lesion directly causes loss of a factor, then all functional systems which include the disturbed factor, are preserved.

The last decade has witnessed the attempts of Reitan (1964) and others to obtain agreements between independent judgments of neuropsychological data and data from the neurological descplines based on individual patient assessments. High positive correlations are found in relation to focal and diffuse differentiation, hemispheric or lobular involvements, actual character of the lesion, and specific lesion categories—tumor, inflammatory degenerative, or demyelinating disease. Recent findings concerning hemispheric asymmetry significantly contribute to the knowledge of brain structures and functional organizations of mental processes and enhance current interpretive efforts.

Halstead's battery (1947), as modified and applied by Reitan (1955), utilizes the major external criterion of lesion localization with or without support of neurologic findings. The multifaceted battery devised originally for adults was extended downward chronologically to be utilized with children as young as five years of age.

Other investigators stress the construction of unique testing situations for each patient in order to detect deviations from average or "normal" functioning in dichotomous fashion. Students were taught to assess children with serious physical impairment and to appreciate the predictive significance of patterns of strengths and weaknesses in brain-injured children. This approach agrees with that of behavioral neurologists, who may utilize varying conceptual rather than operational definitions of behavior. The child is viewed as a biologic system with disturbed functions and the role of the neurologist is to determine whether the disturbances disclosed are likely to be associated with central nervous system. lesions. Properly focusing on optimal treatment potentials, the behavioral neurologist is urged to delineate relatively normal input systems and thereby indicate the instrumentality through which language can be developed in the most fruitful way for the individual.

Discriminant function analysis has been employed in order to obtain the best linear combination of variables in a test battery for the purpose of predicting criterion group membership. Utilizing various mathematical procedures, further progress is being accomplished by attempting to explicate and objectify the decision rules based on neuropsychological batteries as well as collating relevant literature material for a manual which would facilitate teaching and validation of neuropsychological techniques.

It is probably naive to hope that a single differential score index will reflect consistent findings or a range of variables as broad as that represented by brain damage. Work with clinical investigation, normative development, and older children illustrates in several ways the utilization of test batteries and the relationships between diagnosis and remediation. Studies have legitimately drawn reasonable inferences regarding brain and behavioral relationship in children who are both seriously and mildly brain dysfunctioned. The effects of earlier incurred lesions and later personality development in older children and various theoretical formulation, particularly those suggesting relationships between MBD and certain neurological and psychological hierarchical patterns resulting from genetic and environmental factors are currently under intensive study.

A study of behavior of an MBD child cannot escape the central fact of language deficit. The literature stresses that various components of language as crucial to the acquisition of skill in reading. Syntactic, semantic, and chronologic cues alert one to critical differences in letters and words. Poor readers in fact may have difficulty both in linguistic references associated with given stimuli. Disordered language or dysphasia resulting from central nervous system dysfunction is a major focus of assessment efforts. Assessment of this condition requires close examination of symbol formation disorders as reflected from behavior in each communicative modality: listening, speaking, reading, writing, and gesturing. Brief screening tests are frequently used to supplement extensive aphasia test batteries allowing quick flexible differentiations between aphasic and nonaphasic patients. The reciprocal relationship between developing language and intelligence is also receiveing much current attention. There are distinguishable groups of aphasics who can understand nonlinguistic cues and may be able to learn other means of symbolic communication. Remedial application of these findings to the MBD child through teaching to strengths is recommended.

Considerable professional effort and study has centered around the sensori-motor and perceptual-motor development of the MBD child. All investigators in this area agree that adequate thinking and conceptualization can occur only when the various perceptual motor systems have been fully developed and integrated. Assessment attempts are concerned usually with the presence or absence of a particular behavior segment, or whether the behavior under study is appropriate for the child's age. The diagnostic findings are ordered in a manner which will lead toward future therapeutic and educational remediation. These methodologies have the justification of urgent need, but have been regarded as oversold and overgeneralized from scant empirical findings. They are described as ignoring the central role of language and academic skills in their approach.

Integration within the rubric of education of potentially helpful approaches to children with minimal brain dysfunction continues to be a paramount challenge. Implicit is the need for interdisciplinary communication and collation of empirical research findings. Meaningful assessment and eventual remediation can proceed best from a firm knowledge base rather than devisive beliefs.

This project was supported by grant No. MCT–000–918–12–0 and MCT 000–912–12–0 awarded by the Bureau of Community Health Services, Health Services Administration, Public Health Service DHEW and grant No. 59–P–25297/5–06 awarded by Region V, Social and Rehabilitation Service DHEW to the University Affiliated Cincinnati Center for Developmental Disorders and the University of Cincinnati Department of Psychology.

REFERENCES

Ayers, A. *Southern California Motor Accuracy Test.* Los Angeles: Western Psychological Services, 1964.

———"Patterns of perceptual-motor dysfunction in children: A factor analytic study." *Perceptual and Motor Skills,* 203, (1965).

———*Southern California Perceptual-Motor Test.* Los Angeles: Western Psychological Services, 1965–69.

———*Southern California Figure-Ground Visual Perception Test.* Los Angeles: Western Psychological Services, 1966a.

———*Southern California Kinesthesia and Tactile Perception Test.* Los Angeles: Western Psychological Services, 1966b.

———"A neurobehavioral approach to evaluation and treatment of perceptual motor dysfunction." (Paper read before the American Orthopsychiatric Association Annual Meeting, Washington, D.C.: March, 1967.)

———*Sensory Integration and Learning Disorders.* Los Angeles: Western Psychological Services, 1972.

Basso, A., E. De Renzi, P. Foglione, H. Scotti, and H. Spinnler. "Neuropsychological evidence for the existence of cerebral areas critical to the performance of intelligence tasks." *Brain,* 96, 715–728, (1973).

Bateman, B. "Three approaches to diagnosis and educational planning for children with learning disabilities." *Academic Therapy,* 2, 215–222, (1966–1967).

Benton, A. *The Revised Visual Retention Test: Clinical and Experimental Application,* 3rd ed. Iowa City: The State University of Iowa, 1963. [Distributed by the Psychological Corporation of New York]

Benton, A. "Constructional apraxia and the minor hemisphere." *Confina Neurologica,* 29, 1–16, (1967).

Bobath, K., and B. Bobath. "The facilitation of normal postural reactions and movements in the treatment of cerebral palsy." *Physiotherapy*, 50, 246–262, (1964).

Boll, T. "Behavioral correlates of cerebral damage in children aged 9 through 14," in R. Reitan and J. Davison, eds., *Clinical Neuropsychology Current Status and Application*, pp. 91–120. Washington, D.C.: Winston & Sons, 1974.

Chalfant, J., and M. Scheffelin. *Central Processing Dysfunctions in Children*. Institute for Research on Exceptional Children. Urbana: University of Illinois; Bethesda, MD.: U.S. Department of HEW, 1969.

Cohen, H., H. Birch, and L. Taft. "Some considerations for evaluating the Doman-Delacato 'patterning' method." *Pediatrics*, 45(2), 302–314, (1970).

Cohn, R. "The neurological study of children with learning disabilities." *Exceptional Children*, 31(4), 179–185, (1964).

Davison, L. "Introduction," in R. Reitan and L. Davison, *Clinical Neuropsychology: Current Status and Application*, pp. 1–46, 325–363. Washington, D.C.: Winston & Sons, 1974.

Delacato, C. *The Diagnosis and Treatment of Speech and Reading Problems*. Springfield, Ill.: Thomas, 1963.

Denny-Brown, D. *The Basal Ganglia*, Chaps. 5, 6, 7. New York: Oxford University Press, 1962.

Diller, L. "Brain damage, spatial orientation, and rehabilitation," in S. Freedman, ed., *The Neuropsychology of Spatially Oriented Behavior*. Homewood, Ill.: Dorsey, 1968.

Doman, R., E. Spitz, E. Zucman, C. Delacato, and G. Doman. "Children with severe brain injuries: Neurological organization in terms of mobility." *Journal of the American Medical Association*, 174, 257–262. (1960).

————"Children with severe brain injuries: Neurological organization in terms of mobility," in E. Frierson and W. Barbe, eds., *Educating Children with Learning Disability*, pp. 363–386. New York, Appleton-Century-Crofts, 1967.

Ernhart, C., F. Graham, P. Eichman, J. Marshall, and D. Thurstone. "Brain injury in the pre-school child: Some developmental considerations: II. Comparison of brain injured and normal children." *Psychological Monographs*, 77, 17–33, (1963).

Fay, T. "Neurophysiologic aspects of therapy in cerebral palsy." *Archives of Physical Medicine*, 29, 327, (1948).

Fernald, G. *Remedial Techniques in Basic School Subjects*. New York: McGraw-Hill, 1943.

Flax, N. "The development of vision and visual perception: Implications in learning disability," in D. Newcomb, ed., *Proceedings of the International Convocation on Children and Young Adults with Learning Disabilities*, pp. 130–135. Pittsburgh: Home for Crippled Children, 1967.

Freeman, R. "Controversy over 'patterning' as a treatment for brain damage in children." *Journal of the American Medical Association*, 202, 385–388, (October 30, 1967).

Gaines, R. "Southern California Figure—Ground Visual Perception Test." in O. Buros, ed., *The Seventh Mental Measurements Yearbook*, Highland Park, N.J.: Gryphon, 1972.

Gainotti, G. "Emotional behavior and hemispheric side of the brain." *Cortex*, 8, 41–55, (1972).

Gallagher, J. "Children with developmental imbalances: A psychoeducational definition," in W. S. Cruickshank, ed., *The Teacher of Brain Injured Children*, pp. 23–43. Syracuse, N.Y.: Syracuse University Press, 1966.

Gazzaniga, M. *The Bisected Brain*. New York: Appleton-Century-Crofts, 1970.

Geschwind, N. "Problems in the anatomical understanding of the aphasias," in A. Benton, ed., *Contributions to Clinical Neuropsychology*. Chicago: Aldine, 1969.

Gesell, A., and F. Ilg. *Infant and Child in the Culture of Today,* New York: Harper & Row, 1943.

Getman, G. "The visuomotor complex in the acquisition of learning skills," in J. Helmuth, ed., *Learning Disorders,* vol. 1. Seattle: Special Child Publications of the Seattle Seguin School, 1965.

Gibson, E. "Perceptual learning and the theory of word perception." *Cognitive Psychology,* 2, 351–368, (1971).

Goldstein, K. *Language and Language Disturbance,* New York: Grune & Stratton, 1948.

Goldstein, K., and M. Schurer, "Abstract and concrete behavior." *Psychological Monographs,* 53, 1941.

Goodglass, H., and F. Quadfasel. "Language laterality in left handed aphasics," *Brain,* 77, 521–548, (1954).

Goodman, K. "The psycholinguistic nature of the reading process," in K. Goodman, ed., *The Psycholinguistic Nature of the Reading Process.* Detroit: Wayne State University Press, 1968.

Hagin, R. "Perceptual training for children with learning difficulties." *Symposium.* Middlesex General Hospital Speech and Reading Clinic, N. J. 1965.

Halgren, B. "Specific dyslexia: A clinical and genetic study." *Acta Psychiatrica et Neurologica,* 65, 1–287, (1950).

Halstead, W. *Brain and Intelligence: A Quantitative Study of the Frontal Lobes.* Chicago: University of Chicago Press, 1947.

Halstead, W., and J. Wepman. "The Halstead-Wepman aphasia screening test." *Journal of Speech and Hearing Disorders,* 14, 9–15. (1959).

Harris, A. "Lateral dominance, directional confusion and reading disability." *Journal of Psychology,* 44, 283–294, (1957).

Hebb, D. *The Organization of Behaviors.* New York: Wiley, 1949.

Hecaen, H. "Cerebral localization of mental functions and their disorders," in P. Vinken and G. Gruyn, eds., *Handbook of Clinical Neurology,* vol. 3, New York: Wiley, 1969.

Hirsch, K. de, J. Jansky, and W. Langford. *Predicting Reading Failure: A Preliminary Study.* New York: Harper and Row, 1966.

Horton, K. "Organic language disorders in children," in C. Haywood, ed., *Brain Damage in School Age Children,* pp. 87–109. Washington, D.C.: The Council for Exceptional Children, 1968.

The Institutes for the Achievement of Human Potential. "Developmental Profile." Philadelphia: 1963.

Itard, J. *The Wild Boy of Aveyron,* New York: Appleton-Century-Crofts, 1962.

Jones, L., and J. Wepman. "Language: A perspective from the study of aphasia," in S. Rosenberg, ed., *Directions in Psycholinguistics,* pp. 237–253. New York: McMillan, 1968.

Kephart, N. *The Slow Learner in the Classroom.* Columbus, Ohio: Merril, 1960.

———— "The Southern California Kinesthesian and Tactile Perception Tests." in O. Buros, *The Seventh Mental Measurements Yearbook,* pp. 1288–1289. Highland Park, N.J.: Gryphon Press, 1972.

Kimura, D. "Dual function asymmetry of the brain in visual perception." *Neuropsychologica,* 4, 275–285, (1966).

Klonoff, H., G. Robinson, and G. Thompson. "Acute and chronic brain syndromes in children." *Developmental Medicine and Child Neurology,* 11, 198–213, (1969).

Landis, D. "The Southern California Perceptual Motor Test," in O. Buros, ed., *The Seventh Mental Measurements Yearbook,* pp. 1290–1291. Highland Park, N.J.: Gryphon Press, 1972.

Lashley, K. *Brain Mechanisms and Intelligence,* Chicago: University of Chicago Press, 1929.

Lerner, J. *Children with Learning Disabilities,* pp. 142–207. Boston: Houghton Mifflin, 1971.

Lezak, M. *Neuropsychological Assessment,* pp. 10, 54, 69–84. New York: Oxford University Press, 1976.

Lord, E. *Children Handicapped by Cerebral Palsy.* New York: Commonwealth Fund, 1937.

Luria, A. "Neuropsychology in the focal diagnosis of brain damage." *Cortex,* 1, 2–18, (1965).

Luria, A. *Human Brain and Psychological Processes,* pp. 71. New York: Harper & Row, 1966.

McDonald, C. "Neurological organization: An evaluative review of the theories and procedures of Doman and Delacato," in H. C. Haywood, ed., *Brain Damage in School Age Children,* pp. 212–225. Washington, D.C.: The Council for Exceptional Children, 1968.

McFie, J. *Assessment of Organic Intellectual Impairment,* pp. 132–144. London, England: Academic Press, 1975.

McGinnis, M. *Identification and Education by the Association Method,* Washington, D.C: Volta Bureau, 1963.

McIntosh, W. "Clinical and statistical approaches to the assessment of brain damage in children." *Journal of Abnormal Child Psychology,* 1, 181–195, (1973).

Milner, B. "Intellectual function of the temporal lobes." *Psychological Bulletin,* 51, 42–62, (1954).

———"Discussion of the subject: Experimental analysis of cerebral dominance in man," in C. Millikan and F. Darley, eds., *Brain Mechanisms Underlying Speech and Language.* New York: Grune & Stratton, 1967.

———"Interhemispheric differences in the localization of psychological processes in man." *British Medical Bulletin,* 27(3), 272–277, (1971).

Myklebust, H. "Psychoneurological learning disorders in children," in S. Kirk and W. Becker, eds., *Conference on Children with Minimal Brain Impairment,* pp. 26–36. Chicago, Ill.: National Society for Crippled Children and Adults, 1963.

Neman, R., P. Roos, B. McCann, F. Menolascino, and L. Heal. "Experimental evaluation of sensorimotor patterning used with mentally retarded children." *American Journal of Mental Deficiency,* 79(4), 372–384, (1974).

Owens, F., P. Adams, and T. Forrest. "Learning disabilities in children: Sibling studies." *Bulletin of the Orton Society,* 18, 33–62, (1968).

Penfield, W., and L. Roberts. *Speech and Brain Mechanisms,* Princeton, N.J.: Princeton University Press, 1959.

Piaget, J. *The Child's Conception of Numbers.* New York: Humanities Press, 1952.

Porch, B. *Porch Index of Communicative Ability.* Palo Alto, Cal.: Consulting Psychologists Press, 1967.

Proger, B. in O. Buros, ed., *The Seventh Mental Measurements Yearbook,* pp. 1291–1292. Highland Park, N.J.: Gryphon, 1972.

Reed, H. "Screening children with cerebral dysfunction," in H. C. Haywood, ed., *Brain Damage in School Age Children.* pp. 109–127. Washington, D.C.: Council for Exceptional Children, 1968.

Reed, H., R. Reitan, and H. Klove. "The influence of cerebral lesions on psychological test performances of older children." *Journal of Consulting Psychology*, 29, 247–251, (1965).

Reitan, R. "An investigation of the validity of Halstead's measures of biological intelligence." *Archives of Neurology and Psychiatry*, 73, 28–35, (1955).

————"Psychological defects resulting from cerebral lesions in man," in J. Warren and K. Ahert, eds., *The Frontal Granular Cortex and Behavior*, pp. 295–313. New York: McGraw-Hill, 1964a.

Reitan, R. "Manual for administering and scoring the Reitan-Indiana Neuropsychological Battery for Young Children." Indianapolis: University of Indiana Medical Center, 1964b.

Renzi, E. De, and L. Vignolo. "The token test: A sensitive test to detect disturbances in aphasics." *Brain*, 85, 665–678, (1962).

Robbins, M. "A study of the validity of Delacato's theory of neurological organization." *Exceptional Children*, 517–523, (April, 1966).

Rood, M. "An interpretation of the approach of Rood to the treatment of muscular dysfunction." *American Journal of Physiological Medicine*, 46, 900–957, (1967).

Ross, A. *Psychological Aspects of Learning Disabilities and Learning Disorders*, pp. 62–84. New York: McGraw-Hill, 1976.

Rourke, B., D. Yanni, G. McDonald, and G. C. Young. "Neuropsychological significance of lateralized deficits in the grooved pegboard test for older children with learning disabilities." *Journal of Consulting and Clinical Psychology*, 41, 128–134, (1973).

Russel, E., C. Neuringer, and G. Goldstein. *Assessment of Brain Damage: A Neuropsychological Key Approach*. New York: Wiley-Interscience, 1970.

Satz, P., and S. Sparrow. "Specific developmental dyslexia: A theoretical formulation," in D. J. Bakker and P. Satz, eds., *Specific Reading Disability*, pp. 17–41. Rotterdam, The Netherlands: Rotterdam University Press, 1970.

Satz, P., K. Achenbach, and E. Fennell. "Correlations between assessed manual laterality and predicted speech laterality in a normal population." *Neuropsychologia*, 5, 295–310, (1967).

Schuell, H. *Differential Diagnosis with the Minnesota Test*. Minneapolis: University of Minnesota Press, 1965.

Seguin, E. *Idiocy and Its Treatment by the Physiological Method*. Clifton, N.J.: Augustus M. Kelley, 1971. [Originally published in 1866.]

Semans, S. "The Bobath concept in treatment of neurological disorders." *American Journal of Physical Medicine*, 46, 732–785, (1967).

Silver, A. "Perceptual training for children with learning difficulties." *Symposium on Speech and Reading*. Middlesex, N.J.: Middlesex General Hospital Speech and Reading Clinic, Middlesex, N.J.: 1965.

Silver, L. "Acceptable and controversial approaches to treating the child with learning disabilities." *Pediatrics*, 55(3), 406–415, (1975).

Sparrow, S., and P. Satz. "Dyslexia, laterality and neuropsychological development," in D. J. Bakker and P. Satz, eds., *Specific Reading Disability*, pp. 17–41. Rotterdam, The Netherlands: Rotterdam University Press, 1970.

Sperry, R. "Problems outstanding in the evolution of brain function." James Arthur Lecture on the Evolution of the Human Brain. New York: American Museum of Natural History, 1964.

Sperry, R. "Cerebral dominance in perception," in F. Young and D. Lindsley, eds., *Early Experience and Visual Information Processing in Perceptual and Reading Disorders*. Washington, D.C: National Academy of Sciences, 1970.

Spreen, O., and A. Benton. "Neurosensory center comprehensive examination for aphasia." Victoria, B. C.: Neuropsychology Laboratory, Department of Psychology, University of Victoria.

Strauss, A., and L. Lehtinen. *Psychopathology and Education of the Brain Injured Child.* New York: Grune & Stratton, 1947.

Taylor, E. *Psychological Appraisal of Children with Cerebral Defects,* pp. 3–37. Cambridge, Mass.: Commonwealth Fund, Harvard University Press, 1959.

Taylor, J., ed. *Selected Writings of John Hughlings Jackson,* J. Landon, Hodder and Stoughton, 1932.

Truex, R., and M. Carpenter. *Strong and Elwyn's Human Neuroanatomy,* 5th ed., pp. 111–112. Baltimore: Williams & Wilkins, 1964.

Valenstein, E. "Aphasia and intelligence." (Paper read before the Second Annual Course in Behavioral Neurology and Neuropsychology, Orlando, Florida, 1976).

Vellutino, F. "Alternative conceptualizations of dyslexia: Evidence in support of verbal deficit hypothesis." *Harvard Educational Review,* 47(3), 334–355, (1977).

Wepman, J. "The interrelationships of hearing and speech, and reading." *The Elementary School Journal,* 9, 325–333, (1960).

Werner, H. *Comparative Psychology of Mental Development.* Chicago: Follet, 1948.

Wheeler, L., and R. Reitan. "The presence and laterality of brain damage predicted from responses to a short aphasia screening test." *Perceptual and Motor Skills,* 15, 783–799, (1962).

Wheeler, L., C. Burke, and R. Reitan. "An application of discriminant functions to the problem of predicting brain damage using behavioral variables." *Perceptual and Motor Skills,* 16, 417–440; 681–701, (1963).

Wohl, T. "Psychologists working with LD children," in K. Donelly, ed., *Communicative Disorders.* Boston: Little, Brown. [1978] in press.

PART SEVEN

Relationship of MBD To Other Concepts of Dysfunction

Chapters 19–22

CHAPTER 19

Hyperactivity

Thomas J. Kenny

An overriding need to demonstrate a direct relationship between the entity called Miminal Brain Dysfunction and the behavior termed Hyperkinesis or the Hyperkinetic Syndrome has taken on an air of desperation that seems to reflect the unsettled status of each condition. This approach has led to the synonymous or interchangeable use of the terms as if each is coexisting proof of the other's legitimacy. This has become such a common practice in the area of MBD-hyperkinesis that people now refer to the diagnosis as an all-encompassing wastebasket that describes everything and defines nothing.

The generally accepted definition of MBD given by Clements (1966) is as follows:

The diagnostic and descriptive categories included in the term minimal brain dysfunction refer to children of near-average or above average general intelligence with learning or certain behavioral abnormalities, or both, ranging from mild to severe which are associated with subtle dysfunctioning of the central nervous system. These may be characterized by combinations of deficits in perception, conceptualization, language, memory and control of attention, impulse or motor function. During the school years a variety of special learning disabilities are the most predominant manifestation.

This definition involves factors that deal with general cognitive ability, neurologic development, specific learning ability, and variations in behavior. Though this is a broad set of criteria, the focus has been on one element, neurologic development, and its relation to another factor—hyperactivity. Interestingly the correlated behavior, hyperactivity, has never been effectively defined or quantified.

The term hyperactivity or hyperkinesis is both nonspecific and subjective. It is used differently by different observers, with the subjective interpretation as a pitfall in its usage. Werry and Sprague (1970) has defined hyperactivity as a chronic, sustained, excessive level of motor activity which is the cause of significant and continued complaint both at home and at school. After many studies, Cromwell, Baumeister, and Hawkins (1963) concluded that hyperkinesis is at best an elusive phenomenon, one which does not lend itself well to objective criteria or measurement. According to Budenhagen and Sickler (1969), hyperactivity describes those aspects of a person's behavior which annoy the observer.

After a considerable investment of time and resources the question, "What is MBD-hyperkinesis?" is still unanswered. We must look critically at what our research efforts have produced in order to discard less productive ideas and to generate new, challenging opportunities. The purpose of this chapter will be to present in a critical manner the traditional approaches that have been used in assessing MBD-hyperkinesis and to attempt to judge the utility of the process.

After reviewing the status of the syndrome with an attempt to reconceptualize the problem, some suggestions for needed research strategies will be offered.

THE NEUROLOGIC TRADITION IN HYPERKINESIS

The presumed relation of MBD and hyperkinesis has several origins. The earliest studies usually cited in the formulation of a neurologic relationship between the two syndromes go back to behavior changes related to demonstrable brain insult. In children, the study of Kahn and Cohn (1934) is a major starting point. The identification of a pattern of organic drivenness as a result of encephalitis in children was a precursor of much of the current theory. It is important to note that the early studies dealt with populations that had demonstrated brain damage and associated behavioral change. The subsequent efforts built on this correlation inferring that, from behavior similar to that of brain-damaged children, one can diagnose brain damage without the historical proof.

There has been a long standing effort in physiology and neurophysiology to map areas of brain function. The process involves relating damage or dysfunction in the brain to corresponding impairment in sensory or motor function. Major areas of the cerebral cortex have been identified as the centers of certain aspects of sensory-motor function. The issues of localization of communication processing in the left temporal hemisphere is a case in point.

Identification of the area of damage or dysfunction in the neurologic system was undertaken in the belief that this information directly determined the course of treatment and the prognosis. This is the so-called medical model which implies that knowledge of the etiology yields a prescription for treatment. There seem to be two factors that have interacted to sustain the medical model approach to MBD-hyperkinesis. First the medical model holds out the promise of a simple, successful treatment or cure. The medical profession has had a long tradition of attacking a physical problem and by virtue of their effort, eliminating it. This approach has worked well in the area of infectious disease, such as malaria, smallpox, yellow fever, polio, and so on. Unfortunately this same zeal has been extended into an area that is not as amenable to either prevention or cure, MBD-hyperkinesis. It would be gratifying to find a virus to explain this problem and then develop an inoculation against it. Such an answer avoids all issues of guilt, emotional deprivation, environmental and educational deprivation, and is certainly more palatable to the American public.

The second factor involved in sustaining the neurologic focus relates to the original definition of MBD. This definition had elements of neurologic, psychologic, and educational deficits, but the prime assessment role seemed to be relegated to the physician. The recommended diagnostic evaluation included a detailed medical history, a physical and neurologic examination, and an electroencephalogram. These procedures seemed designed to identify the underlying etiology of the problem while the psychological or educational evaluation was only useful in describing the symptom manifestations or consequences of the problem. In the attempt to gain acceptance of the existence of MBD-hyperkinesis, a great effort was made to alert physicians to the problem and to have them accept a role in its diagnosis. In the early years of this stage of the MBD controversy, it became routine for the physician to assume the controlling role in the process with educators, social workers, and psychologists quietly abandoning their expertise to the physician or functioning as extensions or agents of the physician. In some states children could not legally be placed in special educational programs without the recommendation or justification by a physician. In some school systems one criterion for placement included the record of an abnormal electroencephalogram. The physician was thus put in the position of translating a dysrhythmic set of scriggly red lines into an educational program or interpreting the meaning of poor finger-to-thumb opposition for a remedial educational plan. This was an unfair demand to make of the physician, it was an abdication of responsibility by the educator, it was disregard for the sophistication of mental health professionals, and it was an unconscionable imposition on the child. One unfortunate result of this approach to the MBD-hyperkinesis problem was the start of a pattern that transformed the numerous problems usually manifested by children into a unitary entity. Barton Schmitt (1977) noted that the children who are brought into the physician's office for ''not minding'' are now brought in because of hyperkinesis. Schmitt goes on to say that in his experience an organic basis for the referral complaint of hyperkinesis can be determined in less than 1% of the children.

BRAIN DAMAGE VERSUS BRAIN DYSFUNCTION

It has been repeatedly pointed out that the phenomena called MBD-hyperkinesis have had a variety of names associated with the syndrome (Bax, 1963). The early terms such as organic behavior syndrome or minimal brain damage came to be unacceptable because the organic or damage aspect of the syndrome had never been clearly delineated. Names for the syndrome proliferated as experts attempted to find an honest and reasonable compromise to explain the state of scientific knowledge about the syndrome. The end result reflects a semantic exercise that might well be considered a scientific cop-out. Lacking any clear proof of damage, the experts created a description that very strongly implies a relationship to damage, but which they suggest obviates the need to document the evidence of the relationship. This maneuver raises the question of the possibility of a continuum of reproductive causality in which gross brain damage represents one pole and neurologic integrity represents the other pole, with Minimal Brain Dysfunction between the two extremes. The idea has merit but there are inherent complications which must be acknowledged. The concept could imply a rigid, one dimensional continuum that would make neurologic status the main factor in human function. In reality neither of these positions is correct. Certainly one must acknowledge many other factors interact with neurologic status to affect human functioning and given the reality of individual difference, the points between normality and pathology represent at best a rubber tape measure that has different gradients for each individual at each age. The point of this discussion is to emphasize that the concept of Minimal Brain Dysfunction cannot be viewed as half-way toward the effects of demonstrable brain damage. The finding that measles encephalitis produces motor drivenness does not justify the assumption that something less, but somehow akin to encephalitis, can produce the same behavior in lesser degree. In the case of brain damage it is understood that factors such as age of onset and extent of neurologic involvement combine to influence the manifestations of the damage. Brain damage is not expressed in one type of sensory-motor behavior, but in various types that are somehow related to all of the factors mentioned above so that brain damage explains not only hyperactivity but also language and communication disorders; learning disabilities; and problems of gait, balance, and coordination in varying combinations. The idea of a continuum ranging from gross brain damage to minimal brain dysfunction to normal development leaves no place for severe emotional disturbance such as schizophrenia. Introducing the issue of severe emotional problems raises the question of all the other factors that can interact to produce behavioral change. Given the accepted idea that emotional dysfunction can produce anorexia nervosa, it is simplistic to think that hyperactivity can only be produced by neurologic dysfunction. It is possible that hyperactive behavior is a symptom that can reflect neurologic dysfunction, emotional disturbance, a language disorder, or a social-environmental deficit. Anxiety may be the key commonality in many instances of hyperactive behavior. Anxiety may relate to a basic emotional insecurity or dysfunction or it may reflect the frustration experienced as a result of a poor learning experience or a learning disability. The inability to use language effectively frequently results in a child becoming motorically active. A poor parent-child relationship may teach the child to make his presence known to society by attention-getting over-activity.

The symptom, hyperactivity, is probably as nonspecific as the symptom, fever. There may be a neurologic basis for some manifestations but it is of limited benefit to attribute all of the symptom manifestations to this single factor.

HYPERKINESIS AS A SYNDROME

The previous section concerned the historical emphasis on neurologic factors to explain the behavior associated with MBD and/or hyperkinesis. Looking again at Werry and Sprague's (1970) definition, we note that:

Hyperactivity has been defined as a chronic, sustained level of motor activity which, because of its excessive degree, is the source of continued complaint from both the child's home and his other environment.

The words chronic, sustained, and excessive clearly suggest that the behavior is easily discriminated from other, more normal motor-behaviors. Unfortunately this is not the case. When brought to critical analysis, the concept of hyperactivity becomes subjective, personally and situationally related, and grossly overlapping with nonhyperactive behavior. Budenhagen and Sickler (1969) has stated that hyperactivity is that aspect of a person's behavior that annoys the observer. Others describe instances in which a child with little motor activity frustrates one person while a more active child is readily accepted by a different person. Dubey (1976) reacts to this problem by writing:

Typically hyperkinetic children are described no more specifically than as being restless, overactive, impulsive, and distractible. Common diagnostic measures, such as Conner's Rating Scale, require no more than global ratings and thus do not provide specific information concerning the topography, frequency, and intensity of the child's behavior. As such, the present diagnostic procedures provide little basis for recognition of the particular behavioral characteristics of the individual child.

In a study of 100 children referred for evaluation with a primary complaint of hyperactivity, Kenny, et al., (1971) found that only 35% of the children were judged to be hyperactive by the majority of those professionals observing them. Less than half the group was felt to be hyperactive by *any* of the observers and only 13% were rated as hyperactive by all observers. This finding can be explained in terms of personal difference in the concept of hyperactivity between the referring persons and the clinic staff or in situational factors that produced the behavior in a particular place. It is questionable whether either of these factors should legitimately affect a population defined by Werry's criteria.

Attempts to improve on global ratings or observer judgment by using precise or quantifiable measures have generally failed to produce reliable differences. Many attempts have been made and the level of technical sophistication has extended from counting objects touched or manipulated, number of grid squares in a room traversed in a time period, the recording of wrist and foot movements using pedometer and converted wristwatches, to a recent attempt to use ultrasonic movement detection beams. The outcome of these studies has led to an explanation that hyperactive children do not differ in amount of motor activity but in the quality or type of activity. That is hyperactive children are not *more* hyperactive than other children, but their activity is more purposeless, nonfunctional, and annoying.

Failing to define the single factor of motor activity as a unique attribute of the MBD-hyperkinetic population, it is useful to look at the efforts to describe or isolate a syndrome. There have been several well conceptualized attempts to establish the hyperkinetic syndrome (Werry, et al., 1972; Routh and Roberts, 1972; Langhorne, et al., 1976). The most usual approach involves a factor-analytic evaluation of a broad list of examination procedures and behaviors to establish some descriptive clustering. At this time these efforts have most often met with what must be considered scientific failure. Werry, et al., (1972) reports on a study of 103 hyperactive children in which 10 factors were extracted that had significant loadings. The major factor identified by this analysis accounted for only 16% of the total variability. The factor loadings ranged from the high of 16% to a low of 8%. The results do not convincingly identify any specific clustering that could reliably constitute a syndrome. Langhorne, et al., (1976) conclude in a study of 94 hyperkinetic boys that the results of factoral analysis in their study showed factor loadings were more source-related than symptom-related. These findings are similar to those reported by Werry in his paper. Routh and Roberts (1972) also report an inability to factor analyze a cluster of factors that could be considered a syndrome.

The approach used in the studies cited range from very broad to reasonably specific. In a 1968 study of hyperactivity Werry began with approximately 150 variables but reduced these to 67 by eliminating those items that had a frequency of abnorality of less than 10%. In his 1972 factor analytic study Werry and co-workers began with 140 signs of abnorality but found that 70 were totally absent in the population. Of the 70 signs that occurred only 17 were present in more than 10% of the children. The import of these data strongly contradicts the likelihood of finding a well-defined symptom cluster to explain hyperactivity. The size of the item sample slso suggests that broadening the evaluation process does not insure that an undetected factor is lurking around the corner.

Even though these studies fail to find a syndrome of hyperkinesis, one must look at some of the methodologic shortcomings. These problems would not improve the likelihood of finding a syndrome but are raised in the hope of laying to rest the effort to produce uniformity out of etiologic diversity.

As has been mentioned by both Werry and Langhorne, et al., (1976) the factors identified by the analysis more usually reflected the sample source rather than symptom complexes. What this indicates is that Werry's Factor 1 largely evolves from the neurologic examination and may well be as much a result of the neurologist's interest or approach as a reflection of a symptom relation. Similarly, the loading in Factor IX reflects items from the psychological examination and probably reflects the psychologist's approach. If the factors were symptom related, it is more likely that they would cross examiner procedures and reflect similar underlying processes being tapped by different examination techniques. In a study of 100 children referred for evaluation because of hyperactivity, Kenny, et al., (1971) found that there was no statistical relationship among the different parts of the medical examination, that is among the medical history, neurologic examination, and electroencephalogram. Children suspected to be hyperactive did not show a tendency to cluster test abnormality so as to indicate an additive effect from each part of the examination. In fact the results showed an unrelated pattern of findings of abnormality so that each part of the evaluation had no less probability of identifying the child's problem than multiple combinations of the procedure.

THE EVALUATION OF THE HYPERACTIVE CHILD

There is an extensive body of reports dealing with the evaluation of MBD-hyperactive children. It is difficult to sort out those papers which primarily focus on MBD from those that deal with hyperactivity. Most often the evaluation approach is basically similar in the study of both factors. This overlap in the literature may make a discussion of the evaluation of hyperactivity similar to that reported in sections of this book dealing with MBD or parts of the evaluation process involved in MBD, nonetheless it seems cogent to review briefly the evaluation procedures. The usual approach to the evaluation of hyperactivity seems to have been taken directly from Clement's (1966) task force's recommendations for evaluating MBD. The features of the evaluation include a detailed medical history, a neurologic examination, an electroencephalogram, psychological assessment, and an educational assessment. A review of the efficiency of the component parts of the evaluation process seems in order.

The Neurologic Examination

The effort to identify a neurologic basis for the observed hyperactive behavior is the most pervasive theme in the research literature. The usual neurologic examination has been used in its classic form, expanded, modified, abridged—everything except automated.

The relative ineffectiveness of the classic neurologic examination in the area of MBD has been acknowledged since the early 1960s. The use of the term, Minimal Brain Damage, was abandoned after a conference of experts agreed that the behavior (syndrome) entity described did not present the accepted definition of brain damage, destruction of brain cells (Bax, 1963). The idea of *minimal* ruled out the use of the traditional approach and required that the examination cover new ground. This decision was part of the process that helped create interest in soft neurologic signs. The traditional examination of neurologic status was modified in ways that were felt to facilitate the diagnosis of this new entity. Studies began to report the incidence of soft signs in an aberrant population without comparison of these signs in a general population or consideration of the maturational factors involved in the sign. The process was almost routinely correlational, that is take an atypical population, assess that population for the presence of the soft signs, and relate this to the outcome behavior. Little effort was exerted to determine if these soft signs were related to MBD-hyperkinesis per se or if they happened to be a characteristic of atypical children in general. Despite these methodologic shortcomings, it is still important to note that the low level correlations in the study did not raise questions about the hyperactive children who did not show soft signs. There seemed to be little concern about the reason for this difference. The unstated assumption was that not enough soft signs were tested to demonstrate the difference of this group. Most of the studies focusing on soft signs find that nearly 40% of the population have no abnormal finding, yet the diagnostic inference is drawn from this marginal finding (Kennard, 1960; Kenny, 1971). In the study by Kenny, et al., (1971) previously mentioned, it is interesting to note that evidence of soft neurologic signs was found in 48% of the population. In those children with soft signs that were seen by two physicians, usually the staff pediatrician and a neurology consultant, there was a consistent tendency for the pediatrician to find soft signs and the neurologist not to identify the signs. This occurrence may represent greater attention by the pediatrician or the fact that the neurologist, acting as a consultant, was more removed from the referring complaint and less influenced by it. There are a number of other methodological flaws in the studies of neurologic evaluation of hyperkinetic children. The neurologic examination was developed on adults and like many other medical procedures was extrapolated to children with no real effort to account for maturational factors. The tacit assumption seems to be that children are miniature adults and that the same standards apply to them. Similarly the "all or none" approach of a manifestation of abnormality in adults is accepted with children, this is in opposition to the finding that signs that appear at one age in children may disappear at a later age. Very few of the studies reporting abnormal findings in children include any data relating to test-retest stability of the findings over a period of time. Greenberg and McMahon (1977) have recently published a study which concludes that there is a lack of reliability of these signs over a time period. In short the usual neurologic examination procedures provide little standardization of criteria for judging abnormality, little evidence of the distribution of soft signs in the general population or in other atypical populations, and limited consideration about the influence of maturation on the stability of manifest signs. The study by McMahon and Greenberg reporting on serial neurologic examinations of hyperactive children concludes:

The clinician must be circumspect in the use of these signs as diagnostic criteria. Furthermore, there is no indication that these signs have any value in assessing course of treatment.

Efforts to refine methods of eliciting and measuring responses, as well as determination of the optimum subject state and ambient conditions, seem unlikely to result in greater reproducibility and usefulness.

These observations raise serious doubt whether testing for these soft neurologic signs has any justification in a clinical setting.

The Electroencephalogram

The use of the electroencephalogram to assess epilepsy is an accepted diagnostic procedure. The extension of this tool to a group of children with behavioral problems is accepted on the basis of the assumption of an underlying continuum of causality. The weakness of this assumption is similar to that discussed in the extension of the hard neurologic examination into the area of soft signs. It is a well accepted fact that the results of an EEG is subject to interpretation and to functional limitations. Authorities accept that normal EEG's occur routinely in abnormal populations and that abnormal EEG records are found in up to 15% of the normal population. Thus experts argue that a normal EEG is not diagnostic of normality but are concerned about interpreting an abnormal EEG as nonsignificant. In addition the EEG is another instance in which adult standards for pathology have been extended to encompass a population of children without adequate concerns about the maturational factors involved. The addition of borderline diagnostic categories of EEG abnormalities closely parallels the status of soft neurologic signs. The studies of abnormal findings in EEG records of hyperkinetic children is usually about the same magnitude as that of positive findings of neurologic abnormality, that is a low correlation. In addition there is a question of the meaning of certain EEG findings in children when assumed from adult standards. Kellaway and Kubola (1967) reports in a large study of children that abnormal findings that are significant in adults have a less reliable meaning when found with children. His findings note that 50% of a group of children who had a specific spike focus in the EEG record—a very realiable sign of damage in an adult population—failed to produce this finding on subsequent records and did not manifest any clinical problem. Similar questions have been raised about the borderline findings, including a special pattern called 14/6 per second spike waves. This pattern has often been called an EEG correlate of behavioral problems, yet studies by Lombroso, et al., (1966) suggest that it may be typical in children and disappear with age.

The studies of EEG abnormalities in children raise an issue that is not usually considered in the effort to identify an etiologic relationship to neurologic dysfunction. Most studies fail to show any evidence that the type or frequency of these abnormalities is particularly related to MBD—hyperkinetic children. On the contrary these studies tend to show that these findings are associated with a broad range of behavioral problems or atypical groups of children. At the other end of the continuum Dubey (1976) states:

> Absence of a relationship between EEG abnormality and hyperkinesis is further suggested by the failure to note differences between those hyperkinetic children who demonstrate the abnormality and those hyperkinetic children who show normal EEG tracings. The failure to find such differences in the areas of clinical symptomatology, severity of disturbance, and psychological test performance suggests strongly that the presence of an EEG abnormality in some hyperkinetic children may be more of an irrelevant association than an etiological factor.

The current state of EEG studies suggests a lack of clear or generalized findings. In clinical practice there is a growing movement away from the use of the EEG as a diagnostic tool. The pragmatic reason is probably more related to the cost of the study rather than its utility, but the result is the same. In addition even most EEG enthusiasts will acknowledge that an abnormal EEG has little value in prescribing treatment. Only in cases in which epilepsy is diagnosed is there any reason to accept the assumption that the EEG will influence treatment. However there is a persistent tendency to use abnormal EEG records as a justification for prescribing medication. This is yet another instance of the medical model constricting the possible treatment approaches to a behavioral problem.

The Medical History

There is a wide belief that complications of pregnancy and birth, such as severe prematurity or anoxia, can be associated with impaired development, cognitive deficits, and behavioral problems. Pasamanick, Rogers, and Lilienfeld, (1956) in their classic study noted a relationship between severity of birth complications and risk for atypical development. As a consequence of this study Pasamanick conceived of a "continuum of reproductive casualty" which related the severity of birth complications to the manifestation of developmental disorders. The work of Pasamanick did not deal with MBD—hyperkinesis but became a convenient means of explaining the probable etiologic origins of the problem. Subsequent efforts to confirm this relationship tended to use the data gained from populations identified by the referral problem of a behavioral abnormality and to question the parents to find an historical explanation, a procedure used in spite of long-standing evidence of the questionable reliability of retrospective data gathered under such circumstances. As in the other studies of discriminate signs of dysfunction in MBD, the studies of the medical history tend to report a number of questionable findings in the population of hyperkinetic children, but these findings are not usually specific to the hyperkinetic population. That is to say that while it is possible to find or identify questionable factors in the history, there is no clear proof that these signs are related to MBD—hyperkinesis rather than being occurrences in a broader population, some of whom manifest hyperactive behavior. Birth anomalies occur with increased frequency in several types of childhood problems, including hyperkinesis; speech problems; learning disabilities; hearing problems; and even major deficits, such as Down's syndrome. The import of this finding may be the demonstration of an underlying, nonspecific developmental vulnerability which combines with environmental, educational, or social stresses to produce a behavioral manifestation.

The same general limitations are to be found in genetic studies of hyperactivity. There is evidence of a clustering phenomenon in families, but the results are nonspecific and have limited treatment potential on their own. The significance of the genetic data may be similar to the history data in suggesting a vulnerability factor which can be used in combination with a mediating release mechanism to express the problem behavior.

Psychological Assessment

The most common expectation of the psychological assessment has been to provide collateral support for the medical diagnosis. Referral for psychological testing was usually made when the physician suspected, but could not demonstrate, evidence of neurologic dysfunction. This procedure resulted in a limitation of the psychological evaluation in that it focused on test signs and scores that were interpreted as evidence of brain dysfunction. The simplest and most common example of this approach is the idea that a 10 point difference in scores on the verbal and performance sections of the Wechsler Intelligence Scales is an indication of brain damage. Various mathematical ratios have been developed to use test data as a means of neurologic diagnosis. The Bender Visual-Motor Gestalt Test and other tests of visual-motor function have also been used with scoring systems to produce an index score reflecting neurologic dysfunction. This approach to using psychological assessment has several important limitations:

1. There is a question of how to establish the validity of the diagnosis. Concurrent validity will only serve to compare the psychological data with another approach which has at least an equal problem in validation, for example the neurological examination or the EEG.

2. Ratios and scores have a tendency to conceptualize neurologic dysfunction as more or less unimodal, for example visual-motor dyscoordination. A low performance score on the Wechsler test may indicate brain damage when the area involved is related to visual-motor function. A low verbal score could as readily indicate brain damage when the area involved relates to aphasic or communication processes.

3. The "all or none" aspect of an index score, ratio, or differential set of scores comes into conflict with possibilities of developmental variance or delayed maturation. Developmental psychologists would readily acknowledge that maturation will vary to yield individual difference in acquisition of specific abilities, so that a single assessment sample may reflect a point of developmental delay rather than an instance of dysfunction.

4. There is presumably a difference between brain damage and minimal neurologic dysfunction. Most of the assessment procedures are geared to identifying damage, usually focal in type and at a cortical level. Minimal dysfunction could represent diffuse or nonspecific problems. In addition minimal dysfunction may represent a dysfunction at a subcortical rather than a cortical level, especially if no intellective processes are affected.

5. The use of psychological assessment for diagnosis, especially neurologic diagnosis, by means of a set of scores has limited potential for translation into a useful treatment approach.

Psychological assessment has a broader potential value than confirmation of a neurologic diagnosis. The psychological test battery should provide information about cognitive ability, developmental status, emotional integrity, and provide a sample of behavioral response to assessment in all those areas. The testing should provide a profile of assets and weaknesses that can be of use in developing a treatment or intervention strategy. To be of maximal utility the psychological assessment should be used as a broad, open-ended consultation which systematically assesses cognitive, developmental, and emotional factors, coupling this with a careful observation of the behavioral system as manifested by the child and family during the evaluation session. A major value of the psychological assessment is the chance for clinical impressions to be added to the test data to supplement the test material. Psychologists should not have to be reminded that naturalistic observation is an accepted and important skill and that skilled interviews often yield unique data which no test was designed to elicit. The integration of test data with clinical observation has consistently proven to be a better approach to assessment than a simple process of mathematical prediction based on test scores. If the psychologist is to benefit the patient fully, then he must use himself as a part of the evaluation as well as using the mechanical parts of the test.

Educational Assessment

As a discipline education has only recently come to be as preoccupied with diagnosis as is medicine or psychology. This is not to imply a special virtue, but rather to reflect a reliance on other sources for diagnosis. The advent of diagnostic and prescriptive teachers is a recent trend and has not fully replaced the reliance on physicians and psychologists for diagnostic services. Educators have had programs for MBD-hyperkinetic children dating back to the early ideas of Strauss and Lehtinen (1947). However in the early years of these programs a medical diagnosis was often required for placement as well as a psychological assessment that indicated eligibility. Seemingly little attention was given the fact that this diagnostic procedure was usually of little benefit in establishing the educational program. In extreme situations some school systems required EEG reports before placing a child in a special program, although it is difficult to see how an EEG report could be used to develop an educational plan. The early educational programing for MBD-hyperkinetic children was conceived on an empirical basis and closely replicated the experiences in the education of the retarded. In that model the watered-down curriculum was a theoretically reasonable, but functionally limited idea. In MBD-hyperkinesis the idea focused on such diverse factors as reduced stimulation, segregated classes, programmed teaching, multisensory training, and so on. One could even argue that educators relinquished management responsibility by referring children for treatment. It was not an uncommon practice to exclude children from school until their behavior was acceptable in the context of existing resources. The usual management strategy was medication. If chemotherapy is excluded from the educational sphere, the major approach to dealing with the MBD-hyperkinetic child is placement in a segregated class. When this approach is examined in light of the current emphasis on educational mainstreaming, there is a seeming conflict in theories. In speaking to this issue, Marcel Kinsbourne (1976) states that grouping ten hyperactive children does not constitute a class. Each child's problem is so unique that the group may actually constitute ten classes. If this logic is followed, Kinsbourne reasons that staffing this group with a teacher and an aide yields a 5 to 1 ratio of teachers to classes. In a mainstreaming situation a class may consist of 25 children with 23 of them relatively similar and 2 hyperkinetic (a proportion near 10% of the population). In this case a teacher and an aide would be dealing with three classes — the 23 relatively similar children and the two individual hyperkinetic children — which produces a staff to class ratio of 3 to 2. Granted both of these examples are simplistically extreme, it becomes evident that our approaches have unwittingly moved to such expediently simple extremes. What must be considered is an educational continuum of programs and services that can be individualized to produce a combination of services for each child. As a final factor it is interesting to consider the increase in reports of hyperkinesis in relation to changes in educational concepts. The role that open-space classrooms, reduced structure, and relaxed discipline play in the reported increase in hyperkinesis is open to speculation. Certainly a heightened recognition of the problem is one factor, but epidemiological studies from other countries fail to replicate the reported incidence in the American population.

A MULTIFACTORIAL APPROACH TO HYPERKINESIS

The efforts to identify a single etiological basis for MBD—hyperactivity have been largely unsuccessful. The evidence reviewed does not convincingly support the premise that organic factors play a significant role in the manifestation of hyperkinetic behavior. Those specialized studies that examine the birth history, electroencephalographic data, or psychological tests have been equivocal and filled with methodologic shortcomings. The most serious limitation of these studies is the strong tendency to a unitary concept of the problem. The evidence repeatedly suggests that many factors may interact to produce the behavior. What may be needed is a determined commitment to change the focus from a single etiologic factor to an emphasis on a multifactorial scheme and at the same time to use the information obtained to formulate management programs. The current situation in the area of MBD-hyperkinesis replicates previous controversies in the area of mental retardation and schizophrenia. In the attempt to eliminate those problems, dedicated researchers pursued genetic, biochemical, physiological, and environmental studies to identify a specific etiology. These earlier efforts were also geared to emphasizing one element as the causative agent to the exclusion of the other factors. It is historically important to note that in all of these conditions —mental retardation, schizophrenia, and MBD-hyperkinesis—the efforts to relate etiology to treatment approach have been less than an outstanding success. It is equally important to note that in schizophrenia and mental retardation the movement away from the so-called medical model has produced management programs that are broader, eclectic, and multidisciplinary. It seems probable that hyperkinesis could follow the same path. The similarities in issues between schizophrenia and MBD-hyperkinesis can be seen by examining the following quote from an article by Paul Meehl, written in 1962, entitled, ''Schizotaxia, Schizotypy, and Schizophrenia'':

Here we run into some widespread misconceptions as to what is meant by SPECIFIC ETIOLOGY in nonpsychiatric medicine. By postulating a 'specific etiology' one does NOT imply any of the following:

1. The etiological factors always, or even usually, produce clinical illness.
2. If illness occurs, the particular form and content of the symptoms is derivable by reference to the specific etiology alone.
3. The course of the illness can be materially influenced only by procedures directed against the specific etiology.
4. All persons who share the specific etiology will have closely similar histories, symptoms, and course.
5. The largest single contributor to symptom variance is the specific etiology.

This quote points out the limitations of a unifactor explanation of hyperkinesis. The issues raised by Meehl about the etiology of schizophrenia should alert researchers to potential problems in looking for the specific etiology of MBD-hyperkinesis. This statement can be used to identify some of the important unanswered questions in hyperkinesis. It would seem that the issue of the incidence of the problem may be understood in light of Meehl's first point. That is it may be that the estimates are so varied because the factors involved may not always express themselves as the clinical problem. This point is closely related to the concept of genetic traits versus genetic illness. The second point can explain the shortcomings of the studies of the neurologic signs, EEG patterns, and so on. The third statement reflects the potential folly of assuming that knowledge of the etiology affects treatment. Taken as a whole Meehl's statement strongly suggests the need for a multifactorial approach to the MBD-hyperkinetic syndrome. The manifest problem, hyperkinesis, may best be understood by seeing it as an interactive, additive process that has a number of factorial elements that combine to produce a similar manifestation.

Using Meehl's basic approach and translating it to MBD-hyperkinesis could produce a multifactorial model that would help in understanding the problem and be more useful in planning treatment. As a point for discussion, the proposed model would include seven factors and would involve three levels of complexity. This attempt at a model is not to be considered definitive nor are the seven factors mutually exclusive or exhaustive. Rather the intent is to examine the value of multifactorial, interactive conceptualization of this problem (Figure 19–1).

The first factor in the proposed model is a genetic predisposition. This factor has great significance for understanding the total problem. A genetic involvement can be considered as a latent vulnerability, which means that the behavior may or may not express itself. Such a concept can help to clarify the confusing array of findings from studies that focus on specific factors, such as neurologic status, and the inability of these studies to discriminate MBD-hyperkinesis from other atypical populations. The genetic predisposition could combine with a variety of other factors which would then lead to the expression of the observed behavior.

The interest in a genetic component in MBD-hyperkinesis has been triggered by observation of the disproportionate number of boys represented in the population as well as anecdotal reports of family patterns of the problem. The usual expression of the problem in families — from father to son — reinforces the interest in a genetic element.

Factor II, a developmental lag, is an effort to account for the group of children who display physical, neurological, or visual-motor lags. This would include children who manifest the soft neurologic signs as well as those with poor motor coordination or atypical findings on psychological testing. There is a growing tendency to change the terminology from neurologic dysfunction to developmental delay. This approach fits with the concept of a continuum of causality which would identify these children as lagging behind, but not as abnormal. This idea

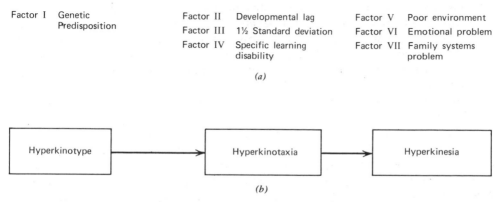

Factor I	Genetic Predisposition	Factor II	Developmental lag	Factor V	Poor environment
		Factor III	1½ Standard deviation	Factor VI	Emotional problem
		Factor IV	Specific learning disability	Factor VII	Family systems problem

(a)

Hyperkinotype → Hyperkinotaxia → Hyperkinesia

(b)

Figure 19–1. A multifactorial model of MBD-hyperkinesis (a) Factors in hyperactivity. (b) Stages of hyperactivity.

would help one understand the failure to find consistently soft signs or to replicate findings over time periods. These children are growing through their problems but they are vulnerable to expressing the problem behavior during the period of delay.

The third factor is the "1 1/2 Standard Deviation Child." This is the child whose overall development is not abnormal, but is below average and at the lower end of the accepted normal distribution. A prime example of this would be a child with a 75–80 IQ whose overall ability puts him at risk in an educational or social system. The normal competition to succeed would be a constant strain on this group of children and in especially stressful situations, such as school, could produce a level of anxiety that would result in a change in behavior.

Factor IV includes those children with "Specific Learning Disabilities." These would include those children with more or less average intelligence, but with problems in school that would include dyslexia, dyscalculia, and so on. As with the "1 1/2 Standard Deviation Group," these children have special problems in school which increase the likelihood of behavioral problems.

The fifth factor involves a "disadvantaged environment" and includes children from lower socioeconomic backgrounds. This group of children tends to be over-represented in many dimensions of atypical development. Their problems repre-sent a combination of physical, educational, and social elements that include a higher rate of premature birth, nutritional deficiency, and poor social support resources, including housing, schooling, recreation, and so on. If children identi-fied as having a behavior problem manifested by hyperactivity are sampled from this population, they will be more likely to display other signs of difficulty, includ-ing delays in physical development, learning problems, or atypical psychological test scatter. The presence of these findings is more apt to be related to socioeco-nomic factors than to be a direct cause of the hyperactive behavior.

Children with emotional problems constitute the sixth group. In the press to find an organic cause for hyperactivity we have ignored the fact that anxiety is an emotional factor that regularly affects a child's behavior. A child's response to a disorganized, stressful, or frustrating environment will involve the displacement of anxiety. This anxiety may be expressed by an acting out of feelings in an open, poorly controlled purposeless manner that will involve increased motor activity. Another less recognized possibility is that hyperactivity may represent a form of childhood depression. The similarity of symptoms of agitated depression in the adult and hyperactivity in the child is striking and includes irritability, poor con-centration, motor excitation, and a negative self-concept. Burks and Harrison (1962) have reported on a group of children who used aggressive behavior as a means of avoiding a clinical depression. In this group they describe a symptom cluster including hyperactivity, impulsivity, emotional lability, poor object rela-tionships, and feelings of worthlessness. Agitated and/or aggressive behavior may be a more developmentally appropriate means of expressing depressive feelings in young children.

The seventh factor is a family systems concept taken from the work of Minu-chin (1974) in the area of psychosomatic or chronic illness. It is not clear why the emphasis in hyperkinesis has been on an acute illness model when the facts strongly suggest that the problem is most usually chronic in nature. Considering hyperactivity as a chronic problem makes it useful to apply the information gained from research in the area. The idea that a chronically ill child can become a family scapegoat may be important in understanding the refractory nature of hyperactivity in some children. Minuchin's work would suggest that the hyperactive child may fulfill a needed role in the family which in the operating system would not allow the child to get well. The family's problems become enmeshed with the child's dysfunction and evolve into a circular pattern that becomes a self-sustaining. This system's approach has been identified in studies of children with anorexia nervosa, diabetes, and asthma. Work by Minuchin with those populations suggests new and potentially useful treatment approaches that could be used with hyperactive children.

The Interactive Model

Using the seven factors that have been described, an interactive model can be constructed so that looking at possible combinations can facilitate understanding of the problem and can help to determine treatment procedures. In the interactive model three levels of the problem are postulated. Borrowing from Meehl's terminology, these are called hyperkinotype, hyperkinotaxia, and hyperkinesia. (Figure 19–1). In this approach a child with a genetic predisposition is a hyperkinotype. When a second factor is added to the genetic predisposition, this is hyperkinotaxia and, in the conceptualization of this model, will express the problem behavior. There are combinations of factors (Figure 19–2) that can produce hyperkinotaxia and can be used to consider a treatment approach. Combining Factors I and II would produce a situation wherein the children would manifest soft neurologic signs and would have a high probability of responding to stimulant medications to relieve the problem behavior. Medication may make these children more acceptable to the teacher but has little potential for facilitating any long term change. At best these children will get through school and still be slow learners. Factors I and IV in combination would probably produce a pattern similar to that of combining I and III, but the added intellectual ability of the child would result in a potential for improved functioning as academic programs become more student selected, as in high school or college.

On the other hand, combining Factor I with either Factor V, VI, or VII would produce pseudohyperkinotaxia and would result in a situation wherein the usual medical treatment would fail or would merely mask the true problem. This is the group of children that Minde, Weiss, and Mendelson, (1972) sees as displaying later socially maladaptive outcomes, including psychosis and delinquency. In treatment these children need a more psychodynamic approach and/or psychotropic medications.

If the genetic factor is not involved and the behavior is a result of the combination of two factors from II to VII, the result is a mixed hyperkinotaxia which would have a variable set of signs and a variable response to medication as a

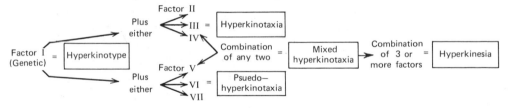

Figure 19–2.   Interactive model of hyperactivity.

treatment. The outcome would depend on the combination of factors involved and could include temporary or partial resolutions of the behavior.

In the proposed model, hyperkinesia represents the third level of the problem and is the result of three or more factors acting in combination. Many of the combinations could give the appearance of having one primary etiology, but the unidentified contributing factors would diminish the prospects of a successful outcome using a unitary treatment approach. It is important in hyperkinesia to be oriented to multifaceted approaches to assessment and remediation. There are a number of intervention strategies that are available to help with the problem behavior characterized by excess motor activity. For those children whose problem involves Factors III and IV, a therapeutic educational program is a critical need. A change in school placement, more individualized instruction, or a teacher who has been taught to handle the child could well result in an amelioration of the problem. Behavior modification is another technique that has great promise in the management of some of the children who display hyperactive behavior. Social intervention strategies, including counseling and psychotherapy, would be appropriate for the children who have Factors V and VI as part of the problem, while Minuchin's family intervention approach would be indicated for those children who have a Factor VII in the problem situation.

The major aim of the proposed model is to stimulate broader thinking about the MBD-hyperkinesis syndrome. There is no magic in seven factors or three levels, but this model can help to produce innovative ways of understanding the problem and as a result lead to a broader range of treatments.

NEEDED RESEARCH

Given that MBD-hyperkinesis is likely to be a multifaceted problem, there is still a need to sort out characteristics of the specific subtypes. There are important factors that have received little study, perhaps due to the unitary approach that has preoccupied researchers. The recommendations to be made in this section are not new or unique, but represent solid scientific methodology that has not been effectively utilized in studying MBD-hyperkinesis. The usual deterrent to these studies has been the time and expense involved in carrying out the procedures. This expense tends to reflect the presence of many procedures that have been less than productive, such as the EEG. The proposed studies could be done by eliminating some of the procedures and substituting different comparison samples. For example it would be helpful to establish a study comparing children identified as hyperactive with a normal control group who were matched for age, sex, and socioeconomic status. These children could be evaluated by a pediatrician and a psychologist without using the EEG or expensive laboratory studies. The key to the study would be a blind evaluation of each child. It would be important to control for the influence of historical data, so that the group would either be examined without history available or the normal controls could have histories borrowed from children who had been diagnosed as hyperactive. In this study one could begin to control for (or evaluate) the influence of behavioral reports to see if they bias the examiner. A significant factor to study would be the number of false positives in the diagnostic categories. This approach might also be helpful to find the positive factors that minimize the behavioral expression of a problem. That is, given that some normally functioning children have similar test findings as hyper-kinetic children, what factors differentiate them from those children who express the problem behavior? Such information would be useful in organizing preventive efforts to avoid the occurrence of the problem.

Two other research approaches warrant consideration for future studies, these are: (1) studies using multiple examiners to establish inter-rater reliability and (2) serial evaluation studies to evaluate test-retest reliability of measures. Yet an-other approach that deserves study would use more than one group of problem children and a normal control group. The measure or measures applied would need to discriminate between the groups. Kenny (1971), in a study using the Cantor Background Interference Procedure with the Bender-Gestalt test, found that this instrument discriminated between children diagnosed as MBD, those diagnosed as emotionally disturbed, and a comparison group of normal children. This study also controlled for age and intellectual level.

There is a need to more carefully evaluate environmental factors in the expres-sion of hyperactive behavior. Studies (Cantwell, 1972; Morrison and Stewart, 1971; Stewart and Morrison, 1973) suggest that the children with MBD-hyperkine-sis have an excessive amount of pathology in their families. The effect of a stressful environment may be an important mediating factor in the expression of the behavior problems. Furthermore the awareness of environmental stress can suggest broader treatment approaches that may prove more effective than a strat-egy that concentrates only on the child. The problem of an MBD-hyperkinesis syndrome is complex, frustrating, and challenging. We should learn from similar situations that existed with schizophrenia and mental retardation and abandon the simplistic, unitary approach that has marked our efforts. If a new feeling about MBD-hyperkinesis were to begin with a multifactorial concept and broader treat-ment approaches, it is likely that some progress could be made in discriminating some of the major subgroups that exist in this heterogeneous group of children. The parochial efforts that have been used to date tend to be protective of the investigator's bias rather than to be focused on the needs of the child, parents, or society. Too great an effort has been directed to producing information that might tell us what happened to a child and not enough concern has been given to the child's future. We are at a point when the emphasis must shift to search for ways to help facilitate the development of the child's potential and to look at the broadest range of treatment resources that can be developed to meet the needs of the heterogeneous group of children identified as MBD-hyperkinetic.

REFERENCES

Anderson, W. "The hyperkinetic child: A neurological Appraisal." *Neurology,* 13, 371–382, (1963).

Bauer, R. and T. J. Kenny. "An ego disturbance model of MBD." *Child Psychiatry and Human Development,* 4(4), 238–245, (1974).

Bax, M., and R. MacKeith, *Minimal Cerebral Dysfunction.* London: Little Club Clinics in Developmental Medicine No. 10, 1963.

Budenhagen, R., and P. Sickler. "Hyperactivity: A forty-eight hour sample plus a note on etiology." *American Journal of Mental Deficiency,* 73, 580, (1969).

Burks, H.L., and S.I. Harrison. "Aggressive behavior as a means of avoiding depression." *American Journal of Orthopsychiatry*, 32, 416–422, (1962).

Cantwell, D. "Psychiatric illness in the families of hyperactive children." *Archives of General Psychiatry*, 27, 414–417, (1972).

Capute, A. E. Niedermeyer, and F. Richardson. "The electroencephalogram in children with minimal cerebral dysfunction." *Pediatrics*, 41, 1104–1114, (1968).

Clements, S. D. *Minimal Brain Dysfunction in Children—Terminology and Identification.* NINDB Monograph No. 3, U. S. Department of EW. Washington, D.C.: 1966.

Clemmens, R., and T. Kenny. "Clinical correlates of learning disabilities, minimal brain dysfunction and hyperactivity." *Clinical Pediatrics*, 11(6), 311–313, (1972).

Connors, K. "A teacher rating scale for use in drug studies with children." *American Journal of Psychiatry*, 126, 884–888, (1969).

Cromwell, R. L., A. Baumeister, and W. F. Hawkins "Research in activity level" in N. Ellis, ed. *Handbook of Mental Retardation.* New York: McGraw-Hill, 1963.

Dubey, D. R. "Organic factors in hyperkinesis: A critical evaluation." *American Journal of Orthopsychiatry*, 46(2), 353–366, (1976).

Greenberg, L., and S. McMahon. "Serial neurologic examination of hyperactive children." *Pediatrics*, 59(4), 584–587, (1977).

Kahn, E., and L. A. Cohen. "Organic drivenness: A brain stem syndrome and experience." *New England Journal of Medicine*, 210, 748, (1934).

Kellaway, P., and M. J. Kubola. "Cerebral concussion in children: A longitudinal EEG profile." *Electroencephalography and Clinical Neurology*, 23, 82, (1967).

Kennard, M. "Value of equivocal signs in neurologic diagnosis." *Neurology*, 15, 883–891, (1960).

Kenny, T. J. "Background interference procedure: A means of assessing neurologic dysfunction in children." *Journal of Consulting and Clinical Psychology*, 73(1), 44–46, (1971).

Kenny, T. J., and R. L. Clemmens. *Behavioral Pediatrics and Child Development: Clinical Handbook.* Baltimore: Williams & Wilkins, 1975.

Kenny, T. J., R. L. Clemmens, B. W. Hudson, G. A. Lentz, R. Cicci, and P. Nair. "Characteristics of children referred because of hyperactivity." *Journal of Pediatrics*, 79(4), 618–622, (1971).

Kinsbourne, M. "School Problems." (Paper presented at the Annual Meeting of the Medical and Chirurgical Faculty of Maryland, Baltimore, April, 1976).

Langhorne, J. E., J. Loney, C. E. Paternite, and H. P. Bechtoldt. "Childhood hyperkinesis: A return to the source." *Journal of Abnormal Psychology*, 85(2), 201–209, (1976).

Lombroso, C. T., I. Schwartz, D. Clark, H. Muench, and J. Barry. "Ctenoids in healthy youths: A controlled study of 14 and 6 per second positive spikes." *Neurology*, 16, 1152–1158, (1966).

Meehl, P. "Schizotaxia, schizotypy, and schizophrenia." *American Psychologist*, 17, 827–836, (1962).

Minde, K., G. Weiss, and N. Mendelson. "Five year follow-up study of 91 hyperactive school children." *Journal of American Academy Child Psychiatry*, 11, 596–610, (1972).

Minuchin, S. *Families and Family Therapy: A Structural Approach.* Boston: Harvard University Press, 1974.

Morrison, J., and M. Stewart. "A family study of the hyperactive child syndrome." *Biological Psychiarty*, 3, 189–195, (1971).

Pasamanick, B., M. Rogers, and A. Lilienfeld. "Pregnancy experience and the development of behavior disorder in children." *American Journal of Psychiatry*, 112, 613–618, (1956).

Routh, D., and R. D. Roberts. "Minimal brain dysfunction in children: Failure to find evidence for a behavioral syndrome." *Psychological Reports*, 31, 307–314, (1972).

Schmitt, B. "Hyperactivity: Myth." *Learning Disabilities: An Audio Journal*, 1(3), (1977).

Stewart, M., and J. Morrison, "The psychiatric status of the legal families of adopted hyperactive children." *Archives of General Psychiatry*, 28, 888–891, (1973).

Strauss, A., and L. Lehtinen. *Psychopathology and Education of the Brain Injured Child*. New York: Grune & Stratton, 1947.

Werry, J. "Studies on the hyperactive child. IV. Empirical Analysis of the Minimal brain dysfunction syndrome." *Archives of General Psychiatry*, 19, 9–16, (1968).

Werry, J. S. and R. L. Sprague. "Hyperactivity," in C. G. Costello, ed., *Symptoms of Psychopathology*, p. 397. New York: Wiley, 1970.

Werry, J. S., K. Minde, A. Guzman, G. Weiss, K. Dogan, and E. Hoy. "Studies on the hyperactive child - VII: Neurological status compared with neurotic and normal Children." *American Journal of Orthopsychiatry*, 43(3), 441–449, (1972).

CHAPTER 20

Learning Disorders

Tanis H. Bryan and James H. Bryan

INTRODUCTION

This is a chapter about the status and findings of children who have trouble learning and who are not obviously stupid or emotionally disturbed. Children having such difficulties are referred to by many names: learning disorders, learning disabilities, specific learning disabilities, educationally handicapped, minimal cerebral dysfunction, and so on. While various terms to describe such children are frequently employed, the empirical basis for the application of any of them to particular children is often obscure. If this is the case, then the presumed differences between children assigned one label and not another remains even more obscure. At the present time the use of the term learning disabilities, learning disorders, or minimal cerebral dysfunction is likely to be more indicative of the educational training and philosophical stance of the user than reflective of any empirically demonstrated characteristics of the population being discussed. The use of the term minimal cerebral disorders may be more assoicated with a labeler's educational background which emphasizes the medical model rather than being reflective of hard evidence for the existence of some brain dysfunction. Likewise the use of such terms as educationally handicapped, learning disabilities, or specific learning disabilities, may be more assoicated with a diagnostician's educational background which emphasizes the educational model approach to deviance, rather than emphasizing specific characteristics of the child. There appears to be no consensus as to significant distinctions which differentiate groups, much less how one goes about measuring these distinctions.

Given this state of affairs, we take certain specific positions. Due to the present difficulties in definition and assessment, empirical distinctions among children labeled as minimally brain damaged, learning disabled, or specific learning disabled have not yet been demonstrated. This is not to say that important conceptual distinctions cannot be made which will in the future be shown as heuristic to science, diagnosis, and treatment. We argue that such distinctions have not yet received empirical support, for instance, are children with only a specific disability, such as delayed reading, markedly different from children who have trouble in learning both reading and writing? Besides differences in their symptoms, are there demonstrated differences in their learning processes, memory functions, susceptibility to remediation techniques or the social or motivational pressures to which they are exposed during their everyday activities? We do not think such evidence exists. While it would be foolhardy to deny that some children have brain dysfunctions, it is unlikely that all learning-disabled children can be so described. Certainly the brain is linked to learning, though it does not necessarily follow that it is appropriate to assume that all learning problems are indicative of some brain dysfunction. Certainly variables external to the individual's brain, such as motivation, parents and peers, teachers and tutors, also affect learning. At this time it is probably easier to remediate the child through attention to external variables than to brain processes. The external variables are certainly easier to study experimentally!

The definitional problems in the area of learning disabilities are great and must eventually be solved through systematic empirical work. Children labeled by one name should share empirically demonstrated similarities which separate them from children labeled by other names. As yet distinctions and commonalities among and between groups have not yet been evidenced. Indeed our conceptual differentiations have prematurely outstripped our empirical knowledge. Labels, such as learning disabilities, specific learning disabilities, and so on, may be serving important political and social aims, but empirically such distinctions are not warranted.

In this chapter we present a summary of the history which we feel has had a marked influence upon the field of learning disabilities, the models of viewing learning disabilities, definitions of learning disabilities, and finally a review of the research related to the field. Throughout we look to a number of studies that have used a variety of types of children as subjects. While we wish that the field could yield an abundant amount of studies on particular and meaningful types of children, such is not the case. Studies related to children with specific learning disabilities, hyperactivity, learning disorders, and brain damage will be included. Admittedly use of such heterogeneous samples introduces a certain amount of chaos, but it is from this fodder that the field of learning disabilities will continue to grow.

HISTORICAL INFLUENCES

The field of learning disabilities originated with teachers, clinicians, and physicians who viewed learning problems as the result of some type of dysfunctioning of the central nervous system. While these pioneers had their own interpretations of what specifically was wrong, they shared the assumption that human behavior reflected central nervous system functions and that learning failures meant something was wrong with the person's brain. While this assumption hardly seems radical, it met with opposition on several grounds. In this section we shall start with the historical basis of the field of learning disabilities and trace these notions to current research, which has sought to prove or disprove the value of these pioneering ideas. We shall see that to understand or discuss the relationship of ideas about learning disorders and minimal cerebral dysfunction it is necessary to keep in mind the substance of the original debate.

While the field of learning disabilities is very young in terms of official (that is legislative) recognition, its history can be dated to the middle 1800s and to the works of Broca, Wernicke, John Hughlings Jackson, Henry Head, and Kurt Goldstein (Bryan and Bryan, 1975). The works of these scientists in the areas of aphasia and perception have had a lasting influence and are reflected in the perspectives of many contemporary professionals. Broca, rejecting phrenology (a method of diagnosis based upon feeling the bumps on the patient's head), did link the loss of speech to a particular part of the brain. Wernicke extended Broca's initial linkage of brain and speech to other forms of speech and other parts of the brain. Hence he linked an inability to understand speech (receptive aphasia) to a specific section of the brain. Jackson furthered the development of modern linguistics with his argument that words did not constitute speech, at least in the sense that: if one could not talk, one could not understand speech. Head argued for and introduced systematic observation to clinical practice and reliable classifications for understanding aphasias. Kurt Goldstein, following in the tradition of Gestalt psychology, linked the brain with perceptual processes—not simply blindness or deafness, but rather to basic understanding of the world around one. *Perceptual impairment,* discriminating the important from the unimportant, the trivial from the necessary, is traceable to the work of Kurt Goldstein. The questions we now ask about learning problems, the interpretations we place on behaviors, the educational techniques developed to aid the learning disabled, and today's research on the topic show many traces of the influence of these early pioneers.

More recently, from approximately 1925 to the 1950s, the works of Strauss, Werner, and Orton have played an important role in the development of the learning disabilities field. Strauss and Werner were among the first investigators to extend the previously stated ideas concerning the brain and learning problems from adult subjects with brain injuries to children with learning problems. Like their predecessors, they felt that brain dysfunctions were critical to learning; unlike their predecessors, they studied this possibility by investigating children rather than adults. Learning problems in children were associated with organic causes and not limited to problems of genes, the unconscious, or demonic possession. They believed, like their predecessors, that brain damage in children was associated with hyperactivity, distractibility, and disinhibition as well as learning difficulties. Children suffering such etiology and associated characteristics were, and still are, referred to as demonstrating the Strauss syndrome. While the original group of children studied by Strauss and his colleagues were considered mentally retarded, the syndrome has become associated with children who have adequate intelligence, but who otherwise are functioning poorly within social or academic contexts. Their work apparently led to the view that: (1) children can have normal intelligence, but be cognitively or behaviorally disabled and (2) such children suffer from some not so obvious brain dysfunction, in other words minimal brain dysfunction. As we shall see, a major area of research in the field of learning disabilities today is the study of hyperactivity.

Samuel Orton, another pioneer in the field of learning disorders, studied language problems, laterality of motor skills, and the relationship of language and motor skills to dominance of one or another part of the brain. He believed that when children had difficulty hearing sounds or writing letters in the correct order, one side of the child's brain was dominant while the other side was dormant. The techniques developed by Orton to remediate such problems have been subsequently found to be effective (Bateman, 1964). Orton was important not only because of his efficacious remedial techniques but also because he was one of the first to associate language deficits with reading problems.

MODELS OF LEARNING DISORDERS

The influences upon the field of learning disability are old, though the formal terms of the definition, the specific institutions designed to render such children exclusive treatment, and the modes of treatment may well be in their infancy (Lilly, 1977). One of the problems of infancy is that of self-identity, and it is to this problem which we now turn. We shall look at the various forms of models that shape the views and actions of the various professionals constituting the corps of the learning disability field.

Efforts to develop classification systems to describe and define learning disabled children have been hampered by two major problems: one conceptual, the other practical. The conceptual problem revolves around which of two disparate models should be adopted in viewing learning-disabled children. The practical problem revolves around the measures and materials available for diagnosis and remediation.

The Medical Model

While there are apparently many medical models within the field of medicine (London, 1972), the disease model has had great influence on the clinical practices of psychologists and educators. The disease model provides the practitioner an approach to a problem which focuses on the afflicted person. The assumption is made that if the problem can be removed from the person, he will be immune to it irrespective of the social context in which it might occur. Within the field of learning disabilities, such a perspective leads to the notion that the child's behavior and achievements, or lack thereof, are traceable to brain processes and where there is a behavioral disturbance, there is a brain disturbance. The medical disease model thus draws attention to biological explanations for problems, and the biological functions deemed important are those intrinsic to the patient. Various parts of the central nervous system have been hypothesized to account for learning, they range from the reticular activating system (Dykman, et al., 1971) to specific points in the left cerebral hemisphere (Geschwind, 1968). This model not only dictates where one should look, but also where and how one should treat. The physician's office, not the classroom, is the remediation center; the pill, not the teacher, a valuable source of cure. The continuing impact of the medical model in learning disabilities is evident in the 1975 learning-disability definition's reference to perceptual handicap, brain injury, minimal brain dysfunction, dyslexia, and development aphasia (Federal Register, 1976).

Virtually all of the assumptions underlying this form of the medical model have been challenged. Here are some of the objections: There is little evidence to demonstrate a biological foundation for many personality and education problems. While a virus produces syphilis, what virus is responsible for reading problems, hyperactivity, or arithmetic difficulties? Is it reasonable to assume that causes of problems transcend situations, so that they can survive in the context of many varying social settings? Many do not believe so. And even if there is a physical base for whatever ails the student, does the disease model yield helpful hints as to the cures for such ailments? The search for the site(s) and dynamics of brain damage which might be predictive of school performance has yielded little useful information, or so some argue. Just how advanced is medical technology, how reliable are the tools? Finally if school failure is the problem, yet the child is being treated for distractibility, the customer may well be getting what he did not ask for. In response to these beliefs, another model of learning disabilities has been generated and that is the education model.

The Education Model

This model dictates an approach to the learning-disabled child which, not surprisingly, is educationally oriented. Within this perspective the focus is on reading, writing, and arithmetic as *the problem,* not as *a symptom.* Diagnosis is directed to forces within the environment that may affect learning. Reinforcements, not neurons; task analysis, not reaction times; teachers as well as children are, or should be, the objects of diagnosis. The classroom, not the clinic, is the setting for diagnosis and cure. Proponents of this model argue that proper understanding of the learning-disabled child's problems is generated through the proper understanding of the child's environment. The cure consists of the removal of the symptom and is generated through the judicious manipulation of the environmental forces affecting the child.

There is no doubt a multitude of reasons why the medical model is losing and the educational model is gaining favor. First there has been a long history of research failure to demonstrate that learning-disabled children have minimal brain damage. This is not to say that many brain-damaged children do not suffer learning problems. But it is quite another to say that all learning problems reflect some central nervous system dysfunction. Second the education model seems to provide a better framework for both the diagnosis and treatment of learning-disabled children (Bryan and Bryan, 1975). It seems to provide more useful information about and more efficient modes to attenuate academic difficulties than does the medical model. It is likely that future research in learning disabilities based on this model will extend our knowledge of reinforcement, tasks, teacher, and peer effects in affecting the child's learning of reading, writing, and arithmetic. However its relative success should not be a rationale for discontinuing efforts to understand those brain and biological processes which underly learning failures. They are there and should be searched for.

DEFINING LEARNING DISABILITIES

Let us look at the definition(s) of learning disabilities. The National Advisory Committee on Handicapped Children (1968) developed the following definition of learning disabilities:

Children with special learning disabilities exhibit a disorder in one or more of the basic psychological processes involved in understanding or using spoken or written language. These may be manifested in disorders of listening, thinking or talking, reading, writing, spelling, or arithmetic. They include conditions which have been referred to as perceptual handicaps, brain injury, minimal brain dysfunction, dyslexia, developmental aphasia, etc. They do not include learning problems which are due primarily to visual, hearing, or motor handicaps, to mental retardation, emotional disturbance, or to environmental disadvantage. [P. 34]

More recently this definition was scrutinized in conjunction with the development of the 1975 *Education for All Handicapped Children Act.* It remained unchanged. Developmental aphasia and dyslexia for example are included as basic learning disability problems. In essence children with learning disabilities have intelligence within the normal range; are not retarded, deaf, blind, or emotionally disturbed; and have problems which are not due to cultural or economic disadvantagement.

There have been several additional efforts to develop classification systems to describe the characteristics associated with learning disabilities. There have been many characteristics associated with this label, all of them aversive. With the exception of stupidity or craziness, ruled out by the definition, any and all negative attributes imaginable have been mentioned as a problem in learning disabilities. The most frequently cited are: hyperactivity, perceptual-motor impairments, emotional lability, general coordination deficits, disorders of attention (that is short attention span, perseveration, distractibility), impulsivity, disorders of memory and thinking, specific learning disabilities (that is reading, mathematics, writing, spelling), speech articulation problems, equivocal neurological signs, and electroencephalographic irregularities (Clements, 1966, p. 13).

By and large, neither the definition nor the classification systems proposed have met with much success, scientifically or politically. McDonald (1968) surveyed teachers, directors of special education, school nurses, social workers, school psychologists and speech therapists concerning their views of the definitions of learning disabilities. He reported a preference for a definition which excludes mention of any brain related disabilities. In the definition preferred by his sample, the learning-disabled child,

is any child who demonstrates a significant discrepancy in acquiring the academic and social skills in accordance with is assessed capacity to obtain these skills. In general, these discrepancies are associated with specific disabilities such as gross motor, visual memory, visual discrimination, and other language related disabilities. [1968, p. 375]

Essentially the preferred definition reduces to an emphasis on the discrepancies between what a child should be, but is not achieving.

Additionally the current definitions of learning disabilities have not been helpful in aiding us to produce a very homogeneous grouping of children. The terms used in the definition are difficult to measure and to operationalize, and the characteristics so specified are not likely, on a priori groups, to be correlated. The definition allows a hodgepodge of children to be placed under one conceptual, albeit leaky, umbrella. Finally evidence concerning the presumed characteristics of these children, that is their hyperactivity, impulsivity, and what have you, has been very limited in amount and not very supportive in results. There is no doubt that some children with some learning problems do share some of the characteristics so often associated with them. That is not the same as demonstrating that most learning-disabled children share most of these behaviors or traits. The characteristics presumably shared by learning disabled children do not appear to be either very common or frequently shared (Bryan, 1974a).

Federal Guidelines for Definitions

While the definition of learning disabilities is still tied to notions concerning brain pathology, the proposed federal guidelines for assessing, placing, and treating children with learning difficulties is more consistent with the views of those surveyed by McDonald (1968). The emphasis is more on educational difficulties and capacity and performance discrepancies in academic matters, than on perceptual impairments and brain dysfunction. The proposed rules and regulations stress the notion that the child must exhibit a rather profound discrepancy between his ability and his achievements in order to be considered learning disabled. The areas in which the child must manifest the discrepancy include: oral and written expression, reading comprehension, basic reading skills, listening comprehension, mathematics calculation, mathematics reasoning, and spelling (Federal Register, 1976, p. 52407). The proposed federal guidelines may well be more important in affecting the treatment, research, and diagnosis of children, than definitions offered by special education specialists. The reason for their special importance is that they reflect those criteria by which the federal government will support educational institutions (that is give money). In the absence of data, money rather than logic is likely to affect contemporary practices in who and how many get defined as learning disabled, educable mentally retarded, and emotionally disturbed.

The proposed guidelines will attenuate the burden of demonstrating or speculating on the role of brain dysfunction experienced by the child with learning problems. Neither money nor respectability will now require it. It is also likely to lessen the anxiety and guilt of parents and children that is generated by concern over the brain's lack of integrity. However Public Law 94–142 indicates that for purposes of funding, not more than 2% of the state's population who are defined as learning disabled will be eligible for federal aid. Given that some professionals have estimated that up to 28% of the elementary school population within the United States suffers from learning disabilities (Bruinincks, Glaman, and Clark, 1971; Clements, 1966), it is likely that adjustments in definitions will be made. Additionally it should be noted that according to the guidelines, the eligible child must demonstrate a relatively large discrepancy between ability and achievement. We anticipate several consequences of the guidelines on the numbers of children and the types of children who can be eligible for aid. The first is that many children with mild learning disabilities will either not be given help or will be diagnosed in such a way as to be aided by monies directed toward other needy children. If funds are abundant for the emotionally disturbed, the mildly retarded, or whomever, one might expect a transfer of some of the bounty towards the service of the mildly learning disabled called by yet another name. Second, the learning-disability specialist is increasingly likely to be dealing with a population of children with rather severe learning problems, children who may indeed have a greater likelihood of suffering from central nervous system dysfunction than those with whom the specialist had previously interacted. Notions concerning minimal cerebral dysfunction and the medical model thus may gain in importance, popularity, and scientific usefulness.

REVIEW OF RELATED RESEARCH

The remainder of this chapter will be devoted to an examination of research related to learning-disabled children. This does not represent a large corpus of information since reseach is of a recent origin. This is to be expected from a field in which a definition of their target population is but ten years old. As previously indicated there is little research concerning how children defined as learning disordered differ from those labeled hyperactive or as suffering from minimal cerebral dysfunction or specific learning disabilities. After a brief discussion concerning some methodological difficulties associated with studying learning-disabled children, we shall review studies of brain processing of information, attention, hyperactivity, perception, language, and social behaviors of such children.

Methodological Problems in Learning-Disabilities Research

As must be self evident from the previous discussion, one problem confronting the researcher is the selection of a sample of children to study. Obviously the definition of learning disabilities would not be likely to yield a very homogeneous sample of children. Most investigators employ as their learning-disabled sample children who have difficulty reading. Indeed about 80% of the research on learning-disabled children have used children's reading scores to define their samples (Torgesen, 1975). The usual definition of the learning-disability sample is that it consists of children reading six months below grade level in the primary grades, and one and one-half grades below grade level in the higher grade levels. Thus research on learning disabilities reduces to research on poor readers. Several problems are associated with this research tradition. First children who are good readers but who demonstrate other school failures are not likely to be included in the research, nor will they be reflected in the "truths" that arise concerning a class of children called learning disabled. Additionally there are problems associated with assessment of reading. Both the reliability and validity of many reading tests are open to criticism (Silberberg and Silberberg, 1977).

A second problem associated with research in learning disabilities is essentially the narrow conceptualization of the processes under study. Whether we are concerned with perception, attention, or social behavior, our conceptualizations rarely match the complexity of the processes as indicated in other investigations. For example children's attention apparently is a very complex process, consisting of several component behaviors. Yet most investigators treat attention as a unitary concept. While it is true that a single research study must of necessity take a narrow perspective, the use of programatic research in any particular area of study is infrequently undertaken.

A third problem confronting the researcher pertains to the notion of ability or intelligence. A pivotal idea concerning learning disorders is that the child demonstrates a normal potential to learn. Normal potential is usually defined by the child having an intelligence test score within the normal range. In fact both the concept of potential and test results pertaining to intelligence raise serious questions. When one argues that one has potential, does he mean for mastering the particular content being taught at that moment, for mastering substantive materials in related areas of concern, or for always being able to master material dictated by the school board or teacher. Noteworthy is the fact that potential is traditionally measured by intelligence tests. But performance on intelligence tests is quite variable for individual children and is affected by the atmosphere of testing, the nature of the testers, the child's motivations, and other external and basically irrelevant factors (Bryan and Bryan, 1975; Masland, 1969). Since 9% of children can be expected to show variations of 30 points or more in their intelligence test scores when repeatedly tested, how is one to know which particular scores reflect the child's potential. In addition, even if we assume that intelligence test scores assess potential, it has been repeatedly found that controlling or matching learning-disabled children and nondisabled children on the basis of IQ scores is extremely difficult (Bryan and Bryan, 1975), and to make matters worse some investigators do not bother to attempt to match the children on this dimension at all (Hallahan, 1975). The failure to match subjects for intelligence is significant insofar as many children defined as learning disordered have intelligence test scores below 90 at the time of the initial labelling (Ames, 1968). Characteristics of behavior assigned differentially to learning-disabled and nondisabled children may frequently reflect group differences in intellectual levels (Browning, 1967; Hallahan, 1975).

In summary the methodological problems associated with research in the field of learning disabilities consists of those associated with selecting an appropriate (representative) sample of learning-disabled children, the lack of programatic research, and the somewhat cavalier disregard of the concept of ability or intelligence. As research progresses in this new field, these problems may dissolve, but perhaps new ones will arise. In the meantime some knowledge of "truths" are being gained, some myths are now being laid to rest. We now turn to the review of research on the learning-disabled child.

INFORMATION PROCESSING

Attention

Deficits in children's attention have long been a central issue in the field of learning disabilities. Attentional problems were included as a characteristic of such children in one of the earliest proposed syndromes, the Strauss syndrome (Torgesen, 1975). This concept remains important to this day. Dykman, et al., (1971), Keogh and Hall (1973) view attentional problems as the core problem experienced by the learning-disabled children. Moreover this view is held by other than professional researchers. Keogh (1973) found that teachers and other professionals still indicate that difficulties in sustaining attention are among the most important problems associated with learning-disabled children.

Do learning-disabled children manifest attentional deficits? First it is important to recognize the complexity of attention. From the teacher's perspective a child's inattention seems like a simple and certainly familiar enough phenomenon. But attention represents a number of complex behaviors. When talking about attentional deficits it is important to look closely at which component of attention is being assessed. Attention is defined as "the degree to which thresholds are selectively lowered for one class of stimuli relative to others" (Kagan and Kogan, 1970, p. 1297). Attention can be subdivided into at least three components: (1) the orienting response (Pick and Pick, 1970); (2) the child's ability or strategy in scanning and focusing upon the appropriate stimulus material (Dykman, et al., 1971; Kawabe, 1976). In this case the child becomes aroused, comes to attention, and then has to focus on the critical features of a task; (3) the ability or motivation to sustain attention, to focus on critical features of the task across a period of time. This is usually referred to as vigilance (Pick and Pick, 1970).

The orienting response is a primitive one, shown by lower as well as higher organisms. There seems to be little research concerning the orienting response of learning-disabled children, even though some clinicians have suggested that defects in such responding may characterize these children. For example Strauss and Lehtinen (1947) and Cruikshank (1975) suggest that learning-disabled children overreact to external stimuli. The hypothesis concerning orienting responses of learning-disabled children remains untested.

Considerably more work has been conducted on the learning-disabled child's ability to scan the stimulus array and to focus upon the appropriate stimuli. There have been two somewhat separate approaches to this area of research, that involving the study of field dependence and that involving the study of impulsivity. Keogh and Margolis (1976) argue that appropriate attention requires not only the arousal of the organism but proper organization of the perceptual field. They suggest that the child must select the correct stimulus from the vast array of stimuli on which to focus and then respond appropriately. Field dependence reflects a child's inability to do this. Field-dependent children become distracted by the irrelevant stimuli, cannot determine which stimulus of the array should be their proper target of focus. The approach which emphasizes impulsivity refers to the performance of a child who believes he has detected the correct stimulus, but who has not done so—and he has acted with relatively great speed (Kagan and Kogan, 1970). While one process may reflect the effect of distractions from irrelevant stimuli and the other the lack of reflection by the subject, both impulsivity and field-independence scores are positively correlated (Messer, 1976). Both processes may play an important part in the child's ability to assimilate correctly the stimulus features of any new task.

Keogh (1973) has stressed the notion that learning-disabled children are likely to have difficulty organizing perceptual inputs and are likely to focus on the irrelevant features of such inputs. She believes that field dependence may characterize these children and argues that learning-disabled children have difficulty in separating the field from the ground. Keogh reports the results of several unpublished studies which support the hypothesis that perceptual organization difficulties might characterize children who do, or will, experience academic difficulties in school. She cites an investigation by Watson which found that reading ability was correlated with ability to ignore irrelevant features of a stimulus display, and one by Becker whose results indicated that high-risk kindergarten children were also less able than low-risk children to ignore irrelevant features of a task. Finally Keogh and Donlon (1972) found mildly and severely disabled groups to perform more poorly on a variety of field-dependence tasks than normal children. The data are sparse, but compelling.

Are learning-disabled children impulsive? Do they fail to reflect upon the possibilities when one of several choices appears to be correct? Impulsivity is usually measured with the Matching Familiar Figures Test (MFFT) (Kagan, et al., 1964). This is a match to sample procedure in which the child must indicate which of six pictures matches the sample or standard. Impulsivity is defined as committing many errors and doing so quickly. Children who are reflective take their time and make fewer errors. Messer (1976), summarizing a series of studies, indicates that impulsive children are less systematic and more global in viewing test items. They apparently fail to scan the distinctive features of the items in the same way reflective children scan. While there have been few studies in which performance on the MFFT is related to academic and cognitive problems, other studies have found that impulsive children have less adequate short-term auditory memory, less adequate short-term visual memory, less competency solving mazes, and even less skillfulness playing the card game Hearts (Messer, 1976).

More relevant to the field of learning disabilities is the study by Keogh and Margolis (1976). They report that learning-disabled boys make a greater number of erroneous judgements on the MFFT than achieving boys. Kagan (1965) reported that scores on the MFFT were predictive of oral reading scores one year later. Keogh and Donlon (1972) found severely learning-disabled children were more impulsive than mildly disabled children, although the mildly disabled group had scores comparable to those obtained by others for normal achieving children. Finally Kagan (1965) reported that impulsive first-grade children were less able than reflective children to match the experimenter's spoken word with one of five words presented visually. The evidence then clearly supports the notion that children who are or might be likely to experience academic failures are also children who give impulsive answers when required to analyze the fine details of a stimulus array.

The third component of attention is vigilance, the child's ability and/or willingness to attend to a task which is long in duration and low in interest. In studies of vigilance the child is usually presented with a task which requires maintenance of interest on some rather monotomous stimulus presentations. Measures of vigilance include the occasions or times the child notices the correct signal or responds to an incorrect signal.

Several studies employing children who might be expected to have school problems and several which used subjects having such difficulties have indicated that vigilance problems may characterize children who experience academic failures. For example Messer (1976) reported that hyperactive children identify fewer correct and more incorrect signals than nonhyperactive children. Children with reading difficulties have slower reaction times to correct signals than nondisabled children (Noland and Schuldt, 1971). Learning-disabled children, particularly those defined as hyperactive, were found by Anderson, Halcomb, and Doyle (1973) to have difficulties maintaining vigilance. In this study learning-disabled subjects were found to make fewer correct detections and more incorrect responses to the stimulus signal than comparison subjects. Doyle, Anderson, and Halcomb (1976) replicated these results. Learning-disabled children again emitted more incorrect responses and again most differences were attributable to the hyperactive learning disabled rather than the hypoactive or normoactive children. In summary there is both direct and indirect evidence to support the hypothesis that learning-disabled children suffer from attentional problems, at least in focusing, scanning, and maintaining attention.

Auditory Perception and Information Processing

One legacy left to the contemporary learning-disability specialists from the early pioneers' work on brain-damaged adults is the hypothesis that learning-disabled children will demonstrate perceptual problems. Perceptual, perceptual-motor, and auditory and visual information-processing problems are frequently considered primary causes of learning disorders (Frostig, 1972; Kephart, 1963; Kirk and Kirk, 1972). Many feel that learning disorders spring from problems of processing sensory information or from making sense of adequately received inputs, and thus being unable to respond to them appropriately. It is not the reception of the input that is faulty, but rather it is the adequate integration of the input. Thus some research has been concerned with how learning-disabled children integrate or process information as received through various sensory modalities. One such modality is hearing, and it is towards that area of research which we now turn.

Clearly learning in the classroom or other settings which demand that children respond to sound, requires the child to sort auditory signals into meaningful units, to order these units across time, to remember them, and then to respond appropriately (Rosner, 1973). This too is a complex process with many points where it may go amiss.

Auditory information processing has been subdivided into a number of processes which include ability to discriminate sounds, sequence sounds, comprehend sounds, assign appropriate meanings to sounds and remember them. It is generally assumed that these processes are interrelated, so that difficulty with one process will affect other processes involved in auditory processing of information. Such defects are expected to affect the child's performance on academic tasks. Finally there has been the assumption that children showing such difficulties can be helped to better integrate auditory inputs and that such remediation efforts will have a positive effect upon their school performance.

Methods employed to study auditory processing involve a variety of techniques and measurements. For example some children may be asked to identify sounds that are presented in isolation and/or that are embedded in more complex auditory stimuli. In other investigations the child might be confronted with the task of determining the correct word when its auditory presentation is incomplete. Yet other studies require the child to order correctly a string of isolated sounds, numbers, or words.

While the idea that learning-disabled children have deficits in auditory processing has been so germane to the development of the field of learning disabilities, there is a paucity of data concerning such children's auditory information processing. Two research studies have focused specifically on children labeled learning disabled, while several others have reported data based upon brain-damaged or aphasic subjects. Connors, Kramer, and Guerra (1969) studied the role of short-term memory and auditory synthesis by comparing the performances of learning-disabled and normal children. Short term memory was assessed by the child's ability to remember numbers presented to him on a dichotic listening task. Auditory synthesis required the child to indicate the correct word that had been previously incompletely presented. The results of the study were that learning-disabled children did not differ from nondisabled ones in their performances on the short-term memory task. Differences between the groups were found however on the word synthesis task with learning-disabled children performing less adequately than comparison children. Connors, et al., (1969) then suggest that short-term memory differences do not appear critical in discriminating the learning disabled from nondisabled peers, but that critical differences do exist in learning-disabled children's ability to synthesize sounds.

Bryan (1972) compared learning disabled and normal children on a task which required subjects to learn a list of words presented by tape recorder and words presented by slide projector. Learning-disabled and comparison children both performed better with the visual than the auditory stimulus and learning-disabled children performed less adequately than normal children under both stimulus conditions.

Insofar as it is often assumed that learning-disabled children suffer from some central nervous system dysfunction, research concerning the auditory information processing of brain-damaged subjects becomes of interest to learning-disability specialists. Rourke and Czudner (1972) compared normal and brain-damaged children in their vigilance to auditory signals. They reported an interaction effect of age and disability on the task. Neither young six- to nine-year-old, nor older 10- to 13-year old normal, nor older brain-damaged children differed in their attentiveness to the auditory signals. They did find however that young children who were brain damaged showed less vigilance to the task than the remaining three groups.

Grassi (1970) compared brain-damaged, behavior-disordered, and normal adolescents on a vigilance task involving auditory signals. Grassi reported that normal children performed best, followed by behavior-disordered children. Brain damaged subjects performed this task least adequately. This study provided evidence that auditory information processing, in this case auditory vigilance, is deficient in brain-damaged adolescents. The finding that behavior-disordered adolescents performed less well than normal peers suggests that other factors are operating in addition to, or instead of, brain processing of auditory information.

Dykman, et al., (1971) conducted a series of studies in which learning-disabled children and those with minimal cerebral dysfunction were required to discriminate auditory signals. The results reveal that brain-damaged children had greater difficulty than their nonbrain-damaged peers in discriminating tones, in following instructions, and in profiting from practice on the tasks. McReynolds (1966) reported that aphasic children between the ages of four to eight years, were less able than nondamaged children to discriminate sounds, particularly when the sounds to be discriminated were embedded in the context of nonsense syllables. Deterioration in the children's performances was directly related to the complexity of the auditory signals.

There does appear to be some evidence that children with brain dysfunction and perhaps children defined as learning disabled may have some difficulties associated with auditory processing. It should be noted that a variety of factors appear to affect performance on some of the tasks employed and these factors are not necessarily related to auditory processes. The age, complexity of the task, type of task, and the responses demanded by the task may all enter into affecting the child's ultimate performance. Moreover there is evidence that sound discrimination depends in part upon the children's verbal skills, and this suggests that general vocabulary level may play an important role in affecting responses to auditory tasks (Wood, 1971). Just how "pure" the measures of auditory information processing are remains to be empirically demonstrated.

Another assumption is that auditory processing difficulties can be remediated through techniques directly addressed to that modality and that such treatment effects will have a beneficial impact upon academic performance. So far studies based upon the notion of specific modality training have not yielded information which would lend support to this assumption (Bruinincks, 1970; Smith, 1971). Indeed Newcomer and Hamill (1975) have challenged the advisability of engaging children and professionals in such remedial tasks.

Visual Perception and Information Processing

Many professionals have hypothesized that learning disabilities are the result of deficits in the development of visual perception and visual-motor skills, the results of which adversely affect the child's academic performance (Barsch, 1967; Cruickshank, 1972; Frostig, 1972; Kephart, 1963). Many characteristics of children experiencing difficulty learning to read, for example reversals of letters and mirror writing, were interpreted as symptomatic of poor or slow development of their capacity to process visual information. This deficiency in turn is believed to be related to brain damage or slow cerebral development.

The research on visual information processing, like that in auditory information processing, finds a wide variety of samples of children have been employed as subjects. The performances of children with reading disabilities, minimal cerebral dysfunctions, and aphasia form the primary bases for our knowledge in this area.

Lyle and Goyen (1968; 1974) and Goyen and Lyle (1971; 1973) are among the few who have systematically studied visual information-processing skills of reading-disabled children. Using tachistoscopic presentations of visual stimuli under various rates of presentation and incentive conditions, these investigators consistently found that young retarded readers (children under 8.5 years) perform less well than older retarded and all young and old readers. The young retarded readers' problems appear to be related to their inefficiency in noting critical details of the visual stimuli and their slowness in responding to the task. Time and knowledge concerning the important features of a stimulus display are factors which discriminate the young poor reader from others. Their findings suggest that visual perceptual problems or visual information-processing problems may be important in young retarded readers, but do not appear to be so for older retarded readers.

Guthrie and Goldberg (1972) have also compared retarded and adequate readers on several tests presumably tapping visual memory. They found that retarded readers performed less adequately on the Benton Visual Retention Test but that children's scores on subtests on the Illinois Test of Psycholinguistic Abilities presumably assessing visual sequential memory were not associated with reading problems.

As in the case of research concerning auditory processing, several studies of visual information processing have involved children with some form of brain damage. We will now turn to these investigations.

Doehring (1960) compared the performances of aphasic, deaf, and normal children on a task assessing short-term visual memory. He reported that aphasic children performed less adequately than did children from the other two groups. However since aphasic children also had lower intelligence test scores than the comparison children, the results might plausibly be interpreted as reflecting general intellectual deficits rather than specific visual information-processing problems.

Poppen, et al., (1969) compared the abilities of aphasic and nondisabled children, between the ages of 7 to 11.6 years, to sequence adequately visual stimuli. In this investigation children were exposed to various sequences of flashing lights and their task was to reproduce the displayed sequence. They found that normal children made fewer errors in reproduction than did the aphasic subjects. It was also found that while delays between the presentation of the stimuli and the children's responses to it would negatively affect the performance of both groups, delays particularly affected aphasic children's performances. While results do support the notion that brain-damaged children may have some difficulties in visual information processing, it should be noted that memory tasks require language processing insofar as such processes aid the individual to code, rehearse, and retrieve the vital information. Thus it is not clear whether the aphasic subjects in this study performed poorly because of a language or a visual information-processing problem.

Dykman, et al., (1971) compared the performances of children with minimal cerebral dysfunction and those without such problems in their impulsivity in responding to visual cues (flashing lights on a panel). Children were instructed to press a lever for certain flashing lights, but to ignore others. The results were that the brain-damaged children committed more errors while responding more slowly to the correct stimuli than did the comparison children. The differences between the groups in their performances was apparently increased with practice. Dykman, et al., also conducted a similar study in which the subjects defined as learning-disabled children were subdivided into three groups: hyperactive, normoactive, and hypoactive. Learning-disabled subjects made more errors than normal children in following instructions and responding to the visual stimuli. The response latency to visual signals, measured under several conditions, was consistently longer for the learning-disabled than the normal children. They further found that the hypoactive learning-disabled group did respond slower than either the hyperactive or normoactive learning-disabled child.

Czudner and Rourke (1970) also investigated brain-damaged children's reaction times to visual signals. One group of subjects consisted of children diagnosed as having minimal cerebral dysfunction, the other group consisted of nondisabled children. The results indicated that the brain-damaged subjects were slower to respond than the nondamaged children, results consistent with those reported by Dykman, et al., (1971).

Before turning our attention from this area of research, mention should be made of two tests which are frequently used, in both research and clinical practice, as devices to assess visual information processing. Their current popularity warrants attention. These tests are the ITPA, Illinois Test of Psycholinguistic Abilities (Kirk, McCarthy, and Kirk, 1968) and the DTVP, Developmental Test of Visual Perception (Frostig and Horne, 1964).

Skepticism concerning these tests for such assessments is increasing. The basis for doubt rests on the findings that the subtests do not correlate with one another as they should, and that subtests which are presumed to measure one ability are in fact highly correlated with tests presumably measuring other abilities. For example Burns and Watson (1973) have found that while the visual processing items in the ITPA were positively correlated with one another, they also were correlated with subtests which are supposed to be independent measures of language ability. In a review of the research literature on the ITPA, Carroll (1972) concluded that the test taps three or four abilities, not the nine hypothesized by the test's authors. Huizinga (1972) found the ITPA subtests on visual processing to be positively related to the children's scores on the Stanford-Binet Intelligence Scale and the Wechsler Intelligence Scale for Children. There is considerable doubt whether the subtests presumed to assess visual processing are not in fact tapping quite different abilities, such as linguistic skills.

New comer and Hamill (1975) have presented a summary of research concerning the Frostig DTVP. Like the studies involving the ITPA, there is little reason to assume that various subtests involving visual processing are in fact assessing different perceptual skills. In sum the tests seem to confound language and/or intellectual abilities with visual-processing skills.

Cross-Modal Information Processing

A second view concerning the information processing of learning-disabled children is that such children have difficulty in integrating information from different modalities (Birch and Lefford, 1963). It is not so much that learning-disabled children have auditory of visual-processing difficulties, but rather that they suffer from an inability to integrate the information received through the visual and auditory channels.

Several methods have been employed to test this hypothesis. For example sometimes the subjects are required to match sounds with patterns of dots and dashes presented visually (Birch and Belmont, 1964, 1965). Others have required subjects to recall information which has been presented at a rapid speed through two modalities (Senf, 1969; Senf and Freundl, 1971; Vande Voort and Senf, 1973).

An early study by Birch and Belmont (1964) stimulated much of the research concerning the learning-disabled child's ability to integrate cross-modal information. In this study the investigators compared retarded and nonretarded readers in the performance of a task which required that they indicate whether the auditory pattern of stimuli was identical to a pattern of visually displayed dots. Birch and Belmont (1964) found that retarded readers performed significantly worse than did nonretarded readers. It should be noted however that Birch and Belmont did find that intelligence test scores were related to adequacy in the children's task performance.

Using an adaptation of the Broadbent dichotic listening task, Senf and colleagues have conducted a number of studies of cross-modal integration of visual and auditory information (Senf, 1969; Senf and Freundl, 1971; Vande Voort and Senf, 1973). While there were procedural differences in these studies, the subjects were presented with information simultaneously in both the auditory and visual channels. The dependent variables were the order and modality in which subjects reported what they had seen and heard. The results of these studies did not support the notion that learning-disabled children have greater difficulties than others in integrating information from auditory and visual channels, rather, the disabled subjects tend to have problems dealing with material within channels, such as the visual-spatial and auditory-temporal dimensions. In addition the learning disabled had particular problems ordering the information, that is recalling the auditory-visual inputs. Organization of the information for recall which is responsive to instructions appears to be more descriptive of the differences among groups than claims about auditory and visual cross-modal information processing. What was striking was that the normal subjects show developmental sequences as their performance improves with age, the disabled population did not.

While there is some evidence that reading-disabled children perform less adequately than nonretarded readers on tasks presumably assessing cross-modal information processing, several methodological problems attenuate support for this hypothesis. First, the data are not clear that differences in performance are not attributable to difficulties in information processing within a single modality. Rarely do investigators control for possible differences between groups in their ability to process within a given modality. Second, attentional differences between groups may account for some of the differences found. Third, information tasks are related to language skills and levels (Freides, 1974). Additionally learning-disabled children may have less skill in adapting appropriate strategies of task analysis given instructions which run counter to the child's mode of organizing information (Torgesen, 1975). Since learning-disabled children appear to have problems on a variety of tasks, in addition to those occasionally found in cross-modal information processing ones, the problems experienced by poor readers cannot be dismissed on the basis of intermodal information processing (Torgesen,

1975). Problems in decoding, memory, attention, and organization of information may well cut across the various experimental tasks used in cross-modal information-processing experiments.

Language Deficits

The hypothesis that children with learning disabilities may have specific deficits or delays in language development has its roots in the early years of the field of learning disabilities. Language disturbances were included in Clements (1966) publication concerning the characteristics of children with minimal brain dysfunction. At that time language dysfunctions were described as aphasia, impaired discrimination of auditory stimuli, slow language development, and frequent but mild speech disorders. Subsequently these ideas were translated in the later definitions of learning disabilities as specific disorders in talking, reading, spelling, and disabilities primarily related to communication processes (Kirk and Kirk, 1972). In spite of the relatively long history of this idea, it has been only very recently that empirical studies of language in learning-disabled children have been conducted. There is accumulating evidence that children without physical evidence of brain damage may show delayed language development, a delay which results in their language being different from, rather than simply slower than, children who do not experience such delays. Menyuk (1969) compared the linguistic competence of language-delayed children, ages three to six years, with comparable nonlanguage delayed children. The results were based on three measures: the children's responses to a projective test, their conversation with an adult and a peer, and their ability to repeat a list of grammatical and nongrammatical sentences. Menyuk reported that linguistically delayed children did not perform as well as the normal children at any age; indeed, the three-, four-, and five-year old delayed children used similar syntactic structures in their verbal productions. Thus the language delayed children formed a homogeneous group and differed from the control subjects in their language productions. Lee (1974) has developed two language tests, one being a screening test to assess syntax development, the other a quantitative method for assessing children's language across a variety of linguistic dimensions. Lee further describes the differences between linguistically delayed and normal children's speech. Among the specific problems that Lee notes are the language-delayed children's difficulty in learning pronouns, using negatives, learning the syntactic forms for posing questions, and slowness in employing infinitives.

The question can be raised as to whether the children studied by Menyuk (1964) and Lee (1974) later become identified as learning disabled. There is some evidence to suggest this may be the case. For example Kirk and Elkins (1975) found that 43% of children being served in learning-disability Child Service Demonstration Centers were receiving remedial help for language development. Owen, et al., (1971) interviewed parents of learning-disabled children and reported that parents describe the learning-disabled subjects as having less adequate verbal skills than siblings and other children. Owen, et al., divided their learning-disabled sample into four subgroups. One group was characterized as having a history of organic or physical abnormality; the second group had high WISC performance scores relative to verbal IQ scores; the third group had relatively low IQ scores; and the fourth had high IQ scores but evidence of emotional problems. Owen, et al., report that the first three groups manifest some kinds of language deficits. The authors also noted that the mothers and siblings of these children also evidenced language problems.

Semel and Wiig (1975) have conducted several studies of language processing, using samples of learning-disabled children which included adolescents. Using Lee's tests of syntax development, Wiig and Semel reported that learning-disabled children were significantly inferior to nondisabled children on measures of language production and language comprehension. The language problems were severe insofar as three quarters of their subjects scored below the tenth percentile in language comprehension. Fry, Johnson, and Muehl (1970) compared the oral language of good and poor second-grade readers. Based on the children's story tellings in response to pictures, three differences between the good and poor readers were found. Good readers had larger speaking vocabularies and were more fluent, used more complex linguistic structures, and used more complex sentence forms than did poor readers.

Vogel (1974, 1977) studied the oral syntax of boys labeled dyslexic. She reported that the dyslexic boys were less competent than nondyslexic ones in detecting whether a sentence heard was a statement of information or a question, in repeating sentences, or in responding to a modified Cloze task (that is filling in a word deleted from a spoken paragraph). In addition Vogel found dyslexics to have less knowledge than the control group regarding the rules of morphology which employed nonsense words. The learning-disabled subjects perform less adequately than the comparison nondisabled children. The learning-disabled children had difficulty with such tasks as forming plural forms of possessives and forming the progressive tense. Learning-disabled children, in this case 8 to 10-year-olds, were unable to respond competently to linguistic tasks which normal 3 and 4-year-olds can typically master. Wiig and Semel (1975) also found learning-disabled adolescents to be less competent than nondisabled peers on naming verbal opposites, formulating sentences, defining and retrieving words; to be slower and less accurate in responding to test items; and to be less able to detect their incorrect responses.

The language problems of learning-disabled children, at least boys, was also found in a study by Bryan and Pflaum (1978). In this study a linguistic analysis is applied to the communications uttered by learning-disabled and normal children while playing a game. Fourth-and fifth-grade learning-disabled males used significantly less complex social communications than nondisabled same sex peers. Language differences between learning-disabled and nondisabled females however were not found. Female learning-disabled subjects differed from male learning-disabled children in employing more complex linguistic utterances. Another noteworthy difference between male and female learning-disabled subjects was found in this study. The analysis of communications included interactions between same age and younger children. The female learning-disabled subjects made linguistic adjustments and used simpler syntax when speaking with the younger child, while the learning-disabled males failed to make such an adjustment.

There is thus considerable evidence that learning-disabled boys, at least, show less linguistic competence in a variety of measures than do normal peers. Unfortunately most researchers on learning-disabled children have limited their samples to male subjects. It is not yet clear that female learning-disabled children would show these same differences relative to their same sex peers.

Hyeractivity

There is probably no area more confused in learning disabilities than that related to hyperactivity. Hyperactivity was one of the 10 most frequently cited characteristics of learning disabilities when the literature in the field first appeared (Clements, 1969; McCarthy and Paraskevopolos, 1969). Yet the current guidelines for defining learning disabilities which is employed for use in the *Education for All Handicapped Children Act* of 1975 makes no reference to hyperactivity or any similar behavioral traits (distractibility, emotional lability, impulsivity). Has hyperactive behavior disappeared as a problem or are we living through an educational version of the emperor's new clothes? It must be acknowledged at the onset of this discussion that we have little empirical knowledge of the incidence of hyperactivity in learning-disabled children. We also do not have an operational definition of hyperactivity. This is not to say that some learning-disabled children are not hyperactive by some definition or another, nor that hyperactive children do not manifest learning problems. However direct information concerning the relationship of hyperactive behavior to learning-disabled children is sparse. As in other areas of research, the samples of children selected for inclusion are defined along a variety of dimensions and include children with brain damage, retardation, as well as children on medication for hyperactive behavior.

Pope (1970) conducted an ingenious study in which brain-damaged children, ages 7 to 11 years, were observed in four different situations:

1. Assigned to a simple task.
2. Assigned to a difficult task.
3. In undirected play.
4. When asked to remain seated in a chair.

The results indicated that hyperactivity of the brain-damaged child was situationally specific. When engaged in undirected play, brain-damaged children did not differ from comparison children in their total motor activity. When performing a simple task, the brain-damaged children again did not show more motor activity than did the control subjects. While performing a difficult task however brain-damaged children did engage in more motor activity than comparison children, although they did maintain their persistence in the task. When requested to sit still, differences between these groups of children were again found. Thus while brain-damaged children did show greater motor activity than the control subjects, this was the case only in some but not all situations.

The subject of hyperactivity is made more complex when we examine an extensive study of institutionalized children in which several dimensions of hyperactivity were assessed. While the subjects are discrepant from those who are the focus of this chapter, the results of the study call for our attention. Schulman, Kaspar, and Throne (1965) investigated the behavior of 11- to 14-year-old children with IQs ranging from 46 to 87. Using several measures of both hyperactivity and distractiblity across a number of situations, these researchers also found that children's activity across situations was not consistent. In addition hyperactivity and distractiblity were not general traits of children nor were they related to one another. Finally these behaviors did not have positive correlations with psychometric measures. The presence of neurological signs for example was correlated with hypoactivity rather than hyperactivity. What is important about this study's findings is that it appears unlikely that there are syndromes of brain damage consisting of both hyperactivity and distractibility.

Hyperactivity and distractibility, as typically viewed by the researcher and practitioner, represent complex multidimensional constructs. It is unreasonable to believe that a single test or measure would adequately capture the various dimensions implicit in current usage of the term hyperactive or distractible. In addition to the characteristics of the child, task demands and other situational and social constraints will affect these complex behaviors.

Let us now turn to research conducted on children defined as hyperactive. These studies have defined hyperactive children on the basis of teacher and parent ratings of the children on scales, by their reports during interviews, or by virtue of the child receiving medication for hyperactivity (Denckla, 1973; Langhorne and Loney, 1976; Solomons, 1971; Whalen and Henker, 1976). By and large the definition of hyperactivity assumed by professionals is that hyperactivity reflects excessive motor activity by a child. The results of the research suggest however that children labeled hyperactive are not engaging in excessive activity levels relative to nonhyperactive children. Whalen and Henker (1976) reviewed the findings pertaining to studies of hyperactivity and reported that there is a failure to find differences in activity level between hyperactive and nonhyperactive children, irrespective of whether the assessment is based on global ratings by teachers and parents, behavioral observations, or electromechanical recordings. If these children are not engaging in excessive motor activity, what is it they do that elicits the label hyperactive? It appears that the differences between hyperactive and nonhyperactive children are related to the quality rather than the quantity of motor movement. When teachers or examiners make demands on children so labeled, they appear to show high levels of motor restlessness. The problems appear to be more related to ability to modulate motor behavior in response to situational and perhaps social demands. Whalen and Henker also suggest that it is not the excessive wiggle and jiggle that constitutes the problem, but rather that hyperactive children seem to be more impulsive and less able to maintain vigilance or attention to the task than do other children.

While excessive motor activity has been the major trait of hyperactive children, a variety of other characteristics have become associated with this term. Hyperactive children are thus considered distractible, clumsy, showing short attention span, antisocial behavior, poor peer relationships, and low self-esteem (Langhorne and Loney, 1976). Research on the relationships among these characteristics have failed to support the notion that these co-occur. Correlations which are found among these traits appear to be associated with the persons doing the judging rather than with the child being judged (Langhorne and Loney, 1976). We are now in the position where physicians agree with physicians, teachers with teachers, and parents with parents on ratings of hyperactivity but these groups fail to have judgments correlated with one another. Since we now have some evidence that hyperactive behavior may not occur across situations (that is that it is unlikely to be a consistent characteristic of the child), it is not surprising that judges who see the children in quite varying circumstances would also view them differently.

There have been attempts to subcategorize hyperactive children. Denckla (1973) devised three categories on the basis of clinical observations that different kinds of hyperactive children respond differentially to various drugs. Solomons (1971) has devised a classification scheme of four categories ranging from low level of energy expenditure to impulsive, distractible, irritable, and hyperexcitable. While these categories are based on clinical observations rather than on empirical data, the fact that these physicians find differential responsiveness to treatments suggests interesting research possibilities.

While we are at a primitve stage in defining hyperactivity and how it might relate to learning disorders, the children being categorized by this label appear to have a rather bleak future. Weiss, et al., (1971) conducted a five-year follow-up study of children labeled hyperactive and found them to show no improvement in academic grades, to have few friends, and that 15% of these children had been referred to the courts for having committed antisocial acts. Mendelson, Johnson, and Stewart (1971) found that parents of hyperactive children reported more than 50% engaged in stealing, fighting, frequent lying; 59% had had some interaction with the police. In sum whatever differentiates hyperactive from other children is more likely to be situationally linked and to involve attentional skills rather than gross motor activity. These children appear to have persistent problems and the employment of drugs does not seem to make a difference once the treatments are discontinued (Whalen and Henker, 1976).

Social Relationships

There has been considerable research now on the social relationships of children labeled as learning disabled (who may or may not be hyperactive). When we use sociometric measures, laboratory studies of social interactions, observations of interactions in the classroom and special education resource rooms, laboratory based studies of learning-disabled children's perceptions of others and others' perceptions of them, the results consistently indicate that learning-disabled children are experiencing difficulties in their social relationships with teachers and peers (Bryan, 1974a, 1974b, 1978; Bryan and Wheeler, 1972).

The results of these studies are consistent in indicating that the learning-disabled child may have pervasive difficulties in relating to others: if their classmates are asked, they indicate that they do not like such children (Bryan, 1974b). Moreover if learning-disabled children are observed in interactions with peers, they give and get more hostile communications than do nondisabled classmates (Bryan, et al., 1976). Within the classroom setting, teachers are more likely to ignore the learning-disabled child than his peers (Bryan, 1974a); within the home setting, parents are likely to indicate that their learning-disabled child is not the preferred offspring (Owen, et al., 1971). While the bases for such rejection are yet undetermined, it has been shown that the learning-disabled child is less adequate in interpreting the nonverbal behaviors of adults (Bryan, 1978). It is reasonable to assume that such a deficiency would also hold true for their understanding of such behavior by other children. It is likely that learning-disabled children are poor people readers and that this factor may hamper their social relationships.

The findings concerning poor social relationships are consistent across methodological approaches and varying samples. These children's apparent lack of social skills suggest that their social problems should not be overlooked in either therapeutic or research endeavors.

SUMMARY, OPINIONS, AND SPECULATIONS

Our knowledge concerning the learning-disabled child is quite primitive. There are many more questions than answers, many more hints than facts. What can be said about our current knowledge? First it does appear that learning-disabled children are more likely than nondisabled ones to score low on tests of intelligence. This is hardly surprising since intelligence tests were designed and are successful in predicting academic performance. There is suggestive evidence that learning-disabled children do have some attentional problems, at least when attention is defined by perceptual organization and vigilance. While there is evidence to suggest that learning-disabled children may have problems in processing auditory and visual information and in integrating information from both these sources, the tasks which are used to assess such processes are likely to involve the language and verbal abilities of the child. While the evidence is sparse, it does seem clear that the learning-disabled child may be particularly deficient in such skills. His linguistic development appears to be markedly retarded. At this time we know that hyperactive children are not hyperactive all the time, but seem to have difficulty in modulating their motor behaviors in accordance with task demands. Moreover the hyperactive child appears to have a wide range of social problems. What we do not know as yet is whether most learning-disabled children are hyperactive by anyone's definition. Finally the evidence is considerable that the learning-disabled child confronts a social world which is relatively hostile to and rejecting of him. Teachers, peers, and parents apparently view such children with less than the usual benevolence. Finally these children appear to have difficulties in understanding the nonverbal communications of adults and are likely to be poor people readers.

The major problem facing the field of learning disabilities is the definition of the target population. The field emerged because of practical problems of training children, it is sustained by the hopes that such problems can be remediated. Progress however ultimately depends upon adequate research, and adequate research requires ever increasing refinements in definitions, measurements, and hypotheses. As yet there has been relatively little success in empirically refining the definition of learning disabilities. Children who now fall under this conceptual umbrella are clearly a heterogeneous group; some are failing mathematics, others reading, others academic life in general. Research is needed that will allow us to form more homogeneous groups, the basis of which will allow a more rapid accumulation of empirically based knowledge. Some attempts in this direction are now being made. Thus Keogh and Hall (1973) and Dykman, et al., (1971) have looked at learning-disabled children categorized across the dimension of hyperactivity. Bruininks (1970) and Smith (1971) have subcategorized learning-disabled children as to modality preferences in learning tasks, while Denckla (1973) and Solomons (1971) have attempted to categorize hyperactive children on the basis of their behavior and responsiveness to medication. Such refinements will, no doubt, continue to be made.

It is also time to realize that many of the tests and measurements prized by the field carry little more than face validity. All tests do not measure what the authors purport them to measure and all must be judged on their predictive power. Simply failing a series of items labeled as assessing auditory information processing does not mean that the failing subject has an auditory problem. The exact nature of what those items assess is defined by the correlations of those items with other bits of behavior. The use of tests, particularly for clinical practices, has clearly outstripped our empirical knowledge concerning them.

It is probably characteristic of any new field or research that the initial views of a behavior are undifferentiated or simplistic. The field of learning disabilities is no exception. It is not uncommon for many professionals to view very complex behaviors as representing a unidimensional factor. It is increasingly recognized that such is not the case. Attention, information processing, hyperactivity, and language, to name but a few, are very complex processes, consisting of various behaviors and constrained and affected by many situational influences. Happily attempts further to refine our knowledge about some of these complex behaviors are being made as in the case of Keogh's (1973) work on attention behaviors. Programmatic research which involves the study of the component parts of these behaviors which comprise the construct awaits much needed further research.

At the present time there are a number of unknowns which are likely to affect seriously the field of learning disabilities in the immediate future. A major recent event is the *Education for All Handicapped Children Act of 1975* (P. L. 94–142). As yet we do not know if the states will subscribe to the currently proposed guidelines associated with this legislation. There are no doubt ways to avoid full compliance with the spirit, if not the letter of the law. A ceiling has been placed on the number of learning-disabled children within a state who are eligible to receive federal funding for educational programs. As the funding is constrained by numbers, it is likely that the criteria for including children within the learning-disability groups will become more stringent. Some learning-disabled children may well become redefined as educable mentally retarded. The definition of learning disabilities embodied within the law emphasizes children's academic performance rather than medical status. The shift towards the educational model is underscored by this law. Hopefully this shift will increase our attention to variables other than those of the child. Teachers, parents, peers, tasks, and various other influences, all produce their share of effects in creating or attenuating learning disabilities. Their influence will certainly be better known in the near future.

REFERENCES

Ames, L. B. "A low intelligence quotient often not recognized as the chief cause of many learning difficulties." *Journal of Learning Disabilities*, 1, 45–48, (1968).

Anderson, R. P., C. G. Holcomb, and R. B. Doyle. "The measurement of attentional deficits." *Eceptional Children*, 39, 534–539, (1973).

Barsch, R. H. "Achieving Perceptual Motor Efficiency." Seattle: Special Child Publication, 1967.

Bateman, B. "Reading: A controversial view," in L Tarnopol, ed., *Learning Disabilities*, pp. 289–304. Springfield, Ill.: Thomas, 1969.

Birch, H., and L. Belmont, "Auditory-visual integration in normal and retarded readers." *American Journal of Orthopsychiatry*, 34, 852–361, (1964).

———"Auditory-visual integration, intelligence, and reading ability in school children." *Perceptual and Motor Skills*, 20, 295–305, 1965.

Birch, H. G., and A. Lefford. "Intersensory development in children." *Monographs of the*

Society for Research on Child Development, 28, 1963.

Browning, R. M. "Effects of irrelevant peripheral visual stimuli on discrimination learning in minimally brain-damaged children." *Journal of Consultant Psychology*, 31, 371–376, (1967).

Bruininks, R. "Teaching word recognition to disadvantaged boys." *Journal of Learning Disabilities*, 3, 28–35, (1970).

Bruininks, R., G. Glaman, and C. Clark. "Prevalence of learning disabilities: Findings, issues, and recommendations." Research Report No. 20, Department of HEW, (June, 1971).

Bryan, T. "The effect of forced mediation upon short-term memory of children with learning disabilities." *Journal of Learning Disabilities*, 5, 605–609, (1972).

Bryan, T., "An observational analysis of classroom behaviors of children with learning disabilities." *Journal of Learning Disabilities*, 7, 26–34, (1974a).

Bryan, T. "Peer popularity of learning disabled children." *Journal of Learning Disabilities*, 7, 304–309, (1974b).

Bryan, T. "Children's comprehension of nonverbal communication." *Journal of Disabilities*, (1978) in press.

Bryan, T., and V. Bryan. *Understanding Learning Disabilities*. New York: Alfred, 1975.

Bryan, T. and S. Pflaum. "Linguistic, cognitive and social analyses of learning disabled children's interactions." *Learning Disabilities Quarterly*, 1, 70–79, (1978).

Bryan, T., and R. Wheeler. "Perception of children with learning disabilities: The eye of the observer." *Journal of Learning Disabilities*, 5, 484–488, (1972).

Bryan, T., R. Wheeler, J. Felcan, and T. Henek. " 'Come on dummy' An observational study of children's communications." *Journal of Learning Disabilities*, 9, 661–669, (1976).

Burns, G. W., and B. L. Watson. "Factor analysis of the revised ITPA with underachieving children." *Journal of Learning Disabilities*, 6, 371–376, (1973).

Carroll, J. B. "Review of the Illinois Test of Psycholinguistics." in O. K. Buros, ed., *The Seventh Mental Measurement Yearbook*, 819–823, Highland Park, N. J.: Gryphon Press, 7, 1972.

Clements, S. D. *Minimal brain dysfunction in children—Terminology and Identification*. NINDS Monograph No. 3, Public Health Service Bulletin No. 1415. Washington D. C.: U. S. Department of HEW, 1966.

Connors, C. K., K. Kramer, and F. Guerra, "Auditory synthesis and dichotic listening in children with learning disabilities." *Journal of Special Education*, 3, 163–170, (1969).

Cruickshank, W. M. "Some issues facing the field of learning disability." *Journal of Learning Disabilities*, 5, 380–388, (1972).

Czudner, G., and B. P. Rourke. "Simple reaction time in brain damaged and normal children under regular and irregular preparatory interval conditions." *Perceptual and Motor Skills*, 31, 767–773, (1970).

Denckla, M. B. "Research needs in learning disabilities: A neurologist's point of view." *Journal of Learning Disabilities*, 6, 441–450, (1973).

Doehring, D. 'Visual spatial memory in aphasic children." *Journal of Speech and Hearing Research*, 3, 138–149, (1960).

Doyle, R. B., R. P. Anderson, and C. G. Halcomb. "Attention deficits and the effects of visual distraction." *Journal of Learning Disabilities*, 9, 48–54, (1976).

Dykman, R. A., P. T. Ackerman, S. D. Clements, and J. E. Peters. "Specific learning disabilities: An attentional deficit syndrome," in H. R. Myklebust, ed., *Progress in Learning Disabilities*, vol. II, 56–93, New York: Grune & Stratton, 1971.

Federal Register, 41, no. 230, (Nov. 1976).

Freides, D. "Human information processing and sensory modality: Cross-modal functions, information complexity, memory and deficit." *Psychological Bulletin*, 81, 284–310, (1974).

Frostig, M. "Visual perception, integrative functions, and academic learning." *Journal of Learning Disabilities*, 5, 1–15, (1972).

Frostig, M., and D. Horne. "The Frostig program for the development of visual perception." Chigago: Follett, 1964.

Fry, M. A., C. S. Johnson, and S. Muehl. "Oral language production in relation to reading achievement among select second graders." in D. J. Bakker and P. Satz, ed., *Specific Reading Disability*, 123–159. The Netherlands: Rotterdam University Press, 1970.

Geschwind, N. "Neurological foundations of language," in H. R. Myklebust, ed., *Progress in Learning Disabilities*, vol. I, pp. 182–198, New York: Grune & Stratton, 1968.

Goyen, J. D., and J. G. Lyle, "Effect of incentives and age on the visual recognition of retarded readers." *Journal of Experimental Child Psychology*, 11, 266–273, (1971).

———"Short term memory and visual discrimination in retarded readers." *Perceptual and Motor Skills*, 36, 403–408, (1973).

Grassi, J. "Auditory vigilance performance in brain damaged, behavior disordered, and normal children." *Journal of Learning Disabilities*, 3, 302–304, (1970).

Guthrie, J. T., and H. K. Goldberg, "Visual sequential memory in reading disability." *Journal of Learning Disabilities*, 5, 41–46, (1972).

Hallahan, D. P. "Comparative research studies on the psychological characteristics of learning disabled children," in W. M. Cruickshank and D. P. Hallahan, ed., *Perceptual and Learning Disabilities in Children*, Syracuse, N. Y.: Syracuse University Press, 1975.

Huizinga, R. J. "The relationship of the ITPA to the Stanford-Binet form L-M and the WISC." *Journal of Learning Disabilities*, 6, 451–456, (1973).

Kagan, J. "Reflection-impulsivity and reading ability in primary grade children." *Child Development*, 36, 609–628, (1965).

Kagan, J., and N. Kogan. "Individual variation in cognitive processes," in P. H. Mussen, ed., *Carmichael's Manual of Child Psychology*, vol. I. New York: Wiley, 1970.

Kagan, J., B. L. Rosman, D. Day, J. Albert, and W. Phillips. "Information processing in the child: Significance of analytic and reflective attitudes." *Psychological Monographs*, (1964). 78 (1), Whole No. 578.

Kawabe, K. K. "Attentional deficits in learning disabled children." *Division for Children with Learning Disabilities Newsletter*, 2, 35–41, (1976).

Keogh, B. K. "Attentional characteristics of children with learning disabilities." (paper presented at the International Symposium on Learning Disabilities. San Diego, California, November, 1973.)

Keogh, B. K., and G. Donlon. "Field dependence, impulsivity, and learning disabilities." *Journal of Learning Disabilities*, 5, 331–336, (1972).

Keogh, B. K., and R. J. Hall. "Functional analysis of WISC performance of children classified as EH and EMR." Technical Report SERP 1973-A9. Graduate School of Education, University of California, Los Angeles, 1973.

Keogh, B. K., and J. Margolis. "Learn to labor and to wait: Attentional problems of children with learning disorders." *Journal of Learning Disabilities*, 9, 276–286, (1976).

Kephart, N. C., *The Brain-Injured Child in the Classroom*. Chicago: National Society for Crippled Children and Adults, 1963.

Kirk, S. A., and J. Elkins. "Characteristics of children enrolled in the Child Demonstration Service Centers." *Journal of Learning Disabilities*, 8, 630–637, (1975).

Kirk, S. A., and W. P. Kirk. *Psycholinguistic Learning Disabilities: Diagnosis and Reme-diation.* Urbana: University of Illinois Press, 1972.

Kirk, S. A., J. J. McCarthy, and W. D. Kirk. "Illinois Test of Psycholinguistic Abilities," rev. ed. Urbana: University of Illinois Press, 1968.

Langhorne, J. E., and J. Loney. "Childhood hyperkineses: A return to the source." *Journal of Abnormal Psychology,* 85, 201–209, (1976).

Lee, L. L. *Developmental Sentence Analysis.* Evanston, Ill.: Northwestern University Press, 1974.

Lilly, M. S. "A merger of categories: Are we finally ready?" *Journal of Learning Disabili-ties,* 10, 115–121, (1977).

London, P. "The end of ideology in behavior modification." *American Psychologist,* 27, 913–920, (1972).

Lyle, J. G., and J. D. Goyen. "Visual recognition, developmental lag, and strepho-symbolia in reading retardation." *Journal of Abnormal Psychology,* 73, 25–29, (1968).

————"Effect of speed of exposure and difficulty of discrimination upon visual recognition of retarded readers." 1974. [Unpublished manuscript].

Masland, R. L. "Children with minimal brain dysfunction—A rational problem," in L. Tarnopol, ed., *Learning Disabilities,* Sringfield, Ill.: Thomas, 1969.

McCarthy, J. M., and J. Paraskevopoulos. "Behavior patterns of learning disabled, emo-tionally disturbed, and average children." *Exceptional Children,* 35, 69–74, (October 1969).

McDonald, C. W. "Problems concerning the classification and education of children with learning disabilities," in J. Hellmuth, ed., *Learning Disorders,* vol. 3, Seattle: Special Children Publication, 1968.

McReynolds, L. V. "Operant conditioning for investigating speech sound discrimination in aphasic children." *Journal of Speech and Hearing Research,* 9, 519–528, (1966).

Mendelson, W., N. Johnson, and M. A. Stewart. "Hyperactive children as teenagers: A follow up study." *Journal of Nervous and Mental Disease,* 153, 273–279, (1971).

Menyuk, P. "Comparison of grammer of children with functionally deviant and normal speech." *Journal of Speech and Hearing Research,* 7, 109–121, (1964).

Messer, S. B. "Reflection-impulsivity: A review." *Psychological Bulletin,* 83, 1026–1052, (1976).

National Advisory Committee on Handicapped Children. "Special education for handi-capped children. First annual report." Washington, D. C.: U. S. Department of HEW, (January, 31, 1968).

Newcomer, P. L., and D. D. Hammill. "ITPA and academic achievement: A survey." *The Reading Teacher,* 28, 731–741, (1975).

Noland, E. C., and W. J. Schuldt. "Sustained attention and reading retardation." *Journal of Experimental Education,* 40, 73–76, (1971).

Owen, R. W., P. A. Adams, T. Forrest, L. M. Stolz, and S. Fisher. "Learning disorders in children: Sibling studies." *Monographs of the Society for Research in Child Develop-ment,* 36 (144), (1971).

Pick, H. L., and A. D. Pick. "Sensory and perceptual development." in P. H. Mussen, ed., *Carmichael's Manual of Child Psychology.,* vol. 1, New York: Wiley, 1970.

Pope, L. "Motor activity in brain-injured children." *American Journal of Orthopsychiatry,* 40, 783–794, (1970),

Poppen, R., J. Stark, J. Eisenson, T. Forrest, and G. Wertheim. "Visual sequencing performance of aphasic children." *Journal of Speech and Hearing Research,* 12, 288–300, (1969).

Rosner, J. "Language arts and arithmetic achievement, and specifically related perceptual skills." *American Educational Research Journal*, 10, 59–68, (1973).

Rourke, B. P., and G. Czudner. "Age difference in auditory reaction time of brain damaged and normal children under regular and irregular preparatory interval conditions." *Journal of Experimental Child Psychology*, 14, 527–539, (1972).

Schulman, J. L., J. C. Kaspar, and F. H. Throne. *Brain Damage and Behavior*, Springfield, Ill.: Thomas, 1965.

Semel, E. M., and E. H. Wiig. "Comprehension of syntactic structure and critical verbal elements by children with learning disabilities." *Journal of Learning Disabilities*, 8, 46 –52, (1975).

Senf, G. M. "Development of immediate memory for bisensory stimuli in normal children and children with learning disorders." *Developmental Psychology*, 1, 1–28, (1969).

Senf, G. M., and P. C. Freundl. "Memory and attention factors in specific learning disabilities." *Journal of Learning Disabilities*, 4, 94–106, (1971).

Silberberg, N. E., and M. C. Silberberg. "A note on reading tests and their role in defining reading difficulties." *Journal of Learning Disabilities*, 10, 100–103, (1977).

Smith, C. M. "The relationship of reading method and reading achievement to ITPA sensory modalities." *Journal of Special Education*, 5, 143 149, (1971).

Solomons, G. "Guidelines on the use and medical effects of psychostimulant drugs in therapy." *Journal of Learning Disabilities*, 4, 420–475, (1971).

Strauss, A., and L. Lehtinen. *Psychopathology and Education of the Brain-Injured Child.* New York: Grune / Stratton, 1947.

Torgesen, J. "Problems and prospects in the study of learning disabilities," in M. Heatherington, ed., *Review of Child Development Research*, vol. 5. Chicago: University of Chicago Press, 1975.

Vande Voort, L., and G. M. Senf. "Audiovisual integration in retarded readers." *Journal of Learning Disabilities*, 6, 170–179, (1973).

Vogel, S. A. "Syntactic abilities in normal and dyslexic children." *Journal of Learning Disabilities*, 7, 103–109, (1974).

————"Morphological ability in normal and dyslexic children." *Journal of Learning Disabilities*, 10, 35–43, (1977).

Weiss, G., K. Minde, J. S. Werry, V. Douglas, and E. Nemeth. "Studies of the hyperactive child: A five year follow-up." *Archives of General Psychiatry*, 24, 409–414, (1971).

Whalen, C. K., and B. Henker. "Psycho-stimulants and children: A review and analysis." *Psychological Bulletin*, 83, 1113–1130, (1976).

Wiig, E. H., and E. M. Semel. "Productive language abilities in learning-disabled adolescents." *Journal of Learning Disabilities*, 8, 578–588, (1975).

Wiig, E. H., E. M. Semel, and M. A. Crouse. "The use of English morphology by high-risk and learning disabled children." *Journal of Learning Disabilities*, 6, 457–465.

Wood, N. E. "Auditory perception in children." Social and Rehabilitation Service Research Grant (RD–2574–S). Los Angeles: University of Southern California, (March 1971).

CHAPTER 21

Emotional Disorders

S. Thomas Cummings and D. Craig Finger

INTRODUCTION

In this chapter we have three goals: (1) to describe the major patterns of emotional disorders of children; (2) to call attention to the overlapping symptomatology of these disorders relative to the primary symptomatology associated with the minimal brain dysfunction (MBD) syndromes; and (3) to discuss issues and questions relevant to the problem of differential diagnosis. Our age focus is on preadolescent and early adolescent children. Our point of view combines aspects of psychoanalytic ego psychology and social learning theory.

Emotional Disorders of Children: An Overview

The emotional disorders of children comprise a broad class of disturbances in adaptive functioning in which the experiences of the child are believed to have caused him to deviate significantly from his peers in the quality, quantity, and modes of expression of his emotions. The accompanying etiological premise is that the child's past experiences are the prime cause of his dysfunctions. Use of the term, emotional disorder, usually implies that the diagnostician is making a judgment about etiology, namely that he views various constitutional factors (brain integrity, maturational lag, somatic illness) as relatively unimportant in the development of the child's pattern of dysfunctions. The term emotional disorders is a nonspecific term. It does not specify that the total or even the primary symptomatology manifested will be in either the experience or expression of feelings. The symptoms may be expressed in deviant sensory or motor patterns, in learning problems, in somatic ailments, as well as in immature forms of interpersonal relationships. But the term does indicate that disturbances in emotional processes are common causal links in the varied symptoms shown and that these disturbances are learned primarily from experience rather than being determined by physiological structure.

Some practitioners prefer the terms psychological or psychiatric in specifying that a disorder is functional, that is, not primarily determined by constitutional factors. However we see merit in using the term emotional, the clinical descriptive term, even though its use most often indicates an etiological emphasis rather than a highly distinctive patterning of emotional expressions unique to this class of disorders. The value lies in emphasizing that *how* and *what* an individual feels about himself and other people are potent determinants of the course of his personality development of which his particular patterns of adaptive dysfunction are but one aspect. In view of the implied constructs about the nature of children's emotional disorders and their principal etiological source, it follows that in treatment efforts, the emphases are on changing the child's feelings (anxious, guilty, angry, erotic, dependent) about himself and about others within his social matrix and on ameliorating the quality of experience he derives from his primary socializers, his parents and siblings.

Children with primary constitutional determination of their adaptive dysfunctions, as in the prototypic MBD syndromes, may also show marked deviations in emotional processes. The most common assumption regarding the origin of these is broadly structural, that is deficient CNS anatomy and/or physiology. Emotional lability, impulsivity, and hyperaggressivity are frequently described emotional symptoms associated with the MBD syndromes which often accompany the perceptual, cognitive, and motor symptoms: perceptual-motor dysfunctions, distractibility, hyperactivity, and learning disabilities. Many MBD specialists describe the emotional disturbances they see in their patients as secondary to the social and psychological stresses of experiencing the hypothesized primary MBD symptomatology, while acknowledging *en passant* a probable compound of structural and functional determinants in their MBD patients. However few practitioners seem to conceive of the possibility of primary codetermination of their MBD patients' symptoms by structure and experience. Our reading of this literature leads us to conclude that many MBD specialists pay little attention to the possible experiential determinants of their patient's symptoms, whether primary or secondary, and minimize these in their treatment planning. We return to this issue in our final section.

Incidence and Prevalence of Children's Emotional Disorders

We are in the early stage of the development of knowledge of children's emotional disorders. This is a result of the relatively recent emergence of the basic disciplines concerned with research on children's adaptive functioning: dynamic psychiatry, pediatrics, child psychiatry, child development, and clinical child psychology. No broadly accepted typology of children's adaptive disorders yet exists, although there is considerable agreement about the existence of the major categories of mental retardation, organic brain damage, neurosis, and psychosis. Characteristic of a young discipline, new typologies appear frequently, reflecting the shifting models of disorder and structural-functional etiological emphases gaining ascendance. Four major revisions of the nosology of children's disorders have occurred in the last thirty years.

No matter by what names the infinite variety of children's emotional disorders are labeled, they comprise a significant component among the adaptive disorders experienced by our population of children. Engel (1972) reported Glidewell's (1968) summarization of a large number of incidence studies of maladjusted elementary-school children. The latter's estimate of the prevalence of maladjustment indicated that in 1960 2.7 million or 9% of these children needed professional help. The report of the Joint Commission on Mental Health of Children (1970) estimated that .6% were psychotic, 2 to 3% were severely disturbed, and another 8 to 10% were in need of specialized services (that is experiencing neuroses and kindred disorders). Of the 10 million young people under the age of 25 estimated to be in need of knowledgeable help, about 5% were actually receiving services in mental health facilities during the late 1960s.

Although limitations of space prevent our including material on the treatment of children's emotional disorders, we find it important to note the continuing national neglect of the critical treatment needs of emotionally disturbed children as pointed out by Rexford (1969) and many others.

Classification of Children's Emotional Disorders

The classification of children's emotional disorders has been a field marked by lively controversy since its inception. The controversies occur at several levels, including not only how and what to classify (surface behavior, referral complaints, personality processes, suspected etiological agents), but also challenges to the value of classifying at all (Hobbs, 1975a, 1975b). Prior to the late 1960s the approximately two dozen classification systems of childhood psychopathology then extant presented a welter of different terms and organizing principles— some directly modeled after the taxonomy of adult disorders, some little more than listings of referral complaints, some attempting to incorporate etiological concepts within their dimensions. Most of them were adultomorphic in essential structure, reflected little of the developmental plasticity characteristic of childhood, and none was widely adopted. The reader who wishes to pursue the history and dimensions of these classification controversies further will find valuable reading in Rie (1971), Kessler (1966, 1971), the Group for the Advancement of Psychiatry's Diagnostic Manual (1966), and Eron (1966).

The two classification systems used most frequently at present in American psychiatry are: (1) the Group for the Advancement of Psychiatry's (GAP) proposed classification which appeared in 1966 and (2) the second version of the American Psychiatric Association's, *Diagnostic and Statistical Manual of Mental Disorders* (DSM-II) published in 1968. Each portrays children's disorders more accurately and comprehensively than had been done previously and incorporates developmental principles.

Other recent developments in the classification of children's emotional disorders that are likely to influence future work in the area include: Anna Freud's (1965) "Developmental Profile" based on psychoanalytic formulations of the development of personality structures; a World Health Organization sponsored multiaxial approach to classification of childhood psychopathology (Rutter, 1976; Rutter, Shaffer, Sheppard, 1973). This provides data on five axes:

1. Clinical psychiatric syndrome.
2. Intellectual level.
3. Etiological biological factors.
4. Etiological psychosocial factors.
5. Developmental disorders.

A similar multiaxial approach has been incorporated in the current draft of the *Diagnostic and Statistical Manual* of the American Psychiatric Association (DSM –III, 1977) now undergoing field trials and scheduled for publication in 1979. This draft extensively revises and enlarges the coverage given to children's emotional disorders in DSM–II, particularly in the areas of conduct disorder and childhood psychosis.

Very few specialists in clinical work with children are satisfied with the diagnostic classification systems available. They point out that the classification systems fail to include enough relevant data about an individual's various personality components to be helpful in choosing appropriate treatment strategies and that they fail to offer comparable information about different patients on a common set of components. It seems likely that classification systems of the future will move increasingly to meet these objections, as progress in the differentiation of personality constructs and their reliable measurement allows. The multiaxial refinements just mentioned are a step in this direction. Others are being developed. Cummings (1964) has outlined a classification of 6 ego-function systems as an approach to understanding the differential impact of parental influences on different components of a child's adaptive behavior. Bellak, Hurvich, and Gediman (1973) describe their schizophrenic, neurotic, and normal subjects by rating them on 12 ego functions, which ratings are then related to prognosis. Below we illustrate the application of 2 ego-function concepts to the understanding and classification of the 3 major classes of children's emotional disorders: neuroses, conduct disorders, and psychoses.

Patterns of Variation in Two Ego Functions in Emotional Disorders

At the risk of leading some readers over highly familiar terrain and oversimplifying some complex ego constructs, we trace some relationships between patterns of ego functioning and forms of emotional disorder. Ego functioning refers to all those behavior systems through which individual adaptiveness is accomplished, that is through which integrations of cognitive and affective experience are transformed into effective actions. While adaptive behavior sequences constitute complex wholes, ego functions are components of these wholes and may be differentiated according to the salient experiential elements and/or psychological processes revealed in these components through observations of the individual's attempts to satisfy different motives under varying environmental conditions. The more commonly described ego functions include: reality testing, impulse modulation, object relating, environmental mastery, and identity synthesis.

We find it useful to conceive of neuroses, conduct disorders, and psychoses as reflecting different levels of development in two principal ego functions: reality testing and impulse modulation. Reality testing comprises that group of psychological operations—perceptual, memory, associative, conceptual—by which self is distinguished from non-self and through which objects acquire accuracy and constancy of meaning. From infancy to adulthood in normal human development, a sequence of stages in the development of the effectiveness of this ego function can be traced which bears directly on the adaptiveness of the individual's behavior and the constancy of his identity organization. The distinguishing ego weakness of psychotic patients is their deficiency in reality testing; this underlies their confused and often fragmented identity organization. Neurotic patients do not typically experience difficulty in this adaptive function, nor generally do patients with conduct disorders experience difficulty in emotionally neutral situations. However under intense emotional arousal, the latter may show brief losses of reality testing followed by quick recovery. On an effectiveness of reality testing continuum, they would stand between neurotics and psychotics.

Impulse modulation concerns the goals of socialization: the development of various controls used to delay impulses and to bind the tension associated with various arousal states, be these from primary drives or from derived drives and affects. The typical developmental progression from infancy to middle childhood reflecting progressive ego development in this function is: from impulsive immediacy of motor expression of arousal states, through a period of gradually acquiring conscious controls accompanied by experiences of conflict with the socializing agent who makes the demands for delay and control, and ultimately to the learning of a set of durable internalized controls, largely unconscious, by which the healthy normal regulates his own behavior. Patients with conduct disorders and neuroses show different deviations from the course of normal development. Those with conduct disorders fail to develop reliable internal controls manifesting combinations of impulsivity and externalization of their conflicts with socializers. We characterize them as displaying externalization disorders. Neurotics on the other hand share the characteristic of having overlearned inhibitory control. They construct intricate networks of inner control structures—defenses bulwarked by neurotic symptoms—monuments to delay, so that their dangerous impulses are not translated into action. They internalize too much, allowing themselves few appropriate action releases of impulse and emotional arousal experiences characteristic of their more normal peers. As a group, we characterize the neuroses internalization disorders. Psychotics as a group are highly variable in the quality and directions of their impulse modulation mechanisms, both interindividually and intraindividually. Overall their impairments in reality testing predispose them towards qualitatively poorer impulse modulation behaviors which are characteristically inappropriate, primitive, and grossly externalizing.

GENESIS OF CHILDREN'S EMOTIONAL DISORDERS: CONSTRUCTS, DETERMINANTS, MODELS, CAVEATS

The emotional disorders of children are primarily a product of their experiences. Constitutional characteristics are considered to play a minor role in the development of neuroses and conduct disorders, but in some childhood psychoses they are accorded a definite role. The major classes of experiential determinants are: (1) environmental influences—the responses to the child of his parents and of other persons valued by him, which modify his experiences of pleasure and pain and define his meaning and value; (2) psychological influences—the child's gradually developing organization of self-representations and self-evaluations; and (3) "traumas"—unique, nonrecurrent, usually sudden threats to the child's security and/or prepotent motive satisfactions, for example floods, wars, death of a loved one. To place the contributions of these to the development of children's emotional disorders in perspective, we briefly review some of the developmental stage concepts, specific experiential determinants, and etiological models which figure prominently in contemporary thinking in this area.

Developmental Stage Concepts

Freud's (1905) theory of psychosexual development was a major step forward in personality theory construction when it appeared. In portraying a sequence of fateful encounters between the need-dominated young child and his socializers, the outcomes of which have determining significance for the personality organization of that child thenceforward, the theory specifies a developmental series of interactions between the child and his parents from which variations in adaptive and defensive behavior patterns can be predicted. Its imprint is clearly visible on most subsequent theories of personality development in such concepts as: the critical period hypothesis which portrays nodal points of development when the timely availability of particular forms of environmental input are crucial to continued development; the concepts of fixation (failure to progress to more advanced motive pursuits and modes of adaptation) and regression (return to less mature motive pursuits and adaptive modes), as definitive characteristics of maladaptive states. Erikson's (1950) theory of ego epigenesis refines some of Freud's developmental stage notions, calling attention to the determining significance of different qualities of parental care needed by the child at different developmental stages. It also specifies the successive stages of object relations and identity organization characterizing progressive developments in personality integration. In latter day applications of these concepts to the classification of children's emotional disorders we find such constructs as: age-or phase-appropriate developmental conflicts; the concept of developmental deviations; and the continuum of stages of ego development from psychosis through conduct disorder and neurosis to relative normality.

Relevant Environmental Determinants

Highly familiar to most readers, the principal classes of environmental determinants will be only briefly outlined. Of overriding importance are the parents' contributions in their roles as need-gratifiers, impulse-modifiers, and models for ego-skill acquisition via the child's identifications with the parents. Thus parental caretaking qualities, behaviors demonstrating their accessibility, sensitivity, responsiveness, consistency, and allocentricity are focal determinants. Related, but distinguished from the preceding, are the prominent parental personality features. These serve more powerfully than any words the parents use as models for their offspring to imitate in developing their defensive styles, object relationship patterns, conscience organization, and adaptive skills. Another set of determinants is found in the relationship qualities of the parents' marital relationship. Here what the parents demonstrate in their quality of caring, reciprocity, stability and as models for interpersonal problem solving, critically affects the child's sense of security about his needs being satisfied. These demonstrations also provide both a definition of the clarity of the boundaries between the child and the older generation and a relationship paradigm for his caring relationships with others. Beyond the parental pair's contributions, the structure of the sibship and of other household members' roles in the family can play important parts in the child's experience of continuity of care; the opportunities for learning various role relationships; and the opportunities afforded him for pairing with more competent seniors in learning ego skills. Friendships with peers, teachers, and adult neighbors are also of importance, particularly when they compensate for lacks in opportunities for relationship-learning and identity-confirming imposed by loss of a parent.

Models for Conceptualizing Effects

Follow-up studies of the personality outcomes in adult life of young children who either had constitutional deficiencies or experienced aversive environmental inputs have largely been inconclusive, except when either set of these etiological agents have been extremes on their respective continua, for example severe brain damage or a childhood characterized by continuous disruption of social ties. While the short-term effects of pathogens are readily demonstrated between adjacent developmental phases, few suspected pathogenic agents show clearcut, long-term effects from early childhood to adulthood. Better conceptual models are needed than that which portrays the continuous flow of influence of a single etiological agent to an individual through major stages of personality development. Models are needed to account for feedback from object to human etiological agent (that is bidirectionality of influences) and to account for ameliorating influences which produce self-righting, positive, long-term outcomes.

Sameroff (1977) and his collaborators (Sameroff and Chandler, 1975; Sameroff and Zax, 1973) have helpfully illuminated the limitations of the main-effects model just described for conceptualizing the majority of pathogenic influences on personality development, that is single agent or influence in unidirectional flow. They recommend replacing the main-effects model with interactional and transactional models. An interactional model portrays outcomes of influence transfer processes, as between parent and child, as a product of the two or more sets of influences interacting simultaneously, for example Thomas, Chess, and Birch's (1968) longitudinal study of outcomes of congruence-incongruence between actual infant primary reactivity patterns and parental preferences for certain infant reactivity pattern types. The transactional model portrays a dynamic reciprocity, through time, of the multiple influences flowing between parent and child which continuously induce reorganizations in each. It appears to be the most realistic model for conceptualizing etiological course in the majority of constitution-environment and parent-child fields of events encountered in childhood personality development. Its application as a research methodology is however extremely complex and demanding. Most of the etiological studies mentioned below are based on the simpler short-term, main-effects model.

Developmental Caveats

A redundant theme of child mental health specialists is the importance of recognizing the underlying differences in behavior patterns in children which may superficially resemble adult patterns or about which similar descriptive terms are used. Only firsthand knowledge of the actual differences in cognitive and language characteristics, styles of emotional expression, modes of interpersonal relations in children at successive developmental stages allows an appreciation of the differences, for example between an unresolved oedipal complex in a five-year-old and twenty-five-year-old, between the bereavement processes of a three-year-old and a thirteen-year-old.

Plasticity of development is the prime characteristic which distinguishes childhood from adulthood. Plasticity implies the contingent characteristics: relative modifiability of structure, capacity for rapid change, sensitivity to influence.

Our language forms inadequately reflect the magnitude of the differences between adult and child personality organization of which the emotional disorder patterns described below are one segment.Oversimplifications are likely to occur especially in abbreviated descriptive accounts such as those which follow. These oversimplifications can obscure the important developmental differences between disorder patterns bearing the same name in adults and children.

PSYCHONEUROSES IN CHILDREN (INTERNALIZATION DISORDERS)

The psychoneurotic disorders comprise the most numerous and varied of any class of emotional disorders of children, while constituting overall the least severe group of disorders of the three broad classes presented here. These are the children who are most heavily represented in the caseloads of the "front line" echelon of children's mental health services, the family physician, pediatric clinic, school special services offices, and community mental health centers. The patterning of their neurotic manifestations and the severity of their disorders are quite varied—from monosymptomatic expressions of sleeping difficulty, sibling antagonism, or speech difficulties which affect only limited portions of their lives to more extensive involvements of most of their social relations in the more severe syndromes resembling the adult neuroses. Although highly diverse in external behavior patterning, these disorders show a number of common structural and psychodynamic features.

The most prevalent emotional characteristic shared by these children is some form of experienced anxiety. Feelings of anxiety may be associated with concrete environmental objects in the child's having specific fears (of dogs, the dark, school) or may be experienced as a sense of nameless dread or as a sense of guilt and badness. The common psychological process characterizing their varied modes of modulating their conflicts and anxiety is *internalization.* Their conflicts are expressed primarily as internal conflicts, usually unconscious, between their sexual and aggressive drives and either their parents' prohibitions of these drives or their own internalized version of these parental prohibitions, that is their consciences. They learn how to quiet the discomfort associated with their conflicts and attendant anxiety by developing new personality structures: defense mechanisms which have a repressive function and symptoms which often symbolize the nature of the underlying conflict elements. Typically some of their symptoms will also be behavioral expressions of anxiety which is not bound (successfully repressed) by either the defenses or the symptoms, for example restlessness, increased startle reactions, difficulties with concentration. Depending on their age and intelligence, these children hurt and are likely to be aware that they hurt, while having little understanding of how, where, or why. Their psychic pain is a positive force towards accepting therapeutic help, as is their characteristically high level of ego functioning.

We understand in only a limited way the patterns of etiological development of various neurotic disorders. While their determinants are believed to be derived primarily from experience, the possibility remains open that some constitutional factors are implicated, such as temperament (Thomas, Chess, and Birch, 1968), intellectual endowment, and individual somatic system vulnerabilities.

Among the neuroses of children, one finds great variation in the type, timing, and combinations of relevant experiential factors, such as losses or illnesses of family members, injuries and illnesses of the child himself, marital conflict between the parents, emotional disturbance in the parents, but also found is a common factor of oversocialization of these children by their parents. Oversocialization means a zealous, fear-inducing style of teaching the child the likely ill consequences of expressing his basic drives, sex and aggression, so that the child begins to experience loss of love at the mere thought of or wish to perform a proscribed activity. Other potent parental determinants of child neurosis include the child's identification with a parent's neurotic personality features as a natural concomitant of his social-learning process as well as two factors which sharpen the triangular competitiveness with the same-sexed parent: (1) open marital conflict between the parents and (2) indulgent parenting by the parent of the opposite sex. Usually the parents of neurotic children provide generally adequate care of the child's primary, drive-derived needs and make a positive emotional investment in the child. In some parents of neurotic children however an ambivalent emotional investment becomes evident when the parent subtly distorts the child's unique identity through unconscious partial identifications of the child in fantasy with a conflict-endowed figure from the parent's past relationships, for example a rival sibling, an angry grandparent.

Our classification of neurotic children groups them in three major subcategories: neurotic trait reactions, neurotic syndromes, neurotic personality patterns. The children within each of these groups will vary considerably in symptom patterning. Each group overlaps slightly with each of the others.

Neurotic Trait Reactions

This extremely diverse category comprises the mildest and usually the earliest forms of neurotic manifestation seen by clinicians serving children. In distinguishing these from normal developmental crisis reactions or from reactive disorders which they resemble, the clinician judges that the level of symptomatic expression exceeds that appropriate to the child's present stress level. Here are found a legion of single symptom disorders: isolated fears of animals, the dark, or certain social situations; nervous habits like nail-biting and nose-picking; mild eating disorders; nocturnal enuresis without additional symptoms; sleep disturbances; speech disturbances like elective mutism and stuttering.

When thorough histories are taken, the origins of many of these mild disorders emerge as interactions between a normal developmental crisis occurring in a child whose anxiety level has been increased by one or more realistic stresses. Often one of these stresses is a temporary lowering in the adequacy of parental care associated with a higher stress level in the parent. With parental guidance and amelioration of the family's overall stress level, these mild disorders usually abate without requiring direct treatment of the child. Although the symptoms found in these maladaptations represent some internal structuring of anxiety and conflict and thus enhance the possibility of the child's repeating them under subsequent stress situations, with early attention the prognosis for most of these disorders is very good. A small percentage will comprise the earliest expressions of more severe disorders, which are virtually indistinguishable from the more benign variety until early treatment efforts have proven unsuccessful.

Neurotic Syndromes

These disorders constitute the approximations during preadolescence and early adolescence of the psychoneuroses commonly found in adults. The developmental plasticity characteristic of childhood, that is the child's great responsiveness to maturational and experiential forces, means that these syndromes in children do not entail the degree of rigidity of symptom pattern found in adult neuroses. While many clinicians support the Freudian dictum that the seeds of the adult neurosis are sown in the infantile neurosis, that is during childhood, few find in their caseloads of neurotic children exact replicas in miniature of one of the classical neuroses of adults.

The neurotic syndromes are a group of maladaptive patterns demonstrating: internalization of unconscious conflict over sexual and aggressive drive pressures, experienced anxiety, and anxiety-reduction serving as a potent defense and symptom reinforcer. The typical sequence of maladaptive emotional development contains these elements: a partial awareness of an impulse which is unacceptable to the ego or to the conscience; repression of the emotional and cognitive representations of this unacceptable drive expression; the development of anxiety as a signal of impending dangerous drive expression; gradual structuring of defenses to contain the anxiety linked with the unconscious drive representations; ultimately, the addition of structured symptoms (phobias, compulsions) to the defensive work. Structured symptoms not only perform defensive functions but also typically offer the child some adaptive advantages: partial satisfaction of a repressed desire (wish) in fantasy; reassurance of parental love through gaining parental attention in occupying the role of the sick person; and often discharge of tension through motor expressions of the symptomatology. The cycle is maintained by the repeated interaction of biological drive forces with dangerous situations in the environment which recreate the possibility of acting out the prohibited drives with ensuing experience of anxiety.

The most frequently presented neurotic syndromes of children are phobic neuroses, hysterical neuroses, obsessive-compulsive neuroses, and depressive neuroses.

Phobic Neurosis

Children with phobic neuroses have persistent unrealistic fears which arise as displacements of their ego-alien feelings toward their parents. Fears of the dark, of animals, of vehicles, and of school are some of the most common. Typically these patterns begin with a pattern of motoric and affective expressions of free anxiety of a more general kind and settle into a focus on a narrow range of environmental objects, with resulting reduction in the amount of the child's moment-to-moment discomfort, but with extreme degrees of fearfulness in proximity to the phobic object(s). Commonly what begins as a phobia limited to one or more concrete objects or events develops into a more extended range of feared objects, conceptually linked by class characteristics or by memory associations to the objects perceived as part of the typical context of an original phobic object or event. Freud's treatment of his five-year-old phobic patient, Little Hans (Freud, 1909), not only illuminated the mechanism of displacement in the development of phobias, but also offered support for the relevance of infantile sexuality in personality development.

School phobias are some of the most common examples of these syndromes in school-age children and have received more research attention than any other phobic syndrome (Waldfogel, Coolidge, and Hahn, 1975; Eisenberg, 1958; Coolidge, et al., 1960). While varying greatly in age of onset, intensity of anxiety, and severity of associated symptoms (restrictions on contact with other common environmental situations and persons; gastrointestinal disturbance), these syndromes have strikingly similar dynamics. Separation anxiety developing from a reciprocal hostile-dependent relationship between parent and child have been determined as important dynamic factors in many cases (Johnson, et al., 1941; Estes, Haylett, and Johnson, 1956).

The importance of unresolved dependency-independence conflicts is highlighted in the development of school phobias, but is not confined to this group. In our experience the developmental histories of many neurotic children present evidence that the pathogenic foundations begin during the infantile period when oral nurturance issues are being negotiated by mother and child. This view contrasts with earlier psychodynamic thinking, which emphasized the child's focal traumatization at only one psychosexual stage, the phallic, and implied generally satisfactory resolutions of conflicts inherent in earlier phases. More recent thinking about the development of severe neuroses points toward a series of partial failures of developmental conflict-resolution beginning in infancy.

Hysterical Neurosis

In this group of neurotic syndromes, conflicts over expression of ego-alien drives and their associated affects and imagery are managed, first by attempts at repression, which proving inadequate, are supplemented by the formation of hysterical symptoms. Hysterical symptoms, as described by Kessler (1966), typically take one of several forms: (1) sudden emotional outbursts; (2) disturbances in sensation and movement; (3) alterations in consciousness, as in somnambulism, fainting, or multiple personality; and (4) temporary losses of the sense of reality, as in hallucinations which are experienced with some insight into their unrealistic nature. Typically where the hysterical symptoms occur regularly (are integrated into the defense organization), the hysteric experiences much of his life with equanimity and even good cheer, implying effectiveness in his defensive efforts when bolstered by his choice of hysterical symptoms.

The most frequent of these symptom patterns is conversion hysteria. Here anesthesias and paresthesias of skin surfaces, lack or distortion of visual or auditory functioning, functional weaknesses or paralyses of limbs, and tics constitute some of the more common sensory and motor dysfunctions. The conversion mechanism entails a conversion of psychic conflict (drive urges, prohibitions against these) into a bodily ailment. Typically the particular conversion symptom chosen permits some partial drive release simultaneously with the defensive binding achieved. Quite often the nature of the bodily ailment provides an indication of the precipitating stressful event which supplied the impetus to symptom adoption. Secondary gain through increased parental attention to the child occupying a sickness role is a further reinforcing condition for many such children.

These syndromes appeared with much greater frequency in both adults and children during the first half of this century than they have over the past 25 years. Some recently trained child mental health specialists have completed their training without encountering a true conversion syndrome. The continued existence of these syndromes is confirmed by periodic reports from investigators whose patients often originate from rural and/or lower socioeconomic environments (Proctor, 1958; Rock, 1971). Proctor's account of the family life experiences of the hysterical children whom he studied emphasizes the marked discontinuity between their sexual-impulse stimulating family living circumstances (parents sleeping with children, observation of parental intercourse) and the severe fundamentalist religious prohibitions against thinking or talking about sex which characterized their lives.

Obsessive-Compulsive Neurosis

In this syndrome class, the other major symptom neurosis of adulthood, only a very small portion of neurotic children (Anthony, 1975) are found to replicate the essential elements of the adult neurosis, while many neurotic children show a symptom or two of this variety, for example a child's frequent repeated checking on the security of his possessions, or their exact arrangement in a container, or repetitious worries and inquiries about the health of a family member.

The hallmark of these syndromes is senseless repetition—repetition of thoughts or acts which have no adaptive function. The repeater typically has some awareness of the senselessness of his repetitions, while lacking the ability to suppress them without experiencing intense anxiety. "Did I put my bike away?", "Where did I leave my homework?", "Will someone trip over the jeans I just dropped on the floor?", are examples of intrusive thoughts of the obsessional child. Repetitious hand-washing and knocking on wood to guarantee good luck are familiar compulsions found in the normal population of adults and children as well as in neurotics. The differences between the obsessive-compulsive neurotic and his normal counterpart are primarily in degree: the number of such repetitious thoughts and habits developed by any given individual, that is the amount of his total life space on which they intrude and the amount of anxiety ensuing from interruption or suppressive control of the symptoms.

The psychoanalytic interpreters of the development of obsessive-compulsive neurosis emphasize fixation on and regression to anal drive phenomena, which become a focus on interaction between the child and his caretakers during the second and third years of life. At this period a large number of new controls are rapidly being acquired by the toddler: excretory sphincter controls, controls over large muscle activity in order to achieve coordinated motility, and verbal controls of the environment during this period of rapid vocabulary expansion. Management of aggressive drives is a concurrent preoccupation during this period and many of the control mechanisms learned at this time acquire a defensive function, relative to the modulation of aggression, predisposing the youngster to obsessive-compulsive styles of functioning and defense usage during subsequent stimulation of aggression (Sandler and Joffe, 1965). Ultimately settling into a defense pattern accentuating the defenses of isolation (of affect from thought), regression, intellectualization, reationalization, undoing, and reaction-formation is usual. Brief episodes of magical thinking and omnipotence of thought, often of a subtle sophisticated variety, are common cognitive regressions in these defenses.

The older literature regarding the early family experiences of children predisposed towards obsessive-compulsive symptom development as adults showed a simplistic emphasis on the traumas of severe and premature toilet training. Latter-day interpreters (Salzman, 1968; Adams, 1973) point to a broad tapestry of interactive determinants between parent and child, many of which achieve the final common function of teaching the child in an authoritarian manner the dangerousness of his aggressive drives. Ambivalence in object relations characterizes these children and frequently their general demeanor is of the conscience-stricken, worry-wart variety. Some more severe reality-testing disorders may first present resembling obsessive-compulsive patterns. The quality of the child's reality testing and object relationships and the intensity of his ambivalence provide the principal diagnostic dimensions for differentiating between the true neurotic patterns and the incipient or borderline psychosis masked by obsessive-compulsive symptoms.

Depressive Neurosis

Recognition that children experience forms of neurotic depression has arrived relatively recently in the annals of childhood psychopathology. Rie's (1966) survey of the literature on childhood depressions of only a dozen years ago found some writers in the recent past unable to accept that depressive conditions in children actually existed. Malmquist's (1972) subsequent review of the more recent literature leaves no doubt about the existence of depressive phenomena in children.

Nowhere else in childhood psychopathology is a developmental point of view more relevantly applied than in understanding the variety of manifestations of depression in children. The manifestations of depression in children are appreciably more varied and variable, compared to the characteristics of adult depression, which are: sad mood; self-depreciation; expressions of guilt, helplessness, and hopelessness; and psychomotor retardation. The differences in depression between adult and child derive from the developmental characteristics of childhood personality organization, which in comparison with adult personality structure show: greater instability in defense organization; less object constancy and greater ease in substituting objects; a more narrow temporal frame of reference, emphasizing the present; and less tolerance for sustaining painful affect. All of these childhood state characteristics combine to influence the manner of expression of childhood depressive reactions towards masked (Glaser, 1967) depression or forms of depressive equivalents (Sperling, 1959), such as sleeping and eating disturbances, somatic symptoms and preoccupations, or hyperactivity (Toolan, 1962) and aggressiveness (Burks and Harrison, 1962). Some children with conduct disorders (reviewed below) reveal underlying depressive symptoms. The overlap between childhood neurosis and conduct disorders appears to be substantial in the more action-oriented children of the depressive neurotic subtype.

The understanding and classification of depressive reactions in children are at an early stage. The psychological determinants of depression most often noted in adults have been: (1) longing for a lost love object; and/or (2) internalized aggression, resulting from external or internal constraints upon the direct outward expression of aggression; and/or (3) the occurrence of narcissistic injury (failure to actualize an ego-ideal) in a personality organization characterized by great vulnerability to esteem loss as the result of continual dependency on other persons for esteem replacement. Object loss experiences are nearly ubiquitous in the histories of psychotic children and of many conduct disorders. While they are present in the histories of some depressive neurotic children, more frequent are the other two categories of loss, especially the intropunitiveness stemming from anger experienced originally at a parent figure and subsequently deflected back towards the self. A study of 14 overtly depressed children and their parents by Poznanski and Zrull (1970) found a high incidence of parental depression and rejection of the children, plus difficulties in handling aggression and hostility in both the children and their parents.

Neurotic Personality Patterns

As the developing child gradually differentiates the various structures of his personality organization (that is his characteristic modes: of attending, perceiving, and thinking; of responding to impulses and feelings; of communicating his representations of himself and other people to himself and to others) and as these systems become more stable and predictable, we come to identify his personality as unique and as distinguishably different from those of his peers. It is commonly held that the adolescent years provide the key set of biological and psychosocial determinants of the essential structures of the child's developing personality, that quasi-stable organization of mechanisms for integrating experience into effective actions with which he will enter early adulthood. However some children begin to stabilize sooner, to show reduced variation in their range of responsiveness prior to adolescence. Within the neurotic range these are the children who are diagnosed as neurotic personality patterns. They differ from neurotic syndromes in showing few acute symptoms of disturbance, but portray their deviance through their styles of relating to others, rigidly imposing a uniform affective definition on the markedly different people and situations which they encounter. Within this neurotic personality pattern subgroup are included: anxious, inhibited, hysterical, compulsive, passive-dependent, and passive-aggressive types.

As we review these patterns, several caveats are in order: (1) again, the developmental one: the stability of personality organization implied in these patterns is less than that found in adolescent and adult patterns; (2) variety in patterning: frequently mixtures of several of these patterns are found in any given child and the labeler conventionally chooses the most prominent pattern as a diagnostic term; and (3) some of these children will reveal externalizing defenses in their interpersonal relationships, making them resemble conduct disorders at times, but their internalization of conflict, self-repudiation, and functioning conscience confirm them as essentially neurotic. (In several other nosologies, the reader will find these patterns classed with personality disorders, a classification practice with which we disagree because of the higher levels of ego functioning shown by these essentially neurotic children.)

Anxious Personality

These children experience anxious discomfort as a continual backdrop to their daily lives. Their anxiety is accentuated in meeting new situations, but seldom peaks to a level which requires them to abandon opportunities for exploring new, unfamiliar social experiences. Their restlessness and hesitance, their requiring longer periods to settle into a new routine, and their greater demands for reassurance from adults imply that their inner worlds routinely contain more dangers than do those of their more normal peers.

Inhibited Personality

These unusually shy children lack spontaneity and are constricted in their responsiveness to many environmental experiences, both in the narrow range of familiar experiences which they tolerate and in their overt behavior, speech, and expressions of feelings. Fearful of doing the wrong thing (sexual and/or aggressive urges) they easily sink into the woodwork and may be quietly, anxiously nonproductive while seated at their desks in school classrooms not daring to bother anyone. They reveal their capacity and eagerness to relate in spite of their avoidant behavior by responding positively to nonintrusive demonstrations of interest from adults.

Hysterical Personality

At the other end of the emotional expressiveness continuum from the two patterns described above are these flighty, attention-getting, emotionally labile, often coy, seductive, and provocative children. Girls outnumber boys in this group by a wide margin. Beneath facades of seeming precocious heterosexual interest, these children are often found to be quite dependent in their strivings towards others. Typically their interests are narrowly focused on people interactions, especially of the romantic variety, reducing their investment in intellectual activities or in potentiation of any latent skill areas which cannot shortly be used to attract others.

Compulsive Personality

These children present in caricature an early twentieth century model of well-behaved children. Conforming, conscientious, practicing careful habits of cleanliness and conduct, they may appear unusually mature to older adult observers. Their deviance gradually becomes apparent when it is observed over time that they are made unduly uncomfortable when there is interference with their rigid patterns for conducting their daily lives, that they deprive themselves of much spontaneous enjoyment in play with normal peers, and that their rigidities and seeming maturity hinder their ease at establishing peer friendships.

Passive-Dependent and Passive-Aggressive Patterns

Admixtures of age-inappropriate dependency claims by children along with various oppositional patterns, primarily passive in nature, are found in these patterns and labeled according to the predominant pattern displayed. The dawdlers and the clingers seldom confront their parents directly with accusations that they have not been given enough nurturance to want to stand on their own feet or to do what they are asked within a reasonable period of time, but the redundant message in their frustrating interpersonal styles often seems to be clearly that. Thus these children reveal more directly conflicts over oral nurturance and early issues of autonomy than do the other neurotic personality patterns.

Symptomatology Common to Neuroses and MBD

The reader of other chapters in this handbook has become aware that we are in a relatively early stage in the development of criteria for distinguishing between the MBD syndromes and other maladaptive syndromes in children. Both the MBD syndromes and emotional disorders of children are characterized by extensive heterogeneity of their symptomatology, as presently described. Substantial overlap appears to occur in several symptom areas between the two major classes of disorders. This overlap appears to be a function of multiple etiological determination of the symptoms in some instances, but is also an indication of our relative ignorance about differential diagnostic cues. At this early stage vulnerability to parochial myopia is great, as MBD specialists, specialists in the emotional disorders of children, and special educators all attempt to serve the maladjusted children referred to them as best they can, yet they are largely uninformed as to the special knowledge of their professional counterparts. No research has yet appeared that clearly distinguishes the neurogenic from the psychogenic components of the overlapping symptoms. Clinicians continue to rely on their second-best inference base, their clinical impressions.

Children's neuroses present a moderate amount of overlap with the following behavioral symptoms associated with the MBD syndromes: hyperactivity, distractibility, impulsivity, and emotional lability. The high levels of anxiety experienced by many neurotic children often result in their being restless, distractible, and having difficulties in concentration. These symptoms, usually in combination with other emotional interferences with learning, frequently lead to poor school performance, the most common referral complaint for all varieties of emotionally disturbed children. Some neurotic children perform adequately in school; seldom do neurotic children with learning problems have as severe learning problems as do those children with conduct disorders and psychoses. A distinguishing feature of the restlessness-distractibility symptoms of the predominantly neurotic child, compared to his predominantly MBD counterpart, is the greater variability of these symptoms in the neurotic child. This variability is associated with his varying levels of anxiety which, in turn, is related to the stimulation of his internal conflicts by external stress.

Impulsivity and emotional lability are also symptoms of some neurotic children, largely those of the hysterical variety. These children's strongly repressive defenses protect them from awareness of their unpleasant emotions and conflict sources, albeit with some sacrifice of the learned process of thinking things through as an adaptive mode, inclining them towards episodes of acting-out. Learning problems with academic subjects are especially likely to occur in these children, whose basic cognitive style deemphasizes verbal conceptual thinking and learning. In our experience their impulsivity and lability are not easily distinguished from those same traits in the typical MBD child. However seldom do these hysterical children reveal as negatively toned self-concepts, particularly in their views of themselves as school learners. Hyperaggressiveness, a common behavioral symptom in MBD children, is rarely a recurrent symptom in essentially neurotic children.

These observations then suggest that some symptomatology is shared by some neurotic children and some children with MBD syndromes. Overall the amount of overlapping symptomatology appears to be less in neurotic children than in either the children with conduct disorders or those with psychoses. In children suspected of MBD on the basis of having some of the overlapping symptomatology described above as well as a learning problem, yet without neurological signs or perceptual-motor symptoms a conservative diagnostic approach would appear to call for considering a primary psychogenic determination of their symptoms.

CONDUCT DISORDERS IN CHILDREN (EXTERNALIZATION DISORDERS)

Childhood psychopathology is a young discipline. In the area of conduct disorders this is revealed clearly in the terminological diversity that has characterized classification efforts. Three different versions of the DSM (1952, 1968, 1977) have each produced a different set of disorder labels in this area. The GAP (1966) classification scheme has yielded yet another group. Most of these terms are still in use in some parts of our mental health enterprise, making statistical comparisons of types of disorder between different data sources ambiguous and unreliable. Character disorder, psychopathic personality, antisocial disorder, sociopath, neurotic character, primary behavior disorder, unsocialized aggressive reaction, impulse-ridden personality—are a small proportion of the terms in recent usage. Juvenile delinquent is a legal and sociological term applied to most of these children, once their infractions of laws and mores come to the attention of the police and courts. Our preference for the term conduct disorder, an old term which was virtually abandoned for many years in the literature, is based on its accuracy and simplicity. We note that the current draft of DSM–III (1977) has also adopted it.

The principal symptomatology found in these disorders includes patterns of lying, stealing, vandalism, aggressive attacks on others, truancy, running away from home, and sexual promiscuity.

Thus the complaints of others about the offensiveness of their acts usually determines these patients being referred to professional attention. Their acting-out causes others to hurt rather than their seeming to experience psychic pain, but this may be more apparent than real. They are almost never self-referred. Males run the gamut of the symptoms indicated. Females show a concentration of less physically aggressive symptoms with lying, stealing, running away, and sexual promiscuity being more frequent.

As the array of symptoms indicated above would suggest, children with conduct disorders are characterized by repetitive misconduct, that is they lack age-appropriate controls over impulses to act out in antisocial ways. Common to the life histories of nearly all patients so described is a pattern of failure in parental socialization efforts, which ends in these children being undersocialized, that is in not controlling those behaviors which a given society believes should be controlled. Common to these patients' modes of defense is an emphasis on *externalization* of the anxiety and conflicts they experience. Externalization is characteristic not only of their defense organizations, but of their perceptual and cognitive styles and action systems as well. No matter what the actuality of circumstances, blame is typically directed outwardly to other persons and objects, producing the effect of making others look bad or feel badly. Often the aggression and blaming are acted out physically by harming someone else or his property.

We describe two major categories and one additional miscellaneous grouping of conduct disorders: conduct disorder, aggressive type; conduct disorder, unaggressive type; and other conduct disorders. The first two are similar to the terms used in the current draft of DSM–III.

Conduct Disorder, Aggressive Type

Children with this disorder pattern, while varying in the forms of their misconduct, show common related characteristics of aggressive destructiveness towards others, impulsivity, and a pronounced lack of conscience. Uniformly they fail to develop close attachments to others, peers or adults.

The DSM–III draft (1977) offers this portrayal of them:

> . . . The lack of concern for the feelings, wishes and well-being of others, is manifested toward peers by bullying, physical aggression and cruel behavior. Towards adults, the individual may be hostile, verbally abusive, impudent, defiant and negativistic. Antisocial behavior takes many forms, including destructiveness, stealing which may be accompanied by physical violence, persistent lying, frequent truancy and vandalism. Peer relationships, characteristically with other youngsters with conduct disorders, lack in closeness and stability. [P.M: 44]

The school adjustments of these children are understandably poor and they typically are retarded one or more grades before completing elementary school. A minor, but significant fraction, are sufficiently restless, distractible, and impulsive to merit the secondary diagnosis, hyperactivity syndrome. Boys outnumber girls many fold in this disorder, with estimates of as much as 12 to 1 for the more severe forms.

Many early studies of children with this form of disorder focused on the determinants of pronounced but limited features of the pattern, that is the aggressivity and resistance to learning behavior controls associated with a relative lack of conscience. However there has gradually developed a view of these children as experiencing deficiencies in a broad variety of ego functions, the origins of which antedate the development of conscience. Aichhorn's (1935) classic early study of some of these children foreshadowed this view in his descriptions of his patient's multiple deficiencies in relinquishing the pleasure principle for the reality principle and in the development of identification. Redl and Wineman (1957) have more fully developed it in describing the aggressive delinquents with whom they worked, enumerating 22 ego-control devices which are lacking in this group, including their developmental delays in time sense, intentionality, and inferential thought.

The concept of this disorder, particularly in its more severe forms, as a broad-gauge, ego-deficiency disorder is partially supported by its poor prognosis. Robins' (1966) 30-year follow-up study of adults who were referred to a child guidance clinic as children indicates considerable continuity between childhood sociopathy and adult sociopathy: 95% of the sociopathic adults had been referred to the clinic as children showing moderate to severe antisocial behavior. A compelling argument for viewing some of these children as other than affectless, as they have sometimes been described, is made by Burks and Harrison (1962), whose study indicated that the timing of aggressive outbursts in their patients was closely related to the surfacing of intense depressive feelings, suggesting that the aggressive displays served as avoidance maneuvers for dealing with painful feelings of loss and hopelessness.

Conduct Disorder, Unaggressive Type

This broad category of disorders refers to children who act-out in highly diverse ways, for example stealing, lying, running away, vandalism. They may also be referred for fighting, temper outbursts, or cruelty, indicating that many readily display hostility. However, in these children, physical aggressiveness toward people does not predominate in their acting-out pattern, as it does in the children discussed above.

This group also contains greater diversity in levels of ego organization and in admixtures of neurotic and psychotic features. Some of these children will eventuate as neurotic personality pattern disorders, some as forms of borderline personality organization (Kernberg, 1975), some milder cases of more recent origin will disappear into the fold of relative normality, but the majority are likely to continue to show some form of antisocial conduct as adolescents and adults. In factor analysis and cluster analysis studies of juvenile delinquent populations (Quay, 1965; Jenkins and Glickman, 1947), these patients tend to be grouped with the disturbed-neurotic or emotionally disturbed groups.

The DSM–III draft (1977) characterizes these youngsters as markedly egocentric and having little concern for the rights and feelings of others, implying ". . . a failure to establish a normal degree of affection, empathy or bond with others." Two subvarieties are described. In the first the children are fearful and timid; emotionally immature, as shown in their temper tantrums and demandingness; and they are likely to show self-protective and manipulative lying. They view themselves as rejected by and unfairly treated by others, and they tend to be mistrustful of other people.

In the other subvariety the children present an ingratiating facade for exploitative purposes with rapid loss of interest in those who do not meet their needs quickly. Affectionless, guiltless, often surreptitious, they tend not to develop social ties and become anxious chiefly in the face of imminent punishment.

The sex ratio in these groups has been described as approximately equal, with the preponderance of conduct disorders in girls falling in this group. In both varieties substandard academic achievement is typical. A pattern of restlessness and distractibility commonly accompanies the syndrome as in the aggressive type of conduct disorder.

Other Conduct Disorders

Other groupings of patients with patterns of externalization and impulsive acting-out in violation of social norms include: group delinquent reactions, sexual deviations, and alcohol and drug-abuse patterns. We believe that these share important common features of personality organization with the two above-described major categories—impulsive acting-out, alienation from parents and peer culture, overt or covert hostility, immature conscience development—such as to merit their being grouped with these. Other classification schemes usually differentiate them into separate syndromes.

Group Delinquent Reactions

Large group studies of juvenile delinquents' behavior and personality features have often delineated a subgroup who are distinguished from other delinquent subgroups by two features: (1) consistent performance of their delinquent acts with one group of other delinquents, that is a gang and (2) expressions of loyalty and other signs of positive social bonds to members of the gang. They are predatory against the major culture or community, while showing some positive social behavior within their delinquent subcultural groups. They typically originate in high delinquency areas of urban communities from families who are ethnic minorities.

Research on delinquent youngsters diagnosed with this label or with its alternatives (subcultural delinquents, dyssocial reaction, socialized conduct disorder) present some evidence of their having some consistent positive interpersonal relationships and approximately age-appropriate moral ideologies (Jurkovic and Prentice, 1977). Whether these youngsters truly develop conduct disorders akin to the forms described above awaits more thorough study of their personality organizations and long-term psychiatric histories.

Sexual Deviations

Beyond the sexual promiscuity characteristic of girl delinquents, disorders during preadolescence in which the principal symptoms are repeated sexual acting-out are very rare. When they occur, more than one deviation is often shown by any one individual deviant: exhibitionism, voyeurism, compulsive masturbation, bestiality, promiscuity, sexual activity with a person of the same sex. These disorders have received little research attention. A research study of lower class adolescent males with sexual deviations suggests that they originate from family contexts characterized by paternal rejection, intense parental conflict, and maternal attitudes reflecting an authoritarian posture and high sex anxiety (McCord, McCord, and Verden 1962). Many normal adolescents will show a single deviant symptom in an isolated episode or two in the process of integrating their ripened sexuality. The syndromes described here involve repetitive patterns of sexual deviance over extended periods of time, that is a year or more.

Alcohol and Drug-Abuse Patterns

The past decade and a half has seen an increasing experimentation with alcohol and soft drugs by adolescents and older preadolescents from widely varying socioeconomic and personality integration levels. Ingestion of illegal drugs per se does not identify any disorder. Children and adolescents who regularly use alcohol and/or soft drugs (for example marijuana) excessively or who are dependent on hard drugs (for example heroin) show substantial similarity in personality features, such as impulsivity, egocentrism, and depression (Braucht, et al., 1973), but they do not constitute independent syndromes in our view. Rather these drug-dependent youngsters resemble youngsters with conduct disorders of the unaggressive type. Admixtures of depressive neurotic and borderline psychotic personality organization are commonly found among them.

The Genesis of Externalization Behaviors and Disorders

We have characterized children with conduct disorders as undersocialized, that is as representing partial failures in parental efforts to teach them controls over impulsive behavior. To gain further understanding of the development of these diverse children who have in common deficiencies in impulse control and prominent externalization defenses, we present a brief synopsis of the socialization process in preschool-age children and then summarize the etiological factors addressed by research on conduct disorders.

The Learning and Unlearning of Externalization Patterns in Young Children

Typical preschool-age children (two and a half to five years) and their parents invest substantial effort in the learning and teaching of behavioral controls. With his basic locomotor, manipulative, and excretory controls rapidly increasing in effectiveness and his life space enormously enlarged by his motor skills and language facility, early in this period the toddler is expected to start learning more mature ways of responding to intense arousal states. No longer tolerated readily are the temper tantrums, marked avoidant behavior, or destruction of property of the preceding age period. During toddlerhood parents, often unwittingly, are teaching a prep course in learning to live in the real social world. Shortly in first grade, the teacher will require of her charges a serviceable set of impulse restraints and emotional controls. First grade peers, also shaky in their integrations of new controls, will offer limited tolerance for babyishness shown in repeated selfish appropriation of playthings or in unmodulated displays of anger.

During the early phase of the preschool period, a youngster is quite ready to take credit for achievements which gain him esteem but seldom is his ego strong enough to accept the responsibility for attempted achievements which fail or for selfish or antisocial acts about which others complain to him. Externalization is a favorite defense of the preschooler: on the playmate who did not throw the ball accurately, making it be missed; on the hammer that did not strike accurately; on the little brother who happened to be near the open purse when the dime was filched. Most children externalize to some extent at this age because they have limited knowledge of their developing capacities; because they experience repeated demonstrations that external powers are nearly always greater than their own; and because they experience themselves as strongly dependent on parental support, having only partial understanding that the loss of love implied in a momentary critical remark by a parent is not forever.

How parents deal with the preschoolers' torrential affects, uncontrolled impulses, and repeated externalizations will critically influence the differentiations of the ego during this period. This is gradually revealed in the internalization of controls and the lessening of the child's egocentrism, aggressiveness, and externalization defenses. In addition to their direct instruction of their children in learning behavior controls, parents possess two other important means for inducing socialization in their offspring, both of them chronologically and psychologically antecedent to their direct socialization efforts: the quality of care which they have been able to provide their children from birth and the models for outer control and inner control which they spontaneously offer a receptive learner in their own behavior. Common to the preschool histories of child patients with conduct disorders are deficiencies in one or more of three important parental inputs which allow children to relinquish externalization for a coherent integration of inner controls, to exchange the law of the jungle for harmonious peer relationships: (1) genuine affection translated into caring; (2) parental models of effective impulse control; (3) parental efficiency in teaching controls, revealed in the consistency, clarity, and coherence among their control-induction messages. The externalization symptoms shown by children with conduct disorders do not represent bizarre depravity, but appear to be determined by their socialization experiences with their caretakers. Again we emphasize the developmental perspective: that externalization behaviors are universal among preschool-age children, being characteristic of relatively undifferentiated beings with immature levels of cognitive development who have had insufficient socialization time and socialization nutriment to enable them to acquire reliable "controls from within" (Redl and Wineman, 1957).

Etiological Factors in Conduct Disorders

The etiological determinants of conduct disorders are currently not known in a scientific sense, although we believe there is cumulative evidence sufficient to suggest that psychogenic factors predominate. Constitutional determinants (essentially genetic) were emphasized in the early studies of the late nineteenth and early twentieth centuries. Sociological factors achieved prominence during the second quarter of this century. The predominant etiological emphasis over the past 30 years has been psychogenic and has focused on parental and family system influences. Before reviewing the salient parental factors predisposing children to the development of conduct disorders, we briefly review some of the constitutional and sociological determinants which studies to date have delineated.

We know the least about the possible constitutional determinants of conduct disorders. The principal factors posited to account for the symptomatology of conduct disorders include the following:

- Unusually strong instinctual (sex and aggression) endowment, which reduces the effectiveness of social influences on impulse expression (Freud, 1937).

- A primary reactivity pattern in infants characterized by intense activity rate, impatience in need-satisfaction behaviors, hypersensitivity to stimulation (Thomas, Chess, and Birch, 1968).

- Muscular (mesomorphic) body-build associated with aggressive delinquent patterns (Sheldon, 1949; Glueck and Glueck, 1956).

- Mild cerebral damage occurring prenatally or perinatally (Knoblock and Pasamanick, 1959).

Our review of the currently available evidence regarding the constitutional contributions to conduct disorders in children leads us to the conclusions that: (1) the evidence is inconclusive and (2) such constitutional variations described to date ard quantitatively essentially within the range of normal variation, that is variations which parents of normal parental competence can effectively respond to with appropriate variations in their socialization practices.

The long-known relationship between low social class status and vulnerability to developing juvenile delinquency has secured a place for investigating possible sociological determinants of antisocial behavior. Deprivation of physical needs, higher incidences of family disruption by death and desertion of the parents, greater availability of criminal models in relatives and neighbors, social rejection by the higher social classes—all of these conditions are characteristic of the lives of the poor, especially the urban poor, and have been classed as determinants of juvenile delinquency. Yet none of these is a necessary, much less sufficient, determinant of antisocial patterns in children. Each is found in some families above the lowest rungs of the social order and not all children experiencing these conditions become delinquent (Scarpitti, et al., 1960). The implication is that these sociological pathogens are modifiable by favorable levels of parental caretaking competence.

In our view a group of psychogenic factors imbedded in parent-child relations bear the strongest weight in determining the multiple ego deficiencies that are labeled conduct disorders. Parents have the prime opportunites to provide their children the emotional nutriment, the models, and the learning situations: for internalizing controls over impulses; for valuing other people sufficiently to withhold destructive and/or exploitative impulses toward them. Numerous clinical studies of the parents of children with conduct disorders are in substantial agreement in indicating the principal ways in which some parents fail to use these opportunities effectively to enable their children to become socialized beings. Most often these parental failures are seen to result from the parents' own inadequate socialization experiences with their parents, leaving them with deficiencies in personality integration and ambivalent about the demands of parental caretaking. A review of research findings delineates the following factors:

- Inadequate maternal caregiving during late infancy which interferes with self-other discrimination, affective development, the reduction of ambivalence, the development of identification, and conscience and ego ideals (Aichhorn, 1935; Friedlander, 1945, 1947; Winnicott, 1960, 1963).

- Maternal inconsistency and/or indulgence in limit-setting, narcissistic preoccupations and direct modeling of impulsive behavior due to unresolved maternal dependency conflicts (Rexford and van Amerongen, 1957; Malone, 1963).

- Parental inconsistency and intolerance for experiencing strong feelings, predisposing them to model acting-out for their children (Reiser, 1963).

- Parental display of unrestrained emotions, flooding the child with excitation which exceeds his immature control structures, resulting in his acting-out (Friedlander, 1945).

- Parental vicarious gratification of their own poorly integrated forbidden impulses through permitting and provoking acting-out in the child with concomitant aggressive release toward the child (Johnson, 1949; Johnson and Szurek, 1952; van Amerongen, 1963).

- Paternal hostility to the child and modeling of aggressive behavior in physical punishment of the child (Bandura and Walters, 1959).

The implications of the above studies for the vicissitudes of a child's socialization course strongly suggest a correlation between defaults in parental caretaking (including abandonment, deprivation, abuse, and/or extreme indulgence of a child) with impairment of a child's capacities to internalize controls and ultimately as a parent himself to teach others to do so.

Symptomatology Common to Conduct Disorders and MBD

Children with conduct disorders as a group are impulsive, distractible, and restless. The majority of them are unsuccessful students, show reading retardation, and are behind at least one grade in school. Many are emotionally labile, readily acting out their feelings rather than verbalizing them or even experiencing them in conscious thought; many are also hyperaggressive. The overlapping symptomatology with some of the prominent behavioral symptoms associated with MBD is clear and appears to be greater in this group of emotional disorders than in either the neuroses or psychoses.

Our review of the etiological factors contributing to conduct disorders has stressed the primary importance of psychogenesis, that is the effects of parental personality features and child-rearing styles on the child's developing ego structures. Some children with conduct disorders probably also experience some form of MBD. The disproportionately large number of infants from the lower social classes who have experienced pregnancy and birth complications, given the over-representation of this same social group among juvenile delinquents, makes this plausible on a statistical basis alone. Such children would be the more difficult differential diagnostic cases and would probably be characterized by poor prognoses in view of their symptomatology being determined both developmentally quite early and by multiple pathogens. No research known to us has studied the courses of such children while making these diagnostic distinctions. Child diagnosticians unfamiliar with either conduct disorders or neuropsychological problems in children are clearly more vulnerable to diagnostic error and to less than adequate treatment planning when they work with children whose primary symptoms are of the kind just described. We shall now elaborate further on this dilemma.

CHILDHOOD PSYCHOSES (Reality Testing Disorders)

This group of disorders is a heterogeneous group of clinical syndromes characterized by severe disturbances in ego functioning. As described above, ego functioning refers to the integration and execution of various aspects of an individual's adaptive behavior, including perceiving and ordering of experiences, assessing reality, controlling and channeling of impulses, and relating to people. Severe impairments of these functions are characteristic of children with childhood psychoses.

Although the course of development and the extent of impairment may vary widely among psychotic children, the most commonly shared symptomatic expressions of psychosis are: (1) impairment of reality testing, (2) impairment of identity formation, (3) extreme anxiety, and (4) vulnerability to severe regression. Psychosis typically develops when the primary mechanisms of defense are unable to reduce the overwhelming experience of anxiety, resulting in severe regression to a psychotic level of functioning.

Attempts to classify and understand childhood psychoses have been hampered by lack of agreement on appropriate terminology. A plethora of terms have been employed almost interchangeably in the literature: childhood psychosis, childhood schizophrenia, infantile autism, atypical child syndrome, symbiotic psychosis, dementia praecocissima, dementia infantilis, and, in the DSM–III draft (1977), pervasive developmental disorder. Attempts at distinguishing among types of severely disturbed children have often not increased conceptual clarity because some workers employ these diagnostic terms without specifying the unique and distinguishing features characteristic of each proposed syndrome.

We review here the three forms of childhood psychosis which have received extensive attention in the literature and which can be distinguished by their onset during different periods of development: early infantile autism, symbiotic psychosis, and childhood schizophrenia. The current state of our knowledge does not yet clarify whether these disorders comprise distinct homogeneous classes or are etiologically related, either to each other or to psychosis occurring in adulthood.

Although not as prevalent in the population as the psychoneurotic disturbances, childhood psychoses command attention because of the profound debilitating effects which they have on children. Treffert (1970) reports that these disorders occur in 3.1 cases per 10,000, while Werry (1972) estimates the occurrence at 6 per 10,000 children in the population. Aug and Ables (1971) indicate that up to one-fourth of the children admitted to mental hospitals are psychotic, while Milt (1963) reports that there may be over half a million psychotic children in the United States. Relative to the prevalence rates among adults, Achenbach (1974) reports that the rates for adult psychotics are nearly 400 times as great as the highest estimated rates for children.

It is relevant to note that the literature in this area typically distinguishes between psychoses caused by or associated with unequivocally demonstrable brain tissue pathology and disorders in which structural changes in the brain have not been demonstrated. The former category includes the toxic psychoses, metabolic psychoses, infectious psychoses, and traumatic injury psychoses (Eisenberg 1966). These disorders often resemble the functional psychoses, those for which brain tissue changes have not been demonstrated.

Early Infantile Autism

Considered prognostically as the most severe of the childhood psychoses, infantile autism was first identified as a behavioral syndrome by Kanner (1943). It has been studied more recently by Eisenberg (1966), Rimland (1964), Rutter (1965, 1976), and DeMyer (1977). The disorder is marked by extreme aloneness from earliest infancy (lack of response to other human beings), impaired communication skills, obsessive insistence on the maintenance of sameness, and bizarre fascination with inanimate objects.

Infantile autism can be differentiated from other psychotic disorders by its early onset, typically appearing shortly after birth and always identifiable prior to 30 months of age. Autistic children presumably never begin to establish normal object attachments. Their failure to begin to develop object ties is typically manifested in infancy by a lack of eye contact and facial responsiveness and by indifference or aversion to physical contact. The infant is often described by the parents as quiet and essentially little trouble to care for. In older children the defect is mainly shown by brief visual attention, by lack of postural accommodation when looking at someone, by a lack of cooperative group play, and by the failure to develop persisting friendships.

Psychogenic theories of etiology have viewed the primary symptom of autism as a defensive maintenance of isolation from human contact. It is hypothesized that the infant's inability to receive and integrate communicative input from his human environment causes the child to sense the world as unpredictable, chaotic, and potentially hostile and unrewarding. Bettelheim (1967) has interpreted autistic behavior as a defense against threats of total destruction from a world perceived as hostile and rejecting. The perception of the human world as hostile and threatening may result from pathogenic elements in the parents' style of caretaking, from constitutional limitations in the child's ability to accurately receive and process information from the environment, or from some combination of constitutional and experiential factors.

A recently advanced theory (DeMyer, 1975, 1976, 1977) holds that autistic children have a neurobiologically based language dysfunction which interferes seriously with the acquisition of expressive speech and abstract language. In addition autistic children are thought to have a visual-motor imitation deficiency akin to dyspraxia which interferes with the acquisition of normal body language and the processing of nonverbal communicative input so important during the preverbal stage of development. Although the precise neurophysiological mechanisms involved have yet to be identified, the long-term result is impairment of communication skills characterized by immature grammatical structure, echolalia, pronominal reversals, nominal aphasia, the inability to use abstract terms, and in some cases a total absence of language. Nonverbal means of communication, such as socially appropriate facial expressions and gestures are also lacking in the autistic child.

The failure of communication skills to develop may in part account for the social isolation of the autistic child as he refrains from attending to other human beings with whom communication is basically impaired and unsatisfying. Alternatively the child turns attention toward the less intrusive, more predictable inanimate objects in his environment, thus accounting for the bizarre responses to various aspects of the environment. These include: attachment to odd objects, resistance to minor changes in the environment, fascination with movement, and ritualistic behavior organized around specific objects or locations.

Within the population of autistic children there is variation in the severity of the four primary symptoms and in the incidence of several associated clinical features. About 40% of autistic children have a measured IQ below 50 and only 30% have an IQ of 70 or above (DSM–III, 1977). It is not unusual for autistic children to show extreme variability in intellectual functioning. They often do poorly on tasks requiring abstract thought, symbolism, or sequential logic, but perform well on those tasks which which demand manual skills and visual-spatial skills.

Autistic children may display hyperresponsivity or hyporesponsivity to sensory stimuli, such as light, pain, or sound. Disturbance in mood and affect is not unusual and may range from unexplained crying spells to inappropriate laughter. There may be lack of appreciation of real dangers, such as moving vehicles and heights. Rocking or rhythmic body movements also may occur.

Infantile autism severely hampers progressive ego development and is chronic. Several follow-up studies have been completed (Eisenberg, 1956; Kanner, 1971; and Kanner, Rodriguez, and Ashenden, 1972). In general, two-thirds of the autistic children remain severely handicapped and unable to live independent lives as adults. About one-sixth are able to obtain regular employment and make a marginal social adjustment. This group of successful children however tend to display residual signs of social inappropriateness. The communication skills of all autistic children remain impaired and fully one-half remain without speech. The single best predictor of positive outcome is minimum impairment in language development.

Symbiotic Psychosis

Margaret Mahler (1952, 1965, 1968) has drawn a distinction between autistic psychosis and symbiotic psychosis, however both syndromes are believed to originate during the early mother-child relationship. In autistic psychosis the child defensively shuts out the human object world, thus preventing the development of an age-appropriate symbiotic attachment to the mother. Without this primitive and basic object attachment the infant cannot learn to associate the mother as an external object with internal need gratification. The child is thus in a constant state of anxiety unable to be comforted, oriented, guided, or taught by the mother from whom most children receive their initial sense of well-being, the precursor of normal ego development. Mahler's autistic psychosis closely resembles Kanner's description of infantile autism. Most authors suggest that in autistic children even the most effective mothering cannot adequately complement or support the inherently defective tension-regulating system of the ego.

Symbiotic psychosis by contrast results from a fixation at, or a regression to, the symbiotic phase of normal development. Development within the first 18 to 24 months may proceed in a relatively normal fashion marked by attachment of the infant to his mother. However Mahler hypothesizes that the child fails to develop a mental representation of the mother as a separate, outside object. The mental representation of the mother remains fused with that of self and continues the child's delusion of omnipotence through attachment to the primary object. The child fails to view himself as a separate and independent person.

The symbiotic disturbance does not become apparent until the second to fourth or fifth year of life when maturation of the ego would normally enable the child to master new aspects of the environment independent of his mother. When challenged by expectations for independent functioning, the child may show intense separation anxiety and clinging and also regressive trends, such as relinquishing communicative speech. The symptom picture commonly includes gradual withdrawal from interpersonal relationships, emotional aloofness, autistic behavior, and distorted perceptions of reality, which in combination approximate the syndrome of infantile autism.

According to Mahler (1965) symbiotic psychosis usually involves some unspecified constitutional predisposition toward inherent ego deficiency. However inappropriate parenting plays a role by interfering with the separation-individuation process which normally ends the phase of symbiotic attachment.

Because symbiotic psychosis has been differentiated from other childhood psychoses relatively recently, little research effort has been devoted to it thus far (Mahler and Furer, 1972).

Childhood Schizophrenia

There is considerable conceptual confusion concerning the parameters of the term childhood schizophrenia. Historically the term is linked to Bleuler's (1911) term, schizophrenia, for adult disorders characterized by a detachment from outer reality. In recent years the term childhood schizophrenia has frequently been employed as a synonym for childhood psychosis. At times it has been broadly interpreted so as to subsume the two syndromes discussed above, infantile autism and symbiotic psychosis.

Childhood schizophrenia refers to a pervasive psychotic disorder involving a decline or arrest in ego development following a period of relatively normal development, occuring in children who demonstrate some degree of useful language and relatedness to others (GAP, 1966). Onset occurs between 6 and 12 years of age. Among children thus characterized however there are wide variations in personality organization, clinical course, intellectual functioning, and identifiable etiological conditions.

The GAP (1966) description for schizophreniform psychotic disorders is as follows:

This reaction ordinarily is not seen until the age period between six and twelve or thirteen years. Onset may be gradual, neurotic symptoms appearing at first, followed by marked and primitive denial and projection, looseness of association in thought processes, concretistic thinking, low frustration tolerance, hypochondriacal tendencies, and intense temper outbursts. Later developments may include marked withdrawal, intense involvement in fantasy, autistic behavior, emotional aloofness, true disorders in thinking, and a breakdown in reality testing. In other instances more acute and sudden eruptions at this developmental phase may involve crises accompanied by intense anxiety, uncontrollable phobias, and marked withdrawal leading to autistic behavior and disoriented reality testing . . . Ideas of reference, dissociative phenomena, somatic delusions, catatonic behavior, paranoid thinking, and other manifestations seen in adults may occur. [pp. 254–255]

Etiological considerations in the development of childhood schizophrenia include constitutional deficiencies in the child, primary deficits in the psychosocial environment, and theories of multiple causation.

A number of studies have demonstrated elevated frequencies of neurological signs and pre- and peri-natal complications in schizophrenic children. On the basis of such evidence Bender and Faretra (Bender, 1942; Bender and Faretra, 1973) hypothesized that schizophrenia is the result of a pervasive inherited vulnerability beginning prenatally and manifested in evident unevenness of development. In spite of the evidence for CNS related impairment in some childhood schizophrenics, the theory does not seem relevant for many others, since any or all of the signs may be absent in a significant number of schizophrenics and, in addition, may occur in nonpsychotic children as well.

Studies of twins reared separately and studies showing high concordance rates among family members of schizophrenics have been cited as evidence for a genetic component in adult onset schizophrenia. However such studies for childhood schizophrenia have not been reported in the literature. In addition Pollin, et al., (1966) have suggested that the high concordance rate for adult twins may derive from greater risk for perinatal CNS damage in twins rather than from similarity in genetic origins.

Among the experiential factors thought to have etiological significance for the development of childhood schizophrenia are: maternal overprotection, maternal rejection, stimulus deprivation during infancy, inconsistent parenting, and severe and repeated emotional trauma experienced by the child. Etiological theories based exclusively on psychogenic determinants fail to account for the significant number of children exposed to apparently schizophrenogenic experiences who do not manifest overt psychopathology. There is no evidence at this time that any uniform set of attitudes, personality characteristics, or behavior patterns characterizes the parents of schizophrenic children.

The heterogeneity of symptom pattern and treatment course observed among schizophrenic children suggest that several patterns of disorder with varying multiple etiological determinant combinations are being observed. A comprehensive theory of multiple causation has been elaborated by Goldfarb (1961, 1974). According to this view, the disordered adaptation of each child reflects the interplay of intrinsic deficits in the child and of deviations in psychosocial organization of the family. "It is presumed that each of these classes of aberration varies dimensionally from none to marked and that the relative contributions of each class of disorder to the functional impairments of the child vary from child to child" (Goldfarb, 1974).

Symptomatology Common to Childhood Psychoses and MBD

The MBD child and the psychotic youngster may share a common sense of uncertainty about the world; the former due to limitations in perceptual and integrative processes, the latter because of poorly defined ego boundaries which result in a distortion of the perceptual process. This uncertainty or inability to predict accurately expectations and responses from parents, parent substitutes, and peers may lead to anxiety and a common set of associated problems including impulsivity, distractibility, emotional lability, and at times hyperactivity. Both the MBD and psychotic youngster may demonstrate learning problems associated with attentional difficulties and both may show a preference for regular routines and simplicity in the environment.

As Goldfarb (1974) has suggested, the diagnosis of brain damage and schizophrenia are not mutually exclusive. Brain impairment is considered a primary etiological agent in many instances. However the diagnostician is not relieved of responsibility for clarifying any relevant psychogenic factors in evaluating psychotic youngsters with manifest brain impairment, for such psychogenic components may provide pivotal access for treatment leverage.

THE PROBLEM OF DIFFERENTIAL DIAGNOSIS: ASKING THE RIGHT QUESTIONS

MBD or Emotional Disorder?

Only a few years ago (more recently than we are comfortable in acknowledging) our training and experience would have led us, the present writers, to accept this as an appropriate question. We would have attempted (and did attempt) to answer it in working with a variety of puzzling maladjusted children, many of whom presented some of the symptoms common to the MBD-syndromes and to emotional disorders.

The perceptive reader of this chapter knows that we no longer view this as an appropriate question. We view it as a non-question today because it does not conceptualize the nature of behavior disorder and its implied etiology in terms appropriate to the levels of knowledge and of concepts presented by contemporary behavioral science, that is, multiple determination of complex adaptive behavioral patterns by successive sets of interacting determinants, constitutional and experiential.

In the sections describing patterns of emotional disorder in children, we have called attention to the overlapping symptomatology of MBD and emotional disorder patterns, covering most of the behavioral symptoms associated with the MBD syndromes: hyperactivity, distractibility and short attention span, impulsivity, emotional lability, and aggressive tendencies. We have focused attention on the psychogenic determination of these symptoms in many children. Compared to the nonbehavioral, presumptively neurogenic, symptoms (that is, perceptual-motor dysfunctions, motor symptoms, and learning disabilities) only in the case of learning problems does the available clinical research literature suggest psychogenesis and/or strong emotional contributions in some children's maladaptive patterns. Some MBD specialists, largely those who are unfamiliar with children's emotional disorders, may find it difficult to accept that the overlapping symptomatology is truly codetermined by the child's psychological organization and functioning, except when these symptoms can be viewed as secondary to MBD. We now present some additional observations, supporting the view that experiential factors exert considerable influence on the symptomatology associated with MBD.

The heterogeneity of symptom patterning in the MBD syndromes is amply demonstrated in the literature, including some chapters of this handbook. Heterogeneity characterizes not only the composition of syndromes, but also quantitative and qualitative variations in the symptom components. While this heterogeneity does not prove the existence of psychogenic components in the behavioral symptoms associated with MBD, it is strongly suggestive of this possibility in some children, given the inexact selection criteria characterizing this early heuristic stage in the development of the MBD concept. An extension of this line of evidence is derived from research which delineates various subgroups within the MBD-hyperkinesis gross class by either factor analysis or logical analysis of developmental, symptomatic, behavioral, educational performance and family history data. By such analyses, one or more subgroups are recurrently found with characteristics which bear minimal resemblance to the nuclear symptom groups with presumptive MBD. Conners' (1973) factor analytic study of 267 children referred to a clinic for hyperactive children produced a large group (53) without any resemblance to the clearly learning-disabled, MBD groups, after having screened out subjects whose families showed severe psychopathology and/or sufficient stress to account for the child's behavior problems, (that is measures were taken to exclude children with psychogenic problems, but a substantial group implicitly slipped through the screening measures). Ney (1974) has described four categories of hyperactive children, labelling them as to type: genetic, MBD, conditioned, reactive. The conditioned type had parents who responded selectively with attention to their children's active distracting behavior. The reactive type occurred in children from homes in which there was little agreement in discipline, or where there was considerable marital turmoil. Werry (1968) factor analyzed the historical, medical, neurological and other diagnostic data on a group of 103 hyperactive children and found nine relevant but essentially independent dimensions in this group of patients, leading him to infer the existence of different etiological factors and to conclude that the notion of a homogeneous brain-damage dimension in these patients was refuted.

Another body of data supporting the conclusion that experiential factors are important in determining learning handicaps derives from studies focusing on the interaction between early neurological impairments in infants and such social-class related variables as maternal child-rearing style, maternal achievement orientation, and cognitive stimulation provided by the mother. Willerman (1973) has summarized a number of studies which suggest that " . . . familial influences may be able to forestall the onset of a proportion of MBD disorders, even in the presence of brain injury." Holden and Willerman (1972) found a relationship between mental retardation at age four and social class, in following neurologically abnormal one-year-old infants with equal levels of impairment. The four-year-olds from lower class homes had a sevenfold greater incidence of mental retardation than did those from middleclass homes (35% versus 5%). In summarizing the literature which they reviewed in this area, Sameroff and Chandler (1975) state:

> The conclusion to which one is led by these studies is that while many persons with later developmental difficulties can be shown, retrospectively, to have had pregnancy and perinatal complications, the majority of infants experiencing such complications are not found to have later difficulties when studied prospectively. . . . Unless the environmental context is also specified, few predictions can be made about developmental outcomes based on perinatal difficulties. [P. 233]

Another relevant source of evidence regarding the contributions of experiential factors to learning handicaps is provided by the voluminous literature on various psychodynamic factors associated with learning problems in children, including such factors as: the disruption of concentration by anxiety; neurotic inhibitions against making contact with anxiety-laden primary-drive derivatives; perceptual impairments associated with unstable self-other discriminations. Heinicke (1972) has systematically surveyed the research hypotheses and results relating to various learning disorders of children and confirmed the etiological variety accounting for these, which includes a substantial segment with a primary psychogenic component.

In sum we conclude that there is much evidence supporting the view that experiential factors are potent influences on the symptomatology associated with MBD, and therefore that remedial efforts which neglect the importance of these will be less than optimal. How meaningfully to relate various constitutional and experiential factors in a developmental model is another issue that bears on asking the right questions.

Towards a Realistic Model of Effects

It is commonplace to observe that our conceptualization of a dilemma determines our ability to solve it. To a considerable extent we are all prisoners of our limited knowledge of events and our concepts of how these events are mutatively interrelated. Despite its age and endless retelling, an old joke continually reappears at conferences of behavioral scientists and, for good reason, never fails to draw laughter:

> At night a drunk searches unsuccessfully for his car keys beneath a lamppost and when asked if he lost his keys in that spot, he replies, "No, but that's where the light is."

Most of us are uncomfortable about how much we look "where the light is." Few would question that we need not only new data about human behavioral processes, but also new models for organizing them conceptually in more meaningful ways.

Over the past dozen years several concepts have appeared which help to advance conceptualization of the determinants of children's behavior disorders and their interrelationships. Pasamanick and Knobloch (1966), using an earlier concept of Lilienfeld and Parkhurst (1951), described a continuum of reproductive casualty in infants, related to pregnancy and delivery complications, which at the less pathogenic end could produce mild forms of neurological insult undetectable by the usual diagnostic techniques, but which would contribute to a wide variety of subsequent maladaptions in children. This has been a fundamental hypothesis supporting investigators of the MBD syndromes. Thomas, Chess, and Birch (1968) have described the varying consequences for the child's developmental outcome of congruence-incongruence in the interaction between actual infant reactivity type and either the type preferred by the parents or one which they could successfully parent. Sameroff and Chandler (1975), in summarizing the implications of the recent developmental outcome literature have posited a continuum of caretaking casualty to account for the widely different outcomes in later life of children who are judged to be equal in level of competence during infancy. Another useful descriptive construct, scapegoating, has emerged from the family systems and family therapy literature to account for the manner in which some parents force one of their children into narrow roles as a behavioral deviant, directing the preponderance of their aversive parental caretaking influence to this child (Vogel and Bell, 1960; Ackerman, 1961). The typical interpretation made of the prime function of this scapegoating procedure is that it diverts attention from marital conflict which the parents find difficult to confront.

What implications have these for the most productive model portraying the determinants of children's maladaptive behavior patterns? As noted in our introduction, Sameroff and Chandler (1975) have pointed out the limitations of the main effects model which portrays a linear relationship between a pathogenic agent and the developmental outcomes of children at various ages. An improvement on this model is the interactive model, which portrays outcomes as a result of the interactions of two or more variables. But in predicting the long-term outcomes in child behavior patterns, the interactive model fails to account for either the changes in child characteristics (constitutional and experiential) or parental characteristics through time, nor does it account for their successive reciprocal influences on each other. These limitations are overcome in the transactional model, which depicts " . . . a continual progressive interplay between the organism and its environment. . . . " Sameroff and Chandler (1975) further state:

Any truly transactional model must stress the plastic character of the environment and of the organism as an active participant in its growth. . . . The child is, in this view, in a perpetual state of active reorganization and cannot properly be regarded as maintaining an inborn deficit as a static characteristic. In this view, the constants in development are not some set of traits, but rather the processes by which these traits are maintained in transactions between organisms and environment. . . . Breakdown from this organismic or transactional point of view is not seen simply as a function of an inborn inability to respond appropriately, but rather the function of some *continuous* malfunction in the organism-environment transaction across time which prevents the child from organizing his world adaptively. . . . [P. 235]

As a research strategy the transactional model presents some methodological difficulties, for example measuring simultaneously occurring reciprocal reorganizations of experiences in parent and child. However, as a depiction of what occurs in nature, it is more realistic than the other models. The clinician who understands it would appear to have a valuable conceptual tool available to him, providing insurance to his child patients and their familes against the hazards of oversimplifying the child's developmental complexity.

Asking the Right Questions

In practical terms the right questions are those which when answered lead to the choice of the most effective treatment strategies for helping any individual child with a maladaptive disorder. If one adopts the premises presented above, regarding the organism-environment transactional processes which originate and sustain a child's disorder pattern, the right questions become both simpler and more complex than they were. They become simpler in that a universe of focal determining processes can be outlined which can account for variations in the child's symptomatic expressions through successive developmental phases. They become more complex in that the diagnostic focus becomes the unique combination of events and processes comprising an individual disordered-child-in-family-in-community gestalt, which requires of the diagnostician greater time, energy, and conceptual versatility. An additional cost of accepting this complexity is the loss of the plausibility of using simplistic unidimensional etiological constructs and treatment modes. No longer can emotional disorder be treated as if it provided immunity from MBD, nor MBD treated as if it provided immunity from emotional disorder or even a limited immunity to only a few forms of emotional disorder (as in the view that the behavioral symptoms in a child with presumptive MBD are essentially secondary to the child's experiencing the frustrations of his integrative efforts imposed by the presumptive MBD). No longer is a trial of medication justifiable as the total treatment effort.

To most readers the general categories of appropriate questions are already familiar:

1. What are all the symptom dimensions of the child's disorder in its present form? What were they in earlier forms? When did they first appear? How have they changed through successive developmental stages; through successive family life-cycle changes and vicissitudes?

2. What processes in the child-environment field (interacting forces, traits, capacities, motives, affects) appear to have determined the emergence of the child's various symptoms?

3. What processes sustain the symptoms in their present forms?

4. What is the optimal hierarchy of treatment interventions for this child and his family, given the determining processes of his symptoms, his adaptive strengths and weaknesses and those of his parents, and the treatment resources of his school and community?

It is not within the province of this chapter to attempt to enumerate the numerous specific questions which a diagnostician might ask in delineating the answers to the general questions indicated above about any individual child patient and his family. Some of the ingredients for such questions are found in the discussions above on determinants of various forms of emotional disorder. The reader who is interested will find readily available useful diagnostic techniques and organizing schema for evaluating children with adaptive disorders (Goodman and Sours, 1967; Simmons, 1969; Group for the Advancement of Psychiatry, 1957; Mennin-

ger Foundation Children's Division, 1969; Kernberg, 1969). A consistent emphasis in these diagnostic manuals is on the importance of thorough examinations,
employing a wide variety of independent assessment methods beyond the usual
combination of medical examination, diagnostic interviews with the child and his
parents, developmental and family histories, and a psychological test battery. In
working with children whose symptom complexes fall within the gray area between hypothetically pure types of emotional disorder and MBD, it is especially
important to extend the diagnostic armamentarium to include neurological exams,
EEG, speech and hearing exams, perceptual modality analyses, educational
achievement surveys, and family diagnostic interviews.

The translation of diagnostic findings into a relevant set of treatment objectives
and modalities for achieving these is often the weakest link in the clinical service
chain. In working with children who have learning problems with accompanying
components of emotional disorder, a coordinated treatment effort on at least three
fronts is likely to prove beneficial: the child's educational program, the child's
feelings about and relationships with himself and others, his parents' experiencing
of him and parenting of him in the context of their marital relationship and
relationships with their other children. The multiple dimensions and determinants
of the majority of children's adaptive disorders urge consideration of applying
several treatment methods simultaneously, including some combination of the
following:

- An individualized special educational program tailored to the child's per-
  ceptual modality profile and educational achievement test performance.
- Individual psychotherapy for the child.
- Parental guidance.
- Family therapy.
- Individual psychotherapy for the parent.
- Marital therapy.
- Consultation with teachers.
- Activity group therapy.
- Occupational and recreational therapy.
- Medication.

Single treatment modality approaches of any variety fall short of most children's treatment needs. Especially when treatment is limited to medication only,
it fails to communicate accurately the complex nature of the child's disorder and
its learned experiential components, and may also impose other risks to the long-
term well-being of the child (Sroufe, 1975; Rie, 1975). Simplistic treatment approaches are likely to remain in use until the outmoded question, "MBD or
emotional disorder?" is laid to rest.

REFERENCES

Achenbach, T. M. *Developmental Psychopathology.* New York: Ronald, 1974.

Ackerman, N. W., ed., *Exploring the Base for Family Therapy.* New York: Family Service
Association, 1961.

Adams, P. L. *Obsessive Children*. New York: Brunner/Mazel, 1973.

Aichhorn, A. *Wayward Youth*. New York: Viking Press, 1935.

American Psychiatric Association. *Diagnostic and Statistical Manual of Mental Disorders*, 1st ed., Washington, D.C.: 1952.

American Psychiatric Association. *Diagnostic and Statistical Manual of Mental Disorders*, 2nd ed., Washington, D.C.: 1968.

American Psychiatric Association. *Diagnostic and Statistical Manual of Mental Disorders*, 3rd ed., Washington, D. C.: Task Force on Nomenclature and Statistics, April 15, 1977. [Draft version]

Amerongen, S. van, "Permission, promotion, and provocation of antisocial behavior." *Journal of the American Academy of Child Psychiatry*, 2, 99–117, (1963).

Anthony, E. J. "Neurotic Disorders," in A. M. Freedman, H. I. Kaplan, and B. J. Sadock, eds., *Comprehensive Textbook of Psychiatry*, 2nd ed., pp. 2143–2160. Baltimore: Williams & Wilkins, 1975.

Aug, R. G., and B. S. Ables. "A clinician's guide to childhood psychosis." *Pediatrics*, 47, 327–338, (1971).

Bandura, A., and R. H. Walters. *Adolescent Aggression*. New York: Ronald, 1959.

Bellak, L., M. Hurvich, and H. K. Gediman. *Ego Functions in Schizophrenics, Neurotics, and Normals*. New York: Wiley, 1973.

Bender, L. "Childhood schizophrenia." *Nervous Child*, 1, 138–140, (1942).

Bender, L., and G. Faretra. "The relationship between childhood schizophrenia and adult schizophrenia," in A. Kaplan, ed., *Genetic Factors in Schizophrenia*. Springfield, Ill.: Thomas, 1973.

Bettelheim, B. *The Empty Fortress: Infantile Autism and the Birth of the Self*. New York: Free Press, 1967.

Bleuler, E. *Dementia Praecox or the Group of Schizophrenias*. New York: International Universities Press, 1950. [Originally published in 1911]

Braucht, G. N., D. Brakarsh, D. Follingstad, and K. L. Berry. "Deviant drug use in adolescence: A review of psychosocial correlates." *Psychological Bulletin*, 79, 92–106, (1973).

Burks, H. L., and S. I. Harrison. "Aggressive behavior as a means of avoiding depression." *American Journal of Orthopsychiatry*, 32, 416–422, (1962).

Conners, C. K. "Psychological assessment of children with minimal brain dysfunction." *Annals of the New York Academy of Sciences*, 205, 283–302, (1973).

Coolidge, J. C., M. L. Willer, E. Tessman, and S. Waldfogel. "School phobia in adolescence: A manifestation of severe character disturbance." *American Journal of Orthopsychiatry*, 30, 599–607, (1960).

Cummings, S. T. "Family influences on children's ego development." 1964. [Unpublished manuscript]

DeMyer, M. K. "Motor, perceptual motor, and intellectual disabilities of autistic children," in L. Wing, ed., *Early Childhood Autism*, 2nd ed., London: Pergamon, 1975b.

———"The nature of the neuropsychological disability in autistic children," in E. Schopler and R. J. Reichler, eds., *Psychopathology and Child Development*, pp. 93–114. New York: Plenum, 1976.

——— "Research in infantile autism: A strategy and its results," in S. Chess and A. Thomas, eds., *Annual Progress in Child Psychiatry and Child Development: 1977*, pp. 393–415. New York: Brunner/Maazel, 1976.

Eisenberg, L. "The autistic child in adolescence." *American Journal of Psychiatry*, 112, 607–612, (1956).

———"School phobia: A study in the communication of anxiety." *American Journal of*

Psychiatry, 114, 712–718, (1958).

———"The classification of the psychotic disorders in childhood," in L. D. Eron, ed., *Classification of Behavior Disorders*, Chicago: Aldine, 1966.

Engel, M. *Psychopathology of Childhood*. New York: Harcourt Brace Jovanovich, 1972.

Erikson, E. H. *Childhood and Society*. New York: Norton, 1950.

Estes, H. R., C. H. Haylett, and E. M. Johnson. "Separation anxiety." *American Journal of Psychotherapy*, 10, 682–695, (1956).

Friedlander, K. "Formation of the antisocial character." *Psychoanalytic Study of the Child*, 1, 189–203, (1945).

———*The Psycho-analytical Approach to Juvenile Delinquency*. London: Kegan, Paul, Trench, Trubner, 1947.

Freud, A. *Normality and Pathology in Childhood*. New York: International Universities Press, 1965.

Freud, S. "Three Essays on the Theory of Sexuality." *Standard Edition*, vol. 7, pp. 135–243. London: Hogarth, 1953. [Originally published in 1905]

——— "Analysis of a phobia in a five-year-old boy." *Standard Edition*, vol. 10, pp. 5–149. [Originally published in 1909] London: Hogarth, 1955.

———"Analysis terminable and interminable." *Standard Edition*, vol. 23, pp. 216–253. [Originally published in 1937] London: Hogarth, 1964.

Glaser, K. "Masked depression in children and adolescents." *American Journal of Psychotherapy*, 21, 565–574, (1967).

Glidewell, C. *The Prevalence of Maladjustment in Elementary Schools*. (A report prepared for the Joint Commission on Mental Health of Children.) Chicago: University of Chicago, 1968.

Glueck, S., and E. Glueck. *Physique and Delinquency*. New York: Harper & Row, 1956.

Goldfarb, W. *Childhood Schizophrenia*. Cambridge, Mass.: Harvard University Press, 1961.

———"Distinguishing and classifying the individual schizophrenic child," in G. Caplan, ed., *American Handbook of Psychiatry*, 2, vol. 2, pp. 85–106. New York: Basic Books, 1974.

Goodman, J. D., and J. A. Sours. *The Child Mental Status Examination*. New York: Basic Books, 1967.

Group for the Advancement of Psychiatry, Committee on Child Psychiatry. *The Diagnostic Process in Child Psychiatry*. GAP Report No. 38. New York: GAP, 1957.

———*Psychopathological Disorders in Childhood: Theoretical Considerations and a Proposed Classification*. GAP Report No. 62. New York: GAP, 1966.

Heinicke, C. M. "Learning disturbance in childhood," in B. B. Wolman, ed., *Manual of Child Psychopathology*, pp. 662–705. New York: McGraw-Hill, 1972.

Hobbs, N., ed., *Issues in the Classification of Children*, vols. 1 and 2. San Francisco: Jossey-Bass, 1975*a*.

———*The Futures of Children*. San Francisco: Jossey-Bass, 1975*b*.

Holden, R. H. and L. Willerman. "Neurological abnormality in infancy, intelligence, and social class," in E. P. Trapp and P. Himelstein, eds., *Readings on the Exceptional Child: Research and Theory*, 2nd ed., pp. 501–511. New York: Appleton-Century-Crofts, 1972.

Jenkins, R. L. and S. Glickman. "Patterns of personality organization among delinquents." *Nervous Child*, 6, 329–339, (1947).

Johnson, A. M. "Sanctions for super-ego lacunae of adolescents," in K. R. Eissler, ed.,

Searchlights on Delinquency, New York: International Universities Press, 1949.

Johnson, A. M., and S. A. Szurek. "The genesis of anti-social acting out in children and adults." *Psychoanalytic Quarterly*, 21, 323–343, (1952).

Johnson, A. M., E. I. Falstein, S. A. Szurek, and M. Svendsen. "School phobia." *American Journal of Orthopsychiatry*, 11, 702–711, (1941).

Joint Commission on Mental Health of Children. *Crisis in Child Mental Health*. New York: Harper & Row, 1970.

Jurkovic, G. J., and N. M. Prentice. "Relation of moral and cognitive development to dimensions of juvenile delinquency." *Journal of Abnormal Psychology*, 86, 414–420, (1977).

Kanner, L. "Autistic disturbances of affective contact." *Nervous Child*, 2, 217–250, (1943).

———"Follow-up study of eleven autistic children originally reported in 1943." *Journal of Autism and Childhood Schizophrenia*, 1, 119–145, (1971).

Kanner, L., A. Rodriquez, and B. Ashenden. "How far can autistic children go in matters of social adaptation?" *Journal of Autism and Childhood Schizophrenia*, 2, 9–33, (1972).

Kernberg, O. *Borderline Conditions and Pathological Narcissism*. New York: Jason Aronson, 1975.

Kernberg, P. F. "The problem of organicity in the child." *Journal of the American Academy of Child Psychiatry*, 8, 517–541, (1969).

Kessler, J. *Psychopathology of Childhood*. New York: Prentice-Hall, 1966.

———"Nosology in child psychopathology," in H. Rie, ed., *Perspectives in Child Psychopathology*, pp. 85–129. Chicago: Aldine, 1971.

Knobloch, H., and B. Pasamanick. "Syndrome of minimal cerebral damage in infancy." *Journal of the American Medical Association*, 170, 1384–1387, (1959).

Lilienfeld, A. M., and E. A. Parkhurst. "A study of the association of factors of pregnancy and parturition with the development of cerebral palsy: A preliminary report." *American Journal of Hygiene*, 53, 262–282, (1951).

Mahler, M. "On child psychosis and schizophrenia: Autistic and symbiotic infantile psychosis." *Psychoanalytic Study of the Child*, 7, 286–305, (1952).

———"On early infantile psychosis." *Journal of the American Academy of Child Psychiatry*, 4, 554–568, (1965).

———*On Human Symbiosis and the Vicissitudes of Individuation*. New York: International Universities Press, 1968.

Mahler, M., and M. Furer. "Child psychosis: A theoretical statement and its implications." *Journal of Autism and Childhood Schizophrenia*, 2, 213–218, (1972).

Malmquist, C. P. "Depressive phenomena in children," in B. B. Wolman, ed., *Manual of Child Psychopathology*, pp. 497–540. New York: McGraw-Hill, 1972.

Malone, C. A. "Some observations on children of disorganized families and problems of acting out." *Journal of the American Academy of Child Psychiatry*, 2, 22–41, (1963).

McCord, W., J. McCord, and P. Verden. "Family relationships and sexual deviance in lower class adolescents." *International Journal of Social Psychiatry*, 8, 165–179, (1962).

Menninger Foundation Children's Division. *Disturbed Children*. San Francisco: Jossey-Bass, 1969.

Milt, H. "Serious mental illness in children." *Public Affairs*, No. 352, (1963).

Ney, P. G. "Four types of hyperkinesis." *Canadian Psychiatric Association Journal*, 19,

543–550, (1974).

Pasamanick, B., and H. Knobloch. "Retrospective studies on the epidemiology of reproductive casualty: Old and new." *Merrill Palmer Quarterly*, 12, 7–26, (1966).

Pollin, W., J. R. Stabenau, L. Mosher, and J. Tupin. "Life history differences in identical twins discordant for schizophrenia." *American Journal of Orthopsychiatry*, 36, 492–501, (1966).

Poznanski, E., and J. P. Zrull. "Childhood depression: Clinical characteristics of overtly depressed children." *Archives of General Psychiatry*, 23, 8–15, (1970).

Proctor, J. T. "Hysteria in Childhood." *American Journal of Orthopsychiatry*, 28, 394–407, (1958).

Quay, H. C. "Dimensions of personality in delinquent boys as inferred from the factor analysis of case history data." *Child Development*, 36, 215–220, (1965).

Redl, F., and D. Wineman. *The Aggressive Child*. Glencoe, Ill.: Free Press, 1957.

Reiser, D. E. "Observations of delinquent behavior in very young children." *Journal of the American Academy of Child Psychiatry*, 2, 50–65, (1963).

Rexford, E. "Children, child psychiatry and our brave new world." *Archives of General Psychiatry*, 20, 25–37, (1969).

Rexford, E., and S. van Amerongen. "The influence of unsolved maternal oral conflicts upon impulsive acting out in young children." *American Journal of Orthopsychiatry*, 27, 75–85, (1957).

Rie, H. E. "Depression in childhood: A survey of some pertinent contributions." *Journal of the American Academy of Child Psychiatry*, 5, 653–685, (1966).

Rie, H. E. "Historical perspective of concepts of child psychopathology," in H.E. Rie, ed., *Perspectives in Childhood Psychopathology*, pp. 3–50. Chicago: Aldine-Atherton, 1971.

Rie, H.E. "Hyperactivity in children." *American Journal of Diseases of Children*, 130, 783–789, (1975).

Rimland, B. *Infantile Autism*. New York: Appleton-Century-Crofts, 1964.

Robins, L. N. *Deviant Children Grown Up*. Baltimore: Williams & Wilkins, 1966.

Rock, N. L. "Conversion reactions in childhood: A clinical study on childhood neuroses." *Journal of the American Academy of Child Psychiatry*, 10, 65–93, (1971).

Rutter, M. "The influence of organic and emotional factors on the origins, nature, and outcomes of childhood psychosis." *Developmental Medicine and Child Neurology*, 7, 518–528, (1965).

——*Helping Troubled Children*. New York: Plenum, 1975.

——"The development of autism," in S. Chess and A. Thomas, eds., *Annual Review of Child Psychiatry and Child Development, 1975*, pp. 327–356. New York: Brunner/Mazel, 1976.

Rutter, M., D. Shaffer, and M. Shepherd. "Preliminary communication: an evaluation of the proposal for a multi-axial classification of child psychiatric disorders." *Psychological Medicine*, 3, 244–250, (1973).

Salzman, L. *The Obsessive Personality*. New York: Science House, 1968.

Sameroff, A. J. "Early influences on development: Fact or fancy?" in S. Chess and A. Thomas, eds., *Annual Review of Child Psychiatry and Child Development, 1976*, pp. 3–33. New York: Brunner/Mazel, 1977.

Sameroff, A. J., and M. J. Chandler. "Reproductive risk and the continuum of caretaking casualty," in F. D. Horowitz, ed., *Review of Child Development Research*, vol. 4, pp. 187–244. Chicago: University of Chicago Press, 1975.

Sameroff, A. J., and M. Zax. "Schizotaxia revisited: Model issues in the etiology of schizophrenia." *American Journal of Orthopsychiatry*, 43, 744–754, (1973).

Sandler, J. and W. G. Joffe. "Notes on obsessional manifestations in children." *Psychoanalytic Study of the Child*, 20, 425–438, (1965).

Scarpitti, F. R., E. Murray, S. Dinitz, and W. C. Reckless. "The 'good' boy in a high delinquency area: Four years later." *American Sociological Review*, 25, 555–558, (1960).

Sheldon, W. H. *Varieties of Delinquent Youth.* New York: Harper and Row, 1949.

Simmons, J. E. *Psychiatric Examination of Children*, Philadelphia: Lea and Febiger, 1969.

Sperling, M. "Equivalents of depression in children." *Journal of the Hillside Hospital*, 8, 138–148, (1959).

Sroufe, L. A. "Drug treatment of children with behavior problems," in F. D. Horowitz, ed., *Review of Child Development Research*, vol. 4, pp. 347–408. Chicago: University of Chicago Press, 1975.

Thomas, A., S. Chess, and H. Birch. *Temperament and Behavior Disorders in Children.* New York: New York University Press, 1968.

Toolan, J. M. "Depression in children and adolescents." *American Journal of Orthopsychiatry*, 32, 404–415, (1962).

Treffert, D. A. "Epidemiology of infantile autism." *Archives of General Psychiatry*, 22, 431–438, (1970).

Vogel, E. F., and N. W. Bell. "The emotionally disturbed child as the family scapegoat," in N. W. Bell and E. F. Vogel, eds., *A Modern Introduction to the Family*, pp. 382–397. Glencoe, Ill.: Free Press, 1960.

Waldfogel, S., J. C. Coolidge, and P. B. Hahn. "The development, meaning and management of school phobia." *American Journal of Orthopsychiatry*, 27, 754–789, (1957).

Werry, J. S. "Childhood psychosis," in H. C. Quay and J. S. Werry, eds., *Psychopathological Disorders of Childhood*, pp. 83–121. New York: Wiley, 1972.

———"Studies on the hyperactive child. IV: An empirical analysis of the minimal brain dysfunction syndrome." *Archives of General Psychiatry*, 19, 9–16, (1968).

Willerman, L. "Social aspects of minimal brain dysfunction." *Annals of the New York Academy of Sciences*, 205, 164–172, (1973).

Winnicott, D. W. "The theory of the parent-infant relationship," in D. W. Winnicott, ed., *The Maturational Processes and the Facilitating Environment*, pp. 37–55. New York: International Universities Press, 1965. [Originally published in 1960]

———"Psychotherapy of character disorders," in D. W. Winnicott, ed., *The Maturational Processes and the Facilitating Environment*, pp. 203–216. New York: International Universities Press, 1965. [Originally published in 1963]

CHAPTER 22

Developmental Variations in Relation to Minimal Brain Dysfunction

Ronald S. Illingworth

DEVELOPMENTAL VARIATIONS AND MINIMAL BRAIN DYSFUNCTION

Felix qui potuit rerum cognoscere causas.[1] The last three words—*rerum cognoscere causas*— form the motto of the University of Sheffield, England. The word *causas* is plural, implying that conditions may have a multifactorial origin. Many doctors feel that once they have put a name to a condition, or applied the adjective idiopathic to it, they know all about it. But if for instance a previously well child, presenting a difficult diagnostic problem, is found to have anaphylactoid purpura or histiocytosis X, one should want to know what has caused him to develop it—to learn the causes.

So it is with the so-called minimal brain dysfunction syndrome. It has become synonymous with minimal brain damage, implying that the cause of the child's symptoms are understood. A pediatrician in a foreign country told me of the frequency with which he sees children with neuro-vegetative dystonia: this included many symptoms which others ascribe to minimal brain dysfunction—a diagnosis which I never make, because to me the words are meaningless.

Most symptoms are the end result of a wide variety of pathological or physiological processes—often operating through a final common pathway reached by the interaction of numerous correlated factors, often with a final trigger which precipitates symptoms. For instance there are numerous causes of convulsions, but convulsions due to completely different causes may be identical in character. A final trigger, such as a flickering television screen, may precipitate the first fit.

All children are different. They differ in all aspects of development. Probably all the symptoms of the so-called MBD syndrome are developmental variations. The purpose of this chapter is to discuss the causes of developmental variations, beginning with relevant prenatal, perinatal, and postnatal factors, and then to discuss variations in the individual fields of development, with particular reference to difficulties in establishing the diagnosis and prognosis—for it is easy to make a gloomy prognosis, only to be found later to have been completely wrong. I shall not discuss advanced development. I shall try to show how these causes of variations in development overlap, and how delayed maturation, in one form or another, is an important factor in almost all the variations. The variations to be discussed include delay in most aspects of development and the principal features

---

[1]*Fortunate is he who can discover the causes of things.* Virgil. *Georgics II*, 490.

of the so-called minimal brain dysfunction syndrome. I shall suggest that most of the symptoms of this syndrome are merely developmental variations with numerous associated and correlated factors, leading through a final common pathway to the symptoms under discussion.

RELEVANT PRENATAL AND PERINATAL FACTORS

In this section I shall summarize those prenatal factors which are relevant to the subject of developmental variations. Table 22–1 lists some of the factors.

Drugs taken in pregnancy deserve a special mention. Forfar and Nelson (1973) in a survey of 911 randomly selected mothers, found that 82% were taking prescribed drugs, averaging 4 per mother; 65% nonprescribed drugs, averaging 1.5 per mother. We know much more about the short-term effects of drugs than we do about long-term effects. Smoking in pregnancy not only lowers the size of the fetus and reduces physical growth in the first few years, but also may cause learning problems (Davie, Butler, and Goldstein, 1972; Butler and Goldstein, 1973). Heroin addiction in pregnancy may lead to overactivity in the infant, poor concentration, tremors, and irritability at least for a year (Wilson, Desmond, and Verniaud, 1973).

There is controversy about the role of psychological factors in pregnancy. It is reasonable to suggest that an unpleasant pregnancy, such as one with hyperemesis, or one with excessive worry about the viability of the fetus, or a very difficult delivery, might affect a mother's attitude toward her child for years. Several works have related psychological stress in pregnancy to psychological problems in the child (Stott, 1962; Taft and Goldfarb, 1964; Pollack and Woerner, 1967; Werner, et al., 1967).

Malnutrition in pregnancy reduces the weight of the fetus and interferes with brain growth. The cerebellum begins growth later than the rest of the brain and completes its growth sooner (Dobbing, 1975). Malnutrition in late pregnancy may affect the number of neurones in the cerebellum and lead to later clumsiness. Malnutrition reduces the overall brain size, the number of brain cells, the lipid content, and enzyme activity causing intellectual deficits, clumsiness, and overactivity in later years.

Low Birth Weight

It is inadequate to relate developmental variations to low birth weight. One must try to determine the reasons for preterm delivery or for the infant being small for dates. The factors preceding these two conditions overlap. They are mainly:

- Unknown factors.
- Genetic factors, including familial tendencies for low birth-weight babies, chromosomal abnormalities.
- Malnutrition and poverty, mixed social factors; advanced maternal age, poor antenatal care.
- Placental insufficiency.
- Toxemia.
- Antepartum hemorrhage.

Table 22–1. Relevant Prenatal Factors

Factors	Association
Genetic	Metabolic diseases; intellectual potential; personality; multiple pregnancy; low birth-weight babies; chromosomal and other diseases.
Social	
Older mother	Mongols; CNS anomalies; multiple pregnancy; preterm delivery; Klinefelter syndrome; congenital heart disease; hare lip and cleft palate.
Older father	Congenital deafness; craniostenosis; CNS deformities; achondroplasia.
Parity	First born—more patent ductus.
Spacing of births	Wider spacing increases mean IQ.
Illegitimacy	Psychological problems.
Parental upbringing and intelligence	Effect on child management.
Poverty and malnutrition	Effect on fetal brain. Small fetus. Predisposition to hypoglycemia.
Seasonal	Certain congenital anomalies, e.g. spina bifida. Multiple pregnancies started in Lapland summer.
Geographical	Incidence of anomalies, e.g. anencephaly. Multiple pregnancy.
Infections	Abnormalities.
Irradiation	Abnormalities.
Intrauterine factors	Abnormalities.
Hyperemesis	
Placentation	
Antepartum hemorrhage	
Relative infertility	
Phenylketonuria	
Premature labor	
Postmaturity	
Abnormality of placenta	
Toxemia	Cerebral palsy; premature labor; small for dates; myopia; later overactivity and learning problems.
Multiple pregnancy	Abnormal delivery; hypoglycemia in second of twins; speech delay.
Drugs taken	
Smoking	Small size; defective physical growth after birth: retardation in reading and mathematics (Butler and Goldstein, 1973).
Alcohol	Fetal alcohol syndrome and clumsiness; mental retardation; tremors.
Diazepam	Elevated serum bilirubin in neonate, with possible results. Irritability, possible effect on infant-mother bonding.
Oxytocin	Elevated serum bilirubin in neonate, with possible results.

Table 22–1.   Relevant Prenatal Factors (con't.)

Factors	Association
Warfarin	Microcephaly; punctate epiphyseal dysplasia; agenesis of corpus callosum; optic atrophy; nasal hypoplasia.
Antidiabetic drugs	Hypoglycemia.
Phenothiazines	Newborn tremors; difficulty in sucking and swallowing; hypertonia.

Phenytoin
Sulphonamides
    Vitamin K
    Salicylates
	Mental subnormality.
	Elevated serum bilirubin in newborn.

Quinine,
    Streptomycin
    Kanamycin
    Gentamicin
    Neomycin
	Deafness.

Anesthetic and
    analgesic drugs in
    labor
	Predispose to anoxia.

- Artificial induction of labor.
- Rubella syndrome and other infections or illnesses in pregnancy.
- Smoking in pregnancy.

   The outlook for the low birth-weight baby is now greatly better than it was 10 or 20 years ago, but the reasons for the improvement are uncertain: they include fetal monitoring, the prevention or better treatment of anoxia, hypogycemia and hyperbilirubinemia, and the prevention of hypothermia and of malnutrition. The outlook is now so much better that much of the previous work on prognosis is irrelevant and only a few papers will be mentioned. Dugald Baird (1959), in his Aberdeen study of 363 primiparae, found a striking excess of low IQ scores in the mothers of babies giving birth to low birth-weight babies: mixed social factors were probably relevant. Douglas (1960) in a long-term study found that low birth-weight babies compared unfavorably with matched controls in mental ability, school achievement, and concentration. Lubcheno, et al., (1963) studied 94 children at around 10 years of age, whose birth weight had been 1500g or less. Even with normal intelligence they frequently experienced difficulty at school, especially in reading and mathematics. Weiner, et al., (1965, 1968) compared 417 low birth-weight children with 405 matched controls, the former were impaired in comprehension, abstract reasoning, and maturity of speech when social classes were equated. Fitzhardinge and Steven (1962) followed 96 small-for-dates babies and found a high incidence of overactivity, poor concentration, clumsiness, and learning problems; Drillien (1972) followed 300 babies weighing 2000g or less, and

Table 22–2. Side Effects of Drugs in Relation to Behavior

Side Effects

Drugs	Aggressiveness	Ataxia, clumsiness	Color vision	Concentration	Confusion	Convulsions	Deafness	Depression	Drowsiness	Dysarthria	Dysphagia	Excitement	Hallucinations	Insomnia	Involuntary movements, tremors, etc.	Irritability	Lachrymose	Memory impaired	Mental deterioration	Myopia	Overactivity	Slow thought	Tics	Vision impaired
Acetazolamide					X							X			X					X				
Actinomycin D						X																		
Alcohol			X									X												
Aminophylline					X																			
Amitriptyline		X			X	X																		
Amphetamine					X							X	X	X	X						X			
Ampicillin						X																		
Antiepileptics	X	X						X										X						
Antihistamines	X	X	X		X			X				X			X									
Antimitotics																								X
Barbiturates	X																X				X			
Bromides			X				X					X				X					X			
Cannabis												X												
Capreomycin		X				X																		
Carbamazepine				X	X																			X
Cephalexin				X																				
Cephalosporins															X									
Chlorambutol																								X
Chloramphenicol																								X
Chlordiazepoxide	X	X			X			X				X				X					X			
Chloroquine					X	X									X									X
Chlorpromazine					X																			
Clonazepam	X	X		X				X	X			X		X										
Colistin	X						X																	
Corticosteroids					X																X			X
Cotrimoxazole					X		X																	
Cyclopentolate	X				X																			
Diazeoxide															X									
Diazepam	X	X		X	X			X	X			X			X									
Digoxin			X		X																			
Diphenoxylate	X				X				X			X												
Ephedrine												X		X										
Erythromycin							X																	
Ethacrynic acid							X																	
Ethambutol			X																					
Ethionamide			X																					
Ethosuccimide			X																X					
Fenfluramine	X	X						X							X									
Fenfluramine withdrawal									X										X					
Frusemide							X																	
Gentamicin							X																	
Griseofulvin			X									X												
Haloperidol								X		X					X									
Hyoscine			X							X														
Ibuprofen						X																		
Imipramine		X			X			X				X	X	X	X									

526

Table 22–2.   Side Effects of Drugs in Relation to Behavior (con't.)

Drugs	Aggressiveness	Ataxia, clumsiness	Color vision	Concentration	Confusion	Convulsions	Deafness	Depression	Drowsiness	Dysarthria	Dysphagia	Excitement	Hallucinations	Insomnia	Involuntary movements, tremors, etc.	Irritability	Lachrymose	Memory impaired	Mental deterioration	Myopia	Overactivity	Slow thought	Tics	Vision impaired
Indomethacin		X			X		X		X															X
Isoniazid						X																		X
Konamycin							X																	
LSD													X											
Medroxyprogesterone								X																
Mepacrine					X							X												
Meprobamate		X							X															
Methaqualone															X									
Methimazole									X							X								
Metoclopromide						X				X	X				X									
Monoamine oxidase inhibitors					X																			
Nalidixic acid					X			X																X
Neomycin							X																	
Niclosamide		X											X											
Nitrofurantoin					X							X					X							
Nitrozepam	X	X			X				X			X												
Nortryptyline									X			X												
PAS									X															X
Phenobarbitone												X		X	X						X			
Phenothiazines						X		X	X						X									X
Phenytoin					X					X					X						X			
Piperazine		X			X																			
Polymyxin		X																						
Primidone					X					X					X						X			
Propranolal								X																
Propylthiourea								X																
Pyrimethamine						X																		
Quinine								X																
Rifampicin								X																
Salicylates								X																
Solvent sniffing		X										X												
Stimulant drugs												X											X	
Streptomycin		X			X																			
Sulfonamides																				X				
Sulthiame					X					X					X									
Terbutaline															X									
Tetracycline																				X				X
Throxidone																	X							
Throxin																	X							
Tobramycin							X																	
Tranquilizers								X																
Tricyclic drugs	X											X									X			
Trifluoperazine																					X			
Vincristine		X					X						X											
Viomycin							X																	

the prognosis was better if the cause of the low birth weight could be related to late pregnancy. Francis-Williams and Davies (1974) applying Wechsler, Gestalt, and reading tests to 105 children who weighed 1500g or less, found that 1 in 5 had learning difficulties. The mean IQ of those whose birth weight corresponded to the duration of gestation was 99.2, as compared with 92.0 for the small-for-dates children. Davies and Stewart (1975) discussed the remarkable fall in the incidence of cerebral palsy and visual and auditory defects when there is good intensive care of the newborn, but the high incidence of CNS defects in infants who had been given positive pressure ventilation is disturbing (Fitzhardinge, et al., 1976; Marriage and Davies, 1977). Neligan, et al., (1976) confirmed that the prognosis was worse for the small-for-dates babies than for the other low-birth-weight infants.

There is abundant evidence that there has been an important relationship between low birth weight and subsequent developmental variations. Time will tell whether present-day methods of intensive care will lessen that relationship.

Anoxia

It is irrational to ascribe developmental variations to anoxia at birth, instead of considering the causes of the anoxia. These include insufficiency or separation of the placenta, toxemia, hypertension, cord tightly round the neck or prolapsed, anesthetics and analgesics, and an underlying cerebral defect in the fetus. Long-term intrauterine anoxia is more harmful to the fetus than acute periods of more complete anoxia during birth (Scott, 1976). For the same reason the prognosis is better if there is a known cause of acute anoxia, than if there is no known cause—that cause may be a structural brain defect.

The difficulty of defining and measuring anoxia and its duration somewhat negates the value of follow-up studies. In general the outlook for normal development is good (Benaron, et al., 1960; Shipe, Vandenberg, and Williams 1968), especially after the early years (Corah, et al., 1965), but these children are at risk of difficulties, such as overactivity, poor concentration, visuo-spatial and learning problems, though the risk is probably only a small one. Long-term follow-up studies alone are of value in this connection.

Famous persons who suffered severe anoxia at birth included Thomas Hardy, Rousseau, Samuel Johnson (said to have been born more dead than alive), and Voltaire who was born half dead, but was slapped to life by the nurses—he was given 4 days to live but survived for 84 years. Picasso was thought to be stillborn and was given up for dead, but his uncle arrived at the vital moment and resuscitated him. Perhaps some cynics who study Picasso's sketches in his cubist phase (such as "The First Steps") might conclude that he had some residual visuo-spatial problems.

Birth Injury

"Birth is the most dangerous experience to which most individuals are ever exposed" (Towbin, 1971). But the importance of brain damage at birth, as a cause of developmental variations, is exaggerated. It is impossible to prove by neurological examination or psychological tests or other special investigation that a living child's handicap is due to brain damage at birth. Yet one commonly hears that a child's mental subnormality or cerebral palsy is due to brain damage at birth because there was an abnormal delivery, such as a breech presentation: but a fetus presents as a breech because he was small-for-dates, because of placental insufficiency or other factors, or because there was another abnormality. The incidence of breech delivery in children with meningomyelocele is five times greater than in the whole population (Stark and Drummond, 1971). Braun, Jones, and Smith (1975) related breech delivery not only to spina bifida, but to congenital dislocation of the hip, hydrocephalus, anencephaly, and familial dysautonomia. Even if there is a cerebral hemorrhage, the cause may be prenatal. Emminger (1956) in his pathological studies suggested that fetal brain maldevelopment was the primary cause of rupture of the tentorium or falx cerebri or tentorial vein. I have repeatedly been impressed by the fact that when one follows the progress of infants who had an extremely difficult delivery, they do not have cerebral palsy. Others (Keith, Norval, and Hunt, 1953; Amiel-Tison, 1969) have made the same observation.

Abnormal delivery is related to social factors. It was shown in Aberdeen that a low IQ score in children who had experienced an abnormal delivery was related to social factors rather than to the abnormal delivery per se.

In the case of cerebral palsy and spina bifida there is often evidence of reproductive inefficiency before and after the affected birth, as shown by a longer than usual period of infertility—or an increased fetal loss (Chefetz, 1965). Furthermore the high incidence of other anomalies provides supportive evidence of a prenatal cause for a handicap. In my study of 702 children with cerebral palsy seen by me in Sheffield, 53 (7.5%) had a major congenital anomaly, which is far higher than the incidence in the whole population; of 1068 mentally subnormal children seen by me, excluding mongols, cretins, and children with hydrocephalus or cerebral palsy, the incidence of major anomalies was 29.3%. Cohen and Diner (1970) showed that dental enamel defects are definitive chronological markers of the probable date of the insult to the developing fetus.

That a child's brain is sometimes damaged at birth cannot be denied, but as a cause of developmental variations the importance should not be exaggerated.

Neonatal Convulsions

The relationship between neonatal convulsions and subsequent development must depend on the cause or preceding factors. The principal preceding factors are:

- Hypocalcemia, perhaps with hypomagnesemia.
- Hypoglycemia.
- Cerebral edema, anoxia, or hemorrhage.
- Cerebral malformations.
- Infections.

Rare causes include:

- The narcotic withdrawal syndrome.
- Leucinosis.
- Kernicterus.

- Pyridoxine dependency.
- Hyponatremia.
- Hypernatremia.
- Hypersarcosinemia.
- Fructosemia.
- Galactosemia.
- Homocystinosis.

Of those hypocalcemia, commonly presenting around the fifth day, carries the best prognosis, but it occasionally presents in the first day or two in connection with low birth weight, placental insufficiency, cerebral malformation, anoxia, birth injury, or maternal diabetes (Brown, Cockburn, and Forfar, 1972), in which case there is a higher risk of developmental variations in later months or years. If the EEG is normal, the outlook for the future is good; if it is abnormal, there is a considerable risk of future handicap (Rose and Lombroso, 1970).

Hypoglycemia

The causes of neonatal hypoglycemia are often uncertain: it may be related to maternal diabetes, maternal malnutrition or toxemia (Raivio, 1958), or to fetal cerebral defects. It is common in the smaller of twins. Hence it is inadequate to ascribe subsequent mental or other handicap to the hypoglycemia, or to compare the prognosis of asymptomatic and symptomatic hypoglycemia, without attempting to define its cause. Apart from underlying causes, hypoglycemia certainly causes brain damage, including infantile spasms.

Postmaturity

The danger of postmaturity is well recognized (Lovell, 1973), and future long-term studies of its effects are unlikely because of the ease with which labor can now be induced. Butler and Alberman (1969) found that a gestation period of over 42 weeks was associated with an increased incidence of reading problems at the age of six. Wagner and Arndt (1968) found that postmaturity was intrauterine anoxia and placental insufficiency.

Infant-Mother Bonding

Many are belatedly realizing that the establishment of a firm bond between infant and mother may depend both on physical contact between mother and baby as soon as he is born and on the early mother-infant interaction. Failure to establish this bond may affect a child's development for months or years (Klaus and Kennell, 1976). If animals, such as sheep or goats, are not allowed to lick their young as soon as they are born, they will reject their young even though they are returned within three or four hours of birth. Some mothers feel the urge to establish physical contact with their baby as soon as he is born. Therefore they want to be conscious at the time of delivery, so that they can put him to the breast. There is evidence that if a mother puts her baby to the breast as soon as he is born, she is more likely to breast feed him (Chateau and Wiberg, 1977). The bond is further established when the baby begins to gaze at her intently as she talks to him and soon after that to smile at her.

Fanaroff, Kennell, and Klaus (1972), Lynch and Roberts (1977) and others have shown that newborn babies managed in an intensive care unit are more likely than others to suffer child abuse later. It has long been the practice at the Jessop Obstetric Hospital, Sheffield, for mothers to tend to their own babies in the intensive care unit; babies not in the intensive care unit are placed at the mother's bedside day and night, so that the mother can pick the baby up when she wants, feeding on demand.

Prolonged separation of an ill or seriously handicapped child, such as one with a meningomyelocele, may lead to rejection with consequent long-term results. I was once asked to see parents of a child who had been kept in a hospital for his first nine months on account of congenital abnormalities. When told that they could take him home, they refused; I was expected to remind them of their responsibilities. They said that they had been heavily pressured to take him. They were astonished when I said that I fully understood their reaction. Freedman (1975) described the problem of a child with an immunological defect who for the first 27 months had been brought up in a plastic bubble to prevent infection; isolated from all contact with anyone, he had never felt a person's skin or an embrace.

The abnormal baby who is apathetic, overactive, irritable, constantly crying, blind, or autistic and therefore unresponsive, may fail to establish the bond with his mother, with consequent rejection and long-term results (Prechtl, 1963).

Many now feel that the establishment of this bond between mother and child immediately after birth, and then in the first few days, is important for the child's future emotional development; failure to establish it may lead to developmental retardation.

SOME POSTNATAL FACTORS

The Quality of the Home: Environmental Factors, Nutrition

A preschool child's basic needs are physical (especially nutrition and the prevention of infection and serious accidents), emotional (especially love and security, wise loving discipline, a good example, good moral values, the gradual acquisition of independence, and the avoidance of unnecessary restraints), and intellectual (the provision of play material with the opportunity and encouragement to learn). At school age additional needs include interest in and recognition of the importance of education; avoidance of unnecessary absence from school; ambition for the child's success, but not overambition which demands more than his intellectual endowment will permit.

Insecurity is caused by unkindness, rejection, sarcasm, criticism, disapproval, punitive discipline or lack of discipline, overprotection, prolonged separation from a parent, severe illness at home, bereavement, domestic discord, alcoholism at home, financial and other socioeconomic problems at home. Insecurity in its broadest sense is the basis of numerous behavior problems such as aggressiveness, nail-biting, thumb-sucking, head-banging, excessive masturbation, excessive fears, shyness or jealousy, regression to infantile behavior, destructiveness, cruelty to animals, bullying, stealing, lying, truancy, incontinence of urine or feces, stuttering, tics, and overactivity—symptoms sometimes included in the syndrome of minimal brain dysfunction. Prolonged emotional deprivation may lead not only to an inability to give or receive affection, but also to language deficiencies and to impairment of abstract thought and general comprehension. It leads to underachievement and is a potent cause of antisocial behavior and delinquency. It is now thought that much of the damage done by emotional deprivation in the first three years is reversible if there is no further deprivation and the child is given love and security and the home is free from domestic discord (Bowlby, et al., 1956; Rutter, 1971).

Proper nutrition is necessary for brain growth not only in utero, but in the early months after birth. There is evidence of a sensitive or critical period for brain growth (and for physical growth), so that failure to thrive for any reason, if not corrected by the time of the critical period, perhaps 2 or 3 years of age, will permanently damage the brain, affecting its weight and size (and therefore the head circumference), the development of cells and enzyme systems, and intellectual potential (Stotch and Smythe, 1967; Winick and Rosso, 1969). Birch, et al., (1971) found that at school age the mean IQ of 37 children who had experienced severe malnutrition in infancy was 68.5, while that of their siblings was 81.5. Various workers have related early malnutrition to learning problems in later childhood (Klein, Forbes, and Nader 1975), but the difficulty in interpreting their findings lies in the fact that malnutrition is usually associated with other adverse factors in the way of poor homes and other socioeconomic deficiencies.

The Sensitive or Critical Period

The sensitive period is that stage of development at which a stimulus is best applied to elicit a particular response; the critical period is that stage of development beyond which the stimulus will no longer elicit the response. There are innumerable examples of this in the animal kingdom. For instance if red squirrels are not given nuts to crack by a certain stage of development, they will never learn to crack them. In a child if a congenital cataract is not removed by a certain age, he will never see. If a squint is not corrected by a certain age, the squinting eye will be permanently blind. If a deaf child is not taught to speak by a certain age, it will be impossible to teach him. If a cleft palate is not repaired by a certain age, the child will never learn to speak well. In the section on dysphagia, I mention the fact that if a child is not given solids to chew when he has recently acquired the ability, at six or seven months unless he is mentally subnormal, it will be extremely difficult to get him to take solids later. Two of us (Illingworth and Lister, 1964) described nine children in whom this problem had arisen: Madame Montessori based her teaching methods on the sensitive period—teaching children subjects as soon as they were developmentally ready to learn them—and so at a time when they would enjoy learning them. She termed this maturational readiness. It has been said that if children are not given appropriate play material in the preschool years, it will be difficult for them to learn when they reach school, but there is disagreement on this. It is reasonable to suggest that every child has his own sensitive period for learning each subject; hence ideally the curriculum should be adapted to each child's needs in every subject, as it is in fact in British Public (fee-paying) Schools.

African natives commonly have certain characteristic visuo-spatial deficiencies. Vernon (1969) described the difficulties in Nigerian Ibos. Hudson (1960) described the difficulties in pictorial depth perception experienced by South African miners and their children. Biescheuvel (1963, 1967) thought that the difficulty experienced by the Bantus in interpreting pictorial and diagrammatic material, making it difficult for them to learn science and technology and to understand diagrams, was due to lack of appropriate stimulation in childhood; it might also be related to early malnutrition. Biescheuvel wrote that:

> Research on perception and psychomotor skills shows that unless the required experience is provided at the appropriate maturational stages, ability potentials will never be fully realised, despite intensive training at a later stage.

He added that there is evidence that the critical period comes at a very early stage of childhood:

> The data seem to suggest that when for one reason or another, children only learn how to look at pictures at a much later stage than is customary in advanced Western societies, they never quite reach the degree of facility that is normal for Western culture groups.

Bantus are said to have a poor color sense, but to excel in sound patterns.

We do not know exactly when the sensitive or critical period is for each skill or subject which is to be learned. It must be expected to vary from child to child, from subject to subject. But it is highly relevant to later learning problems.

Biochemical Factors

Recent knowledge is providing a new insight into the biochemical basis of behavior (Shaw, 1973). In adult depressive and maniacal states there are alterations in tryptamine excretion and in intracellular potassium and sodium. Eccleston (1973) suggested that the tricyclic antidepressants may potentiate biogenic amine transmitters after their release; monoamine oxidase inhibitors may prevent the breakdown of the neurotransmitters 5-hydroxytryptamine, noradrenaline, and dopamine by monoamine oxidase. Wender and Wender (1976) suggested that the fact that overactive children respond to drugs which affect the brain monoamines and respond to the tricyclic antidepressants which have no effect on normal children, suggests a genetically transmitted variant in monoamine metabolism. Shaywitz, Cohen, and Bowers (1977) demonstrated changes in brain monoamine activity in these children by estimating the CSF homovanillic acid and 5-hydroxyindoleacetic acid. Rats, when dopamine depleted, exhibit increased motor activity. There is a close similarity between the symptoms of amphetamine addiction and schizophrenia, in which much is now being learned about biochemical changes.

Conners, et al., (1976) conducted a double-blind trial of 115 overactive children on an ordinary diet and on a diet from which artificial coloring matter and flavors had been eliminated. Those on the special diet were found by teachers and parents to be significantly less overactive. The commonly used yellow tartrazine coloring agent may sensitize children and cause chronic urticaria, wheezing, or angioneurotic edema (Delaney, 1946). Further investigation of the role of food additives in relation to behavior are indicated.

It is obviously critical to determine whether a child is responding to medicines at the time of diagnosis.

The Relationship of Certain Handicaps to Developmental Delay

Physical, intellectual, or emotional handicaps (or handicaps in any given sphere) have a profound effect on development in other spheres.

Epilepsy may cause considerable psychological disturbance and therefore interfere with progress at school. The child may feel different from others—and this is particularly important at puberty and adolescence. He may feel isolated from others; he may be afraid of having a fit; he may feel inadequate and frustrated. He suffers from the attitudes of others particularly if the teachers treat him differently from other children, preventing him from taking part in sport, such as swimming. The effect of the epilepsy depends not only on its cause, but also on the site of the epileptic focus (Stores, 1971). A focus in the left temporal lobe may delay reading, especially in boys; a temporal lobe focus in the hemisphere dominant for speech may impair verbal ability, learning, and memory; a lesion in the nondominant hemisphere may cause visuo-spatial problems; a focus in the centroencephalic area may impair concentration. Subictal activity and petit mal status both impair concentration. The effect of anoxia in major fits may itself impair intellectual functioning. Ounsted, Lindsay, and Norman (1966) wrote that the worst complication of temporal lobe epilepsy is overactivity. The drugs used for treatment themselves cause symptoms similar to those resulting from the epilepsy: phenobarbitone may impair memory and cognitive functioning and cause aggressiveness, insomnia, irritability, and difficult behavior. Ethosuccimide may impair verbal ability

Head injuries are common in children, but sequelae are rare. Otto (1960) wrote that the salient factors which will decide the occurrence or severity of sequelae are mainly the quality of the home, the child's previous personality, prolonged hospital stay, and parental attitudes. Nylander and Hjern (1964), in a study of 305 children with head injuries, found that 10% had mental sequelae and all came from disturbed homes. They added that children with behavior disorders were more likely to suffer head injuries and were more likely to experience sequelae. The usual sequelae are mainly headaches, impaired memory, and concentration.

Anderson (1976) found that the mean IQ of hydrocephalic children was around 80; those children were presumably untreated, for the outlook for those treated promptly by a Spitz-Holter valve is better. Hydrocephalic children tend to be happy and facile, their talkativeness leads to an overestimate of their overall intelligence. Their comprehension and appropriate use of language is poor and there are commonly defects of visuo-spatial function, difficulties with mathematics and writing, and poor concentration (Anderson, 1973).

The mean IQ of boys with the Duchenne type of muscular dystrophy is around 80 (Allen and Rodgin, 1960). It is said that they are more likely than others to have difficulty with reading and mathematics (Worden and Vignos, 1962). The mean IQ of 97 treated children with phenylketonuria, followed to the age of 2.5 years or more was 90.4, compared with a figure of 105 for parents and unaffected siblings

(Hudson, Mordaunt, and Leahy, 1970). Siegel, et al., (1968) compared 13 treated children with 13 controls—matched for age, sex, race and IQ—and found that the children with phenylketonuria were more clumsy and overactive and concentrated less well.

Other handicaps, such as hemophilia, diabetes mellitus, fibrocystic disease of the pancreas, and metabolic diseases requiring a special diet, present particular psychological problems in adolescence, leading to a variety of behavior problems and poor school performance.

DEVELOPMENTAL DELAYS

General Retardation

By far the commonest cause of general retardation is mental subnormality. The mentally subnormal child, who was retarded from birth (or before), is late in all aspects of development, except occasionally gross motor development, sitting and walking, and very rarely sphincter control. The features of mental subnormality include lateness in smiling, responding to sound, visual attention, and eye following; lateness in chewing and in the inhibiting of the mouthing of objects, casting and of slobbering; lateness in speech, sphincter control, and reading. Outstanding and unfortunately unscorable features include defective interest in surroundings, concentration and responsiveness, and frequently aimless overactivity when the child is able to walk. These children are later than other children in growing out of the normal excessive activity of the young child. The head circumference is usually small in relation to the weight because of defective brain growth; there is a high incidence of congenital anomalies. All this suggests that the diagnosis should be easy; so it is, usually, but there are important snares for the unwary. For many years I followed up to school age all babies and young children with unusual development. A few surprises resulted.

The Slow Starter: Overall Delay in Maturation

An occasional child, for no discoverable reason, is uniformly retarded in the early weeks and then makes unexpected progress reaching a low average, average, or superior level. The following four children all had an uneventful delivery after a normal pregnancy:

1. Seen at 13 weeks, she had complete head lag in ventral suspension and on being pulled to the sitting position. She did not follow with her eyes till 17 weeks or smile till 18 weeks, when she "woke up" and made rapid progress. At 25 weeks her head control was that of a 16-week baby. She sat normally at 32 weeks and walked without help at 13 months. At 5 years her IQ was 122 and there was no disability.

2. Seen at 22 months. I wrote to the family doctor:

The immediate impression was that she was normal mentally. Yet she has been backward in all aspects of development. She is not walking or talking. She has no sphincter control and cannot feed herself. She cast one-inch cubes like a 14-month child. But her head is of normal circumference.

She walked without help at 25 months, at 33 months she joined words together and on the simple formboard was at the 36-month level. At 49 months her speech was advanced, she was normal in all respects, and could count up to 130 without error.

3. Seen at 18 months for uniform retardation. I wrote to the family doctor:

I think that he is a normal boy, but I am not quite sure and will see him again in 6 months. The difficulty is that he has been backward in everything. He did not sit till 1 year; he is not nearly walking; he was late in reaching out for objects (9 months) and imitating (bye-bye at 18 months); and he is not holding his arm out to help his mother to dress him. Yet he is a bright little boy, alert, and interested. I think that he is merely a late starter. It is always a difficult diagnosis to make, and time will tell whether I am right.

At 24 months he was speaking in sentences and his performance on the simple formboard was at the 36-months level. At 48 months he was uniformly advanced on all the Gesell tests.

4. This girl took no notice of her surroundings until 26 weeks, when she began to smile: she reached out and got objects at 9 months, began to say single words at 23 months, but at 33 months she was still slobbering and casting objects like a 12- to 15-month baby. She joined words together at 38 months. At school her IQ was 110 and she was normal with no disability except slight clumsiness.

I have records of seven other children, all of whom had a normal full-term delivery, all grossly retarded in the first 6 to 12 months with a developmental quotient of less than 20, who at school age had an IQ of 75 to 90—three had cerebral palsy, but the others had no other disability. Two other children were grossly retarded for several weeks after neonatal convulsions. In one of them the air encephalogram showed a large amount of air on the surface of the brain, suggesting cortical atrophy. He was discharged with a diagnosis of severe mental deficiency. But after 4 months he began to catch up, at 10 months he was normal, and at 9 years his IQ was 122, he had no disability, and no further fits. The other 9-year-old had an IQ of 88, again with no disability. Two further children had a proved cerebral hemorrhage in the new-born period and were grossly retarded in the early weeks. They caught up and both had a normal IQ at school age, but one with an IQ of 100 had a single fit at 8 years of age, but no further ones in the next five years, after which I did not see her again. Three other children were grossly retarded for several months after encephalitis in the first 4 months, so that a confident diagnosis of mental deficiency was made. All proved to be normal by school age.

Infantile spasms, characteristically developing at around 5 or 6 months of age with the EEG picture of hypsarrhythmia, are the end result of about 20 different diseases mainly structural (cortical defects, neurodermatoses), metabolic (phenylketonuria, hypoglycemia, lipidoses, pyridoxine dependency), infective (toxoplasmosis, cytomegalovirus, syphilis, chickenpox or measles, encephalitis, immunization against pertussis or smallpox), and cerebral vascular. The causes are so diverse that it is irrational to investigate the subsequent intellectual prognosis after ACTH, nitrazepam, or other treatment as if it were a single condition; the prognosis must depend on the cause, but the cause cannot always be determined. I followed a boy who started to have infantile spasms of undetermined origin at the age of 8 months. He was grossly retarded when I saw him. At 13 months he was unable to chew and made no attempt to sit or reach out for objects. He walked without help at 19 months, joined words at 36 months; at 7 years he had had no further fits in the previous 6 years and his IQ was 100, but he had severe visuo-spatial and learning problems in a normal school.

Considerable retardation may result from emotional deprivation and when the pediatrician is consulted about a retarded infant who has suffered such deprivation, it is difficult for him to decide how much of his retardation is of environmental origin. I have assessed many hundreds of babies for adoption, and in the early days I was frequently faced with the problem of emotional deprivation when I assessed them at 6 months, for then illegitimate babies were placed in an institution and placed for adoption only after 6 months. Retardation was usual. In the last 15 years or more it has been the British practice to place children in a foster home at the age of about 10 days with a view to adoption, so that the problem no longer arises.

When faced with a generally retarded child, there are several features to be considered in arriving at the prognosis. One must know whether there is a family history of slow maturation. The developmental history may indicate that the child is already catching up. A normal head circumference in relation to the child's weight should make one very cautious about giving a confident bad prognosis. One remembers that a previously normal brain may recover from a cerebral insult. Arnold Gesell's "insurance factors" are of the utmost importance. They consist of the child's alertness, responsiveness, interest in surroundings, concentration (for example trying to get a toy placed out of reach), and the glint in the eyes—all unscorable items, but all items which the experienced pediatrician knows are of much more importance than almost all other aspects of development, especially sitting and walking.

Generalized delay in maturation can well lead a pediatrician to give a hopeless prognosis for a child who will turn out to be average or well above average.

Cerebral Palsy

I have included cerebral palsy in this chapter because of its effect on other aspects of development. Cerebral palsy is of all degrees of severity and of particular relevance to 'minimal brain dysfunction' syndrome are the very mild trivial forms causing no more than slight clumsiness. In the sections on prenatal and natal factors I have discussed some of the preceding factors; other causes are unknown. Cerebral palsy is associated with many handicaps, especially intellectual, visuo-spatial, visual and auditory problems, delay in speech, convulsions, defective concentration and distractibility, obesity in the spastic form (not in the athetoid form), slobbering, and deformities if not prevented (notably dislocation of the hips, shortening of the tendo Achilles). The speech defects are due to low IQ, spasm or incoordination of muscle, partial deafness, and/or the cortical defect.

Cerebral palsy leads to many psychological problems: the result of dependence on others for daily needs (in severe cases); overprotection, rejection, jealousy of normal siblings; jealousy of the affected child on the part of normal siblings because of the favoritism and attention shown to him; attitudes of others; the feeling of being different, having to go to a special school; periods in hospital, prolonged treatment; loneliness; and later sexual problems and the difficulty of obtaining work. Limitation of normal sensory and other stimulation in itself leads to visuo-spatial and other problems. Education may suffer from time devoted to physiotherapy or other treatment.

Parents naturally want to know the prognosis, but it can be very difficult to answer their questions. In the first place developmental testing for intellectual potential can be extremely difficult, and it is easy grossly to underestimate the intelligence, especially in athetoids. Secondly delayed maturation may occur, so that unexpected intellectual improvement occurs. I have mentioned four such cases in the section on general retardation and I shall mention another in the section on swallowing difficulties. Thirdly changes occur in the neurological status. Many affected children develop deformities, if not properly treated, and these add to their problems. It is not commonly realized that, rarely, signs of cerebral palsy may disappear.

The more carefully one examines the new-born baby and young infant, the more conversant one becomes with the wide variations in muscle tone which they exhibit and with the frequency with which apparently abnormal physical signs, including asymmetry, disappear. If a child is grossly spastic and also shows signs of mental subnormality, including a small head circumference in relation to his weight, one can confidently give a bad prognosis: I would be much less confident if there were no signs of mental retardation. The diagnosis of cerebral palsy must never be made on a single sign, but only on a combination of signs. One has several times seen such gross hypertonicity that there is spontaneous limb clonus or a sustained clonus if the sole of the foot is merely touched. A colleague of mine, C. Harvey, showed a child whose clonus had been noted by the mother. The slightest touch on the sole of the foot, particularly in the direction of dorsi-flexion, started prolonged clonus in the whole leg. This disappeared by the age of 5 weeks and the child walked without support at 8 months, having no abnormal neurological signs. This is rare, but I have seen enough examples to enable me to give a good prognosis for normality provided that there are no other abnormal signs. One must always follow such children to make sure that the opinion was correct.

Even unequivocal cerebral palsy may disappear. I have described one such case in the section on dysphagia. I had taken a film record of his neurological signs for teaching purposes, only to find that the signs later disappeared. Another child filmed by me had a severe life spastic hemiplegia with an almost useless left arm. I was able to follow him for 15 years. By the age of 5 or 6 years the arm was normal and from that time until I last saw him at 15 the only remaining abnormal sign was a left extensor plantar response.

In France Thomas André and Madame Saint-Anne Dargassies (1952) described several examples of the disappearance of signs of cerebral palsy, especially spastic hemiplegia. Amiel-Tison (1969) followed 41 babies who had abnormal neurological signs at birth and found that at the age of two to five years 15 were normal. Minkowski (1956) found that 22 of 43 infants with minor neurological abnormalities in the newborn period were subsequently normal, and that 3 of 6 who had gross neurological abnormalities had only trivial signs in later years.

In America Solomons, Holden, and Denhoff (1963) described 12 infants with abnormal neurological signs at 12 months, who had lost all the signs one to three years later. Of those with spastic hemiplegia, 4 of 5 recovered completely.

These cases are rare. It is hoped that future studies will consist of long-term follow-up to exclude visuo-spatial and learning problems in later years.

Sucking and Swallowing Delays: Dysphagia in the Newborn

Neonatal dysphagia is the end result of a wide variety of pathological processes—anatomical, infective, and neuromuscular (Illingworth, 1969). The neuromuscular group is caused by the following conditions:

- Delayed maturation of the swallowing mechanism.
- Incoordination of tongue, soft palate, upper pharynx.
- Cerebral palsy; bulbar or suprabulbar palsy.
- Cranial nerve lesions.
- Mobius syndrome and myotonic dystrophy.
- Prader Willi, Cornelia de Lange, Klippel Feil, Riley's syndrome of familial dysautonomia.
- The hypotonias.
- Myasthenia.
- Unknown.

Nearly all of this neuromuscular group could be termed cerebral dysfunction and ascribed to brain damage. In the great majority of those described in the world literature which I reviewed comprehensively and in my own series of 18 cases, there was a notable absence of birth difficulties, but hydramnios was a common feature, as one would expect. Most are probably examples of delayed maturation of the swallowing mechanism. De Carlo, Tramer, and Startzman (1952) investigated the swallowing mechanism of 100 new-born babies with iodized oil: 13 aspirated the oil in the first 24 hours and 2 continued to aspirate it for 12 days. Avery (1964) noted the frequency with which some new-born babies aspirate their feeds in the first few days only, due to pharyngeal incoordination. Morgan (1956) and others found no naked eye or histological abnormality in the brain at autopsy.

After full neurological and developmental examination as well as special investigation by the visual techniques, such as laryngoscopy, esophagoscopy, X-ray, and cineradiography, it is usually impossible to give a prognosis, unless there is microcephaly, indicating severe mental subnormality. It is very easy to make the mistake of giving a serious prognosis, since many severely affected babies make a full recovery after varying periods, ranging from 2 weeks to 4 years or more (Frank and Gatewood, 1966; Matsaniotis, Karpouzas, and Gregoriou, 1967). Bellmaine, McCredie, and Storey (1972) described a child with pharyngeal incoordination from birth, resulting in recurrent bronchopneumonia, who completely recovered by the age of 3.6 years. Occasionally some incoordination remains, but the child learns to circumvent it by trick movements of the tongue. However severe a bulbar or suprabulbar palsy, recovery may be complete. Here is a case report of a baby seen by me at birth, with severe suprabulbar palsy and spastic quadriplegia, who made a complete recovery. His signs and progress were recorded on film, the follow-up period being 10 years.

The mother had hydramnios. The baby had gross swallowing difficulty from birth, a weak hoarse cry, palatal palsy, hyperextended legs with crossing of legs because of adductor spasm, grossly exaggerated knee jerks, and sustained ankle clonus. The eyes were constantly rolling and there were constant unwanted movements resembling athetosis, though he had spastic quadriplegia. He had to be sucked out every 15 to 20 minutes, required a special nurse day and night (relieved only by the mother), and he had to be tube-fed for 4 months. At 8 weeks he was less spastic and began to smile. At 26 weeks he had to be sucked out only about four times a day. He had begun to transfer objects, but only with the characteristic splaying out of hands typical of spasticity. At 8 months he sat without support. At 11 months he still had to be sucked out three times a day, but by about 15 months sucking out became unnecessary. At 8 years he was clumsy with some tremor, but there were no other signs. On the Goodenough draw-a-man test, the Goddard formboard, and repeating digits he was average. At 10 years there was no disability; he was doing well at school; the palate, speech, and plantar responses were normal; and there was no clumsiness.

Another child had to be tube-fed for 8 months. Cineradiography at 16 months showed incoordination of tongue and swallowing. At 27 months there was no more feeding difficulty and her developmental quotient was 85. At 7 years she was a bright normal girl doing well in a normal class for her age, but was slightly clumsy and without other disability.

Many children with neonatal dysphagia recover completely, and some only partially. It is impossible to predict the prognosis. Those with the Mobius, Riley, or Prader Willi syndromes are expected to lose their dysphagia at varying ages, though continuing to suffer the symptoms of the underlying syndrome. Factors which might militate against complete recovery include bonding difficulties because of prolonged hospitalization and problems arising from the sensitive or critical period. In the first of the two cases described above we caused the mother to take an active part in tube-feeding and sucking out. She was grateful to feel that she had taken a major part in the boy's recovery. The swallowing difficulty may make it difficult or impossible to give the child solid foods to chew at the critical period when the ability has been recently acquired, with resulting problems later.

Delayed Smiling

The age of onset of smiling is an important milestone, though it cannot be defined precisely because it is not an all-or-none feature. Long before a real smile begins, the baby watches his mother intently as she speaks to him, opening and closing his mouth, bobbing his head up and down, and often splaying the toes. Then gradually the smile begins, about a week later he vocalizes as well as smiles. All mentally subnormal children are late in beginning to smile. In a series of 42 mongols I found that the average age of beginning to smile was 17 weeks.

The most common cause of lateness to smile is mental subnormality. Very rarely does it occur as a feature of generalized late maturation in a child who will prove to be normal, but it is unusual for a normal child not to have begun to smile by 8 weeks (corrected, as always for pre-term delivery). The blind child is late in smiling. According to Peifer (1963) if blindness is present at birth, the muscles around the eye (that is the orbicularis oculis, corrugator supercilii, and frontalis muscles) are not involved in a facial expression, but remain rigid and motionless. If the child becomes blind some time after birth, the facial expression is normal.

An autistic child is very late in beginning to smile. A child with myotonic dystrophy or the Mobius syndrome cannot smile; I have seen errors made in assessing such a child as a result. Smiling is late in emotional deprivation. In an examination paper for medical students consisting of multiple short questions, I set the following question, "Discuss the reasons why an eight-week-old baby has not yet begun to smile at his mother?" A student replied, "His mother may be no laughing matter."

The bonding between infant and mother is considerably affected by the baby's responsiveness. Delay in smiling makes this bonding difficult; he responds less to her and so she responds less to him.

Delayed Visual Maturation

Rarely an otherwise normal baby appears to be blind but on ophthalmoscopic examination there is no abnormality and there is no nystagmus. Then in a period of weeks he begins to show evidence of seeing and soon his vision becomes normal. I have termed this delayed visual maturation (Illingworth, 1961). Gordon (1968) used the term visual agnosia; Duke-Elder (1974) used this term for adults who had the "inability to recognise or orientate objects perceived, although the reception of their sensory impression is intact." A search of the literature on the subject was singularly unrewarding. Doyne (1930), on the basis of experience at the Hospital for Sick Children, Great Ormond Street, London, wrote that "In some cases development of sight is only delayed." He described a 3-month-old baby who appeared to be blind and who showed no sign of vision till 7 months; by 18 months vision was normal. Doggart (1957), from the same hospital, referred to other cases and suggested that it was due to delayed myelination of the optic nerve. Jan (1977) in Vancouver, followed a boy who was apparently blind until 6 months of age, when he rapidly recovered and acquired normal vision. At 4 years of age there was some language disability and other perceptual weaknesses.

Here are case reports of two children seen by me.

1. I saw this boy at the age of 3.6 months. His birth weight was 2500g after a normal pregnancy and delivery. There was no significant family history. His parents said the boy could not see: he took no notice of anything, did not focus his eyes and did not smile, and did not watch them as he talked to them. But he had begun to turn his head to sound at 12 weeks and had been vocalizing from 7 weeks.

On examination he looked normal. The head circumference in relation to weight was average. The hands were open. Motor development and manipulation were normal. He took no notice of a bright light, but the pupils reacted normally. There was no nystagmus and on ophthalmoscopy no abnormality was found.

I told the parents that though it was impossible to be sure, the outlook was good and that mental development was normal.

He began to show signs of seeing at 5 months and at 6 months he followed a light or a dangling ring or bell, but not as far as an average baby. He opened his mouth when the bottle approached. At 10 months he made immediate attempts to pick up an 8mm. pellet. In all respects, visual and otherwise, he was now average. At school age, he was normal.

2. This girl had spasmus nutans beginning at 3 days of age. For the first 6 months she showed no sign of seeing anything and her mother thought that she was blind. She had turned her head to sound at 3 months and at 4 months played with a rattle placed in the hand. She took no notice of the approaching feeding bottle, but in all other aspects of development she was normal. At 6 months she first began to smile at her mother and to reach out for objects and get them. At 11 months she held her arms out for clothes and at 16 months she was speaking in sentences and was most interested in her surroundings. A 33 months she was well above average in Gesell tests. She was a normal child with normal vision. She was followed well into school age.

One often sees children who are thought to be blind (and/or deaf), but who on developmental assessment are found to be mentally subnormal. The optic disc of young babies is usually pale and it is easy to understand that a diagnosis of blindness is readily made. Then in weeks or months it becomes obvious that the child can see. In some of these children the visual difficulty is out of proportion to the degree of general retardation; this may well be due to delayed visual maturation. Gordon (1968) wrote that many children thought to be blind are later found to have normal vision, though are mentally subnormal. He wrote, "Some have a severe specific impairment of visual function, quite out of context with other aspects of their development, and they can be said to be centrally blind." Like children with gross auditory agnosia, those children with particularly marked disorders of visual perception are likely to improve with increasing age. We cannot say whether those children can see, but are unable to interpret what they see.

The condition of delayed visual maturation in mentally normal babies is extremely rare and we do not know the causes. It is so rare that it is impossible to give a confident prognosis. If there is no ophthalmological abnormality, no nystagmus, and the baby on development assessment is otherwise normal, it is reasonable to hold out the hope that vision will become normal. As with all other forms of delayed maturation, it is impossible to be sure that even if vision is otherwise normal, there will not be residual visuo-spatial difficulties.

How far the defect interferes with the bonding between infant and mother one cannot say, but one suspects that the failure of the baby to smile at the mother when she smiles at him must affect her attitude toward him. Neither can one say whether the child's ability to see normally in the early weeks will have a permanent psychological effect.

Blindness

The mean IQ of blind children is less than average and they often have additional handicaps. A blind child is liable to suffer pseudoretardation—to become backward because of lack of the normal stimulation and later because of overprotection resulting from the fear that he will harm himself (for example by feeding himself or trying to walk). A child with bilateral anophthalmia presents a further problem. The mother often cannot tell whether he is awake or asleep, unless he is crying. The developmental assessment is one of considerable difficulty and it is particularly easy to underestimate the child's real potential when various factors have contributed to pseudoretardation.

Other Eye Defects

Trevor-Roper (1971) in a fascinating book on art in relation to visual defects *(The World Through Blunted Sight)* suggested that variations in visual function may affect the personality. Myopic children are likely to be studious, withdrawn, poor at sport, and to please the teacher; hypermetopic children are likely to be extroverts, mischief makers, inattentive, overactive, and truants.

Delayed Auditory Maturation

By far the most common cause of delayed response to sound, apart from hearing loss, is mental retardation. But an occasional child appears to be deaf in the early weeks and later to hear normally. Whether he hears but does not understand what he hears—congenital auditory imperception—we do not know. These children are often late in acquiring speech.

Ingram (1964) wrote that:

Many of the children with 'central deafness,' or 'auditory imperception,' behave as if they are deaf in early life, and only after prolonged observation and as the result of special techniques of testing can it be shown that hearing is present. Inevitably patients are misdiagnosed as suffering from peripheral deafness. Other children who suffer from developmental auditory imperception behave as if they live in a world of their own, and are much more interested in their immediate environment and play than in people in their surroundings.

They are liable to be called autistic or mentally retarded. The autistic child commonly appears to be deaf, certainly to the human voice, and it can be extremely difficult to determine whether he can hear or not.

Psychogenic deafness, regarded as a perceptual defense, has been described by Reed (1961) and others.

Delay in Gross Motor Development—Sitting and Walking

Late development of sitting and walking is usually part of general retardation, but isolated delay is fairly common. If it is an isolated retardation, it cannot be due to mental subnormality, for a mentally subnormal child is late in all aspects of development, except occasionally gross motor development (and very rarely sphincter control). Children with isolated retardation may legitimately be termed unusual, but not necessarily abnormal. I disagree with the statement that the chart in the Denver screening system (Frankenburg and Dodds, 1967; Frankenburg, et al., 1971) "vividly shows the range of normal variations," and "it enables the examiner to determine whether he (the child) is within the normal range." The chart shows no such thing because it is impossible to draw the line between normal and abnormal. The Denver scheme gave the 25th, 50th, 75th, and 90th centile for 105 test items standardized on 1036 presumably normal children aged 2 weeks to 6 years, thought to be representative of Denver children, but excluding pre-term, breech deliveries, and all children with gross physical defects. For that reason alone the children were selected and not representative of the population as a whole. Neligan and Prudham (1969) went further and gave the 3rd, 10th, 25th, 50th, 75th, 90th, and 97th centile for walking, sitting, and other skills: their figures for 3 of those centiles were as follows:

	3rd	50th	97th
		centiles	
		Age in months	
Sitting	4.6	6.4	9.3
Walking	9.7	12.8	18.4

It would be totally wrong to suggest that because 97% of children were walking without help at 18.4 months, those walking later are abnormal. I have seen dozens of normal children who could not walk alone by 18.4 months and at least 16 who could not walk alone until 24 months or later. On follow-up these children were proved to be normal. For example, the following 4 children were followed from infancy to school age, one for 15 years. All had a normal delivery after a normal pregnancy; in nine was there abnormality of muscle tone or other abnormal physical signs.

1. Sat, no support—11 months. Walk, no help—30 months. IQ at 5 years—104.

2. Sat, no support—9 months. Walk, no help—48 months. IQ at 5 years—125.

3. Sat, no support—23 months. Walk, no help—50 months. IQ at 8 years—118. Her teachers reported that she was doing well at school, running and playing games, but "not really nimble on her feet."

4. Sat, no support—12 months. Walk, no support—36 months. A little awkward with her hands. At age 15 could run fast, ride a bicycle, play hockey, but tumbled frequently in the gymnasium. Top of her class in a technical school, but could type only 50 words per minute. I would regard her as a slightly clumsy child.

A child who is unusually late in walking is not always late in sitting.

The factors preceding isolated delayed gross motor development therefore, excluding mental subnormality or cerebral palsy, are as follows:

- Familial, possibly familial late myelination.
- Environmental factors—emotional deprivation.
- Illness, keeping a child lying down.
- Personality, lack of confidence. After a bump, a baby may be afraid to walk alone.
- Shuffling or hitching—on one hand and one buttock.
- Hypotonia (including lower limb paresis in spina bifida).
- Muscular dystrophy, Duchenne type.

For unknown reasons, affected boys are retarded in motor development long before signs of muscular dystrophy develop. Dubowitz (1968) found that 34 of 65 affected boys were unable to walk until 18 months, and 29 not till 2 years of age or later. This is not due to the low IQ (mean IQ in muscular dystrophy around 80). Of 30 with an average or above average IQ, 9 and possibly a further 3 had delayed motor development; of 14 with a low average IQ, 8 were delayed; and of 21 retarded children, 11 and possibly a further 4 were late in walking.

Blindness is liable to delay walking, especially if there is overprotection; neither obesity nor untreated congenital dislocation of the hip delay walking.

When an otherwise normal child is significantly retarded in gross motor development and no physical abnormality is found nor is there a helpful family history, it is difficult to forecast the age at which he will walk and impossible to be sure that there will not be some residual clumsiness, but in my experience that is exceptional. One can only be guided by the degree of weight-bearing on examination. It would be wise to eliminate Duchenne muscular dystrophy by a creatine phosphokinase estimation.

Delayed walking is both a nuisance and source of anxiety for the parents and may be difficult psychologically for the child. It often leads to diagnostic errors, such as mental subnormality, cerebral palsy, or brain damage. A common error is to diagnose ataxia in the case of a late walker. Whereas a child who walks alone at 10 months will probably walk well with little falling by 20 months, a child who first walks without help at 20 months may not be walking well, with little falling, till 40 months; in the meantime a wrong diagnosis of ataxia may be made.

Hypotonia

The numerous causes of hypotonia have been reviewed by Paine and Fenichel (1965) and Dubowitz (1968). Paine (1963) attempted to discuss the prognosis with regard to walking by studying 133 floppy infants. He picked out by process of elimination, including muscle biopsy, those children who might have benign congenital hypotonia and who would eventually learn to walk. He thought that this diagnosis was more likely if tendon jerks were normal, joints were hyperextensible, and there was a family history of delayed walking with hyperextensible joints. He suggested that such children would develop normal motor function for adult life, but retain hyperextensible joints. I have seen several of these children who were otherwise normal and who were able to walk by the age of three to six years. As Paine (1963) wrote, the prognosis must depend on accurate diagnosis of the cause.

Delayed Sphincter Control

Hundreds of articles have been written about urinary incontinence. A comprehensive review was that of Kolvin, MacKeith, and Meadow (1973). Sir Martin Roth in his introduction wrote that enuresis is associated with a poor home, domestic friction, delinquency in siblings and family, and other manifestations of social adversity. He added "a network of causes which may at first glance appear to have a simple underlying pattern tends to prove a maze in which the investigator becomes lost and disorientated."

Primary enuresis, delay in acquiring control, is commonly familial and genetic and probably an example of delayed maturation. MacKeith in the above symposium suggested that parents cannot accelerate the process of maturation, but they can retard it by mismanagement at the sensitive period when control is being acquired; other psychological factors at the sensitive period have the same effect. MacKeith wrote that in the first four years maturation is occurring, independent of training or learning, and it may be inhibited by unsuitable training:

> It appears that what the growing child is sensitive to in the second or third years of life, so far as concerns the. emergence of nocturnal bladder control once maturation has occurred, is not positive factors like teaching or training, but the absence of negative influences which can inhibit the emergence of nocturnal bladder control. [1973]

Delayed maturation is probably the main reason for the delayed control of the sphincter in mental subnormality. Secondary enuresis—incontinence after acquiring control—is usually due to psychological causes or the development of polyuria particularly at the sensitive period. A variety of organic causes may lead to incontinence, notably spina bifida, sacral lipoma, ectopic ureter in the girl, urethral obstruction in the boy, ureterocele, diastematomyelia, and epispadias. Miller, in the symposium (Kolvin, MacKeith and Meadow, 1973) found that 17% of Newcastle children were wetting at least occasionally at 5 years, 11% at 11 years, and 2% at 15 years.

Speech Delay

Lateness in speech development is common and causes distress to parent and child. Amongst famous people whose late speech development caused anxiety were Alessandro Volta (of voltage fame) who said his first word at four and Albert Einstein who at four was feared to be mentally retarded because he could not speak. He was still not speaking well at nine. The subject of delayed speech was fully reviewed by Ingram (1963), Renfrew and Murphy (1964), Morley (1972) and Rutter and Martin (1972), and will therefore by discussed only briefly here.

In her Newcastle study, Morley (1972) found that 73% of children were using single words by 12 months (range 8 to 30 months), 40% were joining words together by 18 months (range 10 to 44 months), and 89% were joining words by 24 months. At 4 years 10% had almost unintelligible speech. Ingram (1963) divided delayed speech into four categories:

1. Mild—dyslalia.
2. Moderate—retarded acquisition of speech with dyslalia, but with normal comprehension of speech.
3. Severe—defective comprehension and expression of speech, congenital word blindness.
4. Very severe—defect of comprehension and failure to perceive the significance of sounds, auditory imperception.

The causes of delayed speech are varied and not all known. It is common for a 12- to 18-month-old child to make no apparent progress in speech development for several weeks and then suddenly to make rapid headway. I have seen two boys who were retarded in speech at 14 months and advanced in speech two weeks later.

Probably the most common cause of delayed speech in a mentally normal child is genetic. There is a family history of it. Environmental causes are evident in that speech tends to be less advanced in the lower social classes—not only because of a lower mean IQ, but also because of reduced parent-child verbal contact, poor speech models at home, and lower parental expectations. Speech is retarded when a child is brought up in an institution, perhaps partly because there is less conversation with him. According to Solomon (1961) parents of late speakers tend to be rigid, overprotective, and disapproving.

The role of laterality is obscure. Zangwill (1968) wrote that handedness and speech are in some way related. Clumsiness or backwardness in reading, spelling, and spatial sense are linked with atypical or inconsistant laterality. Annette, Lee, and Ounsted (1961) found that mixed handers are more likely to have delay in speech than fixed handers.

Twins are commonly late in speaking. The mother of twins has less time to speak to the children than the mother of a singleton. The delay is commonly ascribed to the theory that twins understand each other's jargon and so do not bother to learn properly. I doubt this. Speech is more retarded in middle-class twins than in the lower classes (Rutter and Martin, 1972). Morley noted that the speech defect is rarely the same in both twins. There may be delay in one, but not in the other; or they may both have a speech defect, but of dissimilar type and degree.

The most common cause of delayed speech is mental subnormality. Speech in mentally retarded children tends to be later than other aspects of development, presumably due to late maturation. Mentally subnormal children often forget words after learning them and several weeks elapse before the words are re-learned. Speech is usually defective in cerebral palsy, especially in athetosis. Because of the importance of deafness as a cause of late or defective speech, it is routine to test the hearing in every child who is late in learning to speak or to speak clearly. Speech is always late in autistic children. Elective mutism is usually a form of hysteria.

Delayed speech is not due to tongue tie, jealousy, laziness, bilingualism, or cleft palate—though children with cleft palate have a lower mean IQ than others. Speech delay is not due to the parents doing everything for the child instead of making him speak.

It may be difficult to state the prognosis. Mild dyslalia, apart from the central lisp, is usually self-limiting, and improvement after speech therapy is almost entirely due to maturation rather than the therapy. But the central lisp may persist into adult life. Amongst famous people who were greatly embarrassed by their early speech defects were Emile Zola and Michael Faraday. The latter had to leave school prematurely because of the teasing he suffered for it.

It is particularly difficult to state the prognosis in a case of aphasia. If a child with normal hearing and IQ is is not able to say any words by the age of three, one would be seriously concerned about the prognosis.

Ingram emphasized that a high proportion of children with delayed speech will later have difficulty in learning to read.

Stuttering

The problem of stuttering has been extensively reviewed by Morley (1972), Andrews and Harris (1964), and Fransella (1976). It will therefore be discussed only briefly here. The factor of maturation is important. It is normal for children to fall over words or to repeat syllables when learning to speak, but most grow out of this provided that the parents do not make the children self-conscious about the speech by drawing attention to the stuttering, making them repeat themselves, or by trying to get them to speak more slowly. Parental attitudes are therefore of great importance. Insecurity and unhappiness are the important factors. Stuttering is three times more common in boys. The mean IQ of stutterers is about 7 points below that of nonstutterers. The rather high family incidence of stuttering may indicate a genetic factor or merely imitation. Ninety-five percent of stutterers begin to stutter before the age of seven and 70% before five. Stuttering is not related to handedness, ambidexterity, or change of handedness (Andrews and Harris, 1964).

Stuttering often responds well to rhythmic methods, such as times syllabic speech, and many grow out of it while others continue to stutter in adult life. Among famous stutterers were Moses, Aristotle, Aesop, Demosthenes, Virgil, Charles I, Robert Boyle, Michael Faraday, Aneurin Bevan, Lewis Carroll, Somerset Maugham, Charles Lamb, and Charles Darwin.

Delay in Other Fields

Manipulation

Unless there is mental subnormality, cerebral palsy, or severe hypotonia, delay in the use of the hands is very rare. I have never seen isolated delay in manipulation, though I have seen several examples of generalized delay in maturation in which delayed manipulation was a feature.

Chewing

Delay in beginning to chew occurs almost exclusively in children with mental subnormality or cerebral palsy, but may occur in generalized delay in maturation. I explained earlier that failure to give a child solids when he has recently acquired the ability to chew will cause severe feeding problems later because the child will vomit or refuse to chew. Hence in cases of esophageal atresia in which anastomosis in the new-born period is impossible, there will be serious problems later unless a stoma is made in the neck and solid food is given by mouth, to emerge in the neck (Illingworth and Lister, 1964). Theoretically similar problems might occur in cases of prolonged intravenous feeding from birth. I have not otherwise seen an example of isolated delay in chewing.

Feeding and Dressing

Unless there is mental subnormality, cerebral palsy, or severe hypotonia, the only cause of lateness in learning to feed and dress is the mother's failure to give the child a chance to learn.

Retardation in More than One Field of Development

Apart from examples of generalized maturational delay, one occasionally sees a mentally normal child who is late in two or three fields of development, often for different reasons.

I saw a boy at 36 months because he was not talking, though hearing was normal. As the father had died when the child was an infant, it was not possible to determine when the father began to talk. The boy had begun to walk at 18 months, but the mother had begun to walk at the same age. He was incontinent of urine; dribbled; and was found to have urethral obstruction, which was successfully treated. He was therefore retarded in three fields of development, but he rapidly made a tower of 10 one-inch cubes, followed by a train with a chimney and a bridge. He immediately identified all 10 objects on the Gesell picture card and neatly copied the 0 and +. He immediately adapted on the simple formboard. He was alert and responsive and his developmental quotient was well over 100.

MINIMAL BRAIN DYSFUNCTION

According to Roger Reger (1965) at least 43 symptoms and according to Schmitt (1975) at least 100 symptoms have been ascribed to minimal brain dysfunction (MBD). Hence it would be impossible to discuss each of the symptoms individually. Therefore I have picked out overactivity, defective concentration, clumsiness, and learning disorders, as being the most important ones, for more detailed discussion and comparison with other examples of delayed maturation.

Overactivity

The causes or preceding factors of overactivity have been mentioned in previous sections and hence can now be collected together and merely listed, apart from a few relevant comments. They are:

- Delayed maturation.
- Normal variation.
- Genetic.
- Maternal toxemia.
- Alcohol addiction in pregnancy.
- Prenatal, perinatal anoxia.
- Prenatal, postnatal malnutrition.
- Neonatal hyperbilirubinemia.
- Insecurity: emotional deprivation, adverse socioeconomic factors, parental alcoholism.
- Smoking by the family.
- Therapeutic drugs.
- Restriction of activity.
- Poor motivation to learning: boredom, fatigue.

- Learning disorders.
- Language difficulties in immigrants.
- Auditory or visual defects.
- Phenyliketonuria.
- Lead poisoning.
- Epilepsy.
- Autism.

Hyperactivity usually decreases as the child gets older and many regard the symptoms as delayed maturation of cortical inhibition of motility (Stone, 1976), hence mentally subnormal children, who are late in all aspects of development, are later than others in losing their overactivity. Cartwell (1975) has discussed the genetic aspects noting that commonly one or both parents were overactive in their childhood and still show residual features of it. Denson, Nanson, and McWatters (1975) studied the smoking habits of 60 mothers of hyperkinetic children. They found that the mothers of overactive children smoked on the average two or three times more than the control mothers. It was not clear whether this was due to features of their personality or to the direct action of the smoke.

Levy's work (1944) on the effect of restriction of movements in animals (causing the head-shaking of hens, the weaving tics of horses, the head-bobbing of bears) may be relevant. Children whose motility is restricted by playpens, plaster casts, and other means, may respond by overactivity. Werry (1976) referred to the strong tendency to alcoholism in the family of overactive children. Ounsted (1955) referred to the overactivity which may result from temporal lobe epilepsy and other forms of epilepsy, except petit mal.

As Johnson and Prinz (1976) wrote "hyperactivity is in the eyes of the beholder." There is no convenient objective test for it. As MacKeith wrote (1974) "overactivity is a complaint made only by teachers and parents, and not by the child." The variations in the reported incidence is therefore striking. Lapouse and Mon (1958) in a survey of 482 children in the city of Buffalo found that 49% of mothers thought that their children were overactive. On the other hand Rutter, Tirard, and Whitmore (1970) found in the Isle of Wight survey that 1.6% of psychiatrically disturbed children aged 9 to 11 years were overactive. Their finding was based on psychological tests, the opinions of teachers and parents, and their own observations at interview.

Werry (1968) discussed the early predictors of school-age overactivity and not surprisingly found that in the pre-school period the children had boundless energy, incessant activity, and needed little sleep. But Laufer and Denhoff (1957) wrote that there is no complaint about these children until they start school.

Overactivity is commonly associated with boredom, poor concentration, distractibility, and sometimes with clumsiness and learning disorders. As those children get older they mostly lose their overactivity, but Laufer (1962) found that they were frequent underachievers in adolescence. Weiss, et al., (1971) followed 64 overactive children for five years: the overactivity decreased, but restlessness, poor concentration, and learning disorders continued.

Lord Beaverbrook, because of his overactivity as a schoolboy with poor concentration, was not expected to achieve much in adult life.

Rutter and Lockyer (1967) followed 63 psychotic overactive children and found that many as they grew older tended to become underactive. The long-term effect of stimulant drugs was discussed by Safer, Allen, and Barr (1972), there was a reduction in the weight and height at first. In the long term, stimulant drugs probably have no permanent benefit (*Drug and Therapeutics Bulletin*, 1977).

It is obvious that overactivity is the end result of a wide variety of preceding factors, physical, emotional, and intellectual.

Clumsiness

The word clumsiness is said to be derived from the Scandinavian clomsen, "to be stiff or benumbed, acting or moving as if benumbed, awkward in action, ungainly, wanting in dexterity." Annell (1959) used the term motorial infantilism. Others have referred to clumsy children as motor morons. Annell regarded the condition as one of delayed maturation. Affected children fall excessively, have more than the usual number of bruises, are awkward with their hands, write badly, and hold the pencil in an unusual way. There are all degrees of severity; it is more common in boys. According to Gubbay (1975) at least 5% of the school population is affected to some extent. The causes or preceding factors can be summarized as follows:

a) Normal variations:
- Genetic factors.
- Delayed maturation.
- Malnutrition.
- Prenatal, postnatal malnutrition.
- Insecurity: emotional problems, unkindness of teacher.
- Hypotonia, hypertonia.
- Hyperextensibility of joint.
- Congenital myopathy: muscular dystrophy.
- Side effect of drugs.
- Drug addiction.
- Hypothyroidism.
- Visual deficiencies.
- Mercury or lead poisoning.

b) Rare syndromes, degenerative diseases of the nervous system:
- Lipoidoses.
- Leucodystrophies.
- Ataxia telangiectasia.
- Klippel-Feil syndrome.
- Agenesis of the corpus callosum.
- Platybasia and allied conditions.
- Cerebral gigantism.

- Familial dysautonomia.
- Abetalipoproteinemia.
- Hartnup disease.
- Argininosuccinicacidemia.
- Phenylketonuria.

There are wide normal variations in manual and motor dexterity, often familial. All infants are clumsy and ataxic in their early purposeful movements, but mature with age and most lose their clumsiness. The ataxia of the late walker has been mentioned. Malnutrition in utero and the early postnatal weeks may affect particularly the cerebellum and cause clumsiness. Emotional problems are important: insecurity or unhappiness may be a factor and unkindness of parent or teacher, with criticism or ridicule, may cause or aggravate clumsiness: the child is expected to be clumsy, and he is. He is poor at sport, worries, and feels inadequate; he becomes an underachiever and develops symptoms of the MBD syndrome. He is blamed for his bad writing, on the grounds that he is careless and not trying. On thorough neurological examination abnormal physical signs may sometimes be found which may include minimal signs of cerebral palsy. I have several times found an extensor plantar response in a clumsy child not known to have cerebral palsy. I was asked to see a girl who had played truant from school for one day and found minimal but definite athetosis, which had been responsible for the bad writing and awkwardness which had led to unkindness at school. Drugs given for epilepsy or other conditions may cause clumsiness. Hagberg and Westphal (1970) described the association of hypothyroidism and ataxia.

Gubbay (1972, 1975) in his extensive studies found that most affected children were mentally normal, had no bodily deformity, had normal physical strength, normal sensation and coordination in conventional tests, but had an impaired ability to perform fine purposive movements. Tests included walking on a ledge, timed bead-threading, hopping, screwing the cap onto a bottle, right-left discrimination and the Goodenough draw-a-man test. He found no correlation with prematurity, postmaturity, abnormal delivery, or neonatal illness.

Walton, Ellis, and Court (1962) described five clumsy children with developmental apraxia and agnosia, all with crossed laterality, all referred for clumsiness: they compared those children with Gerstmann's syndrome of parieto-occipital damage to the dominant hemisphere. Cohen, et al., (1967) referred to overflow involuntary movements in the resting extremity (presumably mirror movements) when the other limb was performing a voluntary act. By nine years this overflow had considerably decreased.

There are often associated difficulties consisting of overactivity, poor concentration, distractibility, visuo-spatial problems, right-left discrimination difficulties, and learning problems. These children tend to fare less well on the WISC performance scale than on the verbal scale.

It should be possible to detect clumsiness in later infancy by observing the tremor and unsteadiness when the child is reaching out for objects and later when building a tower of cubes.

The prognosis must depend on the cause and is therefore often uncertain. Assuming that the clumsiness is not due to one of the examples of organic disease mentioned, the clumsiness will probably decrease with maturation, having been partly compensated, or it may disappear completely. Amongst famous people who were clumsy as children were Oscar Wilde, G. K. Chesterton, and Johann Pestalozzi. The latter was described as an awkward, clumsy boy who was bad at spelling, writing, and mathematics and his teacher confidently predicted future failure. Napoleon was always clumsy; as for Beethoven, it was said that nothing was safe in his hands.

Mellsop (1972) investigated the after history of clumsy children referred to the psychiatric clinic of the Royal Children's Hospital in Melbourne and found that their referral rate as adults to the Victoria Mental Health Department was more than three times the expected rate.

Like overactivity, clumsiness is the end result of a wide variety of preceding factors, functional and organic.

Defective Concentration and Day-Dreaming

The causes or preceding factors of defective concentration are many and include normal variation, mental subnormality, various congenital anomolies, diseases, trauma, effects of drugs, emotional difficulties, and school problems including learning disorders.

Many famous people caused anxiety in their childhood on account of poor concentration. They included Gauguin, Edouard Manet, Sibelius, Isaac Newton, and Einstein. Hans Christian Andersen and Honoré de Balzac caused particular difficulties on account of day-dreaming.

Delayed Reading and Other Learning Problems

The most common cause of delayed reading, spelling, and allied problems, including visuo-spatial difficulties is mental retardation, but I shall confine this section to difficulties in the mentally normal child. In association with difficulties in reading and spelling, there are overactivity, clumsiness, defective concentration, and distractibility. I have mentioned most of the causes and correlates in previous sections. (I am uncertain whether difficulties in mathematics, languages, or other subjects should be included in this group of problems.)

It is probable that in most cases several factors operate. The problems are multifactorial. The genetic factor is an essential one in the so-called specific dyslexia, or specific learning problem, in which there is almost always a family history of at least part of the syndrome and in which, apart from the difficulty in reading, there is ambidexterity or left-handedness, reversal of symbols, reading from left to right, reversal of words, and similar defects. Smoking in pregnancy has been related to difficulties in reading and mathematics (Davie, Butler, and Goldstein, 1972). Stewart, Walker, and Savage (1970) followed 150 survivors of rhesus hemolytic disease and found a high incidence of visuo-spatial problems presumably related to the hyperbilirubinemia. Delayed maturation is an important factor. It is normal for children when learning to read to reverse symbols, but they grow out of it while children with reading difficulty commonly continue to reverse symbols much longer. Dykman, et al., (1971) wrote that defective attention is the main problem.

The neurological results suggest that the main cause of learning disabilities is a developmental lag. The child is neurologically immature.

Others have suggested that children are taught to read too early, but that idea presupposes that the sensitive period is the same for all children. It is not.

Denhoff, Hainsworth, and Hainsworth (1972) emphasized the importance of psychosocial problems. Mattis, French, and Rafin (1975) described three syndromes in dyslexia: language disorder, articulation and graphomotor discoordination, and visuo-spatial deficiencies. He said that those three factors explain the difficulties in 90% of dyslexic children.

Fabian (1955) suggested that reading difficulties may be "the protest of an infantile child against growth, by refusing to learn." Psychological problems may not only cause or aggravate a child's difficulties, but also may be caused by the learning problems. Learning difficulties often present as behavior problems, such as truancy. Makita (1969) made the surprising observation that dyslexia is rare in Japan, despite the thousands of characters which the child has to learn, and that it is 10 times more common in Western countries. He added,

It is unthinkable that the Americans and the Europeans have 10 times the population with maldevelopment or malformation of cerebral gyoi than do the Japanese. It is hardly believable that the prevalence of hemispheral dominance—conflict or split laterality is 10 times less frequent in Japan.

He thought that dyslexia was most frequent in English-speaking countries, less in German-speaking and less still in Latin-speaking peoples (Italy and Spain). The reasons for this, if it is true, is obscure.

Many famous persons experienced some of these problems. Jan Smuts could not read until he was 12 and the famous British physician, John Hunter, could not read until he was seventeen. Froebel had a similar problem. Yeats was late in learning to read and spell. Auguste Rodin had difficulty in reading and writing and was described as the worst pupil in the school. His father said, "I have an idiot for a son." Auguste's uncle said he was ineducable.

Boder (1971) made the point that the diagnosis of learning problems is made partly by exclusion: excluding mental subnormality, audiovisual and visuo-spatial defects, emotional disorders, adverse social circumstances, and poor teaching; and partly by positive signs: crossed laterality, right-left discrimination errors, clumsiness, overactivity, Goodenough, WISC and Bender-Gestalt tests, and by an analysis of reading and spelling for reversals, extraneous letters, omission of letters, and errors in letter order. Visuo-spatial difficulties are shown by poor performance on formboards, pattern copying, drawing, poor body image, difficulty in estimating size and depth, and in estimating distance between objects.

Various attempts have been made to predict reading and allied learning problems in children with normal intelligence (Gesell and Amatruda, 1956; Denhoff, Hainsworth, and Hainsworth, 1972; de Hirsch, Jansky, and Langford, 1966; Brenner and Gillman, 1966). In the first place lateness in speaking, clumsiness, overactivity, and adverse socioeconomic factors would place the child in the risk category for later learning disorders and a family history of specific dyslexia would make it likely that the child would be affected. It is questionable however whether it is helpful to place a child in the risk category before he starts school (Alberman, 1963)—the danger is that of the self-fulfilling prophecy if he is labeled (Silberberg,

Iverson, and Goins, 1973). Furthermore there is little that can be done about it. But it can be argued that it is better for the teachers to know that the child has a special difficulty, so that he will not be accused of being lazy, careless, and not trying. It is important that the correct diagnosis should be made, so that the teachers understand that the child's reading, spelling, and writing difficulties are outside his control.

The prognosis must depend on the cause. If it is only a matter of delayed maturation, it will cure itself and it is unlikely that remedial teaching will accelerate the maturation (Silver, 1975; Snyder, 1975). Though it is standard practice to arrange remedial teaching for the various learning disorders, its value is open to doubt. Lovell, Byrne, and Richardson (1963) followed children who had had remedial teaching and found that after a mean period of three and one-half years from the time of referral, there was no difference in the mean reading ages from the controls. Weinberg, et al., (1971) and Belmont and Birch (1974) found the same.

It must be recognized that some of the learning problems will persist throughout life; it is often impossible to predict this. Silver and Hagin (1964) followed 24 cases into adult life. Though improvement had occurred, specific perceptual problems persisted. Numerous famous people retained their learning problems. Napoleon never learned to spell. Joshua Reynolds, Yeats, Henry Ford, Harvey Cushing, Thomas Edison, General Patton, Woodrow Wilson, William James, Paul Ehrlich, Gertrude Bell, Auguste Rodin, and Hans Christian Andersen all had residual difficulties. Picasso never lost his difficulty in remembering the sequence of the alphabet. Henri Poincaré, probably the most famous mathematician France has produced, was never able to draw, scoring a zero for drawing in his school entrance examination. He was ambidextrous, clumsy, awkward with his fingers, and never lost his visuo-spatial difficulties, which made geometry impossible for him.

Like defective concentration, clumsiness, and overactivity, learning disorders are multifactorial in origin.

Some Other Symptoms of the MBD Syndrome

I have remarked that it is impossible to consider individually each of the dozens of behavior problems bunched by some into the MBD syndrome. The underlying factors and causes in nearly all of them are the same, in most cases several factors interacting to cause individual problems. It is a mystery why some children and adults react to emotional stress by one symptom and others by a different symptom. Almost all behavior problems represent a conflict between the child's developing mind and personality and the personality and attitudes of his parents and others in the environment, resulting in insecurity in the broadest sense and so in outward manifestations in the form of a behavioral variation. A child's personality (and intelligence) are partly inherited and partly environmental. It would be unreasonable to suppose that the childhood of Percy Shelly, Vincent Van Gogh, or Henri Cezanne were purely environmental in origin.

The prognosis of these behavior problems must depend on their cause. Some will persist into adult life. Perhaps some of the present-day children with behavioral variations termed by some minimal brain dysfunction will be tomorrow's hippies, dropouts, or eccentrics—amiable and amusing, or otherwise; perhaps some will become members of society's lunatic fringe; most will probably mature and become what society will accept as normal. But it may be said of others that as adults they are immature and have never grown up.

Rutter (1970) found that the prognosis of most childhood neuroses was good, but that the prognosis for aggressive disorders was poor. Earlier Robins (1966) had investigated the adult status of 524 child-guidance patients, comparing them with controls of comparable sex, age, race, IQ, and neighborhood. For antisocial boys there was a 71% risk of future arrest and a 50% risk of divorce; for antisocial girls the risk of divorce was 70%. The boys' later occupation and army records were poor and there was a high incidence of alcoholism.

Pessimism is not justified for the great majority of behavioral symptoms included in the so-called MBD syndrome. All children (and all parents and all teachers) have behavior problems. There is nothing special about those included in the MBD syndrome. They are just a part and parcel of normal human beings with all the differences and variations which make mankind so interesting.

DISCUSSION

In this chapter I have discussed the causes, diagnosis, and prognosis of developmental variations in each case emphasizing that the prognosis must depend on the underlying factors. The developmental variations discussed included overall delay; motor delay; delay in sucking and swallowing, in vision and hearing, in sphincter control and speech, in muscle coordination, and in certain features commonly ascribed to the minimal brain dysfunction syndrome—notably clumsiness, poor concentration, and learning disorders. Some of these variations, especially clumsiness, may have an organic basis. The great majority have no known organic basis, though some, such as overactivity and aggressiveness, may have a biochemical basis interacting with various environmental factors. There is much overlap between these variations with one variation leading to another and almost all have psychological correlates. There is nothing to distinguish the symptoms of the so-called MBD syndrome from all the other variations. Nearly all the variations have several causes in common, especially prenatal and genetic, socioeconomic and psychological—all leading by a final common pathway to one predominant symptom, such as delayed reading, though there may be an associated less important symptom, such as dyscalculia. Underlying nearly all the variations is one major factor, delayed maturation. Peifer (1963) suggested that maturation may consist of myelination, neurofibre formation, maturation of ganglion cells, and biochemical changes, including those involving enzyme systems.

Throughout this chapter I have emphasized the importance of trying to trace the various causes and underlying factors to their origins. Often we do not know enough to define these, but it is totally inadequate to ascribe developmental delay to birth injury, for instance, just because there was an abnormal presentation, premature labor, or anoxia at birth, without going much further to try to determine the causes of the abnormal presentation, prematurity, anoxia, or other feature.

When there are so many factors and causes, it is inevitable that the prognosis must depend on the causes and preceding factors. Often it is impossible to be certain of the prognosis. A learning disorder, for instance, may disappear completely with maturation, or only partly, some improvement having occurred as a result of compensation.

In recent years several experts have expressed their disapproval of the whole concept of the MBD syndrome. Reger (1965) wrote that:

Most of what is assumed to be known about the brain-injured child is folk-lore. The fact that many children are distractible and hyperactive is no reason to assume that the concept of the brain-injured child is worth retaining. There is no justification whatsoever to continue to call children brain-injured if there is no reason to assume that those children have injuries to the brain.

Kinsbourne (1973) wrote that the diagnosis of MBD is based on findings that are abnormal only in relation to age and that the relative delay is a problem of neurological maturation. Masland (1973) wrote that MBD is not a disease, but merely a group of individuals with certain characteristics in common. Schmitt (1975) referred to MBD as an "all encompassing waste-paper basket diagnosis for any child who does not quite conform to society's stereotype for normal children," and wrote that there is no neurological sign or test that distinguishes the child with MBD from normal children. It would hardly be likely that because the syndrome is 10 times more common in boys, 10 times more boys than girls suffer brain damage. Rutter (1977) wrote that "the behavior stereotype of the brain-damaged child must be firmly rejected."

Apley (1976), writing about recurrent abdominal pain in children, said that "the more sophisticated the country, the more belly-achers it will have, large or small." So it is with the MBD syndrome. The syndrome is not a problem of developing countries. Teachers' or parents' complaints about the child's symptoms of overactivity, aggressiveness, and other features stated by some to indicate the MBD syndrome depend on their attitudes, prejudices, and their views as to what is normal. That which is normal in one country may be abnormal in another. It is never possible to draw the line between normal and abnormal. In South Africa I was shown in a centre for brain-damaged children a boy who was said to be overactive and therefore to have been brain-damaged, requiring treatment. To me he was just a bright delightful ebullient normal boy. There is an analogous situation with regard to tonsillectomy (and certain other operations). Muller (1953) conducted a survey of the throats of 640 German school children and found that only 14% had normal tonsils. One feels that he should revise his idea of normality.

There are many other reasons why the term minimal brain dysfunction should be dropped. It is distressing to parents. If a tragedy occurs, it is far better to feel that it could not have been avoided: the statement that the child has suffered brain damaged implies totally unjustifiable blame on the obstetrician or whoever delivered the baby. The suggestion that there is something wrong with the child's brain causes anxiety, depression, and perhaps a feeling of guilt, and it alters the parent's attitude toward the child. Eisenberg (1964) felt that the term conveys the feeling or irreversibility and hopelessness. The term minimal brain dysfunction is bad for the child, for it attaches a label which is difficult to remove. It may cause him to be put into a special class for brain-injured children (Bakwin and Bakwin,

1972); the teacher places him in a special category with all the risks of the Rosenthal and Jacobson (1968) type of self-fulfilling prophecy. The child feels different, and he becomes different. It may lead to play-acting, notoriety-seeking, and to his being the subject of ridicule (Birch, 1964). He is given totally unnecessary medical treatment—perhaps bogus treatment—with its risk of side effects (Barkley, 1977).

It is time that the term minimal brain dysfunction is dropped. Perhaps in its place one might use the term NDSSA—the nondisease syndrome stressful to adults.

REFERENCES

Alberman, E. "The early prediction of learning disorders." *Developmental Medicine and Child Neurology*, 15, 202, (1963).

Allen, J. E., and D. W. Rodgin. "Mental retardation in association with progressive muscular dystrophy." *American Journal of Diseases of Children*, 100, 208, (1960).

Amiel-Tison, C. "Cerebral damage in full-term newborns. Aetiological factors, neonatal status and long-term follow up." *Biologia Neonatorum*, 14, 234, (1969).

Anderson, E. M. "Cognitive deficits in children with spina bifida and hydrocephalus. A review of the literature." *British Journal of Educational Psychology*, 43, 35, (1973).

————in D. Bergsma and A. E. Pulver, eds., *Developmental Disabilities. Psychological and Social Implications*, New York: Alan R. Liss, 1976.

André, T., and St-A. Dargassies. *Etudes Neurologiques sur le Nouveau—Ne et le Jeune Nourisson*. Paris: Masson and Perrin, 1952.

Andrews, G. W. Harris. "The syndrome of stuttering." *Clinics in Developmental Medicine*, No. 17, (1964).

Annell, A. "Motor disorders and difficulties at school." *Seelische Gesundheit*. Berne: Verlag Hans Huber, 1959.

Annette, M., D. Lee, and C. Ounsted. "Intellectual disability in relation to lateralised features in the EEG." *Little Club Clinics in Developmental Medicine*, No. 4, (1961).

Apley, J. in J. A. Dodge, ed., *Paediatric Gastroenterology*, London: Pitman Medical, 1976.

Avery, M. E. *The Lung and Its Disorders in the Newborn Infant*. Philadelphia: Saunders, 1964.

Baird, D. "The contribution of obstetrical factors to serious physical and mental handicap in children." *Journal of Obstetrics and Gynaecology of the British Empire*, 66, 743, (1959).

Bakwin, H., and R. M. Bakwin. *Behavior Disorders in Children*. Philadelphia: Saunders, 1972.

Barkley, R. A. "A review of stimulant drug research with hyperactive children." *Journal of Child Psychology and Psychiatry*, 18, 137, (1977).

Bellmaine, S. P., J. McCredie, and B. Storey. "Pharyngeal incoordination from birth to three years, with recurrent bronchopneumonia and ultimate recovery." *Australian Paediatric Journal*, 8, 137, (1972).

Belmont, I., and H. G. Birch. "The effect of intervention on children with low reading readiness scores." *Journal of Special Education*, 8, 81, (1974).

Benaron, H. B. W., B. E. Tucker, J. Andrews, B. Boshes, J. Cohen, E. Fromm, and G. and K. Yacorzynski. "Effect of anoxia during labor and immediately after birth on the subsequent development of the child." *American Journal of Obstetrics and Gynecology*, 80, 1129, (1960).

Biescheuvel, S. "The growth of abilities and character: symposium in current problems in the behavioral sciences in South Africa." *South African Journal of Science*, 375, (August, 1963).

———*The Development of African Abilities.* Faculty of Education Occasional Papers, No. 8. Salisbury, Rhodesia: University College of Rhodesia, 1967.

Birch, H. G. *Brain Damage in Children.* Baltimore: Williams & Wilkins, 1964.

Birch, H. G., C. Pineiro, E. Alcalde, T. Toca, and J. Cravioto, "Relation of kwashiorkor in early childhood and intelligence at school age." *Pediatric Research*, 5, 579, (1971).

Boder, E. "Developmental dyslexia: Prevailing diagnostic concepts and a new diagnostic approach." in H. Myklebust, ed., *Progress in Learning Disorders*, vol. 2, 293–321, New York: Grune & Stratton, 1971.

Bowlby, J., M. Ainsworth, M. Boston, D. Rosenbluth. "Effects of mother child separation: A follow-up study." *British Journal of Medical Psychology*, 29, 211, (1956).

Braun, F. H. T., K. L. Jones, D. W. Smith. "Breech presentation as an indicator of fetal abnormalities." *Journal of Pediatrics*, 86, 419, (1975).

Brenner, M. W., and S. Gillman. "Visuomotor ability in school children. A survey." *Developmental Medicine and Child Neurology*, 8, 686, (1966).

British Medical Journal. "Chronic urticaria." 2, 68, (1976). [Lead article]

Brown, J. K., F. Cockburn, and J. O. Forfar. "Clinical and chemical correlations in convulsions in the newborn." *Lancet*, 1, 135, (1972).

Butler, N. R., and E. D. Alberman. *Perinatal Problems. The Second Report of the 1958 British Perinatal Mortality Survey.* Edinburgh: Livingstone, 1969.

Butler, N. R., and H. Goldstein. "Smoking in pregnancy and subsequent child development." *British Medical Journal*, 4, 573, (1973).

Carlo, J. De, A. Tramer, and H. H. Startzman. "Iodized oil aspiration in the newborn." *American Journal of Diseases of Children*, 84, 442, (1952).

Cartwell, D. P. "Genetics of hyperactivity." *Journal of Child Psychology and Psychiatry*, 16, 261, (1975).

Chateau P. de, and B. Wiberg. "Long term effect on mother infant behaviour by extra contact during the first hour post-partum." *Acta Paediatrica Scandinavica*, 66, 145, (1977).

Chefetz, M. D. "Etiology of cerebral palsy. Role of reproductive inefficiency and the multiplicity of factors." *Obstetrics and Gynaecology*, 25, 635, (1965).

Cohen, H. J., and H. Diner. "The significance of developmental dental enamel defects in neurological diagnosis." *Pediatrics*, 46, 737, (1970).

Cohen, H. J., L. T. Taft, M. S. Mahadeviah, and H. G. Birch. "Developmental changes in outflow in normal and aberrantly functioning children." *Journal of Pediatrics*, 71, 39, (1967).

Conners, C. K., C. H. Goyette, D. A. Southwick, J. M. Lees, and P. A. Andrulonis. "Food additives and hyperkinesis. A controlled double-blind experiment." *Pediatrics*, 58, 154, (1976).

Corah, N. L., E. J. Anthony, P. Pointer, J. A. Stern, and D. L. Thurston. "Effects of perinatal anoxia after seven years." *Psychological Monographs*, 79, 1–34, (1965).

Davie, R., N. R. Butler, and H. Goldstein. *From Birth to Seven.* London: Longman, 1972.

Davies, P. A., and A. L. Stewart. "Low birth weight babies: Neurological sequelae." *British Medical Bulletin*, 31, 85, (1975).

Delaney, J. C. "Response of patients with asthma and asp idiosyncracy to tartrazine." *Practitioner*, 214, 285, (1976).

Denhoff, E., P. K. Hainsworth, and M. L. Hainsworth. "The child at risk for learning disorders." *Clinical Pediatrics*, 11, 164, (1972).

Denson, R., J. L. Nanson, and M. A. McWatters. "Hyperkinesis and maternal smoking." *Canadian Psychiatric Association Journal*, 20, 183, (1975).

Dobbing, J. "Maternal Nutrition and Neurological Development," in *Modern Problems in Paediatrics*, vol. 14, Basel: Karger, 1975.

Doggart, J. H. "Infantile fundus lesions in relation to mental capacity." *British Medical Journal*, 2, 933, (1957).

Douglas, J. W. B. "Premature children in primary school." *British Medical Journal*, 1, 1008, (1960).

Doyne, P. G. "Amaurosis in infants." *Practitioner*, 125, 174, (1930).

Drillien, C. M. "Aetiology and outcome in low birth weight infants." *Developmental Medicine and Child Neurology*, 14, 563, (1972).

Drug and Therapeutics Bulletin. "Stimulant Drugs for Hyperactive Children." 15, 22, (1977).

Dubowitz, V. "The floppy infant—A practical approach to classification." *Developmental Medicine and Child Neurology*, 10, 706, (1968).

Duke-Elder, W. S. *Textbook of Ophthalmology*. London: Kimpton, 1974.

Dykman, R. A., P. T. Ackerman, S. D. Clements, and J. E. Peters "Specific learning disabilities: An attentional deficit syndrome" in H. R. Myklebust, ed., *Progress in Learning Disorders*, vol. 2, 56–93, New York: Grune & Stratton, 1971.

Eccleston, D. "The biochemistry of human moods." *New Scientist*, 57, 18–19, (1973).

Eisenberg, J. L. in H. Birch, ed., *Brain Damage in Children*. Baltimore: Williams & Wilkins, 1964.

Emminger, E. "Prenatal lesions and birth trauma." *German Medical Monthly*, 1, 58, (1956).

Fabian, A. E. "Reading difficulties: An index of pathology." *American Journal of Orthopsychiatry*, 25, 319, (1955).

Fanaroff, A. A., J. H. Kennell, and M. H. Klaus. "Follow up of low-birth weight infants—the predictive value of maternal visiting patterns." *Pediatrics*, 49, 287, (1972).

Fitzhardinge, P. M., and E. M. Steven. "The small for dates infant. Neurological and intellectual sequelae." *Pediatrics*, 50, 50, (1972).

Fitzhardinge, P. M., K. Pafe, M. Arstikaitis, M. Boyle, S. Ashby, A. Rowley, C. Netley, and P. Swyer. "Subsequent development of mechanically ventilated low birth weight infants." *Journal of Pediatrics*, 88, 531, (1976).

Forfar, J. O., and M. M. Nelson. "Drugs and the unborn child." *Clinical Pharmacology and Therapeutics*, 14, 619, (1973).

Francis-Williams, J., and P. A. Davies. "Very low birth weight and later intelligence." *Developmental Medicine and Child Neurology*, 16, 709, (1974).

Frank, M. M., and O. M. Gatewood. "Transient pharyngeal incoordination in the newborn." *American Journal of Diseases of Children*, 111, 178, (1966).

Frankenburg, W. K., and J. B. Dodds. "The Denver developmental screening test." *Journal of Pediatrics*, 71, 181, (1967).

Frankenburg, W. K., B. W. Camp, P. A. Van Natta, J. A. Demers-Seman, and S. E. Voorhees. "Validity of the Denver developmental screening test." *Child Development*, 42, 475–485, (1971).

Fransella, F. "Stuttering. Some facts and treatment." *British Journal of Hospital Medicine*, 16, 70, (1976).

Freedman, D. A. "Congenital and perinatal sensory deprivation. Their effect on the capacity to experience affect." *Psychoanalytic Quarterly*, 44, 62, (1975).

Gesell, A., and C. S. Amatruda. *Developmental Diagnosis*. London: Hoeber, 1956.

Gordon, N. "Visual agnosia in childhood." *Developmental Medicine and Child Neurology*, 10, 377, (1968).

Gubbay, S. S. "The Clumsy Child" (M.D. diss., University of Western Australia, 1972.)

——— *A Study in Developmental Apraxia and Agnosic Ataxia*. Philadelphia: Saunders, 1975.

Hagberg, B., and O. Westphal. "Ataxic syndrome in congenital hypothyroidism." *Acta Paediatrica Scandinavica*, 59, 323, (1970).

Hirsch, K. de, J. J. Jansky, and W. S. Langford. *Predicting Reading Failure*. New York: Harper & Row, 1966.

Hudson, F. P., V. L. Mordaunt, and I. Leahy. "Evaluation of treatment begun in first three months of life in 184 cases of phenylketonuria." *Archives of Disease in Childhood*, 45, 5, (1970).

Hudson, W. "Pictorial depth perception in African groups." *Journal of Social Psychology*, 52, 183, (1960).

Illingworth, R. S. "Delayed visual maturation." *Archives of Disease in Childhood*, 36, 407, (1961).

——— "Sucking and swallowing difficulties in infancy: Diagnostic problem of dysphagia." *Archives of Disease in Childhood*, 44, 665, (1969).

Illingworth, R. S., and J. Lister. "The critical or sensitive period with special reference to certain feeding problems in infants and children." *Journal of Pediatrics*, 65, 839, (1964).

Ingram, T. T. S. "Delayed development of speech with special reference to dyslexia." *Proceedings of the Royal Society of Medicine*, 56, 199, (1963).

——— in Renfrew, C., and K. Murphy, eds., *The Child Who Does Not Talk*, Clinics in Developmental Medicine, No. 13, (1964).

Jan, J. E. *Personal Communication*, 1977.

Johnson, C. F., and R. Prinz. "Hyperactivity is in the eyes of the beholder." *Clinical Pediatrics*, 15, 222, (1976).

Keith, H. M., M. A. Norval, A. B. Hunt. "Neurological lesions in relation to the sequelae of birth injury." *Neurology*, 3, 139, (1953).

Kinsbourne, M. "Minimal brain dysfunction as a neurodevelopmental lag." *Annals of New York Academy of Science*, 205, (1973).

Klaus, M. H., and J. H. Kennell. "Parent to Infant Attachment," in D. Hull, ed., *Recent Advances in Paediactrics*. Edinburgh: Livingstone, 1976.

Klein, P. S., G. B. Forbes, P. R. Nader. "Effects of starvation in infancy on subsequent learning abilities." *Journal of Pediatrics*, 87, 8 (1975).

Kolvin, I., R. C. MacKeith, S. R. Meadow. "Bladder control and enuresis." *Clinics in Developmental Medicine*, Nos. 48–49 (1973).

Laufer, M. W. "Cerebral dysfunction and behavior disorders of adolescents." *American Journal of Orthopsychiatry*, 32, 501, (1962).

Laufer, M. W., and E. Denhoff. "Hyperkinetic behavior syndrome in children." *Journal of Pediatrics*, 50, 463, (1957).

Lapouse, R., and M. A. Monk. "An epidemiologic study of behavior characteristics in children." *American Journal of Public Health*, 48, 1134, (1958).

Levy, D. "On the problem of movement restraint." *American Journal of Orthopsychiatry*, 14, 664, (1944).

Lovell, K. E. "The effect of postmaturity on the developing child." *Medical Journal of Australia*, 1, 13, (1973).

Lovell, K. E., C. Byrne, and B. Richardson. "A further study of the educational progress of children who had received special education." *British Journal of Educational Psychology*, 33, 1, (1963).

Lubchenco, L. O., F. A. Horner, L. H. Reed, I. E. Hix, D. Metcalf, R. Cohig, H. C. Elliott, and M. Bourg. "Sequelae of premature birth." *American Journal of Diseases of Children*, 106, 101, (1963).

Lynch, M. A., and J. Roberts. "Predicting child abuse: Signs of bonding failure in the maternity hospital." *British Medical Journal*, 1, 624, (1977).

McClelland, H. A. "Psychiatric Complications of Drug Therapy." *Adverse Drug Reaction Bulletin*, No. 41, 132 (1973).

MacKeith, R. C. "High activity and hyperactivity." *Developmental Medicine and Child Neurology*, 16, 543, (1974).

Makita, K. "The rarity of reading disability in Japanese children." in S. Chess, and A. Thomas, eds., *Annual Progress in Child Psychiatry and Child Development*, vol. 2, 231–251. New York: Brunner/Mazel, 1969.

Marriage, K. J., and P. A. Davies. "Neurological sequelae in children surviving mechanical ventilation in the newborn period." *Archives of Disease in Childhood*, 52, 176, (1977).

Masland, R. "Minimal brain dysfunction," in F. F. de la Cruz, B. H. Fox, and R. H. Roberts, eds., *Annals of New York Academy of Sciences*, 205, 81–396, (1973).

Matsaniotis, N., J. Karpouzas, M. Gregoriou. "Difficulty in swallowing with aspiration pneumonia in infancy." *Archives of Disease in Childhood*, 42, 308, (1967).

Mattis, S., J. H. French, and I. Rafin. "Dyslexia in children and young adults: Three independent neuropsychological syndromes." *Developmental Medicine and Child Neurology*, 17, 150, (1975).

Mellsop, G. W. "Psychiatric patients seen as children and adults. Childhood predictions of adult illness." *Journal of Child Psychology and Psychiatry*, 13, 91, (1972).

Morgan, J. "Neuromuscular incoordination in the swallowing in the newborn." *Journal of Laryngology*, 70, 294, (1956).

Morley, M. E. *The Development and Disorders of Speech in Childhood.* Edinburgh: Livingstone, 1972.

Muller, E. "The large tonsil." *Deutsche Medizinische Wochenschrift*, 78, 1017, (1953).

Neligan, G., and D. Prudham. "Norms for four standard developmental milestones by sex, social class and place in family." *Developmental Medicine and Child Neurology*, 11, 413, (1969).

Neligan, G., D. McL. Scott, I. Kolvin, and R. C. Garside. "Born too soon or born too small." *Clinics in Developmental Medicine*, No. 61, (1976).

Nylander, I., and B. Hjern. "Acute head injuries in children." *Acta Paediatrica Scandinavica*, Supplement 152, (1964).

Otto, U. "Postconcussion syndrome in children." *Acta Paedopsychiatrica*, 1, 6, (1960).

Ounsted, C. "The hyperkinetic syndrome in epileptic children." *Lancet*, 2, 303, (1955).

Ounsted, C., J. Lindsay, R. Norman. "Biological factors in temporal lobe epilepsy." *Clinics in Developmental Medicine*, No. 22, (1966).

Paine, R. S. "The future of the floppy infant. A follow-up study of 133 patients." *Developmental Medicine and Child Neurology*, 5, 115, (1963).

Paine, R. S., and G. M. Fenichel. "Infantile hypotonia." *Clinical Proceedings of the Children's Hospital of Columbia*, 21, 175, (1965).

Peifer, A. *Cerebral Function in Infancy and Childhood*. London: Pitman, 1963.

Pollack, M., and M. G. Woerner. "Pre and perinatal. complications and childhood schizophrenia." *Journal of Child Psychology and Psychiatry*, 7, 735, (1967).

Prechtl, H. "The mother-child interaction in babies with minimal brain damage," in B. Foss, ed., *Determinants of Infant Behaviour*, vol. 2, 53–66. London: Methuen, 1963.

Raivio, J. O. "Neonatal hypoglycaemia." *Acta Paediatrica Scandinaviea*, 57, 541, (1958).

Reed, G. F. "Psychogenic deafness, perceptual defence and personality variables in children." *Journal of Abnormal and Social Psychology*, 63, 663, (1961).

Reger, R. *School Psychology*. Springfield, Ill.: Thomas, 1965.

Renfrew, C., and K. Murphy. "The child who does not talk." *Clinics in Developmental Medicine*, No. 13, (1964).

Robins, L. N. *Deviant Children Grown Up*. Baltimore: Williams & Wilkins, 1966.

Rose, A. L., and C. T. Lombroso, "Neonatal seizure states." *Pediatrics*, 45, 404, (1970).

Rosenthal, R., and L. F. Jacobson. "Teacher expectations for the disadvantaged." *Scientific American*, 218, 19, (1968).

Rutter, M. L. "Psychosocial disorders in childhood and their outcome in adult life." *Journal of the Royal College of Physicians of London*, 4, 211, (1970).

Rutter, M. "Parent-child separations." *Journal of Child Psychology and Psychiatry*, 12, 233, (1971).

Rutter, M. "Brain damage syndromes in childhood." *Journal of Child Psychology and Psychiatry*, 18, 1, (1977).

Rutter, M., and L. Lockyer. "A 5 to 15 year follow up study of infantile psychosis." *British Journal of Psychiatry*, 113, 1169–1183, (1967).

Rutter, M., and J. A. M. Martin. "The child with delayed speech." *Clinics in Developmental Medicine*, No. 43, (1972).

Rutter, M., J. Tizard. and K. Whitmore. *Education, Health and Behavior*. London: Longman, 1970.

Safer, D., R. Allen, and E. Barr. "Depression of growth in hyperactive children on stimulant drugs." *New England Journal of Medicine*, 287, 217, (1972).

Schmitt, B. D. "The minimal brain dysfunction myth." *American Journal of Diseases of Children*, 129, 1313, (1975).

Scott, H. "Outcome of very severe birth asphyxia." *Archives of Disease in Childhood*, 51, 712, (1976).

Shaw, D. M. "Biochemical basis of affective disorders." *British Journal of Hospital Medicine*, 10, 609, (1973).

Shaywitz, B. A., D. J. Cohen, and M. B. Bowers. "Cerebrospinal fluid monoamine metabolites in children with minimal brain dysfunction. Evidence for alteration of brain dopamine." *Journal of Pediatrics*, 90, 67, (1977).

Shipe, D., S. Vandenberg, and R. D. B. Williams. "Neonatal Apgar ratings as related to intelligence and behavior in preschool children." *Child Development*, 39, 861, (1968).

Siegel, F. S., B. Balow, R. O. Fisch, and V. E. Anderson. "School behavior profile ratings of PKU children." *American Journal of Mental Deficiency*, 72, 937, (1968).

Silberbeg, N. E., I. A. Iverson, and J. T. Goins. "Which remedial reading method works best?" *Journal of Learning Disabilities*, 6, 547, (1973).

Silver, A. A., and R. A. Hagin. "Specific reading disability." *American Journal of Orthopsychiatry*, 34, 95, (1964).

Silver, L. B. "Acceptable and controversial approaches to treating the child with learning disorders." *Pediatrics*, 55, 406, (1975).

Snyder, R. D. "How much reading?" *Pediatrics*, 55, 306, (1975).

Solomon, A. L. "Personality and behavior patterns of children with functional defects of articulation." *Child Development*, 32, 731, (1961).

Solomons, G., R. H. Holden, and E. Denhoff. "The changing pattern of cerebral dysfunction in early childhood." *Journal of Pediatrics*, 63, 113, (1963).

Stark, G., and M. Drummond. "Spina bifida as an obstetric problem." *Developmental Medicine and Child Neurology*, Supplement 22, 157, (1971).

Stewart, R. R., W. Walker, and R. D. Savage. "A developmental study of cognitive and personality characteristics associated with hemolytic disease of the newborn." *Developmental Medicine and Child Neurology*, 12, 16, (1970).

Stone, F. H. *Psychiatry and the Paediatrician*. London: Butterworth, 1976.

Stores, G. "Cognitive function in children with epilepsy." *Developmental Medicine and Child Neurology*, 13, 390, (1971).

Stotch, M. B., and P. M. Smythe. "The effect of undernutrition during infancy on subsequent brain growth and intellectual development." *South African Medical Journal*, 41, 1027, (1967).

Stott, J. H. "Abnormal mothering as a cause of mental subnormality." *Journal of Child Psychology and Psychiatry*, 3, 79, (1962).

Taft, T. L., and W. Goldfarb. "Prenatal and perinatal factors in childhood schizophrenia." *Developmental Medicine and Child Neurology*, 6, 32, (1964).

Towbin, A. "Organic causes of minimal brain dysfunction." *Journal of the American Medical Association*, 217, 1207, (1971).

Trevor-Roper, P. *The World through Blunted Sight*. London: Thomas and Hudson, 1971.

Vernon, P. E. *Intelligence and Cultural Environment*. London: Methuen, 1969.

Wagner, M. C., and R. Arndt. "Postmaturity as an etiologic factor in 124 cases of neurologically handicapped children." *Clinics in Developmental Medicine*, No. 27, (1968).

Walton, J. N., E. Ellis, S. D. M. Court. "Clumsy children: Developmental apraxia and agnosia." *Brain*, 85, 603 (1962).

Weinberg, S. A., E. C. Penick, M. Hammerman, and M. Jackoway. "An evaluation of a summer remedial reading program." *American Journal of Diseases of Children*, 122, 494, (1971).

Weiss, G., K. Minde, J. S. Werry, V. Douglas, and E. Nemeth. "Studies on the hyperactive child: Five year follow up." *Archives of General Psychiatry*, 24, 409, (1971).

Wender, P. H., and E. H. Wender. "Minimal brain dysfunction myth." *American Journal of Diseases of Children*, 130, 900, (1976).

Werner, E., K. Simorian, J. M. Bierman, and F. E. French. "Cumulative effect of perinatal complications and deprived environments on physical, intellectual and social development of school children." *Pediatrics*, 39, 490, (1967).

Werry, J. S. "Developmental hyperactivity." *Pediatric Clinics of North America*, 15, 581, (1968).

———"Medication for hyperkinetic children." *Drugs*, 11, 81, (1976).

Wiener, G., R. V. Rider, W. C. Oppel, L. K. Fischer, and P. A. Harper. "Correlates of low birth weight. Psychological status at 6 to 7 years of age." *Pediatrics*, 35, 434, (1965).

Wiener, G., R. V. Rider, W. C. Oppel, and P. A. Harper. "Correlates of low birth weight. Psychological status at 8 to 10 years of age." *Pediatric Research*, 2, 110, (1968).

Wilson, G. S., M. M. Desmond, and N. M. Verniaud. "Early development of infants of heroin-addicted mothers." *American Journal of Diseases of Children*, 126, 457, (1973).

Winick, M., and P. Rosso. "Head circumference and cellular growth of the brain in normal and marasmic children." *Journal of Pediatrics*, 74, 774, (1969).

Worden, D. K., and P. J. Vignos. "Intellectual function in childhood progressive muscular dystrophy." *Pediatrics*, 29, 968, (1962).

Zangwill, O. L. "Language and language disorders," in A. Dorfman, ed., *Child Care in Health and Disease*. Chicago: Year Book Publishers, 1968.

CHAPTER 23

Educational Intervention

Selma G. Sapir

Many controversial issues about the education of handicapped children remain unsolved. Changes in philosophy, programming, and educational methodology have been rapid, causing confusion and controversy in the field. How one views these crucial issues will determine how the learning-disabled child is defined, how his deficits are conceptualized, and on what basis the remediation has been predicated.

The concept of brain damage first began to make an impact on the educational scene with the work of Alfred Strauss (1947), Laura Lehtinen (1947), Heinz Werner (1957) and Newell Kephart (1968). The brain damaged era began slowly with the publishing of Strauss and Lehtinen's book in 1947 and did not emerge full blown until the early 1960s. In the late 1950s and early 1960s many research physicians became aware of a population without frank brain damage, but with many of the same symptoms.

In 1962 Sapir and Wilson (1967) began their research in a normal public school setting. As psychologists they had become aware of increasing numbers of children with uneven and deviant cognitive, social, and emotional growth patterns. Early identification screening with the Sapir Developmental Scale (1967) highlighted widely divergent patterns of deficits in youngsters of normal to superior intelligence with gross imbalance of developmental milestones. Boys seemed to have many more difficulties than girls.

As the body or research developed, many disciplines began to coalesce in the emergence of a significant educational concept. At the same time parents began to exert their efforts to develop educational programs suitable for children having severe problems in school. Children were described along a continuum, from seemingly normal with reading problems to profoundly disabled with many dysfunctions. Attempts to integrate the disciplines of education, medicine, and behavioral science were unsuccessful because of the difficulties and differences of definition and goal.

The necessity of defining a vastly diverse population has led to some arbitrary differentiations about the children now described as having learning disability, minimal brain dysfunction, minimal cerebral dysfunction, developmental deficit, aphasia, specific learning disability, dyslexia, strephosymbolia, and about 50 other arbitrary designations. In no other area of special education has so much effort and controversy gone into the refinement of a definition. In 1966 a task force on terminology and identification of the child with minimal brain dysfunction was cosponsored by the National Institute of Neurological Diseases and Blindness of the National Institutes of Health. They defined it as follows:

The term 'minimal brain dysfunction syndrome' refers to the children of near average, average or above average general intelligence with certain learning or behavioral disabilities ranging from mild to severe which are associated with deviations of function of the central nervous system. These deviations may manifest themselves by various combinations of impairment in perception, conceptualization, language, memory and control of attention, impulse or motor function. Similar symptoms may or may not complicate the problems of children with cerebral palsy, epilepsy, mental retardation, blindness or deafness.

By 1968, with a change in terminology to learning disability, the Bureau of Education for the Handicapped, Office of Education, provided the following definition:

Children with specific learning disabilities exhibit a disorder in one or more of the basic psychological processes involved in understanding or in using spoken or written language. These may be manifested in disorders of listening, thinking, talking, reading, writing, spelling or arithmetic. These include conditions which have been referred to as perceptual handicaps, brain injury, minimal brain dysfunction, dyslexia, developmental aphasia, et cetera. They do not include learning problems which are due primarily to visual, hearing or motor handicaps, to mental retardation, emotional disturbance or to environmental deprivations.

Definitions and descriptions of children are many and varied because no learning-disabled child is like another. Symptoms occur in clusters and vary from child to child. MBD is a variable clinical syndrome which changes with age. In the normal child there are primary modes of processing at different ages and stages. As soon as competence is reached in one stage, there is a shift of function to another, for example:

Piaget distinguishes four major stages in the development of intelligence: first, the sensorimotor period before the appearance of language; second the period from two to seven years of age, the pre-operational period; third the period from seven to twelve years of age, a period of concrete operations (which refer to concrete objects); and finally after twelve years of age, the period of formal operations. [Sapir-Nitzburg, 1973, p. 4]

Kephart (1968) using different terms discusses the motor stage in which the child develops the tools for environmental encounters: the motor-perceptual stage during which perceptual information is matched to the previously developed motor information which remains the controlling factor; the perceptual-motor stage during which perceptual exploration becomes the dominant mode of operation; the perceptual stage during which perceptions are manipulated against each other; the perceptual-conceptual stage during which similarities of perceptions are compared and can be combined into an abstracted concept; the conceptual stage during which the child manipulates one concept against another and may become highly verbal; and the conceptual-perceptual stage during which the child depends less and less on perception as a primary source of information and depends more and more on conceptual manipulation of information. At this last stage perceptions are fit into conceptual relations. Thus the old adage, "We see not what is there, but what we want to see."

It is a common occurrence that when one has a record of a child diagnosed as

MBD over a long range of time, one discovers that at three the child may have had speech lags; at seven, the perceptual problem (visual-motor or auditory) is primary; at nine, with the shift of function, the syndrome becomes more language oriented and it is common to find children having difficulty in word finding (substituting words with a category) or word usage (unable to shift the meaning of a word such as hole and whole) or the syntactical problem of shift to another part of speech (block from a noun to a verb); and much later, the difficulty manifests itself in written work with a disability appearing in writing a sentence or a paragraph in an appropriate form.

The message is clear. A diagnostician or educator must always put into context the normal stages of development and look at the degree of deviation from the normal. The dysfunction relates to the primary mode of functioning at that particular time in the child's life and may well disappear as the child moves from one stage to another. This does not necessarily imply a developmental lag or maturational problem. It might be possible to circumvent the problem by helping the child compensate through another mode of performance and it is just this type of educational intervention that is advocated here.

Deviant behavior, learning disabilities, speech disorders, and poor coordination are the most common presenting complaints along with pervasive disabilities in one or more of the cognitive functions. The U. S. Department of HEW in *Minimal Brain Dysfunction in Children*—Terminology and Identification (Clements, 1966) lists 10 characteristics most often cited:

- Hyperactivity.
- Perceptual-motor impairments.
- Emotional liability.
- General coordination deficits.
- Disorders of attention (short attention span, distractibility, perseveration).
- Impulsivity.
- Disorder of memory and thinking.
- Specific learning disabilities in reading, arithmetic, writing, and spelling.
- Disorder of speech and hearing and equivocal neurological signs.
- Electroencephalographic irregularities.

MBD is a mystifying handicap in many ways. It obviously encompasses a wide variety of problems. Just as there are children who fit into such characteristic patterns as have been described, there are others who do not. Some are passive and withdrawn; some are well coordinated; some appear to have excellent emotional strengths and health in spite of their serious handicaps in language and/or reading; and some are well motivated and struggling to succeed.

The term learning disability means many different things depending on how and where it is used. The designation and treatment therefore represents a vast array of etiologies and methodologies. To some it signifies all children who have achieved well below their developmental norm (some say one standard deviation, others two grades below expectation, and so on). To some it means those children who represent some neurophysiological deviation from the norm; for others it means a clustering of symptomatology of minimal brain dysfunction (soft signs such as hyperactivity, poor attention and concentration, small muscle motor dysfunction, visual or auditory perceptual problems).

Probably the only acceptable description of the characteristics of the MBD child is one that is specific to that child, that is one that considers the child's temperamental and cognitive style and particular behavior pattern in a variety of situations. The child has his own particular set of cluster syndromes. It is the number, degree of, and deviation from the norm that is currently used as the determinant for the MBD label. Gallagher and Bradley (1972) state:

> Children with learning disabilities are defined in varying ways but are often identified as children with specific defects in processing information or properly interpreting information from their environment. Such a problem would be revealed by developmental imbalances within the individual child. The key indication of trouble is wide variations and fluctuating strengths and weaknesses of this child against his own developmental norms.

The problems of terminology are complicated by the need to satisfy many diverse demands of clinicians who diagnose, prescribe, or treat; researchers concerned with validity, reliability, and preciseness; educators who are held accountable; and parents and others personally involved with the child. This is further complicated by the fact that the MBD children can manifest varying degrees of severity, from mild to profound, in one or more of specific areas such as sensory, motor, perception, language. These children reveal varying behavior patterns from hyperactive to hypoactive, from excellent motivation to little motivation, from perseverance to short attention span and high distractibility.

CURRENT TRENDS IN MBD EDUCATIONAL PROGRAMS

As there has been confusion in definition and description, so has there been in treatment and programming. It is only natural that as a new field emerges much trial and error has to occur.

At first MBD programs adopted principles and practices used in work with the brain damaged, for example children were provided with special class placement and individual carrels for minimization of visual and auditory stimulation. Such special modifications proved ineffective because they did not help MBD children learn to organize the environment so that they could process stimulation comfortably. A movement in the field toward prescriptive or precision teaching brought with it a need for early identification procedures that could be translated into strengths and weaknesses in basic areas of functioning: motor and body, perception, and language and thought. Screening tests were developed to define remedial procedures in terms of the child, teaching only what was tested. Many programs for MBD children use behavioral objectives and behavior modification techniques, implying that change takes place through reinforcement principles. This is a very questionable theory which also raises issues about the application of these principles in a free society.

Depending on how the term is defined and which children we are discussing, methodology flows. Treatment procedures may be based on behavioral, psychoanalytic, self-aspiring or developmental-interacting theories. Methodology reflects the particular philosophical base in which one believes. Research has seldom compared these different methodologies.

In the late 1950s and early 1960s Bruner attempted to contrast the nature of a theory of instruction with a theory of learning. He pointed out that while a theory of learning is descriptive, a theory of instruction is prescriptive in the sense that it sets forth rules specifying the most effective way to achieve knowledge or mastery of skills. A theory of learning describes the conditions under which such competence is acquired. A theory of instruction sets up criteria of performance and then specifies the conditions required for meeting them. Skinner in the course of his interest in the technology of teaching made the development of procedures for prescribing conditions for learning almost indistinguishable from a theoretical description of learning. Piaget however has continued to make the point that children pass through normative stages of cognitive development, and he has repeatedly insisted that, specific training notwithstanding, the child reaches these stages of development with normal maturation of his specific constitutional endowments, providing he has been exposed to the normal experiences of childhood.

It becomes immediately evident that there is a dichotomy between the Skinnerian and Piagetian approach which needs careful consideration and that the flow of research about these diverse theoretical positions needs to be fed directly to the teacher-practitioner. It also may be possible that both Piaget and Skinner have something to offer for very different situations and this too requires specific research.

John Dewey in his presidential address before the American Psychological Association (1899) expressed concern about developing a linking science between psychological theory and practical use. The decisive matter, according to Dewey, is the extent to which the ideas of the theorist actually projected themselves into the conciousness of the practitioner. It is the participation by the practical man in the theory, through the agency of the linking science, that determines at once the effectiveness of the work done and the moral freedom and personal development of the one engaged in it. It is, in reverse, the teachers' inability to regard on occasion both themselves and the child as objects working upon each other in specific ways that compels them to reach for purely arbitrary measures. They tend then to fall back on mere routine traditions of school teaching or to fly to the latest fad of pedagogical theorists.

If one is concerned with the development of a link between research and practical application, one must consider those theorists who tried to do just this in the past. Certainly B. F. Skinner (1968) is one example of a theorist who tried to work through this linking structure via programmed learning and teaching machines. Why has this failed? Is it possible that as the field became more popular it took on a superficial momentum that separated it from the implicit theory that generated it? Is it also possible that the basic tenet of behavioral systems and operant conditioning fail to consider the myriad of complexities in the human behavioral patterns?

Teachers have in the past been confused or frustrated by diagnostic information that fails to translate into effective instruction. In their desperation they grab at gimmicks and commercially made materials, failing to realize that what is significant is what happens between two people: how well the instructor understands the process of the learner, how capable and flexible he or she can be to adjust to the needs of the child, and how well he or she can on the instant create a new task through which the student may achieve success. There is need for a systematic study of the complexities inherent in instructional interactions. Taxonomies may be well constructed from a theoretical point of view, but have only limited practical application. Theorists like Piaget (1961) and Hunt (1969) have focused on the important match between experiential variables and the child's present developmental level—the closer the match, the more probable the desired behavioral change. Developmental readiness (Bloom, 1964) is seen as the child's internal readiness to benefit and learn from an experience. Developmental pressure is seen as just the right amount of pressure to exert beyond what the child can infer himself as well as what is needed to move the child to the next step of integration. As a result of this concept one group of educators emphasized homogeneous grouping and the use of self-instructional programmed workbooks; another group deemphasized structure and sequencing, encouraging instead many varied experiences to act as catalysts for learning which, they thought, would evolve as a natural consequence. Soon these two separate approaches were discarded because of their obvious lack of balance.

Bloom (1956) identified taxonomies in the cognitive, affective, and psychomotor domains. Learning was assumed to occur in an orderly sequence from the simple to the complex. Gagne's (1971) learning hierarchy attempted to classify several kinds of learning postulates by classical and contemporary psychologists (Pavlov, Watson, Hull, Skinner, Osgood, Bruner, Ausubel). Unfortunately taxonomies were of limited educational value because they failed to provide adequate foundations for generating instructional programming based on theoretical hierarchies. The effective integration of different experiences was lacking (White, 1973). These inadequacies led to the consideration of task analysis in the development of individualized instruction. Task analysis involves the separation and organization of each learning task into its smallest component parts. Task analysis requires an intuitive practical base, involving trial and error experimentation, flexibility of instruction based on observation, and a critical and frequent use of individualized, informal evaluation which constantly is checking hypothesis and hunches. One problem of task analysis is the tendency of special educators to focus on immediate short-term programming. As a result of this approach new criterion-referenced assessment techniques were developed, which according to their developers had ethical appeal as well as instructional legitimacy for the handicapped population. The problem here is that the assessment is short ranged, paying more attention to product than process. Task analysis has value only when it leads the way to an understanding of the process used by each individual. This then leads the learner to long-range planning of strategies for success.

Just as theorists have developed theories of learning and instruction, many special educators have presented models for teaching exceptional children. One attempt to bring a greater degree of coordination and integration to the process of individualization has been the diagnostic-prescriptive model. This model has its roots in systems theory and is based on the behavioral philosophy. Most of these models prescribe linear sequences (Minskoff, 1973; Lerner, 1973; Cartwright, Cartwright, and Ysseldyke, 1973; Adelman, 1971) and imply direct applicability in the classroom. They incorporate task analysis, behavioral objectives, and criterion-referenced testing in a total package equated with individualized instruction.

This model suggests that one can pinpoint diagnosis; indicate exactly where a child is, along a linear line of achievement; and proceed on in such linear fashion with a mechanical conception of the learning process which according to these theorists leads to higher and higher orders of learning. It does not consider the child's complexity of maturation—his own hierarchical patterns as well as his unique, uneven development. It further suggests that one can use the paradigm of pretest, instruct, and posttest. Evaluation in this diagnostic-prescriptive model assumes the child is either correct or incorrect with the focus on the outcome (product), not on the differing ways a child may have used to arrive at a specific outcome (process). The author considers this a rather limiting informational system, which pays little attention to the way children develop schemata, assimilate and accommodate new learnings to their already integrated schematic system. Examples of this model are represented by precision teaching and other programmed instructional forms. In this model, generally clinical diagnosis is separated from educational treatment. One person performs the diagnosis and then prescribes activities that form the basis of a treatment plan. The diagnostician in this model is responsible for recommending or designing appropriate educational environments and procedures for each child based on the child's strengths and weaknesses. You can then end up with two bodies of information in which remedial procedures take on an importance related only to and are limited to the information gathered from a particular testing experience. Mann (1973) has indicated that the diagnostic-prescriptive methodology that programs children based on the strengths and weaknesses of the child's performance on particular tests (ITPA, Frostig, and so on) has little validity. Only too often have we found that children who have performed poorly on certain subtests of the ITPA or Frostig are able to do the tasks of a similar nature and in reverse. Children may have done well on other subtests and yet seem unable to translate that knowledge to a particular task.

Ysseldyke (1973) suggests "there is little support for claims that instruction can be differentiated on the basis of diagnostic strengths and weaknesses." He points out that the match between a child's level of functioning and the selected instruction is seldom realized because procedures used for evaluation (ITPA, Frostig, Early Identification Scales) lack the sensitivity to reflect the dynamic nature of the child-teacher-instruction interaction. He advocates two alternatives: (1) develop more reliable assessment instruments with demonstrated validity, or (2) stop the use of standardized tests and focus on the systematic collection of observational data.

Instructional decisions make little sense when they are divorced from clinical diagnosis, what is needed is the coordination of treatment and diagnostic processes. Unitary study is needed of the child, of his or her environment, and of the transactions occurring in the child's total life space. According to Sameroff and Chandler (1973):

It is apparent that if developmental processes are to be understood, it will not be through continuous assessment of the child alone but through a continuous assessment of the transactions between the child and his environment to determine how these transactions facilitate or hinder adaptive integration as both the child and his surroundings change and evolve.

We seem to be heading in just the opposite direction. The present diagnostic procedures (when the teacher or parent suspects a child has a learning problem) refers the child to a psychometrician or a child-study team for evaluation. The evaluation usually occurs out of the child's classroom in a one-to-one situation with an evaluator who usually presents items from standardized tests. In most cases little consideration is given to studying the school, the home, and the environment as well as the child. In some cases interdisciplinary teams agree on a diagnosis, prescribe a program which is then turned over in written form to the practitioner to be put into effect. Here, communication, language, and understanding of what is meant can become a real problem. Interpretation differs depending on the level of knowledge, particular bias, and experience of the teaching person. Another serious flaw is that the model fails to account for the child's rapid maturing system, one that is in constant flux, changing day by day as a natural developing process. This alone makes it difficult to prescribe because by the time the prescription becomes operable the child may have shifted his primary mode of processing and may well know more or less of what had been indicated. In addition we know that the same individual is different in different environments and with different people and on different days. Who is to say whether the particular examiner has in effect tapped the highest potential of this individual? The conceptual problem is even greater when we consider that we are dealing in large part with developmental problems in a complex culture, rather than with defects in the common cure-seeking framework.

The prescription that results from this evaluation seldom considers the following essential factors:

1. Critical contextual variables present in the classroom which directly affect the child's ability to learn—grouping policies, methodology teacher uses, multisensory nature of presentation, pace, repetitions, number of children, levels of other children, noise, evaluation tools, and so on.
2. Semantic differences of language used in presenting prescription.
3. Differences in experiential level of evaluator and teacher involving ways the teacher puts the prescription into operation.
4. Differences in interaction between child-evaluator as compared to child-teacher.

Rarely does such a strategy produce valid starting points for educational efforts on behalf of children. The whole system breeds bad habits and tends to diffuse responsibility for the education of the child.

A second approach is the ecological model which attempts to integrate the individual and his environment (Carroll, 1974; Posner, 1974). Here contextual, inter- and intra-personal characteristics are identified and classified as a means of systematically assessing their effects on rate and style of learning. Diagnosis based on direct observation within and outside the classroom involves identification, classification, and synthesis of conditions under which the child can and cannot learn (Semmel, 1974). Such diagnostic analysis seems potentially more productive, both from an instructional and a research perspective; results and benefits may be quickly realized; relevance and validity of observational data may be self-evident; the teacher becomes the recipient of immediately useful information and becomes an active participant in the treatment and research process. It enables the teacher, with time, to identify specific learning styles so that optimal instructional patterns can emerge. This approach requires individualized instruction in single or clusters of sequences in which the teacher identifies which unit is a logical next step in programming for a specific child. Each unit may contain one or several objectives; the teacher identifies how much and what kind of information the child must acquire to reach criterion. In this approach there is a test-operate-test (in case the child needs more information), and if objective is reached: exit to terminate instruction. The responses the child makes provides the teacher with needed data with which to make instructional adjustments. These changes may be qualitative and/or quantitative and reflect consideration of interactions among variables. The interrelationships among learner, teacher, and context suggests program changes and permits inferences about underlying psychological processes, such as perception and conceptualization. With this approach the dynamic continuous nature of learning is more easily recognized and more importantly the probability of long-range individualized programming is enhanced.

Shavelson (1975) has proposed a decision-making model. Are teachers aware of the child's states of nature (learning, affect, situational) that may affect selected outcomes for any given child? Are teachers aware of the number of options/strategies available at any given time? The use of the decision-making model has interesting implications: (1) it is possible over time for the teacher to generate a dynamic pattern of conditions under which a child learns best, (2) the dimensions of interest are not based on some arbitrary taxonomy, but on the teachers personal perception of relevant, functional, and variable categories, (3) the teacher is always cued to consider probable states, rather than the absolute state of the child, (4) the procedure leads to continuous reevaluation of options available to the teacher based on personal subjective perceptions of state changes, (5) the teacher will anticipate instructional needs rather than react to instructional failure.

This too has its limitations. A major problem can be the effectiveness and accuracy of the teacher's observational tools as decisions about instructional options are made based on these observations. The teachers ability to isolate, summarize, and make inferences about which instructional options will yield the best results for a given child is critical. The teacher's ability to make decisions, probably more than any other variable, affects how and what a child will learn.

Glaser (1972) has recommended a complete shift of emphasis from input-output variables to process related ones. This requires the integration of contemporary theories of child development, learning, and human performance. The emphasis here is to foster learning-to-learn skills; to recognize that basic strategies can be developed; to design flexible instructional sequences in which the entry point in one sequence is determined by the capability of the child. It recognizes that with sufficient time and optimal circumstances all children are capable of learning. Underachievement is no longer viewed solely as a result of some inadequacy within the child, but may instead reflect the inadequacy of the interactive process between learner characteristics and variables within the instructional system. Individualization must be based not only on the child's unique information processing system but also on task analysis and the child's own communication system.

Doris Johnson speaking at the American Psychological Association Meeting (1976) stated that there can be no simple response or treatment program for the learning-disabled population because of the variability and complexity of their problems. These children need expectations to learn, adjustment of goals, appropriate placements, tutoring in specific school subjects, and teaching to their strengths as well as work on their deficits. She recommended an exploration of the individual modes of input to facilitate change. To help the child learn, it is usually necessary to break down complex tasks into subsystems and to create end products that will be satisfying.

Three methodological questions which concern practitioners are: (1) Can specific cognitive deficits in children's learning be isolated in such a way that they can be assessed and provide a basis for curriculum planning? Such presumption is the foundation of the notion of prescriptive teaching, but there is much question that such fractionalizing is possible or fruitful. It would seem more valuable to analyze tasks as well as interactions between teachers and children; (2) Should teachers teach to the strengths or train the weaknesses of children? On a broad conceptual level one has to teach through the child's strengths, but this does not preclude measures to deal with interfering deficits. The child should be encouraged to become an active collaborator in diminishing his own weaknesses by developing an awareness of his problems and his intact effective compensatory mechanisms. Often the child can be helped to use his conceptualization, for example to tackle consciously a difficult perceptual problem. Such mobilization of the child's strengths would seem to be more effective than training a perceptual skill and hoping for transfer; (3) Should an attempt be made to teach directly the processes of thinking strategies (learning how-to-learn) rather than an assortment of facts? Learning experiences must be structured in a way to enable children to discover and integrate knowledge about the world. Intellectual operations are acquired through interaction between the organism and the environment in lawful sequences.

The Clinical-Diagnostic Teaching Model

Attempting to integrate the most effective approaches with basic child development theory, Sapir and Nitzburg (1973) propose a clinical diagnostic teaching model based on a developmental-interaction point of view. It is practiced in the learning lab, a center for learning-disabled children, at Bank Street College of Education. Basic to its more than 58-years' work with children, Bank Street believes that children grow and function as total beings with the emotional, social, physical, and intellectual dimensions interacting with each other as well as with the human and physical environments which surround the children. Bank Street views learning as part of the maturation process which depends on constant, sensitive, reciprocal interaction between cognitive and affective spheres. In the introduction of their book, Sapir and Nitzburg (1973) state the need to relate knowledge about normal development to children with learning disorders:

Important concepts about cognitive, social and emotional growth need to be considered. At a conference on "The Roots of Excellence," sponsored by the Bank Street College of Education, Barbara Biber stated that: . . . there is a very fundamental relation between learning and personality development. The two interact in what we speak of as a "circular process." According to Dr. Biber, mastery of symbol systems (letters, words, numbers), reasoning, judging, problem-solving, acquiring and organizing information and all such intellectual functions are fed by and feed into varied aspects of the personality for relatedness, autonomy, creativity and integration. The school has a special area of influence for healthy personality because it can contribute to the development of the ego strength. How a child is taught affects his image of himself, which in turn influences what he will dare and care to learn. The challenge is to provide opportunities that will make the most of this circular growth process toward greater learning powers and inner strength.

The acquisition of developmental milestones will be considered within the framework of a developmental-interactive system. Here developmental refers to the emphasis on indentifiable patterns of growth and modes of perceiving and responding, which are characterized by increasing differentiation and progressive integration as a function of chronological age. Interaction refers: (1) to the emphasis on the child's interaction with his environment and (2) to the interaction between neurological, cognitive, and affective spheres of development.

The complexity of this whole process of developing systems is such that it defies understanding. It forever amazes observers that children have such resiliency and inner strength that even with small amounts of nurturance and support they learn, grow, and prosper.

The basic philosophy is to build on an "island of health." One must understand the complexity of organization, that is know not only which factors play a determining role in the course of the individual's growth, but also *how* these factors interact to influence that course. The goal is to maximize positive growth and development of a learning, coping child.

The child is a complex organism with all systems in constant interaction, constantly changing. The developmental point of view sees the child as an ever evolving organism passing through stages, each of which is relevant to earlier and later development. Stimulation of any kind affects all parts of the organism. Children have biological strengths and weaknesses which interact with their environment, helping or hindering growth. The child needs to develop emotional strength that allows for trust and autonomy and permits freedom of play and exploration before symbolic knowledge is possible. A problem for a child in one area will hinder, stunt, or skew growth in other areas. Too often one sees emotionally disturbed youngsters who have distortion of perception and language as well as children with central nervous system damage who have difficulty in ego development and social responses to other children. With an understanding of normal development, one can maximize the child's strengths and develop a program that will foster the greatest overall growth.

To understand the developmental milestones of childhood, we must look for the common patterns shared by all children as they grow and mature. Werner and Kaplan (1963) tell us that as the child matures he moves from a state of global perception and reaction to increasing differentiation and hierarchical organization. The infant initially perceives his world in a global fashion. As the child increasingly learns to differentiate between himself and other objects and people, he becomes less dominated by the stimulus field around him and more able to define himself. He develops concepts about himself and his world. In this way he achieves freedom to organize and control behavior in himself and the world about him. He begins to experience that he has power over his environment.

There are those theorists, Noam Chomsky (1964) among them, who feel that the progression of differentiation and hierarchical integration and the acquisition of certain skills, such as language, are so steady, so rapid, and so complex that they must be based upon innate qualities of the human species and perhaps proceed in maturational patterns that are age appropriate. Others such as Luria (1961) emphasize other aspects of this developmental process, such as the role of speech and perception to produce conception formation. Still others deal with the "why" of development—the motivational aspects of learning. All, I am sure, would agree that it takes the nurturing and supportive environment to allow these processes to emerge.

Jean Piaget (1961) has probably made the most impact on the educational scene in the past decade. He has been preoccupied with the question of how we come to know our world, and he has tried to find the answers through scientific but natural observation of children. Central to Piaget's position is the concept of the organism passing through cognitive stages derived from motor action. The child is continually adding to his cognitive repertoire through the process of assimilation and accommodation. Piaget distinguishes four major stages in the development of intelligence: (1) from birth to about 2 years, the sensorimotor period before the appearance of language; (2) from about 2 to 7 years, the preoperational period; (3) from about 7 to 12, a period of formal operation—all in quest of universal truths. The sensorimotor stage as a whole carries the child from inborn reflexes to acquired behavior patterns. It leads the child from a body-centered (that is self-centered) world to an object centered one. During this period of the development of object constancy, the various sensory spaces of vision, touch, hearing, and the rest are coordinated into a single space and objects evolve from their separate sensory properties into things with multiple properties, permanence, and spatial relationships. The pre-operational stage (from around 2 to 7 years) covers the important period when language is acquired. This permits the child to deal symbolically with the world replacing direct motor action, though his problem-solving still tends to be action ridden. The child is himself still the focus of his own world; space and time are centered around him. Time is only before now, now, and not yet, and space moves as the child moves. When the child is taken for an evening walk, he thinks the moon follows him. Children during this stage learn gradually to conceive of a time scale and of a spatial world which exist independent of themselves. During this stage, when dealing with objects, quantities, and words, children pay attention to just one attribute, neglecting all others. They conclude, for example, that there is more water in a glass graduate than a beaker—though they have seen the water poured from one vessel to the other—because in the graduate the column of water is taller and children of this age and stage neglect to pay attention to the other attribute, the reduction in diameter. The stage of concrete operation, at about age 7, reveals a child less dependent upon his own perceptions and motor actions, and showing capacity for reasoning, although only on a concrete level. Among their logical acquisitions at this stage are classifying, ordering in a series, and numbering. Asked to put a handful of sticks in order by length, they need no longer make all the pair comparisons, but can pick out the longest, then the next longest, and so on. At about 11 or 12 years the child can handle abstract relationships—dealing with symbols, instead of things; with the form of an argument, while ignoring its content.

A discussion of educational milestones cannot be complete without mentioning the language continuum, as it is one of the major contributions to readiness for academic growth. Language, as we know, grows with the child in quantity, quality, size of vocabulary, sentence length, degree of abstraction, and in all kinds of multidimensional ways. It is generally believed that inner language is acquired first, receptive language next, and expressive language last. A child does not first learn words and then meaning; meaningfulness and experience precedes the acquisition of words. Only after children have begun to make sense out of their world, do they begin to understand the words that represent experience. When inner language has been established to a minimal degree, the child begins to comprehend auditory verbal symbols (words), that is receptive language. Reciprocal relationships between processes are evidenced by the fact that with an increase in receptive language, inner language is also increased. Finally after minimal inner and receptive language have been established, the child acquires expressive language, he begins to talk. As he speaks, he enhances both his receptive and inner language. The verbal mediator begins to become a factor in the development of higher order perception and concept formation.

This process of language growth continues throughout life. With new and broader experiences we add new meanings and new words to our vocabularies. Moreover with the acquisition of new symbols, the potential for creating new thoughts and ideas is increased.

Inner language can be evaluated by carefully observing a child's play and noting the appropriateness of his behavior and his ability to make sense out of his environment. If the child is presented with a series of toys, one can observe the ways the child uses and organizes them. For example the little girl may feed her baby doll, comb her hair, and so on. Receptive language, the ability to comprehend spoken words of others, can be observed when the child responds to verbal cues the adults offer. Typically the young child will respond to verbal directions ("Get me your sweater." "Run to the door." "Can you find the pencil?") by motor action—pointing, gesturing, and so on.

Lastly we come to expressive language. Although a disturbance in comprehension will affect expression, we see children who understand but cannot speak. Expressive language can be thought of in three ways: word retrieval, articulation of words, and the syntax of the language. On the development of word retrieval or word naming, there are those children who can remember words for the purposes of recognition when spoken to, but not for spontaneous usage. These children with word finding difficulties have speech full of word substitutions, hesitancies, and often a large flow of words. When shown a comb, they might say: "brush," "thing," "you know what it is, you use it on your hair," or "that thing with points on it." Many children with reading problems manifest word retrieval problems. These are often difficult to detect because children tend to be verbose. It is only after some time that you begin to understand that the language is not specific to the target word, and in fact may be used for a very different object, as in the case of brush for comb. Another aspect of speech development requires a well-defined motor patterning system so that words can be articulated clearly. Children with problems in this area may be unable to enunciate specific sounds. These must be distinguished from those children with auditory processing problems who tend to mispronounce words or misplace syllables, such as "sagetti" for "spaghetti," "aminal for animal."

Finally we come to the syntax of the language, the formulation of sentences— the rules for putting words together to make sense and say exactly what is meant. An example of difficulty in this area is heard when the child says, "The dog pulled the wagon with the boy." He means, and the action shows, that "The boy pulled the dog in the wagon." Another example is the child who does not understand that words can be used in many different ways, for example such a child cannot make the shift from "I rode down the block." to "I build with blocks." to "I block that pass."

An extension of speaking includes the related symbol system, reading and writing. The developmental sequence begins with auditory verbal comprehension (listening) and progresses to oral expression (speaking)—reading and writing. The normal child first learns oral language; later he learns to read and write. He superimposes a visual symbol system on an auditory one. If there is a problem in the auditory oral communication system, there is bound to be difficulty when one has to learn to read or write. But if children have normal growth patterns, they will have two systems for input (listening and reading) and two systems for output (speaking and writing). A disturbance can occur at any point along this developmental continuum.

Some time in the first year of life, we anticipate that most children will say their first intelligible word. If that is reinforced by a smile, praise, or pat, the child will continue to add to his repertoire. A few months later children are saying many words; some children go about the house naming things (table, dog, ball), saying action words (play, see, come), and an occasional quality word (blue, bad, and so on). At about 18 months children are apt to construct two word utterances, such as "push car." The beginning utterances are not said as communications systems, but as reinforcers or stimulants for action. Gradually, at about three years, children with normal development are so advanced in the construction process as to produce all the major variables of English simple sentences up to a length of 10 or 11 words.

Behavior is simultaneously determined by the inborn structure, past experiences, and the particular present situation. Ideas tend to be incorporated into a complex system of thought schemata. The way one organizes the environment to allow for certain appropriate experiences will determine whether the child can build a cognitive structure on which he can achieve age-appropriate intellectual mastery. An optimal environment should provide the structure that will enable children to develop feelings of competence and self-esteem as they master cognitive and social skills necessary to their functioning. To do this the child must perceive his/her competence as valid and must be able to use it in effective interaction with people and work. Furthermore the ingredients of ego strength and the associated competence fostered by the school must be appropriate to the child's developmental stage. On their developmental-interaction approach, Shapiro and Biber (1972) state:

The school also promotes the integration of functions, rather than, as is more often the case, the compartmentalization of functions. Thus, the school supports (with this approach) the integration of thought and feeling, thought and action, the subjective and the objective, self-feeling and empathy with others, original and conventional forms of communication, spontaneous and ritualized forms of responses. . . . generally stated, it is the goal of the school to minimize the gap between capacity and performance by providing an environment that allows and encourages children to do what they are capable of. . . . It is a basic tenet of the Developmental Interaction approach that the growth of cognitive functions—acquiring and ordering information, judging, reasoning, problem solving, using systems of symbols—cannot be separated from the growth of personal and interpersonal processes—the development of self-esteem and a sense of identity, internalization of impulse control, capacity for autonomous response, relatedness to other people. . . . Educational goals are conceived in terms of developmental processes, not concrete achievements.

How can these goals be translated into an effective integrated program for exceptional youngsters? The Bank Street College learning-disability program suggests that White's (1959) definition of competence is central to its goals. Competence is seen as the totality of being—a feeling that one has been able to master certain skills which will promote cognitive power and intellectual mastery, nurture self-esteem and understanding, encourage differentiated interaction with people, and strengthen the commitment to and pleasure in work and learning. Sapir and Nitzburg (1973) state that children are developing organisms, constantly changing. Current approaches fragment the understanding and treatment of the child. They do not allow for treatment on all levels simultaneously—cognitively, emotionally, experientially. The tendency is to do visual-perceptual training in one place with one person, reading instruction with another, language training with a third, and psychotherapy detached from the learning environment with a fourth. It is not possible to isolate learning problems from every other aspect of the growing child. Needed are child specialists who understand therapeutic procedures within a framework of diagnostic teaching and who understand the child's feelings as well as his thinking processes. They need to develop skills to enable them to analyze a cognitive task, determine a child's learning style, and relate it to the child's personality and temperament. This is an attempt to reintegrate the child and to establish the view that all children, including those in trouble, have normal developing processes. Such a program emphasizes:

1. Listening, understanding, and sharing with the child how he feels and where he is cognitively, emotionally, and socially.

2. Providing a program of clinical-diagnostic teaching which is predicated on the principle that diagnosis proceeds from observing the child's attempts to solve tasks, being able to analyze the tasks in terms of what processes are involved, discovering together those parts of the task with which the child can be successful and those parts that are causing problems. The goal is a precise match between the cognitive style of the learner and the cognitive demand of the task.

3. Working with the child's strengths, providing success and building self-esteem that will allow for the development of more pleasure, motivation, and persistence.

4. Through discussions helping the child discover his own compensatory mechanisms, those mechanisms which will enable him to help himself proceed more successfully through his developmental stages.

5. Rearranging the child's environment at home and school so that it provides support systems to help him with the numerous life experiences with which he will continue to have difficulty.

Skills, of necessity, need to be taught as they are needed experientially and in an integrated way so that reading, writing, perception, and conception can be seen as a unified whole. Emphasis needs to be placed on a schemata that fosters thinking processes and encourages the development of strategies that will be effective regardless of the circumstances. An example of this unified approach might be:

• Children become interested in alphabet letters.

- They can be encouraged to sort them, hear likenesses and differences, match them, think of children's names and how they write them.
- Where do the letters go and why?
- Which children's names begin the same way and why?
- Listen to sounds about them; reproduce the sounds.
- Do they sound like any letter sounds?
- What shapes have meaning to them?
- Do the letters remind them of something?
- What concrete object might they think of when they think of a letter?
- What words have special meaning for them?
- Do they want to know what they look like?
- Do they want to put something down with letters (maybe from one of their pictures) so that others can know what they are thinking?

Where there is a deficit at a lower order of thinking or perceiving, it is not possible to retrace one's steps and retrain the individual as though he were back at the younger stage of development. When dealing with multilevel development of great complexity such simplistic thinking is often ineffective. A child of 12 who has a visual-perceptual discrimination problem cannot be taught the same way as the normal child of 4 or 5 years. Many of the current programs do not account for this difference. In no way does this imply that the child does not have to be taught. The mere presentation of an interesting worksheet or exercise is not necessarily teaching. New experiences must be provided, carefully timed and paced at the child's level. Many exceptional children become frustrated and overwhelmed with the introduction of new material. Developmental pressure describes the educational task of providing a balance between experiences that help consolidate the child's understanding and those that provide desirable, growth-inducing challenge.

This model implies a linking of treatment and diagnosis, so that the continually emerging patterns of the child lead to the refinement of diagnosis and revision of strategies. It demonstrates that professionals working together from many disciplines can share their expertise and form a common body of knowledge, skill, and a communication system that can provide better service to children. It provides a commitment that only a totally integrated intervention program assists the child to become independent of his handicaps and allows for his natural compensatory mechanisms to emerge.

The goal of such a program is to develop children who can become adaptable, coping, competent people with educational and social skills that enable them to learn and function effectively in normal settings. It accepts the fact that one of the most important facets of the success of such a program is the child-teacher interaction and the necessary attributes the teacher must have in order to provide successful experiences for children. The teacher must be sensitive and perceptive; have fine observational and decision-making skills; allow for the child's natural exploration of ways to succeed; have knowledge of task analysis, information processing systems, and child development theories. The teacher must also provide the back-up support systems (both cognitive and emotional) that will allow the child to proceed. The teacher must be able to translate for the child, in simple language, the process the child uses that is successful, so that the strategies that work for him can be encouraged and translated to others (family, friends, teachers). Then they too can support and encourage the successful strategies.

The philosophical and methodological base of this model considers growth as an integration of social, cognitive, and emotional development. Education means learning for life. The curriculum for learning-disabled children must provide an organizational structure that allows for the expression of thoughts and feelings about a large variety of experiences and permits the child to discover his own learning processes. The strength he gains will help him to share with his parents and teachers those things that he can do that will help him learn. The planned educational intervention uses a diagnostic teaching paradigm with continual communication among children, teachers, and parents.

This model is complex and requires commitment and dedication of personnel, but it is one which provides many challenges and satisfactions. It involves retraining and reorientation of teaching personnel. This is best accomplished on the job by having a resource person (regardless of discipline in which trained) who can encourage, support, make suggestions and demonstrate, who can be patient, persevering, and generally knowledgeable; and who can be sensitive and perceptive to the needs of both teachers and children. Change is slow and takes effort. It is far easier to follow what someone tells us to do than to be a keen observer, task analyzer, decision-maker, and curriculum-developer. But given time to explore, teachers with the help of supportive resource persons will become autonomous, capable, and responsible for the individual need of each of their learning-disabled children.

At the very least teachers should be allowed to develop their own tools for studying children. If they use tests of developmental scales and if they can understand that tasks, tests, or scales are only as good as the observations they elicit, they will then evolve a scientific method of taking hunches (hypotheses), testing them out, and drawing conclusions to see if they bring success. Such a type of teacher training develops creative, thinking, responsible, and accountable personnel who eventually will be better able to teach children and take leadership in the training of others.

The teacher who puts into operation a set of linear sequential steps that is prescribed for a child, will forever need to have others direct her efforts. It is far more effective in a school to create teams of teachers sharing ideas, studying problems, suggesting ways to solve them, and helping each other become more effective. It is usually helpful to plan the teams in a way that within each there is one leader and a complement of skills among the others on the team. Essential to the team effectiveness is the inclusion of a child specialist who can act as a resource and support person for teachers and children.

Many educational principles have been stated that are important for all children. It is just that for the MBD child it becomes even more critical. We know that in general education the classes in public schools give lip service to individualization and respect for the child. But we also observe that those children who do not fit into the lock step of the curriculum are labeled a problem. There is a mechanistic approach that makes it mandatory that children enter school at a certain age, on the assumption that all children are ready and that if they are not, the school can provide individual programs that will enable the child to succeed. Much of this is a myth. In general education we now hear of open classrooms, team teaching, nongrading—all of which would be excellent in principle for all children and, in particular, would provide a framework in which MBD children could find a niche of meaningful and individual activity that would encourage the development of skills in all areas. But in reality the terms are misunderstood; children are either left to flounder on their own or in some cases nongrading is seen as departmentalization which compartmentalizes the child and increases his sense of failure (Sapir-Wilson, 1978).

An important organizational issue presently being argued is that of special classes versus mainstreaming. Modern thought favors mainstreaming but, as always in the acceptance of any educational solution, there are concommitant dangers in the loss of options for different children. We would all favor the intent of the new federal law, PL 94-142, The Education of the Handicapped, and its emphasis on the least restrictive environment.

To have special education be an integrated part of the mainstream of all education has always been an inspiration of special educators. The current vigorous emphasis on mainstreaming in the United States is supported as never before by legislation and mandated accountability in the schools. The mainstreaming of children can be satisfactory only if it is accompanied by genuine acceptance and mutual understanding. This movement will have achieved its ultimate success when exceptional children do not have to be restored to the mainstream because they will never have been excluded from it.

Narrow separate specialization in special education preparation is unlikely to promote either successful mainstreaming or effective segregated special education. Special education makes the assumption that children differ markedly in important attitudes or other attributes which, in turn, indicate different instructional programs for their maximal education. In the extreme cases of psychotic or sensorily impaired children (deaf and blind), it is obvious that adjustments of curricula must be made. It is also imperative that we understand the need when there are even more subtle differences.

The notion that any specific educational intervention program would be suitable for all MBD children is erroneous. A Frostig (1961) program may help a particular child with a visual motor skill; an Ayres (1972) program might increase the flow of body movement; a program of optometrics might assist another child to become more visually competent. Noné are panaceas and their use are validated only when there is an expressed and specific need for a child. In addition, any claim for transferability is questionable. There is little substitute for a well-planned individualized approach, one which teaches through the integration of all areas and focuses on strategies (learning how-to-learn) and embodies learning in functional and meaningful living experiences. The child must feel and see the need to know something or do something. It may be difficult for the child, for example, to write a letter, but the teacher can set the stage so that it becomes important enough to enable the child to persevere, regardless of his problems and the huge amount of energy expended. The task must be important and worthwhile for the child.

Many persons are concerned that with the new mandated laws many school districts may initiate programs for handicapped children which provide neither education nor recognition of the child's individual needs. In fact they may become a way to victimize children by labeling and adapting programs just for the sake of meeting the government mandates. It has finally been recognized that inappropriate assessment procedures have caused many children (those who are poor; of low social status; or of minority, racial, or ethnic groups) to be incorrectly labeled retarded, disturbed, or socially maladjusted, and thus to be placed in special education classes. There is also evidence that when these children are mainstreamed the results can be disheartening. It becomes obvious then that the success or failure of a program rests on more than methodology or an organizational plan; in part it depends on the willingness and ability of people to make it work, on the knowledge and skills of the personnel, and on the child-adult interaction.

The criteria for evaluating any program has to be assessed on how well it provides for the children under its care:

- Is the program honest and respectful of children?
- Does it provide for a reasonable amount of choices for the child?
- Does it account for the child's individual needs?
- Does it provide for pleasure in work and play?
- Is the child provided with experiences in which there are developmental pressures, but through which he can succeed and learn and grow in self-esteem and cognitive mastery?
- Does the program allow for a range of activity for all the children—in skills, social participation, and creative arts?
- Do the children succeed and become competent human beings?

Some suggested elements may be fruitful in working out a program for MBD children. It is possible to utilize to a large degree existing personnel and resources within the school and to involve regular teachers, which in effect promotes the idea that they are capable and ready to provide services for the MBD child within the regular classroom.

It is possible to establish a materials resource center where the regular classroom teacher can be supplied with specialized teaching materials and share ideas without going through the usual administrative delay. It is possible to create the role of child specialist, one who can provide the support system for the teachers and children. Such a person can translate new ideas and methods to the teachers as well as provide additional service to the child. Such a child specialist, to be effective, can work maximally with 15 teachers and be responsible for about 350 children, assuming that 10 to 20% of these youngsters will need much special help. After all the primary success or failure of a program rests with the child.

We are concerned ultimately with the child's adaptation—his capacity to use to the fullest his internal and external resources in order to function optimally under any circumstances in which he is placed. Successful adaptation is possible only when some degree of homeostasis exists among the many variables considered. With this model, learning can be viewed as a complex adaptive phenomenon influenced by any or all of the factors presented. Because such a conceptual framework emphasizes the interaction of various factors as they affect learning, it permits a logical organization of our knowledge in this area in a way that related the various data within an overall perspective. Walzer and Richmond (1973) wrote:

The challenges are many. Let us hope they will inspire us to create new and more effective models; to learn more about ourselves and the children with whom we are working; to keep an open mind to new ideas; and to constantly explore, critique, stimulate, and above all to share with others. Our thoughtfulness, honesty, and concern for the child and our respect for what the child has to tell us should be our first and most important priority.

REFERENCES

Adelman, H. S. "Remedial classroom instruction revisited." *Journal of Special Education*, 5(4), 311–322, (1971).

Ayres, J. A. *Sensory Integration and Learning Disorders*. Los Angeles: Western Psychological Services, 1972.

Biber, B. Conference on the "Roots of Excellence," Bank Street College of Education, New York, 1957.

Bloom, B. S., ed. "Taxonomy of educational objectives," *Handbook I: The Cognitive Domain*. New York: McKay, 1956.

————*Stability and Change in Human Characteristics*. New York: Wiley, 1964.

Bruner, J. *Toward a Theory of Instruction*. Cambridge: Harvard University Press, 1966.

Carroll, A. W. "The classroom as an eco-system." *Focus on Exceptional Children*, 6, 1–11, (1974).

Cartwright, G. P., C. A. Cartwright, and J. E. Ysseldyke. "Two decision models: Identification and diagnostic teaching of handicapped children in the regular classroom." *Psychology in the Schools*, 10, 4–11, (1973).

Chomsky, N. "Recent contributions to the theory of innate ideas," in *Boston Studies in the Philosophy of Science*. vol. 3, *Proceedings of the Boston Colloquium for the Philosophy of Science*, The Netherlands: D. Riedel, 1964.

Clements, S. D. *Minimal Brain Dysfunction in Children—Terminology and Identification*. NIWDB Monograph No. 3, Washington, D.C.: U.S. Department of HEW, 1966.

Frostig, *Developmental Test of Visual Perception*. Palo Alto, Cal.: Consulting Psychological Press, 1961.

Gagne, R. M. *Conditions of Learning*, 2nd ed. New York: Holt, Rinehart & Winston, 1971.

Gallagher, J. S., and R. Bradley. "Early identification of developmental difficulties," in I. Gordon, ed., *Early Childhood Education*. Chicago: National Society for the Study of Education, 71st Yearbook Part II, 1972.

Gardner, R. W. "Evolution-brain injury." *Bulletin of Menniger Clinic*. 35(2), (March 1971).

Glaser, R. "Individuals and learning: The new aptitudes." *Educational Researcher* 1, 5–13, (1972).

Hunt, J. McV. *The Challenge of Incompetence and Poverty*. Urbana: University of Illinois Press, 1969.

Illinois Test of Psycholinguistic Ability, rev. ed. Urbana: University of Illinois Press, 1968.

Johnson, D. (Paper presented at the 85th Annual Convention of the American Psychological Association, Washington, D.C., September 1976.)

Kephart, N. C. *Learning Disability: An Educational Adventure*. The Kappa Delta Pi Lecture Series, 1968.

Luria, A. R. *The Role of Speech in the Regulation of Normal and Abnormal Behavior*. Oxford, England: Pergamon Press, 1961.

Lerner, J. W. "Systems analysis and special education." *Journal of Special Education*, 7, 15–26, (1973).

Mann, L., and D. Sabatino, eds. *The First Review of Special Education*. Philadelphia: JSE Press, 1973.

Minskoff, E. H. "Creating and evaluating remediation for the learning disabled." *Focus on Exceptional Children*, 5, 1–11, (1973).

Piaget, J. "The stages of intellectual development of the child." *Bulletin of the Menninger School of Psychiatry*, (March 6, 1961).

Posner, G. J. "The extensiveness of curriculum structure: A conceptual scheme." *Review of Educational Research*, 44, 401–407, (1974).

Samerroff, A. and M. Chandler. "An editorial on the continuum of caretaking causality." *American Psychological Association Newsletter.* (Division on Developmental Psychology). Washington, D.C.: APA, 3, (Winter, 1973).

Sapir, Selma G. "Learning disability and deficit centered classroom training." in Jerome Hellmuth, ed., *Cognitive Studies, Vol. 2: Deficits in Cognition,* pp. 324–37. New York: Brunner/Mazel Publishers, 1971.

Sapir, S. G. and A. Nitzburg. *Children with Learning Problems.* New York: Brunner/Mazel, 1973.

Sapir, S. G. and B. Wilson. "A developmental scale to assist in the prevention of learning disability." *Educational and Psychological Measurement*, 27, 1061–1068, (1967).

Sapir, S. G. and B. W. Wilson. *A Professional Guide to Working with the Learning Disabled Child.* New York: Brunner/Mazel, 1978.

Semmel, M. I. *Application of Systematic Classroom Observation to the Study and Modification of Pupil-Teacher Interactions in Special Education.* Bloomington: Bloomington Center for Innovation in Teaching the Handicapped, Indiana University Press, 1974.

Shapiro, E., and B. Biber. "The education of young children: A developmental-interaction approach." *Teachers College Record*, 74(1), 55–79, (September 1972).

Shavelson, R. *Decision Analysis of Teaching.* Los Angeles: University of California Press, 1975.

Skinner, B. F. *The Technology of Teaching.* New York: Appleton-Century-Crofts, 1968.

Strauss, A. A., and L. E. Lehtinen. *Psychopathology and Education of the Brain-Injured Children*, vol I. New York: Grune & Stratton, 1947.

Walzer, S. and J. Richmond. "The epidemiology of learning disorders," in H. Grossman, ed., *Pediatric Clinics of North America,* vol. 20, No. 3, August 1973.

Werner, H. *Comparative Psychology of Mental Development.* New York: International Universities Press, 1957.

Werner, H., and B. Kaplan. *Symbol Formation: An Organismic-Developmental Approach to Language and Expression of Thought.* New York: Wiley, 1963.

White, R. T. "Learning hierarchies." *Review of Educational Research*, 43, 361–375, (1973).

White, R. W. "Motivation reconsidered: The concept of competence." *Psychological Review*, 66(5), 297–333, (September 1959).

Ysseldyke, J. E. "Diagnostic-prescriptive teaching: The search for aptitude treatment interactions," in L. Mann and D. Sabatino, eds., *The First Review of Special Education.* Philadelphia: JSE Press, 1973.

CHAPTER 24

Drugs and Medical Intervention

Dennis P. Cantwell

INTRODUCTION

The chapters in this handbook discuss minimal brain dysfunction from a variety of vantage points. This chapter will focus on a medical approach to diagnosis and treatment of this disorder. Prior to attending to the central focus of this chapter however, some discussion must be made of the medical model and its relevance to psychiatric disorders of childhood in general and to this particular syndrome specifically.

THE MEDICAL MODEL IN PSYCHIATRIC DISORDERS OF CHILDHOOD

There has been a continuing controversy over the value of the medical model in psychiatry (Szasz, 1974; Torrey, 1974). Blaney (1975) notes that the term *medical model* is often used as if it stands for one framework, while he feels there are four separate medical models. Three of these are relevant to our present discussion. These might be labeled as the organic, symptomatic, and classification medical models. Each of these in turn has had another model arise in opposition to it.

In the organic medical model, psychiatric disorders are viewed as organically based disease entities. The opposing psychological model, in its simplest form, states that not all psychiatric disorders are organically based disease entities.

In the symptomatic model, the manifestations of a psychiatric disorder are considered symptoms of some underlying condition which need not be organically based. For most proponents of the symptomatic medical model, the underlying conditions are not felt to be organic. In opposition to the symptomatic model, a social learning theory model has arisen which takes the view that symptoms are not manifestations of any underlying problem and can thus be treated directly.

It should be noted that psychoanalysts and learning theorists would be united in opposition to the organic medical model, but would be on opposite sides of the fence with regard to the symptomatic model.

Finally the classificatory medical model states that psychiatry will progress only when recognizable disease clusters are carefully delineated and described. All fevers were once treated with quinine and only some responded until Sydenham delineated different causes of fever. Proponents of the classificatory model construe the present state of psychiatric treatment as similar to the pre-Sydenham era in medicine. A disease or a disorder in this classificatory model is simply a cluster of symptoms or signs that has a reasonably predictable natural history (Guze,

1972). An anti-labeling school has arisen in opposition to the classificatory model. It is the opinion of this school that no useful purpose is served by placing a patient in a diagnostic category. Rather they feel that giving a patient such a diagnosis applies a pejorative label to the patient and leads to significant problems in and of itself. Moreover proponents of this viewpoint argue that emotional disorders cannot be classified in this manner and that any attempt to do so is necessarily arbitrary and not useful for treatment purposes (Szureck, 1956).

Siegler and Osmund (1974) describe three medical models: clinical, public health, and scientific. In each of these models the doctor-patient relationship is somewhat different. In the clinical medical model, the doctor-patient relationship is a dyad of healer to patient. In the public health model, the patient is replaced by population and the doctor becomes a public health official or officials. In the scientific medical model, the patient becomes an experimental subject and the doctor is a scientific investigator.

This discussion will focus on the clinical and the scientific medical models as they relate to the psychiatric disorders of childhood. Some comments will also be made about the organic, symptomatic, and classificatory medical models.

The basic question is: Does the medical model have value to the practicing clinician and to the scientific investigator? Is it a useful framework for organizing clinical and research data about the psychiatric disorders of childhood?

A MEDICAL MODEL FOR CLINICAL AND INVESTIGATIVE WORK WITH THE PSYCHIATRIC DISORDERS OF CHILDHOOD

The medical model described here has been developed by the author for clinical and research work with the psychiatric disorders of childhood. The author has found the model to be clinically useful as a framework for integrating the data obtained from various aspects of the evaluation of a child referred for psychiatric evaluation as well as for integrating research data. The model has six stages and in its use an investigator begins with an index population of children and carries out studies that can be grouped under the other five stages. The six stages of the model are:

Clinical Description

A careful clinical description of the behavior problem with which the child presents is the starting point for investigative work in this model. Obtaining this requires detailed, systematic, yet flexible questioning of the parents; obtaining reliable information from the school; and performing a reliable and valid diagnostic interview with the child. It also requires taking into account age appropriateness of behaviors, sex of the child, race, social class, and other factors that may affect the clinical picture.

Physical and Neurologic Factors

A systematic physical and pediatric neurologic examination should be performed and the results recorded in a standardized fashion. Special attention should be given to the evaluation of neurodevelopmental abnormalities. It is important to inquire systematically about events in the history suggesting possible CNS involvement.

Laboratory Studies

Included here are the results of all types of laboratory investigations: blood, urine, spinal fluid, EEG, neurophysiological, and so on. Valid, reliable psychometric studies can also be considered as laboratory investigations in this context.

Family Studies

Included in this stage are two different types of investigations: (1) studies of the prevalence and types of psychiatric disorders in the close relatives of a clinically defined index group of child patients and (2) studies of the relationships and interactions occurring among the members of a family.

Longitudinal Natural History Studies

Prospective and retrospective follow-up studies to trace the course and outcome of the disorder help determine whether the original index population of children formed a homogeneous diagnostic category. These studies also provide a standard against which to judge the effectiveness of various forms of treatment.

Treatment Studies

At our present level of knowledge marked differences in response to adequate trials of the same treatment, such as between complete recovery and marked deterioration, can be considered as evidence that the original group of children did not form a homogeneous group. Thus differential treatment response can also be used to subdivide the original index population of patients.

APPLICATION OF THE MEDICAL MODEL TO THE MBD SYNDROME

Clinical Picture

Categorization of clinical pictures in medicine, as well as in psychiatry, are divided into three distinct levels of comprehension (Spitzer, et al., 1975). At the first and simplest level there is an isolated sign or symptom which is noted to occur without any reference to the context in which it occurs. Examples (from internal medicine and psychiatry) are the cough or depressed mood which may occur in many clinical conditions. At the next and higher level a distinctive clinical syndrome occurs, that is a group of signs or symptoms which cluster together and covary over time. Examples (from internal medicine and psychiatry) are cough, fever, and chest pain as seen in pneumonia; rapid speech, elevated mood, and psychomotor excitement as seen in mania. At the third and highest level of sophistication a specific etiologic factor or specific pathophysiology is known to explain and account for the distinctive clinical picture. Examples (from clinical medicine and psychiatry) are pneumococcal pneumonia and amphetamine psychosis.

With most psychiatric disorders of childhood, the clinical pictures are at the distinctive clinical syndrome level. This is true of the minimal brain dysfunction syndrome.

Within the syndrome level of classification in medicine, two distinct categories are recognized: monothetic categories and polythetic categories. These two types of categories have been used by Wender (1971) to describe the syndrome of minimal brain dysfunction. Polythetic categories are categories in which there is no single manifest clinical characteristic shared by all people presenting with the disorder. However individuals who have the greatest number of shared features are grouped together in polythetic categories, while no single feature is essential to group membership or is sufficient to make a person a member of a certain diagnostic group. There are a number of core characteristics which make up the total and complete syndrome. For example Wender considered the classical symptoms of minimal brain dysfunction to be: difficulties in motor behavior, including increased level of activity and impaired coordination; attentional difficulties; cognitive difficulties; learning difficulties; difficulties in impulse control; difficulties with interpersonal relationships; and alterations of emotional behavior, including increased lability, altered reactivity, increased aggressiveness, and dysphoria. None of these symptoms are found in their complete form in all children who are considered to have the MBD syndrome. Thus it can be seen that there are several characteristics that Wender considers to occur together more frequently than they may be expected by chance. However among four individuals, one person might possess characteristics 1, 2, and 3; another characteristics 2, 3, and 4; a third 1, 2, and 5; and the last 1, 3, 5, and 7. No two children share three traits, no individual has all seven traits, and no single trait is common to all of the individuals. However any pair of individuals shares at least two traits of the syndrome. No single trait defines the entire group, rather it is the high intercorrelation of the traits that defines the group. Wender points to other polythetic categories in medicine, such as rheumatic fever. Thus it has been found empirically that patients who have at least two major or one major and two minor signs or symptoms of rheumatic fever have a high probability of possessing an underlying tissue pathology which characterizes the disease of rheumatic fever.

The analogy to minimal brain dysfunction is an apt one and has theoretical value. From the practical standpoint however we have no specific underlying pathology of any type which is unique to the diagnosis, and thus the underlying pathophysiology is inferred for all people who meet the clinical picture of minimal brain dysfunction as a polythetic category defined by Wender.

Monothetic categories on the other hand are categories in which all people who are considered to have this syndrome share a set of core operational diagnostic criteria. Subscribers to this type of category in the minimal brain dysfunction literature usually tend to use behaviorally descriptive terms like the hyperactive child or the hyperkinetic child syndrome to describe this disorder. The new DSM III (1977) diagnostic category for this disorder will be Attentional Deficit Disorder with Hyperactivity (ADDH).

The primary symptoms of this syndrome include attentional difficulties, excessive motor activity, and impulsivity. Children with this disorder are described as having a short attention span in school, as being impulsive and distractible, as failing to follow through on instructions and complete work, and as being disorganized and inattentive. In addition the children are reported to be fidgety, restless, overactive, overdemanding of the teacher's attention, and disruptive of others at play and at work (APA, 1977).

Attentional problems at home are characterized by a failure to follow through on parental requests and instructions or by the inability to engage in most activities for periods of time appropriate for age.

In young children hyperactivity is manifested by excessive gross motor activity, such as running or climbing. In older children and adolescents hyperactivity may be indicated by extreme restlessness and fidgeting. Often the impression obtained is that the quality of the motor behavior is what distinguishes this disorder from ordinary overactivity. The activity tends to be haphazard, poorly organized, and lacking in clear goal orientation. However in situations in which a high level of motor activity is expected and appropriate, such as the playground, children with this disorder do not obviously display more activity than others.

The behavior of children with this disorder is extremely variable. Typically symptoms fluctuate across as well as within situations, and inconsistent functioning is a very common characteristic. A child's behavior may be well organized and appropriate on a one-to-one basis, but become disorganized in a group situation or in the classroom. Home adjustment may be satisfactory and difficulties may emerge only in school. In addition the child's level of motor activity may vary considerably within any situation. The usual pattern is an inconsistent one. It is the rare child who displays uniform, constant symptoms of hyperactivity either within or across settings.

In addition there are many associated symptoms which often change with age. These include obstinacy, stubbornness, negativism, bossiness, or bullying; increased lability of mood, low frustration tolerance or temper tantrums; low self-esteem, lack of response to discipline; and antisocial behavior, especially in adolescence. Specific developmental disorders such as reading and other learning disabilities are also common (APA, 1977).

ADDH children are often not brought to professional attention until the advent of school when the demands imposed by the classroom create symptomatology which leads to a referral. And many of the children are referred not for the primary symptoms of the disorder but rather for associated symptoms such as learning disabilities or acting out behavior. A careful developmental history will reveal the presence of a typical ADDH syndrome from an early age.

Thus in selecting a population of children who chronically manifest the core symptom pattern in both the home and school settings, an investigator or a clinician surely would begin with a heterogeneous group of children. Some attempts can be made to obtain a more homogeneous population by adding other specific inclusion criteria, such as male sex, a specific age range, normal IQ, and tested normal vision and hearing. Adding exclusion criteria, such as any form of definite organic brain damage, would also restrict the population. However the population remaining after application of these inclusion and exclusion criteria will still be a rather heterogeneous one. If this is so, subgroups of the original population should be formed when studies in the other five stages of the medical model are carried out with this index population. This chapter will discuss the possible subgroups that might be formed by application of the medical model and what information this gives us about the natural history and treatment of children with the ADDH syndrome.

Specific questions that we shall attempt to answer by the use of this model are:

1. How can children with the ADDH syndrome be divided into meaningful subgroups whose conditions differ in etiology, prognosis, and response to treatment?

2. Do ADDH children contribute more than their fair share to the pool of psychiatrically ill and maladjusted adults? If so, what specific types of adult psychiatric disorders does the syndrome predispose to?

3. What are the factors within the child, within his family, or within his social milieu that predict which ADDH child will develop into a healthy adult and which child in later life will manifest social or psychiatric pathology?

4. Which children with the syndrome will respond positively to stimulant drug treatment and why do they do so?

Natural History of the ADDH Syndrome

Some evidence of the later life outcome of children with the ADDH syndrome is available from three types of studies: (1) prospective and retrospective follow-up studies of children with the syndrome (Weiss, et al., 1971; Mendelson, Johnson, and Stewart, 1971; Minde, et al., 1971; Minde, Weiss, and Mendelson, 1972; Riddle and Rapoport, 1976; Laufer, 1971; Denhoff, 1973; Menkes, Rowe, and Menkes, 1967; Borland and Heckman, 1976); (2) studies of the childhood histories of adult psychiatric patients with a variety of conditions (Goodwin, et al., 1975; Quitkin and Klein, 1969; Tarter, et al., 1977; Morrison and Minkoff, 1975; Shelly and Reister, 1972; Wood, et al., 1976); (3) family studies of parents of children with the syndrome (Morrison and Stewart, 1971; Cantwell, 1972).

These studies paint the following picture of the ADDH child and adolescent. Hyperactivity, per se, seems to diminish with age, but the children are still more restless, excitable, impulsive, and distractible than their peers. Attention and concentration difficulties remain as major problems. Chronic severe under-achievement in school in almost all academic areas is a characteristic finding. Low self-esteem, poor self-image, depression, and a sense of failure are common. Antisocial behavior occurs in up to 25% of ADDH children, 10 to 15% have had actual police contact or court referral.

While the adult outcome is less sure than the outcome in adolescence, the data from the studies cited do indicate that the ADDH syndrome is a likely precursor to alcoholism and sociopathy in males and to hysteria in females. There is some question that the ADDH syndrome may also predispose to the development of psychosis in later life (Menkes, et al., 1967). There are also data to indicate that the ADDH syndrome may predispose to personality disorders and to other psychiatric disorders characterized by symptoms of anxiety, dysphoria, mood lability, impulsivity, and chronic difficulty in interpersonal relations (Wood, et al., 1976).

Two psychiatric studies of the parents of children with the syndrome have been carried out, one by Morrison and Stewart (1971) and one by Cantwell (1972). Morrison and Stewart (1971) found that 12 parents of 59 ADDH children (9 fathers and 3 mothers) were felt to have been hyperactive themselves as children. Of these 9 fathers, 5 were diagnosed as alcoholics as adults; 1 was a sociopath; 1 had multiple depressive, phobic, and compulsive symptoms; and 2 were heavy drinkers but not alcoholic. Of the 3 previously hyperactive mothers, 1 had a depressive illness as an adult, 1 qualified for both a diagnosis of alcoholism and a diagnosis of hysteria. One father and 1 mother of the normal control children were thought to have been hyperactive as children. As adults the father was an epileptic with psychosis who had a drinking problem and the mother was manic-depressive.

In a similar study Cantwell systematically evaluated the parents of 50 ADDH children and 50 normal control children. Eight of the fathers of the ADDH children were thought to be hyperactive as children themselves. Six of these were given a diagnosis of alcoholism, 1 was given the diagnosis of sociopathy and 1 had an undiagnosed psychiatric illness with heavy drinking as one of the symptoms. One father of a normal control child who was thought to be hyperactive as a child was given a diagnosis of alcoholism as an adult. Of the 2 mothers of the ADDH children who seemed to have been ADDH children themselves, 1 was felt to be a definite hysteric and 1 was given a diagnosis of probable hysteria as an adult. Thus the findings of the family studies support the findings of the retrospective studies of the childhood histories of adult psychiatric patients and the prospective and retrospective studies of follow-up studies of ADDH children.

Treatment Studies

The ADDH syndrome is considered to be a condition par excellence for the use of psychotropic drugs among childhood disorders. Clinical reports dating back to Bradley's original reports (1937) have suggested that central nervous system stimulants such as amphetamines and methylphenidate are effective for a significant number of children who present with this particular clinical syndrome. There are now a number of well-controlled clinical studies attesting to the value of stimulants with this disorder. In Barkley's comprehensive review of stimulant treatment in children with the ADDH syndrome (1977), 15 studies of children treated with amphetamine revealed an improvement rate of about 74%, 14 controlled studies with methylphenidate produced an improvement rate of 77%, and 2 controlled studies involving pemoline produced an improvement rate of 73%. Thus about 75% of children with the ADDH syndrome can be expected to improve after treatment with one of the three major groups of stimulants: amphetamines, methylphenidate, and pemoline. Clearly for this particular condition in childhood, the ADDH syndrome, these three major classes of stimulants are the drugs of choice for this condition.

Whether or not there are other children who fall under the general rubric of MBD, but who do not meet the operational criteria for the ADDH syndrome, and who might be equally likely to respond to central nervous system stimulants, or indeed to other psychotropic medications, is an open question at the moment. As reviewed elsewhere (Cantwell and Carlson, 1978) there is a suggestion that children with attentional problems without hyperactivity, children with conduct disorders and possibly some other specific diagnostic categories might respond to central nervous system stimulants. However this remains a question for future research.

What is meant by improvement from stimulant medication? This has been reviewed in detail elsewhere (Cantwell and Carlson, 1978). Briefly the effect of stimulants on children with the ADDH syndrome may be characterized as fol-lows: they have a consistent positive effect on behavior which is perceived by teachers as disruptive and socially inappropriate. The effect on activity level is not clear because of varying usage of the term and from different measurement tech-niques being used to quantify activity level. In addition differences can arise depending on the type of motor activity being measured (for example ankle move-ments or seat movements) and also due to the situation in which the activity is being measured (for example during the performance of laboratory tests or out on the playground). During performance on laboratory tasks which are designed to measure attention, cognitive style, and concept attainment, the stimulants consistently decrease the activity level, particularly task irrelevant behavior. In free-field situations, such as in the playground, there are suggestions that children who have behavioral improvement, as reported by parents and teachers, actually have an increase in activity level. Thus in the usual clinical situation stimulants have a positive and desired effect on activity level and affect the quality as well as the quantity of activity level.

Cognitive functions, such as perception, attention, and memory are positively influenced by the use of stimulants in ADDH children. Likewise stimulants influ-ence cognitive style and they improve laboratory measures of learning. Con-versely there is no clear evidence that performance on general cognitive meas-ures, such as tested intelligence, complex learning, language skills, and academic achievement are improved by the use of stimulants. In laboratory settings requir-ing sustained performance, stimulants lead to greater reduction in errors of omis-sion. In laboratory tasks which require immediate and delayed perceptual judg-ment and in tasks which require vigilance, stimulants produce an increase in accuracy. They also reduce response latency, and they increase the speed of reaction time in tasks where rapid responses are required in the laboratory. How-ever in the laboratory tasks in which a more deliberate response is desired, the stimulants lead to less impulsive responding.

Finally in reaction time tasks, stimulants reduce variability and they positively affect performance on both simple and choice reaction times.

Barkley's review (1977) strongly suggests that there is little or no evidence to support the view that stimulants positively affect classroom learning, reasoning, or problem-solving ability. While this may be the case for a variety of learning problems, a proper study evaluating the effect of stimulant medication alone on academic achievement of children selected explicitly because they satisfy the criteria for the ADDH syndrome has not been done. Effects on mood and person-ality have been little studied in children. There are reports of children being happier when they are on medication, and there are also reports that stimulants may produce a depression rather than elevation of mood in children who are chronically treated.

Clinically it is a well-recognized fact that there are children who respond posi-tively in some areas, but the parents feel the personality is changed in a negative fashion.

In summary the stimulants have clinical effects in many areas. The observed changes are not a unitary phenomenon. Few studies have tried to correlate im-provement in one area with improvement or lack of it in another area.

Other stimulants such as Deanol and caffeine while touted as being effective in uncontrolled studies have not stood the test of well-controlled rigorous studies

(Cantwell and Carlson, 1978). All of these studies suggest that only a certain percentage of children with the ADDH syndrome will respond positively to central nervous system stimulant medication. Following the medical model, these data would lead to two testable hypotheses: (1) these two groups of ADDH children, the central nervous system stimulant responders and the central nervous system stimulant nonresponders, have similar phenomenological conditions with different etiologic factors and (2) central nervous system stimulant responders and the central nervous system stimulant nonresponders have the same conditions etiologically, but (a) either there are mitigating factors which facilitate the response to central nervous system stimulants in the responders or (b) there are factors present in nonresponders which mitigate against response to the medication. Both of these propositions can be examined in the use of this six-stage medical model.

Clinical Predictors

Since it is accepted that people with the ADDH syndrome are a diagnostically heterogenous group, it would be helpful if one could divide this heterogenous population clinically and predict drug response on that basis. While there have been attempts to divide the population clinically into those with organic and nonorganic hyperactivity, results are inconclusive with regard to this distinction as relevant to response to central nervous system stimulant medication. For example Satterfield and coworkers (1974a) found that while two clinicians were able to reliably differentiate constitutional from psychogenic hyperactivity in 85% of the cases, the psychogenic group actually got a better response to central nervous system stimulants than did the constitutional group, although the differences were not statistically significant. These results are in opposition to the findings of Conrad and Insel (1967). Fish (1971) feels that children with the ADDH syndrome can be subdivided into three major subcategories: those with pure hyperactivity (i.e. without other associated symptomatology), those who are hyperactive and also have the conduct disorder of the unsocialized aggressive nature, and those who have hyperactivity but are primarily overanxious children. She felt that in her population those with primarily neurotic mechanisms were the best responders to central nervous system stimulant medication. Likewise, Arnold and coworkers (1973) found that those ADDH children who also demonstrated a conduct disorder of the unsocialized aggressive type responded well to both d- and l-amphetamine, whereas d-amphetamine was found to be more effective than l-amphetamine with the other two groups: the pure hyperactive and the overanxious group. However Werry and Aman (1975) were able to find no differences between pure hyperactive children and those hyperactive children who also had a conduct disorder on the laboratory tests of vigilance and memory.

Both Satterfield, et al., (1974a) and Loney, et al., (1978) have found that older children have a better response to methylphenidate, as do children who have more hyperactive symptoms reported by the teacher. However Barkley's review (1977) reveals that ratings of severity of hyperactivity by parents, clinicians, or teachers have been equivocal in predicting response to treatment. In contrast he feels that the literature supports the notion that the degree of inattentiveness, however measured, seems to be the best clinical predictor (Barkley, 1977).

In summary there are few valid, reliable clinical predictors reported in the literature that enable one to predict which ADDH children are most likely to respond to central nervous system stimulant medication.

Physical and Neurologic Predictors

If one excludes ADDH children with demonstrable organic brain damage from the index patient population, the physical examination is usually completely normal. In a minority of children defects of vision or hearing may be found (Stewart, et al., 1966) as well as abnormalities of speech (de Hirsch, 1973). One group of investigators (Waldrop and Halverson, 1971) has reported a high incidence of minor physical anomalies in ADDH children such as: epicanthus, widely spaced eyes, curved fifth finger, adherent ear lobes, and so on. Their findings were more consistent for boys than for girls with the syndrome. These authors have suggested that the same factors operating in the first week of pregnancy led to both the congenital anomalies and the behavior disorder.

In a study of 76 ADDH boys, Rapoport, Quinn, and Lamprecht (1974), confirmed this increased incidence of physical anomalies. If an index population of ADDH children is divided into those with minor physical anomalies and those without minor physical anomalies, do these two subgroups differ in other stages of this model? The evidence indicates that those ADDH children with the minor physical anomalies are also characterized by differences in: the clinical picture— earlier onset of the disorder, greater severity of hyperactivity, and more aggressive behavior; other physical factors—history of obstetrical difficulties in the mother; laboratory studies—higher level of plasma dopamine betahydroxylase activity; and family studies—history of hyperactivity in the family (Rapoport, Quinn, and Lamprecht, 1974; Quinn and Rapoport, 1974).

Moreover those fathers of the ADDH children with minor physical anomalies who were themselves hyperactive in childhood also had higher plasma dopamine betahydroxylase activity. Finally it is notable that within the group with minor physical anomalies there is little overlap between those with a history of hyperactivity in the father and those with a history of obstetrical difficulties in the mother. This suggests that there may be two distinct subgroups of ADDH children with minor physical anomalies—a genetically determined one and one determined by adverse events occurring early in pregnancy. If so, comparing the genetic with the obstetrical group should result in finding differences between the two groups in clinical picture, laboratory findings, natural history or response to treatment. The finding that the ex-hyperactive fathers also had high plasma dopamine betahydroxylase levels would support the idea of a genetic subgroup. However there does not seem to be an association between the presence of these minor physical anomalies and response to drug treatment.

Again, if one excludes children from the index population who have demonstrable organic brain disease, hard neurological signs are likely to be absent. There is a general concensus that certain soft neurological signs are more frequent among behaviorally defined ADDH children (Werry et al., 1976), however the results are not conclusive. While there has been a tendency to infer brain pathology from these soft signs (Kennard, 1960; Laufer and Denhoff, 1957), the evidence for doing so is lacking (Werry, 1972; Rutter, Graham, and Yule, 1970). One study compared carefully matched ADDH neurotic and normal control groups of children using a standardized neurological examination of demonstrated reliability

(Werry et. al., 1976). The ADDH children did have an excess of minor neurological abnormalities indicative of sensorimotor incoordination. However the ADDH group did not have an excess of major neurological abnormalities, of EEG abnormalities, or histories suggestive of trauma to the brain.

The relevant question then is *not:* Do ADDH children have an excess of soft neurological signs compared to normal children or compared to children with other deviant behavior? The more important question is: Do those ADDH children with soft neurological signs differ from those ADDH children without soft neurological signs?

Evidence on this is limited. However there are some data indicating that those ADDH children with soft neurological signs are distinguished from those with no such neurological signs by a greater likelihood of response to stimulant drug treatment (Satterfield, 1973; Millicap, 1973), suggesting that they form a meaningful subgroup.

Laboratory Predictors

Laboratory findings are generally more reliable, more precise, and more reproduceable than are clinical descriptions. If some laboratory measure could be found that is uniquely and consistently associated with the ADDH syndrome, it would make diagnosis easier and would permit possible subgrouping of the syndrome. No such laboratory study exists at the present time. However it is possible that there are some relevant laboratory findings which might be used to divide the children with the syndrome into meaningful subgroups whose condition differs in etiology, prognosis, or in response to treatment. Some relevant laboratory studies will now be summarized.

Electroencephalographic Studies

Electroencephalographic findings with ADDH children are quite variable. Studies have reported that 35 to 50% of ADDH children have abnormal EEGs (Satterfield, 1973; Werry, 1972), with an increase in slow wave activity being the most common finding. There are no EEG abnormalities specific to the syndrome. There is even some question whether ADDH children have a greater number of EEG abnormalities than carefully matched normal and non-ADDH emotionally disturbed children (Werry, 1972; Eeg-Olofsson, 1970; Petersen, Eeg-Olofsson, and Sellden, 1968).

Again in the context of this model, the question we are interested in is: Do ADDH children with an abnormal EEG differ in other areas of the model than those ADDH children with a normal EEG? The evidence suggests that those with an abnormal EEG have been found to differ from those with a normal EEG in the clinical picture: greater anxiety at home and school, greater motor restlessness in the classroom (Quinn and Rapoport, 1974; Satterfield, et al., 1974b); laboratory studies: significantly higher WISC full scale and performance IQ, significantly lower Bender perseveration scores (Satterfield, et al., 1974b); and treatment: greater likelihood of response to stimulant drug therapy. Thus the EEG also seems to select out a meaningful subgroup of the index population of ADDH children.

Neurophysiologic Predictors

Neurophysiologic studies of ADDH children have been limited in scope and number and have reached somewhat different conclusions. Satterfield and his associates (1974b) have suggested that ADDH children can be divided into two subgroups based on neurophysiological data: those with evidence of low central nervous system arousal and those with normal or high central nervous system arousal. In a series of four studies they first identified a subgroup of ADDH children who had low central nervous system arousal levels as measured by skin conductance level. They also found that methylphenidate raised the central nervous system arousal levels in ADDH children to a normal or near-normal level. In their second study these authors replicated both of these findings using two additional indicators of central nervous system arousal: (1) the auditory-evoked cortical response and (2) the EEG with the child at rest. In this second study excessive slow wave activity (as measured by power spectral analysis of the EEG) indicated low central nervous system arousal in the subgroup of ADDH children who obtained a positive response to methylphenidate. In a third study the authors found that a low central nervous system arousal level in a population of ADDH children was associated with a greater degree of behavioral disturbance in the classroom as well as with a positive clinical response to central nervous system medication. In a fourth study it was shown then that those ADDH children with excessive EEG slowing (another indication of low central nervous system arousal) obtained the best response to the central nervous system stimulant medication.

In summary Satterfield, et al., (1972) found that ADDH children had lower skin conductance level, larger amplitude, and slower recovery of evoked cortical responses than normal children. These measures together with high amplitude EEG and high energy in the lower frequency (0–8 Hz) band of the resting EEG also distinguish ADDH children who responded best to stimulant drug treatment from those who obtained a poor response. In all the Satterfield group found eight laboratory measures associated with a positive response to methylphenidate. All of these are consistent with the hypothesis that there is a subgroup of ADDH children who have lower levels of basal resting physiological activation than age-matched normals. This subgroup differs from other ADDH children in two areas of the model: the clinical picture: more restlessness, distractibility, impulsivity, and attentional problems in the classroom; and treatment: a greater likelihood of positive response to stimulants (Satterfield, et al., 1972; Satterfield, Cantwell, and Satterfield, 1974c).

However not all neurophysiologic studies of children have produced such consistent results. Many of the differences may be due to different patient populations and diagnostic criteria and to differing experimental stimulus conditions.

Biochemical Predictors

The positive response of many ADDH children to central nervous system medications such as the amphetamines and to the tricyclic antidepressants, both of which affect the biogenic amines, offer indirect evidence that a disorder in monoamine metabolism is an etiologic factor in some ADDH children. There are several other lines of evidence to support this hypothesis. Dextroamphetamine is thought to be 10 times as potent as its isomer, levoamphetamine, in inhibiting catecholamine uptake by norepinephrine terminals in the brain. The two isomers are of approximately equal potency in inhibiting catecholamine uptake by dopaminergic terminals (Snyder, et al., 1970). There is a suggestion that these two isomers have a differential effect on the aggressive behaviors and hyperactive behaviors of ADDH children (Arnold, et al., 1973). These data offer indirect evidence that some symptoms of ADDH children are mediated by dopaminergic systems and others by norepinephrinergic systems.

Most direct studies of a possible metabolic abnormality have been limited. Wender, et al., (1971) failed to detect any differences in metabolites of serotonin, norepinephrine, or dopamine in the urine of ADDH children compared to a group of normal children. However the study population was very heterogeneous. Wender (1969) did find very low concentrations of serotonin in the blood platelets of three children with the syndrome, all of whom were from the same family. In the rest of the study population the platelet serotonin levels were normal or in the borderline range. Coleman (1971) demonstrated low platelet serotonin concentrations in 88% of 25 children with the syndrome. In a group of ADDH boys Rapoport, et al., (1970) found an inverse relationship between the degree of hyperactive behavior and urinary norepinephrine excretion. In addition there was an inverse relationship in response of the hyperactivity to dextroamphetamine and urinary norepinephrine levels (Shekim, et al., 1977).

All of these studies are suggestive of a possible disorder of monoamine metabolism in the ADDH syndrome. However urinary and platelet data only imperfectly reflect brain monoamine metabolism. Since direct measurement of central nervous system monoamine metabolism is not a possibility, the measurement of monoamine levels and turnover in cerebro-spinal fluid, as has been done in adults with affective disorders (Goodwin and Bunney, 1973), might offer a more fruitful approach. Shaywitz and associates (1975) have reported a study suggesting that HVA is reduced in cerebro-spinal fluid of children with the ADDH syndrome following probenecid blockade.

Thus there does seem to be an emergent body of evidence that at least in some ADDH children there may be an abnormality of monoamine metabolism. Moreover the limited studies that have been done suggest that laboratory studies in this area may pick out children with somewhat different clinical pictures with regard to hyperactivity and aggression and that urinary norepinephrine excretion may be related both to the degree of hyperactivity and to response to stimulant medication.

Thus, children selected by biochemical laboratory studies in one stage of this model may differ somewhat in two other areas of the model: clinical picture and response to stimulant medication.

Psychometric Predictors

Psychometric tests which have been shown to be reliable and valid can also be considered to be laboratory studies in the same vein as a biochemical finding (Robins and Guze, 1970). However no single test or battery of tests has been adequately standardized to insure discrimination of an *individual* ADDH child from a child suffering from other psychiatric learning disorders (Conners, 1967). Surprisingly few efforts have been made to use clustering of ADDH children on certain physiological test variables to see if they form meaningful subgroups. Conners' factor analysis of a battery of test scores by ADDH children (1973) yielded five factors:

(1) general IQ

(2) achievement

(3) rote learning

(4) attentiveness

(5) impulse control

He next identified six separate patterns of factor scores or cluster types. The validity of this grouping procedure was then demonstrated by showing that the six groups of children differed significantly from each other on other laboratory studies, such as the Lincoln-Oseretsky test of motor development, and evoked cortical responses (Conners, 1973). They also differed in response to drug and placebo treatment. Thus groups of ADDH children classified on the basis of one set of laboratory studies (cluster types of psychological functioning) differed in other areas of this model: other laboratory studies and response to treatment. This suggests that they may be homogeneous groups of children sharing disabilities of certain underlying psychological and physiological process and perhaps common etiologies.

These laboratory data suggest that in the future EEG, neurophysiologic, biochemical, and psychometric data (along with other laboratory data) may be linked with behavioral data to permit greater subdivision of the heterogeneous group of children with the ADDH syndrome.

Familial Predictors

Two studies of biologic parents of ADDH children revealed increased prevalence rates for alcoholism, sociopathy, and hysteria (Morrison and Stewart, 1971; Cantwell, 1972). One of these studies also reported a high prevalence rate for these same psychiatric disorders in the biologic second-degree relatives of ADDH children (Cantwell, 1972). In both studies it was noted that the ADDH syndrome also occurred more often in the biologic first- and second-degree relatives of ADDH children than in the relatives of control children. Two further studies of the nonbiologic relatives of adopted ADDH children revealed no increased prevalence rates for psychiatric illness or the ADDH syndrome (Morrison and Stewart, 1973; Cantwell, 1975b). These data suggest that genetic factors may be important in the etiology of the syndrome. They also suggest that ADDH children may be at risk, for both genetic and environmental reasons, for the development of significant pathology in adulthood (Cantwell, 1976).

Do family factors play any role in the outcome of children with the syndrome? Mendelson, et al., (1971), and the Montreal group (Minde, et al., 1971, 1972; Weiss, et al., 1971a) found certain familial variables to be associated with an antisocial outcome. Those children with the most antisocial behavior at follow-up in the Mendelson study were more likely to have fathers who had learning or behavior problems as children and who had been arrested as adults. Weiss found that the families of the ultimately antisocial children had been rated as significantly more pathological in initial evaluation. Three specific items on the rating scale, poor mother-child relationship, poor mental health of the parents, and punitive child-rearing practices, distinguished the families of the ultimately anti-social children from the rest of the group. Minde, et al., (1972) found that one of the four factors associated with poor outcome of the ADDH children in their group included more unfavorable ratings of their family environment. Thus certain aspects of family interaction and family pattern of illness do seem to be related to a specific type of outcome in ADDH children.

Do these familial factors play any role in affecting response to stimulants among ADDH children? Few studies have attempted to look at family variables in any systematic way. Conrad and Insel (1967) found that children whose parents were rated as grossly deviant or socially incompetent were less likely to respond positively to stimulant medication even in the face of other factors which tended to predict a good outcome. Their criteria for grossly deviant and socially incompetent indicate that most of these parents were either alcoholic or sociopathic.

Studies of family interaction in relation to drug response have been limited and inconsistent. The Montreal group (Weiss, et al., 1968; Werry, et al., 1966) found that the mother-child relationship and the quality of the home were unrelated to drug therapy, but in a later study (Weiss, et al., 1971b) there was a positive association between response to stimulants and the quality of the mother-child relationship. Others authors (Knobel, 1962; Kraft, 1968) have noted that the attitude of the family to the child taking medication is likely to affect treatment response.

THE ROLE OF THE PHYSICIAN WITH THE ADDH CHILD

Given the above review of the utility of the medical model with this particular syndrome in childhood, what can be considered the proper role of the physician in the diagnosis and treatment of this disorder? It should be noted that the physician is often the first to see the child in an official capacity and the first to make an official diagnosis of some type of problem. Thus the first role of the physician is to do a comprehensive diagnostic evaluation of the child. In essence this role is to answer two questions: Does this child have any type of psychiatric disorder? and Does the child's psychiatric disorder meet the criteria for the ADDH syndrome? Any psychiatric diagnosis in childhood is essentially a clinical one based on a specific clinical picture. The components of the evaluation to make this diagnosis includes a detailed interview with the parent, a detailed psychiatric evaluation of the child, and obtaining information from the school. Using these three diagnostic procedures should enable one to perform a thorough evaluation and answer the question as to whether or not the child has a clinical condition that meets the criteria for the ADDH syndrome.

The physical and neurological examinations, laboratory studies, and family studies as reviewed above generally offer very little to the diagnosis of the ADDH syndrome. However in appropriate cases they should be done to rule in or rule out certain conditions, such as learning disabilities or some medical or neurological problems which may coexist with the ADDH syndrome. Moreover as reviewed above they are helpful in defining subgroups of the population whose condition may differ in etiology, and do seem to differ in prognosis, especially in regard to response to central nervous system stimulant medication.

With regard to the making of the clinical diagnosis of the ADDH syndrome, the interviews with the parents and children have been described in detail elsewhere (Cantwell, 1975a). Some points are however worth emphasizing. It is mandatory in the interview with the parents to make sure that one covers systematically all behavioral manifestations of the psychiatric disorders of childhood. While parents should be allowed to present their own story in their own way, after they are finished a systematic coverage must be completed of all the areas of the child's behavioral and cognitive functioning. The reason for this is obvious. Parents may bring in a child for evaluation for one set of symptoms (such as short attention span and increased activity level) which are very disruptive both in school and home settings. However the child may be actually manifesting much more severe pathology, such as severe depression, hallucinations, or delusions of which the parents or teachers may be unaware and thus fail to report.

Likewise the interview with the child must be systematic. The clinician must attempt to complement what is gleaned from the parental interview and the material obtained from the school. The interview with the child can be considered to provide two different types of information: (1) observations made of the child during the interview setting and (2) verbal reports of the child made during the interview. Likewise the interview with the child can be considered to consist of two major parts: (1) a structured and (2) an unstructured part. The interview with the child should not be considered a one-shot procedure, but each child must be seen two or three times to assure that one is getting a reliable picture of the child's behavior. Following the interview with the child, some systematic method or recording should be used, such as the psychiatric rating scale developed by Rutter and Graham (1968) or the psychiatric rating scale developed by the Early Clinical Drug Evaluation Unit (ECDEU) Committee.

There are a number of ways of obtaining information from the school: a visit to the school which is probably not practical in many cases, a phone call to the teacher, and the use of a systematic teacher rating scale such as that developed by Conners. In a busy office practice, a combination of the use of the Conners rating scale and phone calls with the teacher will be quite sufficient and quite helpful.

As mentioned above physical and neurological examinations are generally done to rule out some treatable medical or neurological problem. A play neurological will allow the physician to make valuable behavioral observations about the psychiatric state of the child. In doing physical and neurological examinations, stress should be placed on recording of baseline height and weight and the screening of all body systems, at least by interrogation of the parent and child.

Laboratory studies are generally not done routinely, but for children who are considered for a stimulant drug treatment, a baseline blood count and urinalysis plus a screening blood battery, such as an SMA 12, are recommended. Other blood testing should only be done if a clear clinical indication exists that the child may have a specific physical or neurological problem or if toxicity develops as a result of drug treatment.

Psychological testing as noted does not contribute as such to the diagnosis of the syndrome. However a psychoeducational assessment should be done with at least an assessment of general intelligence and academic achievement. It is important to have some measure of learning and academic achievement as one way of assessing the effect of any stimulant that might be used. There is evidence that a low dose of a stimulant may improve both behavior and learning in some children, a higher dose may continue to improve behavior, but may impair learning (Sprague and Sleator, 1975).

Whatever diagnostic assessment instruments are used, it is important to be sure that at the baseline period proper assessments have been made of all target functions that are likely to be affected by the use of stimulant medication or any other treatment modality. The various types of assessment instruments that have been found useful in this regard are the Conners Parent Rating Scale, the Conners Teacher Rating Scale, and Physician Rating Scales of behavior and side effects combined with parent and patient side-effects rating scales. All of these may be found as part of the ECDEU package. Once the physician has completed his diagnostic evaluation, he should be able to answer the following questions:

1. Does the child have a psychiatric disorder which meets the clinical criteria for the ADDH syndrome? (Assuming the answer to that is yes, the following questions then are also important.)
2. In addition to the ADDH syndrome, does the child have any other condition which may potentially be important, such as psychosis or depression?
3. In this individual case, what are the likely etiologic factors?
4. In this individual case, what therapeutic modalities are most likely to be effective for what aspect of the child's disorder?

It is important to recognize for treatment purposes that the child with the ADDH syndrome is a multi-handicapped child, thus any *one* treatment modality used alone is unlikely to be effective. A multiple modality treatment approach is probably going to be necessary for any child with this disorder. Each child and his family must have a treatment program designed for their needs, based on an individual comprehensive assessment of their assets and liabilities.

From the standpoint of the physician who evaluates the child, therapeutic interventions can be divided into those which he may provide himself, those which he would recommend be carried out by other professionals, and those "magical" cures which he should be aware of as being touted without solid evidence as being effective for this disorder. In the latter case, the physician's role is to explain to the parent the lack of evidence for effectiveness of these "magical" cures.

The first issue for the physician to decide in the treatment of the ADDH child is whether this particular child will respond to central nervous system stimulant medication. Since we know that about 75% of the children with this syndrome show a positive response (Barkley, 1977), and since we know that there are very few predictors of response which are reliable and valid for individual children, it would seem the children who meet the criteria for this disorder, in the absence of any significant contraindication, should be given a trial on central nervous system stimulant medication.

If the physician has decided to make a trial of stimulant medication, the next step is to involve both the child and his parents in the treatment process. This is often a most neglected part of the use of stimulant medication. Too often medication is prescribed by the physician and given to the parents without any attempt to help the child understand the nature of his difficulties and how the use of the stimulant is intended to help the child help himself. What should the parents be told regarding the use of medication?

It should be explained that the dosage of the stimulant or the type of stimulant may have to be changed to obtain the proper therapeutic effect. The physician should explain in great detail exactly what the positive and negative effects of the medication might be. The parents should be told that in those children who do respond positively stimulant medication seems to affect the attentional process. Thus the children perform better on tests requiring sustained vigilance and attention. During these tests, task irrelevant motor activity is decreased. Parents should also be told that stimulants have a positive effect on that type of behavior which is usually perceived by teachers as disruptive and not socially appropriate.

Finally it should be explained that there is good evidence suggesting that stimulant medication positively affects such cognitive functions as attention, perception, and memory as well as influencing cognitive style and laboratory measures of learning. However there is no evidence to suggest that stimulants alone positively affect classroom learning and academic achievement.

Parents should also be alerted to the possible side effects that might develop as a result of stimulant medication. Short-term side effects include insomnia and decreased appetite, weight loss, abdominal pain, and headaches. Side effects occur only in a minority of children and tend to be minor and temporary.

There is also a paucity of evidence about significant long-term side effects. The one long-term side effect that parents frequently ask about is a possible depression of height and weight growth rate. A recent review of all published literature by the FDA panel (Roche and Jackson, 1978) suggests that any height and weight suppression occurs only for the first year or two of therapy; there does not seem to be any long-term effect on ultimate growth. There also does not seem to be any clear tendency for children who have been treated with stimulants to become abusers of drugs in later life (Beck, et al., 1975). However caution in this area is still necessary since most of the studies have failed to locate a significant number of subjects for follow-up (Cantwell and Carlson, 1978).

If the child does not respond to any of the stimulant medications, it might be worthwhile to give a trial of a tricyclic antidepressant, such as imipramine. Studies indicate that imipramine is effective with ADDH children, but probably less so than stimulants (Cantwell, 1977). These tend to be more poorly tolerated and over a year's period of time more children will drop out of drug treatment with imipramine than with the stimulants. If the child does not respond to either stimulants or to a tricyclic, in the author's experience it is unlikely that any other class of medications will prove effective except in rare cases.

Certain aspects about clinical monitoring of the medication are worth noting. Within a group of drugs such as the stimulants, there is little in the current literature to select one over the other. ADDH children seem to respond about equally well to methylphenidate, the amphetamines, and magnesium pemoline. However there are idiosyncratic children who respond better to one than they do to another or who may respond about equally well to two drugs but get less side effects with one than they do with the other.

As a general rule an older drug which has the value of having been used for a number of years should be used in place of a new drug, unless there is overwhelming evidence for clinical superiority of the newer drug.

Regardless of which drug is used, the author believes that the smallest available dosage should be tried initially; the duration of action of the medication being used will determine how often it has to be prescribed. Short-acting amphetamines and methylphenidates generally have a duration of action of about four hours, while long-acting spansule forms of the amphetamines and pemolines have a longer duration of action and can often be prescribed only once a day. Currently in general practice there is no real way to monitor the medication other than by clinical judgment. Starting with a low dose the physician will titrate the dosage upward looking for a clinical improvement, clinical worsening, or side effects. If clinical improvement occurs, it probably is worthwhile pushing the dose up slightly to see if additional benefit can be obtained without any deleterious effects. Paired associate learning paradigms such as that described by Swanson and Kinsbourne (1978) are probably a better way and also a shorter way to determine the appropriate dosage, at least for the stimulant medications. However these are in their infancy at the moment and have generally been used only in research settings.

There are no hard guidelines available to the physician in determining the optimal dosage of an individual drug for each child. While broad guidelines can be given on a miligram per kilogram basis of body weight, this is a very controversial area as regards the stimulants (Cantwell and Carlson, 1978). We do know from blood level studies of drugs we can measure (such as the tricyclics) that individual children may require a great deal more medication than would be expected on the basis of their body weight. This is due to large individual differences in blood levels of medication per comparable dosage of the same drug in children with the same body weight.

If one does obtain improvement and the improvement seems to disappear, the dosage may have to be increased. The question of tolerance to the stimulants in ADDH children is still an open one. There are clinicians who feel that regular increases in dosage are generally not necessary, while there are others who feel that as time goes by children do require more medication to get the same effect. Generally the stimulants are prescribed five days a week when the child is in school and drug holidays are used for weekends, summer vacations, and other holidays.

However, while there may be theoretical reasons for using drug holidays, their efficacy has never been systematically established. Generally clinicians who use drug holidays feel that the less medicine the child takes the less likely he will become tolerant to it and also the less likely he will develop side effects. Again while this sounds good theoretically, to the author's knowledge there has never been a systematic study of children on and off medication for drug holidays, either for the development of tolerance or for the occurrence of side effects. Most importantly a cost benefit study considering possible detrimental effects of leaving children off medication on the weekends and for summer holidays has not been done. There are investigators such as Swanson and Kinsbourne (1978) who feel for example that methylphenidate tablets should probably be given three times a day and seven days a week. They base this on their studies of the effects of stimulants on learning where they demonstrated a state-dependent learning effect, that is the child did not retain material as well in the nonmedicated state as he had during the medicated state. Thus children may learn something during the day and not be able to apply it to homework at night. Moreover they argue that a good deal of child learning occurs outside the classroom situation, and if a child requires stimulant medication for enhancement of learning purposes, it should not be limited to the school day. This is still however a controversial area.

Once a child is on a stable dose of medication, monitoring should be done carefully. The child should be seen on at least a monthly basis, and the same ratings of behavior and learning that were taken at baseline should be made at regular intervals. The sources of this information would include the parents, the teachers, and the child himself. Evidence of positive or negative effects of the drug should be obtained from all sources. Any other appropriate assessments, such as measurements of learning, height, and weight also need to be done on a regular basis. The general consensus is that, in the absence of clinical evidence of toxicity, blood studies need not be done more than once a year. Something that should be done during the course of every year is a drug-free trial. The best way to do this (if one can) is to substitute a placebo with the parents' knowledge, but without the knowledge of the patient or teacher. The same ratings of behavior and learning can then be obtained and, if there is a deterioration, it can be assumed that the medication is still needed. For many private practitioners, a placebo is not available. Thus the child will simply have to be taken off the medication. The teacher can still rate the child blindly. This is where objective tests are useful.

As a general rule, except for unusual cases, the child should probably start school each September with no medication. After several weeks in a new class with a new teacher, the same ratings can be obtained that were obtained at the end of the previous school year when the child was on active medication. If it appears that medication is no longer necessary, the child should be followed closely to see if behavior and academic performance deteriorate over time. While it used to be thought that this syndrome would somehow be outgrown at puberty, it is now quite clear that in some cases there are adults who are grown-up hyperactive children, who still respond to stimulant medication in adulthood. This has been graphically demonstrated by the study of Wood and Wender and their colleagues at the University of Utah (Wood, et al., 1976).

At the present time clinical judgment is the only thing that can be used to determine when a child should be taken off medication completely. Medication should be stopped only when the clinical picture indicates that the child no longer requires it, not because a certain magic age is reached.

Any physician, whether he is a psychiatrist or a primary-care physician, will also be heavily involved with the family if he is treating children with the ADDH syndrome. As a bare minimum parents should be told about the nature and phenomenology of the syndrome. A primary-care physician may offer family counseling along the lines of basic social learning theory. The author has found that providing parents with reading materials, such as the book by Stewart and Olds (1973), *Raising a Hyperactive Child,* and the book by Wender (1973), *The Hyperactive Child: A Handbook for Parents,* are quite helpful in giving the parents techniques on how to deal with specific aspects of their child's behavior. The use of such books as *Families* by Patterson (1971) and *Living with Children* by Patterson and Gullion (1968) both of which are programmed texts, are quite helpful in teaching principles of structuring the child's environment so that there are regular routines and firm limits on the child's behavior. Also these are helpful in teaching parents to focus on certain specific problem areas such as temper tantrums, peer relationships, self-confidence, fighting with sibs, and so on.

Something which is often neglected in dealing with parents of children with this disorder is referring the family to groups of other parents whose children suffer from this disorder or from other learning disabilities. Organizations such as the

National Association for Children with Learning Disabilities have local branches in almost every major city. Getting together with other parents who have similar problems, allows the parents to give each other mutual support. Moreover these parents are also probably the best source of information regarding community resources, school funding, other parent organizations, and other practical issues.

As noted however a significant number of parents of ADDH children have psychopathology themselves. In some cases there is a great deal of family discord and turmoil, which may result from parents' psychiatric illnesses, other problems, or from the effect of the ADDH child on the family; a more dynamic family therapy approach may be necessary, and/or parents may need to be referred for their own psychopathology. In these instances, the primary-care physician will probably refer the family for such treatment. If the treating physician is also a psychiatrist, he may wish to take this on himself.

For some reason solid, systematic studies of the families of ADDH children are lacking in the clinical literature. It is the author's opinion that this is due to the now outmoded assumption that ADDH children are brain-damaged children and that family discord and other familial factors play no role in their development. In truth the ADDH child because of his intrinsic problems is not only as likely but probably more likely to be sensitive to the effects of psychosocial and familial factors, such as parental mental illness, parental criminality, family discord, and broken homes. Limited evidence reviewed above does in fact suggest that the ultimate outcome of the ADDH child may rest on some of these familial factors.

The primary-care physician will also need to make an assessment of the probable utility of individual or group therapy with the child as part of the total treatment program. The primary-care physician again will probably not be the one directly to offer this type of therapy. If the treating physician is a psychiatrist, particularly a child psychiatrist, he may take the child for individual therapy.

In many cases self-image problems, depression, and other areas outlined by Gardner (1973) who is one of the pioneers in the field of psychotherapy with this problem, will not respond to other treatment modalities. The child may be given an adequate dose of medication to which he responds in terms of improved attention and decreased distractibility. He may be given academic help and make some progress. Family counseling may be used, and yet certain problems remain, which can only be handled on an individual basis with the child.

The evaluating physician also will assess the need for a program of educational therapy or cognitive training. If the child is failing academically or is not performing up to expected grade level, then some type of intervention in this area is necessary. There are a number of cognitive training programs outlined by Douglas and her colleagues (1977) which suggest that children with the ADDH syndrome can in fact be trained to overcome some of their difficulties.

In the author's opinion the obtaining of special educational help in whatever form is often the most difficult, particularly if parents do not have the resources to afford private care or if they live in an area where little is available. The question of whether a child should be placed within a self-contained special class in the public school setting or for that matter in a private setting depends on many factors. Not all of these are directly related to the child's disorder. In some cases in the public school system, special education programs are nothing more than babysitting classes, and the only thing special about the class is that it has 8 to 10 of the toughest children in the district. It may or may not have a special teacher.

Finally there are a variety of other therapeutic modalities that have been advocated for children with this disorder. These include such things as elimination diet, hypoglycemic diets, megavitamin therapy, patterning, neurophysiological retraining, optometry, and sensory integrative therapy (Silver, 1975). In the author's opinion there is no hard scientific evidence for the efficacy of any of these therapies used individually. They are far outstripped by the material which promotes them than by the material which supports their claims. In handling individual cases one or more of these therapeutic modalities is likely to come up and parents will ask about them. It behooves every physician who evaluates ADDH children to be aware of the latest fads and of the evidence, or lack of it, which supports them.

SUMMARY AND CONCLUSIONS

The ADDH syndrome is a very common behavior disorder of childhood. The evidence suggests that untreated these children do quite poorly, and even more sobering is the thought that the long-term outcome of treated groups of ADDH children has not been shown to be all that good. However most of the studies that have been reported thus far have been of children who have been treated with medication alone, and then not consistently used. In a recent study Satterfield and the present author (Satterfield, Cantwell, and Satterfield, 1978) have found improvement on parent ratings of behavior, teacher ratings of behavior, physician ratings of behavior, physician ratings of behavior at the end of one year and at the end of two years, as well as significant changes in academic achievement in mathematics, reading recognition, and reading comprehension. In this long-term study of children treated with a multimodality treatment program offering each child what was felt to be necessary for his optimal development, modalities included the use of medication; family counseling; parent training; individual, group, and family therapy; and individual and group educational therapy. More long-term outcome studies of this disorder and its treatment by various modalities are sorely needed.

This chapter has attempted to outline a medical approach to the diagnosis and treatment of this disorder. The medical model and its value in psychiatry in general, and particularly in child psychiatry, has come under increasing attack (Torrey, 1974; Szasz, 1974). Major criticisms about the medical model however tend to be based on misconceptions. One misconception is that according to the medical model the psychiatric disorders of childhood are all organically based entities. However the medical model does not assume that all psychiatric disorders of childhood are organically based entities. It only assumes that a child who presents with one type of disorder may have a different etiologic condition from a child who presents with another disorder. It should be possible to characterize these two conditions and differentiate them from each other as outlined in the six-stage medical model presented at the beginning of this chapter.

The second misconception, which flows from the first, is that the medical model implies that the preferential method of treatment, in fact the *sole* method of treatment in some cases, is drug treatment. However with treatment modalities as with etiology, the medical model is not an organic one, but is best described as an agnostic one (Woodruff, Goodwin, and Guze, 1974). Without hard evidence proponents of the medical model do not necessarily assume that pills are better than play therapy, nor that play therapy is better than pills. Proponents of the medical model do however require evidence for the suitability of a treatment modality or combination of modalities for a given child with a given disorder.

In recent years an antilabeling school has arisen in opposition to the medical approach to psychiatric diagnosis. Proponents of the antilabeling school suggest that the process of diagnosis in childhood is merely a form of labeling the child, that it is meaningless for clinical purposes, and that the labeling process itself is directly harmful to the child.

The proper answer to this misconception is that a psychiatric diagnosis as described here does not result in applying a label to a child, but it does result in applying a label to a psychiatric disorder the child presents with. The child may have measles at one age, pneumonia at another age, and be perfectly well at the third age. Thus he may present with one psychiatric disorder at one time in his life, with another at a second time, and be perfectly well at a third time.

For research as well as clinical purposes, a valid diagnostic classification scheme is a vital necessity. It is only when people with different orientations have a common language with which they can communicate that we shall be able to compare findings from different centers and from different investigators with different theoretical backgrounds regarding etiology and treatment of this disorder or any other.

A final objection to the medical model is that it is somehow antihumanitarian. It is difficult to see how a tough-minded scientific approach in the study of psychiatric disorders is incompatible with a warm, compassionate, humanitarian approach in therapeutic work. While it is true that the medical model focuses on the patient's disorder as a focus of scientific inquiry rather than on the patient himself, it is difficult to see how more knowledge about a patient's disorder makes one less effective in dealing with the individual patient. Any physician can use this knowledge in a warm compassionate way or in a cold unsympathetic way, quite independently of the model he uses to conceptualize psychiatric disorders (Cantwell, 1975b).

A final comment needs to be made concerning the viewpoint that *no* medication of any type should be used with ADDH children or with children with other types of psychiatric disorders. There is a very vocal antimedication body in the United States, which generally makes itself heard in the public media. Their argument runs along lines suggesting that stimulants are nothing but chemical straightjackets and that oppressive school systems, parents, and certain physicians are in collaboration to turn bright, exuberant, active children into robots because they come into conflict with our system of education. While no one would suggest that serious thought shouldn't be given to the long-term use of stimulants or any medication in children, the idea that a proper use of stimulants produces controlled robots is based on a great deal of ignorance about the effect of these medications on children with the ADDH syndrome. Every therapeutic endeavor in medicine, whether it is giving digitalis for heart disease, operating on appendicitis, or immunizing against diphtheria, attempts to control something. The use of stimulant medication to control negative aspects of a child's behavior and to enhance his learning is no different from these other types of therapeutic controls. The decision whether to use stimulants with ADDH children should be based on the severity of the condition, what is known about its untreated outcome and what is known about the clinical efficacy and safety of the stimulants.

As we have seen this condition can be quite severe and untreated leads to significant social problems and psychopathology in adulthood. A great deal is known about the clinical efficacy of stimulants in particular and their effect on these children. While less is known about the safety over the long-term, there is certainly no evidence to suggest a definite occurrence of significant long-term side effects. The decision to use medication with children with this disorder is a medical one, not a moral or philosophical one, and should be made by physicians and not philosophers.

REFERENCES

American Psychiatric Association. *Diagnostic and Statistical Manual of Mental Disorders,* 3rd ed., Washington, D.C.: Task Force on Nomenclature and Statistics, April 15, 1977. [Draft version]

Arnold, L., V. Kirlcuk, S. Corson, and E. Corson. "Levoamphetamine and dextroamphetamine: Differential effect on aggression and hyperkinesis in children and dogs." *The American Journal of Psychiatry,* 130, 165–170, (1973).

Barkley, R. A. "A review of stimulant drug research with hyperactive children." *Journal of Child Psychiatry,* 18, 137–165, (1977).

Beck, L., W. Langford, M. MacKay, and G. Sum. "Childhood chemotherapy and later drug abuse and growth curve. A follow-up study of 30 adolescents." *The American Journal of Psychiatry,* 132, 436–438, (1975).

Blaney, P. H. "Implications of the medical model and its alternatives." *American Journal of Psychiatry,* 132, 911–14, (1975).

Borland, B. L., and H. K. Heckman. "Hyperactive boys and their brothers: A 25-year follow-up study."*Archives of General Psychiatry,* 33, 669–675, (1976).

Bradley, C. "The behavior of children receiving benzedrine." *American Journal of Orthopsychiatry,* 94, 577–585, (1937).

Cantwell, D. P. "Psychiatric illness in families of hyperactive children." *Archives of General Psychiatry,* 27, 414–417, (1972).

———*The Hyperactive Child: Diagnosis, Management and Current Research.* New York: Spectrum, 1975a.

———"A model for the investigation of psychiatric disorders of childhood: Its application in genetic studies of hyperkinetic children," in E. J. Anthony, ed., *Explorations in Child Psychiatry,* pp. 57–79. Plenum, 1975b.

———"Genetic factors in the hyperkinetic syndrome."*Journal of the American Academy of Child Psychiatry,* 15, 214–223, (1976).

———"Psychopharmacologic treatment of the minimal brain dysfunction syndrome," in Jerry M. Weiner, ed., *Psychopharmacology in Childhood and Adolescence,* pp. 119–148. New York: Basic Books, 1977.

Cantwell, D. P., and G. A. Carlson. "Stimulants," in J. S. Werry, ed., *Pediatric Psychopharmacology—The Use of Behavior Modifying Drugs in Children,* pp. 171–207. New York: Brunner/Mazel, 1978.

Coleman, M. "Serotonin concentrations in whole blood of hyperactive children." *Journal of Pediatrics,* 78, 985–990, (1971).

Conners, C. K. "The syndrome of minimal brain dysfunction: Psychological aspects." *The Pediatric Clinics of North America*, 14, 749–766, (1967).

———"Psychological assessment of children with minimal brain dysfunction." *Annals of New York Academy of Sciences*, 205, 283–302, (1973).

Conrad, W., and J. Insel. "Anticipating the response to amphetamine therapy in the treatment of hyperkinetic children." *Pediatrics*, 40, 96–99, (1967).

Denhoff, E. "The natural life history of children with minimal brain dysfunction." *Annals of the New York Academy of Sciences*, 205, 188–205, (1973).

Douglas, V. I., P. Parry, P. Marton, and C. Garson. "Assessment of a cognitive training program for hyperactive children." *Journal of Abnormal Childhood Psychology*, 4, 389–410, (1976).

Eeg-Olofsson, O. "The development of the electroencephalogram in normal children and adolescents from the age of 1 through 21 years." *Acta Paediatrica Scandinavica*, Supplement, 208, (1970).

Fish, B. "The 'one child, one drug' myth of stimulants in hyperkinesis." *Archives of General Psychiatry*, 25, 193–203, (1971).

Gardner, R. A. "Psychotherapy of the psychogenic problems secondary to minimal brain dysfunction." *International Journal of Child Psychotherapy*, 2, 224–256, (1973).

Goodwin, D. W., F. Schulsinger, L. Hermansen, S. B. Guze, and G. Winokur. "Alcoholism and the hyperactive child syndrome." *The Journal of Nervous and Mental Disease*, 160, 349–353, (1975).

Goodwin, F., and W. Bunney. "A psychobiological approach to affective illness." *Psychiatric Annals*, 3, 19–56, (1973).

Guze, S. "Psychiatric disorders and the medical." *Biological Psychiatry*, 3, 221–224, (1972).

Hirsch, K. de "Early language development and minimal brain dysfunction." *Annals of the New York Academy of Sciences*, 205, 158–163, (1973).

Kennard, M. "Value of equivocal signs in neurologic diagnosis." *Neurology*, 10, 753–764, (1960).

Knobel, M. "Psychopharmacology for hyperkinetic child—dynamic considerations." *Archives of General Psychiatry*, 6, 198–202, (1962).

Kraft, I. "The use of psychoactive drugs in the outpatient treatment of psychiatric disorders of children." *American Journal of Psychiatry*, 124, 1401–1407, (1968).

Laufer, M. "Long-term management of some follow-up findings on the use of drugs with minimal brain dysfunction." *Journal of Learning Disabilities*, 4, 55, (1971).

Laufer, M., and E. Denhoff. "Hyperkinetic behavior syndrome in children." *Journal of Pediatrics*, 50, 463–474, (1957).

Loney, J., R. Prinz, J. Mishalow, and J. Joad. "Hyperkinetic/aggressive boys in treatment: Predictors of clinical response to methylphenidate." *American Journal of Psychiatry*, 35, 1487–1491 (1978).

Mendelson, M., N. Johnson, and M. A. Stewart. "Hyperactive children as teenagers: A follow-up study." *Journal of Nervous and Mental Disease*, 153, 273–279, (1971).

Menkes, M., J. Rowe, and J. Menkes. "A twenty-five year follow-up study on the hyperkinetic child with minimal brain dysfunction." *Pediatrics*, 39, 393–399, (1967).

Millichap, J. "Drugs in management of minimal brain dysfunction." *Annals of the New York Academy of Sciences*, 205, 321–334 (1973).

Minde, K., G. Weiss and M. Mendelson. "A five-year follow-up study of 91 hyperactive school children." *Journal of the American Academy of Child Psychiatry*, 11, 595–610, (1972).

Minde, K., D. Lewin, G. Weiss, H. Lavigueur, V. Douglas, and E. Sykes. "The hyperactive child in elementary school: A five-year, controlled follow-up." *Exceptional Children*, 38, 215–221, (1971).

Morrison, J. R., and K. Minkoff. "Explosive personality as a sequel to the hyperactive child syndrome." *Comprehensive Psychiatry*, 16, 343–348, (1975).

Morrison, J. R., and M. A. Stewart. "A family study of the hyperactive child syndrome." *Biological Psychiatry*, 3, 189–195, (1971).

———"The psychiatric status of the legal families of adopted hyperactive children." *Archives of General Psychiatry*, 28, 888–891, (1973).

Patterson, G. *Families*. Champaign, Ill.: Research Press, 1971.

Patterson, G., and E. Gullion. *Living with Children*. Champaign, Ill.: Research Press, 1968.

Petersen, I., P. Eeg-Olofsson and U. Sellden. "Paroxysmal Activity in EEG of Normal Children." In P. Kellaway and I. Petersen, eds., *Clinical Electroencephalography of Children*, pp. 167–187. New York: Grune and Stratton, 1968.

Quinn, P., and J. Rapoport. "Minor physical anomalies and neurologic status in hyperactive boys." *Pediatrics*, 53, 742–747, (1974).

Quitkin, F., and D. Klein. "Two behavioral syndromes in young adults related to possible minimal brain dysfunction." *Journal of Psychiatric Research*, 7, 131–142, (1969).

Rapoport, J., P. Quinn, and F. Lamprecht. "Minor physical anomalies and plasma dopamine-beta-hydroxylase activity in hyperactive boys." *American Journal of Psychiatry*, 131, 386–390, (1974).

Rapoport, J., I. Lott, D. Alexander, and A. Abramson. "Urinary noradrenaline and playroom behavior in hyperactive boys." *Lancet*, 2, 1141, (1970).

Riddle, K. D., and J. L. Rapoport. "A two-year follow-up of 72 hyperactive boys." *The Journal of Nervous and Mental Disease*, 162, 126–134, (1976).

Robins, E., and S. Guze. "Establishment of diagnostic validity and psychiatric illness: Its application to schizophrenia." *American Journal of Psychiatry*, 126, 983–987, (1970).

Roche, A. F., and T. Jackson. "Hyperkinesis, autonomic nervous system activity and stimulant drug effects." *Journal of Child Psychology and Psychiatry*, [1978] in press.

Rutter, M., and P. Graham. "The reliability and validity of the psychiatric assessment of the child. I. Interview with the child." *British Journal of Psychiatry*, 114, 563–579, (1968).

Rutter, M., P. Graham, and W. Yule. *A Neuropsychiatric Study in Childhood*. Philadelphia: Lippincott, 1970.

Satterfield, J. H. "EEG issues in children with minimal brain dysfunction." *Seminars in Psychiatry*, 5, 35–46, (1973).

Satterfield, J. H., D. P. Cantwell, and B. T. Satterfield. "The pathophysiology of the hyperkinetic syndrome." *Archives of General Psychiatry*, 31, 839–844, (1974c).

———"Multi-modality treatment: A one-year follow up of 84 hyperactive boys." *Archives of General Psychiatry*, [1978] in press.

Satterfield, J. H., D. P. Cantwell, L. I. Lesser, and R. L. Podosin. "Psychological studies of the hyperkinetic child: I." *American Journal of Psychiatry*, 128, 1418–1424, (1972).

Satterfield, J. H., G. Atoian, G. C. Brashears, A. C. Burleigh, and M. E. Dawson. "Electrodermal studies of minimal brain dysfunction children," in *Clinical Use of Stimulant Drugs in Children*, pp. 87–97. The Hague: Excerpta Medica, 1974a.

Satterfield, J. H., D. P. Cantwell, R. Saul, and A. Yusin. "Intelligence, academic achievement and EEG abnormalities in hyperactive children." *American Journal of Psychiatry*, 131, 391–395, (1974b).

Shaywitz, B. A., D. J. Cohen, and M. B. Bowers, Jr. "CSF amine metabolites in children with minimal brain dysfunction (MBD)—Evidence for alteration of brain dopamine." *Pediatric Research*, 9, 385, (1975).

Shekim, W. O., H. Dekirmenjian, and J. L. Chapel. "Urinary catecholamine metabolites in hyperkinetic boys treated with dextroamphetamine." *American Journal of Psychiatry*, 134, 1276–1279, (1977).

Shelley, E., and A. Riester. "Syndrome of minimal brain damage in young adults." *Diseases of the Nervous System*, 33, 335–338, (1972).

Siegler, M., and H. Osmund. *Models of Madness, Models of Medicine.* New York: Macmillan, 1974.

Silver, L. B. "Acceptable and controversial approaches to treating the child with learning disabilities." *Pediatrics*, 55, 406–415, (1975).

Snyder, S., K. Taylor, J. Coyle, and J. Meyerhoff. "The role of brain dopamine in behavioral regulation and the actions of psychotropic drugs." *The American Journal of Psychiatry*, 127, 199–207, (1970).

Sprague, R., and E. Sleator. "What is the proper dose of stimulant drugs in children?" *International Journal of Mental Health*, 4, 75–104, (1975).

Spitzer, R., J. Endicott, E. Robins, J. Kuriansky, and B. Gurland. "Preliminary report of the reliability of research diagnostic criteria applied to psychiatric case records." in A. Sudilovsky, S. Gershon, and B. Beer, eds., *Predictability in Psychopharmacology: Preclinical and Clinical Correlations.* New York: Raven, 1975.

Stewart, M. and S. Olds. *Raising a Hyperactive Child.* New York: Harper and Row, 1973.

Stewart, M., F. Pitts, A. Craig, and W. Dieruf. "The hyperactive child syndrome." *American Journal of Orthopsychiatry*, 36, 861–867, (1966).

Swanson, J. M. and M. Kinsbourne. "Should you use stimulants to treat the hyperactive child?" *Modern Medicine*, 47, 71–80, (April 15, 1978).

Szasz, T. S. *The Myth of Mental Illness.* New York: Harper and Row, 1974.

Szureck, S. A. "Psychotic episodes and psychotic maldevelopment." *American Journal of Orthopsychiatry*, 26, 519–543, (1956).

Tarter, R. E., H. McBride, N. Buonpane, and D. U. Schneider. "Differentiation of alcoholics according to childhood history of minimal brain dysfunction, family history and drinking pattern." *Archives of General Psychiatry*, 34, 761–768, July, 1977.

Torrey, E. F. *The Death of Psychiatry.* Radnor, Pa.: Chilton, 1974.

Waldrop, M., and C. Halverson. "Minor physical anomalies and hyperactive behavior in young children," in J. Hellmuth, ed., *The Exceptional Infant.* pp. 343–380. New York: Brunner/Mazel, 1971.

Weiss, G., K. Minde, V. Douglas, J. Werry, and D. Sykes. "Studies on the hyperactive child. V. The effects of dextro-amphetamine and chlorpromazine on behavior and intellectual functioning." *Journal of Child Psychology and Psychiatry*, 9, 145–156, (1968).

Weiss, G., K. Minde, J. S. Werry, V. I. Douglas, and E. Nemeth. "Studies on the hyperactive child. VIII. Five-year follow-up." *Archives of General Psychiatry*, 24, 409–414, (1971*a*).

Weiss, G., K. Minde, V. Douglas, J. Werry, and D. Sykes. "Comparison of the effects of chlorpromazine, dextro-amphetamine and methylphenidate on the behavior and intellectual functioning. *Canadian Medical Journal*, 104, 20–25, (1971*b*).

Wender, P. H. "Platelet serotonin level in children with 'minimal brain dysfunction.'" *Lancet*, 1012, (1969).

———*Minimal Brain Dysfunction in Children.* New York: Wiley-Interscience, 1971.

———*The Hyperactive Child: A Handbook for Parents.* New York: Crown, 1973.

Wender, P. H., R. Epstein, I. Kopin, and E. Gordon. "Urinary monoamine metabolites in children with minimal brain dysfunction." *American Journal of Psychiatry*, 127, 1411–1415, (1971).

Werry, J. S. "Organic factors in childhood psychopathology," in H. Quay and J. Werry, eds., *Psychopathological Disorders of Childhood*, pp. 83–121. New York: Wiley, 1972.

Werry, J., and M. Aman. "Methylphenidate and haloperidol in children." *Archives of General Psychiatry*, 32, 790–795, (1975).

Werry, J. S., G. Weiss, V. Douglas, and J. Martin. "Studies on the hyperactive child. III. The effect of chlorpromazine upon behavior and learning ability." *Journal of the American Academy of Child Psychiatry*, 5, 292–312, (1966).

Werry, J., K. Minde, A. Guzman, G. Weiss, K. Dogan, and E. Hoy. "Studies on the hyperactive child. VII. Neurological status compared with neurotic and normal children." *American Journal of Orthopsychiatry*, 42, 441–450, (1976).

Wood, D. R., F. W. Reimherr, P. H. Wender, E. L. Bliss, and G. E. Johnson. "Diagnosis and treatment of minimal brain dysfunction in adults: A preliminary report." *Archives of General Psychiatry*, 33, 1453–1460 (December, 1976).

Woodruff, R., D. Goodwin, and S. Guze. *Psychiatric Diagnosis*. New York: Oxford University Press, 1974.

CHAPTER 25

Psychological and Environmental Intervention: Toward Social Competence

Donald K. Routh and Gary B. Mesibov

The purpose of this chapter is to describe and evaluate psychological and environmental approaches aimed at helping children with MBD (minimal brain dysfunction) prepare for competent adult lives. For purposes of the present discussion MBD is taken to include a very heterogeneous group of childhood problems of behavior and performance. In the absence of general intellectual impairment, these are commonly understood to include in various combinations: hyperactivity; disorders of attention; impulsive behavior; difficulty with specific academic tasks, such as reading, arithmetic, handwriting, and drawing; and other problems such as clumsiness and speech and language difficulties (Clements, 1966). Whether or not one finds the evidence compelling that MBD is a clinical entity, the problems described under the heading are certainly real and are serious for the children involved.

Previous chapters in this book have dealt with different treatment approaches, for example medical and educational ones. The focus of the present chapter is, in contrast, psychological and environmental. The chapter begins with a review of some follow-up studies of ex-MBD adolescents and adults in order to discover the nature of their continuing difficulties. It next attempts to describe the dimensions of social competence, which can be measured as well as used as positive goals for evaluating intervention programs for children.

We then discuss both behavior modification procedures for use in the classroom and at home and attempts to restructure the classroom environment to foster better learning in these children. Finally we discuss parent counseling and the problems of coordinating the treatment plan for the MBD child.

FOLLOW-UP STUDIES

Do we know the long-term prognosis of the difficulties of the MBD child in the absence of effective treatment? In our review of follow-up studies it is convenient to consider one diagnostic subgroup at a time, because that is the way the literature is organized.

[1] The preparation of this chapter was supported in part by U. S. Public Health Service, Maternal and Child Health Service Project No. 916 and by National Institutes of Health Grants HD-03110 and ES-01104.

Hyperactive Children

Follow-up studies of hyperactive children seem to agree that the hyperactivity as such becomes less of a problem, but that a multitude of other difficulties continue or appear in its place. Menkes, Rowe, and Menkes (1967) followed up a group of 8 hyperactive children an average of 24 years after they were initially examined. Only 3 were still considered to be hyperactive as adults, however 4 of the group were institutionalized, and 2 others were completely supported by their families. Quitkin and Klein (1969) found that among a group of adolescents in a psychiatric hospital, those with a history of childhood hyperactivity tended to show a syndrome of impulsive and destructive behavior. Mendelson, Johnson, and Stewart (1971) found that of 83 teenagers who had been hyperactive as children, 58% had failed one or more grades in school, low self-esteem was common, and several had been involved in delinquent behavior. Their parents typically complained about their rebellious attitudes. Weiss, et al., (1971), in a five-year follow-up study of hyperactive children, found that 70% had repeated at least one grade, as compared to 15% of matched control subjects. The chief complaints of their mothers concerned distractibility and poor concentration, although hyperactivity itself had declined. Minde, Weiss, and Mendelson (1972), in a five-year follow-up, found that although all target symptoms had declined, all of these symptoms, including restlessness, were still significantly higher than in control subjects. In summary childhood hyperactivity seems often to be predictive of continued academic failure, poor concentration and impulsivity, low self-esteem, poor conduct, and sometimes failure to become a self-supporting member of society.

Reading Disability

There are only a few follow-up studies concerning children with specific reading disabilities. Research concerning adult illiteracy rates is easier to locate. Vogt (1973), reporting on a U. S. government testing program on a national probability sample of youths 12 to 17 years old, concluded that the rate of illiteracy in this age group was 4.8%. Illiteracy was defined as a level of tested reading comprehension below that of the average child at the beginning of the fourth grade. This would of course include persons with physical handicaps, mental retardation, or educational disadvantage, as well as those who would be regarded as having MBD or specific reading disabilities, but at least it establishes an upper limit on the estimated prevalence of continued serious reading problems in adulthood.

The follow-up studies which exist of children with specific reading disabilities typically do not include control groups, provide objective test scores, or give sufficient information on the general social adjustment of adults who had reading problems as children. From what research there is however, it is clear that the possible range of outcomes is great. Hermann (1954, cited by Herjanic and Penick, 1972) examined a register of 541 adults who as children had been aided by the Word Blind Institute of Copenhagen. He found remarkable the proportion of occupations such as domestic work, unskilled labor, and errand-running that existed in this group, and he stated that low self-esteem and depression were common among them. At the other extreme in terms of favorability of outcome are the subjects of Rawson's (1968) study. The children she followed up were of superior intelligence (mean IQ 131), came from high social class backgrounds, and if necessary were given highly individualized tutoring in reading. The dyslexics in this study actually had higher educational attainment at follow-up than did controls. All of the former dyslexics completed high school, all but one completed four years of college, and half achieved postgraduate degrees. In terms of vocational and social adjustment, the history of dyslexia hardly seemed associated with any handicap among this group. Silver and Hagin (1964), in one of the few follow-up studies with carefully matched control subjects, found that poor readers as adults came to have somewhat lower IQs than controls. Of 24 subjects followed up in this study who were poor readers as children, 9 were still inadequate readers as adults. Significant predictors of adult status included the presence of neurological findings, the degree of reading retardation, and the type of specific findings on perceptual tasks.

Arithmetic Disabilities

There is little objective information regarding the outcome of children with specific difficulties in arithmetic. Cohn (1971) reported follow-up information on a group of 31 children with arithmetic disability reexamined after a 10-year period. Only 8 of the 31 were able, at follow-up, to accomplish correct multiplication of a three-digit number by a two-digit number. However these children had many disabilities other than that in arithmetic. On the basis of his own experience, Cohn stated that deficits in arithmetic in children are almost always benign, *if* other language functions are intact. Such specific arithmetic deficits, according to Cohn, could in most cases be easily corrected by drill. In any case Cohn stated arithmetic difficulties are not greatly handicapping to adults, who can overcome them by using calculating machines or by hiring an accountant or tax expert.

Visual-Motor Problems

The authors are not aware of even a single study investigating the adult outcome of children with specific difficulty in the visual-motor skills of drawing, copying, or handwriting. This lack may be considered surprising in view of the long existence of standardized tests of human figure drawing (Goodenough, 1926) and copying (Bender, 1938). Perhaps researchers have been interested in children's performance on such tasks not for itself, but because of a hypothesized relationship to some other, more clinically significant attribute of the child. Thus Strauss and Lehtinen (1947), who made extensive use of visual-motor tasks, may have regarded them mainly as a way of diagnosing brain injury or exogenous mental retardation. Similarly others have used the presence of a perceptual handicap (as indexed, for example by poor copying skills) as a diagnostic cue to the hypothesized MBD syndrome. If it becomes the common view that a child's skills of drawing and copying need be neither an index of neurological impairment nor a sign of MBD, (Dreger, 1964; Paine, Werry, and Quay, 1968; Rodin, Lucas, and Simson, 1963; Routh and Roberts, 1972; Werry, 1968) interest in these functions may decrease.

Deficits in Fine Motor Skills

There is also not much information about the adult status of persons with a childhood history of clumsiness or subtle motor difficulties short of overt cerebral palsy.

Speech and Language Problems

What about the prognosis of children with specific speech and language difficulties? Few relevant studies have been carried out. Griffiths (1969) reported a follow-up of 49 children who had attended Horniman School, which was established in Worthing, England in 1958 "for children with severely delayed development of speech and language which may be attributed to minimal cerebral dysfunction" (Griffiths, 1969, p. 46). At the time of follow-up the children ranged from 7 to 16 years of age. Considering only children with average IQ or above, it could be stated that those with the best language outcome were the group of 8 children with severely defective articulation and normal or near normal language development. These children all had normal articulation and normal language at follow-up, although 3 of the 8 were considered to have poor social development and 6 of 8 to be emotionally maladjusted. Another group of 11 (of average intelligence and normal hearing) were originally characterized by both defective articulation *and* delayed or abnormal language development. At follow-up, 8 of these 11 children still had delayed language and 5 still had defective articulation. Six were considered to show poor social development and 3 to show emotional maladjustment. In Griffiths' study, the group of children with the poorest language outcome were those with auditory abnormalities and speech comprehension difficulties. These 6 children, though of average intelligence, at follow-up were all in schools for the deaf or hearing-impaired. All continued to have delayed language and all but 1 to have defective articulation. On the other hand all were considered to show normal social development and only 1 was felt to be emotionally maladjusted.

There is at least one other follow-up study, Garvey and Gordon, (1973) and there are a few surveys of children with speech and language problems, but unfortunately most of these do not distinguish between children with specific speech and language difficulty and those who are deaf, mentally retarded, cerebral palsied, and so on. It is of interest nevertheless to know the overall prevalence of speech and language problems at different ages. The general view is that by the age of 5 most children have acquired fully intelligible speech and language. A few children continue to have minor errors of pronunciation which spontaneously disappear by the age of 7. Speech problems still present at 7 are more likely to persist into adulthood. This was the rationale for selecting age 7 for a national survey of speech defects among children in England, Scotland, and Wales (Peckham, 1973). In this survey teachers reported 10.7% of the children to be "difficult to understand because of poor speech," and physicians found 13.5% to be "other than fully intelligible" upon examination. But by the time these children had attained the age of 11 years, the rate of speech difficulty found by medical officers had dropped to 4.2% (excluding stammer or stutter). Gillespie and Cooper (1973), studying a sample of over 5000 junior and senior high school students in Alabama in the United States, found an overall incidence of speech problems of 5.5%. For articulatory disorders the incidence found was 2.1%.

Summary

To conclude this brief survey of follow-up studies of ex-MBD adults, the range of possible outcomes is extreme. Some recover, apparently completely, from their hyperactivity, reading problems, speech and language disability, or whatever and go on not only to high educational and vocational attainment but also to good social and emotional adjustment as well. For others not only do the specific difficulties such as attentional problems, which may have earned them the MBD label continue, but also other serious problems emerge in addition. Some few are institutionalized; many more have low educational attainment and are employed in jobs beneath their capabilities; low self-esteem and conduct problems are not uncommon. Thus there is good reason for intervention programs to focus not only on the specifics of children's referral problems, but also on fostering social competence as well.

Having examined what is known about the actual outcomes of ex-MBD children, we shall now consider what the positive goals for intervention programs might be.

SOCIAL COMPETENCE

The term social competence refers to those attributes of an individual which are generally considered desirable, both in others and in oneself. It is related to a number of concepts, such as positive mental health, self-actualization, and the like, which have so far received more speculative attention than empirical study. At the risk of seeming to jump boldly into an area of controversy, we would like to begin this section by stating a set of dimensions which we believe capture many of these desirable attributes in a form which is accessible to psychological measurement:

1. Intelligence versus skill deficits.
2. Responsible behavior versus conduct problems.
3. Social participation versus personality problems.

Intelligence versus Skill Deficits

We would define intelligence broadly to include not only scores on traditional measures of intelligence, such as the Stanford-Binet or the Wechsler tests, but also the kinds of achievements which intelligence tests have always been used to predict, that is academic skills (reading, arithmetic, knowledge of course content, and so on) and occupational skills (those needed in professional and technical jobs with high educational requirements).

Responsible Behavior versus Conduct Problems and Social Participation versus Personality Problems

In the field of personality assessment over the last several years, parent rating scales, teacher rating scales, peer-rating procedures, and self-report questionnaires have been developed in bewildering variety. Until recently the set of dimensions measured by such personality assessment devices has seemed rather ill-defined and even chaotic. However thanks to the integrative efforts of such researchers as Kassebaum, Couch, and Slater (1959) and Schaefer (1961, 1975), one can begin to have some confidence in describing the most salient dimensions underlying both ratings of oneself and others. These dimensions seem to be useful in characterizing the behavior of both children and adults. Even more important in the present context, these dimensions refer to positive or desirable behavior (social competence) as well as to psychopathology.

Perhaps the single best known personality dimension is Jung's (1924) concept of Introversion versus Extraversion. According to Jung the extravert is most responsive to stimulation from the outside world, including other people; the introvert tends to be more responsive to subjective thoughts and feelings. Jung's concept carried no implication that the introvert or the extravert was either more adjusted or more maladjusted than the other. Eysenck (1953) later appropriated Jung's terminology to describe a similar dimension measured by his personality inventory. In Eysenck's theory the dimension of Neuroticism corresponded to the *degree* of maladjustment (normal to disturbed), while the orthogonal dimension of Introversion-Extraversion corresponded to the *type* of maladjustment for example extraverted neurotics were more likely to be hysterics or psychopaths, while introverted neurotics were more likely to suffer from obsessions or anxiety. Eysenck never discussed extensively the meaning of scores at the positive or nonpathological end of his Neuroticism dimension.

Kassebaum, Couch, and Slater (1959) did a factor analysis on the Minnesota Multiphasic Personality Inventory (MMPI), which added a new meaning to Eysenck's system. They included not only the usual clinical and validity scales of the MMPI, but also additional scales, mostly from the California Psychological Inventory (CPI), which had been developed to tap positive rather than pathological aspects of personality. Kassebaum, Couch, and Slater found, as had previous researchers, that two major factors captured most of the common variance of the MMPI scales. They presented convincing arguments that their first factor could be indentified with Eysenck's Neuroticism, but with better definition of its socially desirable pole, for example persons scoring opposite the neurotic end of the factor were found to be high on the CPI and MMPI scales of Lp (Leadership), To (Tolerance), Es (Ego-Strength), and Ie (Intellectual Efficiency). Rejecting Eysenck's label (Neuroticism) and Welsh's label A (Anxiety) for this factor, they preferred to call it Ego-Strength versus Ego-Weakness.

The second major MMPI factor found by Kassebaum, Couch, and Slater was labeled Introversion versus Extraversion. It was similar to Welsh's R (Repression) scale, with persons high on the Si (Social Introversion) scale appearing at the Introversion end and those high on Ma (Mania) and Sy (Sociability) scales at the Extraversion end.

Kassebaum, Couch, and Slater, (1959) did not stop there. Pointing out the arbitrariness of the procedure of locating particular reference axes on plane, they rotated the axes 45 degrees. Now instead of the factors of Ego-strength versus Ego-Weakenss and Introversion-Extraversion, the reference axes were so-called fusion factors halfway in between. The nature of these intermediate factors was just what one might have predicted from Eysenck's theory. They called one of the fusion factors Social Withdrawal versus Social Participation (that is Maladjusted Introversion versus Well-adjusted Extraversion). Persons at the Social Withdrawal end were those scoring high on the MMPI and CPI scales Si (Social Introversion), D (Depression), and Fm (Feminine Masochism), while persons at the Social Participation end of the dimension scored high on CPI scores Sp (Social Presence), Sy (Sociability), and St (Capacity for Status). The second fusion factor was called Impulsivity versus Intellectual Control (that is Maladjusted Extraver-

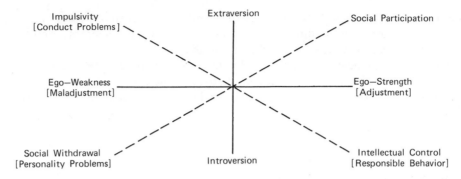

Figure 25–1. Dimensions of personality identified by the Kassebaum, Couch, and Slater (1959) study. The terms in brackets are those used by the present authors in labeling the corresponding dimension.

sion versus Well-adjusted Introversion). Persons at the Impulsivity end of this factor scored high on the CPI and MMPI scales Im (Impulsivity) and Ma (Mania), while persons at the Intellectual Control end scored high on the CPI scales Re (Social Responsibility) and Ac (Achievement via Conformance). Figure 25–1 shows the factorial dimensions of the MMPI identified by Kassebaum, Couch, and Slater in graphic form. It is easy to see from examination of Figure 25–1 that either set of dimensions (the original ones or the fusion factors) is sufficient to provide a description of personality; the choice between them is arbitrary.

Schaefer (1961) found a similar set of dimensions in data from the Parent Attitude Research Inventory (PARI). Of course the content of the items had to do with parent-child relations rather than psychopathology or socially desirable behavior in general. Thus the parental Adjustment-Maladjustment dimension Schaefer found was appropriately named Love versus Hostility (the well adjusted parent showing love and the more maladjusted parent showing hostility toward the child). The parental Extraversion-Introversion dimension on the PARI was called Autonomy versus Control (with the more extraverted parent exerting more control than the more introverted parent allowing the child more freedom). Like Kassebaum, Crouch, and Slater (1959), Schaefer also examined the factors lying at intermediate angles, so to speak. In fact, Schaefer pointed out that a circumplex could be constructed in two dimensional factor space, with each two neighboring variables on the circle sharing more variance in common with each other than with others, and concepts at 180-degree angles from each other being psychological opposites. Thus, for example the combination of Love and Control translates into overprotectiveness. The combination of Hostility and Control is an overdemanding parental style. The combination of Hostility and Autonomy Produces a neglecting approach to child rearing, the combination of Love and Autonomy a democratic one.

In the same chapter Schaefer reviewed the work of many other researchers and suggested that behavioral ratings of children would also lend themselves to the same kind of conceptual arrangement. It was not long before research by others confirmed Schaefer's hypothesis. Becker and Krug (1964) reanalyzed a set of ratings they had previously collected from parents and teachers of normal kindergarten children and found that the resulting factorial dimensions could be organized in circumplex fashion, with the major axes being identified as Emotional

Stability versus Emotional Instability and Introversion versus Extraversion. Becker and Krug's work suggested that earlier research on clinical samples of children could be reinterpreted within this dimensional system. Thus the factor traditionally called Conduct Problems (Ackerson, 1942) or Unsocialized Agression (Hewitt and Jenkins, 1946) can be seen as simply an extraverted type of child maladjustment. And the factor traditionally called Personality Problems (Ackerson, 1942) or Over-Inhibition (Hewitt and Jenkins, 1946) can be viewed correspondingly as an introverted type of child maladjustment. The socially desirable as well as the negative poles of these dimensions were also clear in the child rating data reanalyzed by Becker and Krug. These are essentially the factors advocated as dimensions of social competence by the authors of the present chapter, namely: Responsible Behavior versus Conduct Problems and Social Participation versus Personality Problems. Similar results concerning the applicability of this system to children were found by Baumrind and Black (1967), using Q sort ratings of three- and four-year-old children by psychologist observers, and by Kohn and Rosman (1972), using several different teacher rating scales with preschool and elementary school-age children.

One criticism we need to address concerns the behavioral reality of dimensions found in rating scale data. Our judgment is that the dimensions may not exist in actual behavior, but that the scales are nevertheless useful in measuring social competence. Osgood, Suci, and Tannenbaum (1957) found that when people are asked to rate practically anything along a large number of verbal rating scales, three dimensions of semantic space usually emerge: Evaluation, Activity, and Potency. When people rather than things are being rated, two dimensions seem to be enough: Evaluation and a coalesced dimension of Activity-plus-Potency. There is little doubt at least to Schaefer (1961) that the Adjustment-Maladjustment factor we have been discussing corresponds to Osgood, Suci, and Tannenbaum's Evaluation dimension, and that the Introversion-Extraversion factor is Osgood's Active-Strong versus Passive-Weak dimension. Thus one may reasonably ask whether the emergence of these dimensions in study after study tells us anything about children's behavior or only about the conceptual apparatus used by raters to describe behavior. A study by Passini and Norman (1966) found that raters acquainted only superficially with each other produced peer ratings with factor structures highly similar to those obtained from well-acquainted raters. The finding that similar dimensions exist in self-report personality test data (Kassebaum, Couch, and Slater, 1959) may only mean that people conceptualize their own behavior along similar semantic dimensions. The question about whether these dimensions correspond in any true way to human behavior (as opposed to ratings of behavior) can ultimately be answered only by more direct behavioral observations. In any case the dimensions are clearly important ones in describing the impact people have on each other. It therefore seems to us quite worthwhile to use these dimensions as part of our definition of social competence.

In summary we define the socially competent child or adult as one who is intelligent and who is likely to be judged by other people as showing responsible behavior and social participation. All of these qualities may be assessed by existing intelligence and academic achievement tests, by rating scales (such as Schaefer's Classroom Behavior Inventory), and by self-report measures (such as the CPI).

APPLICATION OF SOCIAL COMPETENCE CONCEPTS TO MBD

Intelligence versus Skill Deficits

Anyone's definition of MBD would surely include such skill deficits as those in reading, spelling, arithmetic, handwriting and drawing, as well as clumsiness and speech and language problems. The psychological treatment approaches to be reviewed are aimed, among other things, at increasing the child's speed and accuracy in the performance of the traditional academic skills of reading, writing, arithmetic, and spelling. Our review of the meager follow-up studies available however suggested that certain skill deficits, such as clumsiness, poor handwriting, and difficulty in spelling or arithmetic had little impact on the lives of ex-MBD adults. Reading skills seemed much more important to these adults, as did residual deficits in speech and language. Also many of the adults seemed to be employed at jobs below their capabilities. Thus one might argue for more emphasis in treatment upon helping the individual explore any special skill areas which might have the potential for development into marketable job skills.

Responsible Behavior versus Conduct Problems

The usual list of MBD symptoms would also include some reference to impulsivity or emotional lability, which carry the implication of disregard by the child of norms for proper conduct in the family and at school. Some of the behavior modification programs to be reviewed have focused on this aspect of behavior, for example Patterson's work with families has emphasized the reduction of aggressive, destructive, and noncompliant behaviors. Almost all classroom behavioral programs have tried to deal with disruptive behaviors (principally talking out without permission). Among certain ex-MBD groups a major problem seems to be their rebellious attitude toward the rules of society, a continued history of delinquency, and other poor conduct. Given the fact that they are at risk for adult antisocial behavior, more treatment emphasis on sensitizing these children to moral and ethical values and on helping them develop self-control seems indicated.

Social Participation versus Personality Problems

The concept of MBD includes very little emphasis upon the emotional and interpersonal adjustment of the child. In accordance with this, the treatment programs to be discussed are focused on bringing the child's behavior under control and remediating skill deficits to the exclusion of much else. And yet follow-up of certain groups of ex-MBD adults reveals low self-esteem, lack of friends, and even depression as common problems. It would seem that we need to correct the imbalance in treatment emphasis and attend to the child's feelings and peer relationships as well as to behavior and academic performance.

Psychological intervention: behavior modification

In this section we review studies of attempts to modify some of the behaviors which are of concern in the MBD child, such as overactivity or out-of-seat behavior at school, disruptiveness in the classroom, short attention span, poor performance on academic tasks, and problems of a similar sort at home. The pros and cons of the use of token reinforcement or material incentives and of punitive procedures, such as response-cost and time-out, will be discussed as well as the problems of generalization across settings and over time. The studies discussed are relevant in that they deal with particular problem behaviors which are of interest. The populations of children studies however are a more mixed group even than children with MBD and include many normal children presenting difficulties in a single situation as well as some children with retardation, severe aggressiveness, or other serious difficulties.

Out-of-Seat Behavior

A number of procedures have been devised for inducing children to stay in their seats in the classroom. Barrish, Saunders, and Wolf (1969), for example, working with a single class of 24 fourth-grade students, demonstrated the effectiveness of what they called the good behavior game. Baseline observations were made of out-of-seat behaviors in the class during math period and reading period over a number of days. Then the class was divided into two teams. First in the math period and later in the reading period as well, each instance of students being out of their seats caused the team to have marks made against it which could result in loss of privileges, such as extra recess, time for special projects, and so on. Both teams could win, if they had few enough marks against them. This procedure makedly decreased the target behaviors, first in math and then in reading period. A reversal condition demonstrated that the experimental manipulation was indeed responsible for the effect.

The workability of the same basic approach was demonstrated by Osborne (1969) with a class of six students at a school for the deaf. In Osborne's version of the procedure, individual students were allowed free time periods during the day contingent upon their remaining seated during regular class time. It was then possible to maintain very low rates of out-of-seat behavior even with noncontingent free time. In order to demonstrate experimental control, Osborne included a condition in which, for a single day the students were given free time only if they *were* out of their seats at least once during the regular class period. Still another experimentally tested version of this same procedure, used with elementary school remedial-class students, is described by Wolf, et al., (1970).

Disruptive Behavior in the Classroom

In the studies under review the most common type of disruptive behavior seems to be talking without permission. The Barrish, et al. (1969) good behavior game dealt with such talking as well as with out-of-seat behavior. Other studies have focused more specifically on reducing this type of disruption. Schmidt and Ulrich (1969) were concerned with the level of classroom noise. They actually set up a sound-level meter near the center of the rear of a regular fourth-grade public school class and defined 42 decibels as too loud. After baseline measures had been taken, students were allowed a two-minute break plus two minutes added to their gym period for each 10 minutes in which the sound-level meter remained at low levels. This procedure produced a marked drop in the average levels of classroom noise. When the contingent rewards were removed, the sound level rose once more; when rewards were reinstituted, the sound level decreased again.

Disruptive behavior in the classroom can of course go beyond just talking out of turn. An example is given by Broden, et al., (1970) in their study of token reinforcement with a junior high school special education class. They mention one teenager, called Rob, who attempted to rebel against the token system. When the system was put into effect, Rob and two others argued that it was childish, said they would not cooperate, and threatened to complain to the principal and the counselor. These remarks were largely ignored and within a day the other two students began to show behavioral improvement. Rob did not. He cursed the teacher, tore up assignments, left the room, fought with other students, and soon had accumulated over 500 minus points. Other students spent increasing time watching Rob and laughing at his antics (it may be that peer reinforcement was maintaining some of his disruptive behavior). The addition of a time-out or isolation procedure in a screened-off area near the principal's office, contingent on refusal to comply with the teacher's requests, was enough to secure Rob's cooperation within a matter of days.

The style as well as the substance of teachers' way of dealing with disruptive student behaviors may be important. O'Leary, et al. (1970), compared the effects of loud, public teacher reprimands with those of soft reprimands communicated to the student in such a way that other children could not hear them. For most children the soft reprimands were much more effective in reducing disruptive behavior. In fact in some cases loud reprimands may have functioned as reinforcers of the behaviors they were intended to inhibit.

A somewhat different, more cognitive, approach to the problem of disruptive behaviors was used by Blackwood (1970) with disruptive children. He required eight-and ninth-graders to write an essay each time they misbehaved. The content of the essay was a definition of the inappropriate target behavior that was performed, its negative consequences, a description of some more appropriate choices, and finally its consequences to the child himself or herself. These essays resulted in fewer disruptive behaviors among the children who had to write them.

Meichenbaum also successfully used a cognitive approach in reducing antisocial behaviors in disruptive children (Meichenbaum and Goodman, 1971). He taught a group of kindergarten and first-grade children several self-instructional techniques. In essence Meichenbaum taught these children a verbal response to certain potentially disruptive situations, hoping they would use these verbal strategies in place of their usually disruptive behaviors. Meichenbaum's data, supported by several later studies, suggest this might be a relevant strategy to pursue.

Spivack and Shure (1974) have used a variant of the Meichenbaum strategy. Spivack and Shure taught children general cognitive, problem-solving strategies so that the children could then think through difficult situations as they confronted them. The ability to think through and solve difficult interpersonal problems should reduce the need for disruptive behaviors, according to Spivack and Shure. The approach is somewhat different from Meichenbaum's in that it stresses having children think through and develop their own individual responses for each problem they confront. The Meichenbaum strategy, in contrast, teaches children one specific alternative behavior that they should always use in problematic situations.

Attention or On-Task Behavior

One major focus of behavior modification studies has been increasing children's ability to pay attention. In a pioneering case study, Allen, et al., (1967) worked with a $4^1/_2$-year-old boy who seemed to have an excessively short attention span. After baseline observations the child's nursery-school teachers began to give attention and approval every time the child remained with any activity for one continuous minute or more. Within a week a number of activity changes the child made went down markedly. When the procedures were reversed and teacher attention made noncontingent once more, the child again began his frequent switching from one activity to another. When contingent social reinforcement began once more, the child's attention span again lengthened. A similar series of experimental demonstrations increasing the amount of study behavior of first-and third-grade students was carried out by Hall, Lund, and Jackson (1968). This was the first article published in the (then) new *Journal of Applied Behavior Analysis* and set the pattern for many other articles in that journal, that is studies using single-subject methodology (an ABAB reversal design) carried out in a field setting with people in the child's natural environment acting as agents of change. In this study records of the behavior of the teacher were presented in addition to presentation of the children's responses.

A novel approach to lengthening children's attention span was presented by Jacobson, Bushell, and Risley (1969). They divided a Head-Start classroom into different activity areas such as the block area, climbing area, and so on and made any child who wanted to move from one area to another perform a switching task to obtain a ticket to go to the other area. One version of the switching task was putting rows of colored pegs on a pegboard. In several single-subject experiments with reversal designs, it was shown that the frequency of switches from one area to another could be shifted upward or downward simply by varying the difficulty or magnitude of the switching task. Thus children would switch more often if a ticket required only one row of pegs than if it required three rows of pegs. They suggested that the switching task could itself be used to introduce academic subjects to the child. Its effectiveness seems to be based on the "Premack Principle" (Premack, 1959) that a high probability behavior (that is going to a different activity area) can be used to reinforce a lower probability behavior (that is performance of the switching task).

Like the research aimed specifically at reducing out-of-seat and disruptive behaviors, a number of studies concerned with increasing students' attention or time-on-task in the classroom use entire groups or classes rather than individual students as the unit of analysis. For example Packard (1970), using token reinforcement contingent on the simultaneous attending of all students in a class, showed that the whole group could be induced to attend 70 to 85% of the time and individual students 90 to 100% of the time. Packard's research was carried out with kindergarten, third, fifth, and sixth-grade classes.

Impulsiveness

Attempts to lessen impulsiveness in children have more often involved training in strategies of self-control than the use of simple reinforcement and have focused on performance on laboratory tasks rather than directly on classroom behavior.

Palkes, Stewart, and Kahana (1968) for example used visual reminder cards to teach hyperactive boys to "stop, look, and listen." The children gave themselves verbal commands out loud before each response on three different training tasks. This procedure significantly improved the performance of the training group relative to the control group on two aspects of the Porteus Maze Tests. This approach was again tried by Palkes, Stewart, and Freedman (1972), who were able to replicate the results only for the Porteus Maze qualitive score and who found the effect rather short-lived. Douglas, et al., (1976) developed a three-month training program involving not only the child but also teacher and parents as well. Relative to the matched control subjects, the children in this study showed reduced impulsiveness (as measured by the Matching Familiar Figures Test), better visual-motor performance, and improvement on other measures. However their hyperactive classroom behavior did not improve.

Performance on Academic Tasks

Behavior modification research has also concerned itself directly with academic task performance. In fact some of the earliest behavioral studies had this emphasis. Thus Staats, et al., (1962) showed that reinforcers such as trinkets, edibles, and tokens could be used to keep four-year-old children at work on a series of somewhat tedious exercises aimed at teaching them to read. Experimental control of these textual responses was demonstrated by reversal procedures.

A recent study by Brent and Routh (1978) demonstrated the utility of behavioral methods in reducing impulsive word recognition errors (that is jumping to premature conclusions about the identity of unfamiliar words). Fourth-graders with average intellectual ability, but poor reading achievement, were given two word-recognition lists, the first one as a pretest and the second list under one of three different conditions: control, positive reinforcement (one nickel for each word read correctly), and response cost (one of 40 nickels taken back for each word read incorrectly). The control subjects showed no change from list 1 to list 2. The positive reinforcement subjects slowed down their time to respond, but did not make fewer errors. Only the response-cost subjects showed a true decrease in impulsive reading style; they not only slowed down but made significantly fewer errors on list 2.

Other research has focused on children's printing and writing skills. Hopkins, Schutte, and Garton (1971), for example, studied the effects of access to a playroom upon the speed with which first- and second-grade children copied printing or writing assignments from the chalkboard. As demonstrated by a reversal design, these children finished their papers faster when this meant an opportunity to spend time in a playroom than under a control condition. Interestingly there was also a trend toward fewer errors in copying under the playroom condition. A similar study with kindergarten children was reported by Salzberg, et al., (1971). In that study a multiple baseline procedure demonstrated that children produced selective reductions in errors in copying certain target letters when access to a playroom depended upon grading of only those letters.

A number of other studies have examined the effects of reinforcement procedures on spelling performance. The study of Benowitz and Busse (1976) had particularly striking findings. Fourteen different fourth-grade classes participated in this study with seven classes randomly assigned to each experimental condition. The study appropriately used class averages rather than individual students' scores as the unit of statistical analysis. For four weeks every class was given a pretest on a spelling list on Monday and then was tested on the same list again on Friday. In classes in the social incentives condition, children who improved their scores over the week received only a good mark on their test paper and a good grade in the teacher's roll book. Children in the material incentives condition learned on an average of more than six new spelling words per week, whereas those in the other groups on the average learned only three new spelling words. The significant advantage of material over social incentives continued over the four weeks of the study.

Generalization of Treatment Effects across Responses

Should the teacher try first to bring students' behavior under control and then concentrate on teaching them, or would it be better to concentrate first on their learning and hope the behavior problems will resolve? Winett and Winkler (1972) wrote a relevant and provocative article, *"Current Behavior Modification in the Classroom: Be Still, Be Quiet, Be Docile."* Their review of the literature suggested to them that behavior-modification researchers were much more interested in keeping students silent and immobile than with the quality of their learning experience. Winett and Winkler contrasted this philosophy unfavorably with that of the British informal or open classroom, which was said to encourage students to move around, to interact with peers, to select learning materials according to their momentary interests, and to learn at a self-paced rate. O'Leary (1972) replied, on behalf of behavior-modification researchers, suggesting that a straw man was being set up and that the informal or open classroom might not be the best approach, particularly for children with marked social and academic problems.

More recent research is beginning to suggest however that it may be better to concentrate on the student's academic performance first rather than automatically expecting the child who is well behaved to learn. Ferritor, et al., (1972), for example, used behavioral contingencies (tokens) to reduce disruptive behavior and increase attending among third-graders who were doing their arithmetic assignments. However these procedures had no effect on arithmetic performance as such. It was only when contingencies were also placed on arithmetic performance directly (not just on attending behavior) that performance improved. Apparently children can give the appearance of attentiveness without actually increasing their quality or quantity of work output.

Ayllon and Roberts (1974) approached the question from the opposite direction. They applied systematic token reinforcement to the reading performance of the five students ranked as the most disruptive in their fifth-grade class. Not only did these boys' reading performance improve, but their disruptive behaviors declined markedly, apparently as a side effect. They were observed to make comments such as, "Shut up, I'm trying to do my work," and "Quit bugging me, can't you see I'm reading?" (Ayllon and Roberts, 1974, p. 75). A reversal procedure demonstrated experimental control over both reading and disruptive behaviors. The recent study by Hay Hay, and Nelson (1977) supports Ayllon and Roberts' interpretation of their findings.

Behavior Modification by Parents

The MBD child of course presents problems in other places besides the class-room. Thus the growing literature on the use of parents as behavior therapists with their own children is relevant. A pioneering study of this type was carried out by Hawkins, et al., (1966). After baseline observations a hyperactive four-year-old boy was given attention, praise, and affectionate contact by the mother for certain defined desirable behaviors, and time-out (isolation) contingent on various objectionable behaviors. The child's behavior improved. An attempt to demonstrate experimental control by a reversal procedure was made, but the mother found it difficult to go back to her previous (baseline) style of interacting with the child.

The researcher best known for carrying out behavior modification in the home is undoubtedly Gerald Patterson at the Oregon Research Institute. Patterson's programs are complex and individualized to fit the specifics of each child's difficulties. An early statement of treatment goals by the Patterson and Brodsky (1966) is worth quoting:

> Our assumption is that the effect of conditioning (or any successful treatment) produces a re-programming of the social environment; the altered program of positive and negative reinforcers maintains the effect of the initial behavior modification. The fact that the peer group now responds by dispensing more social reinforcers also means that the effect would 'generalize' to any social setting in which one would find members of this peer group. In effect the term 'stimulus generalization' is an oversimplification. For this reason. . .we use the phrase 're-programming the social environment' [instead]. [P. 292]

The above quotation also introduces the problem of generalization across set-tings to which we shall return repeatedly. Although it may be true that the child's initial behaviors are similar at home and at school, it is often found that the modification of behaviors in one setting does not generalize to the other. Wahler (1969) found that a child trained (by means of differential attention and the use of time-out) to be cooperative at home did not generalize this behavior to school until it was specifically programmed there as well. A second child was given training in study behavior at home (and later at school also) with essentially similar results.

For some kinds of situational behavior difficulty, it may be sufficient to repro-gram the child's behavior in the setting in which the problem occurs. Barnard, Christopherson, and Wolf (1977) carried out experimental demonstrations with three 5- to 6-year-old children in which they were taught appropriate shopping behavior. At the outset of the study these children caused problems by running up and down the aisles of a supermarket and picking up or otherwise disturbing merchandise in the store. Using token reinforcement, with response cost added, the parents taught these children first to stay in close proximity to them (the parents) at the store and then to refrain from disturbing merchandise. The multi-ple baseline design demonstrated experimental control of the children's behavior.

It may be useful in certain cases to forge a link between home and school in order to use home reinforcers to maintain school behaviors. Bailey, Wolf, and Phillips (1970), working with predelinquent boys in a group home, showed how daily report cards on children's behavior and academic performance at school could be used to determine their privileges at home. A reversal design was used to show experimental control.

There seem to be many more technical problems in doing behavior-modification research at home than at school. School research is probably more relevant to the treatment of MBD children in any case, since their problem is most evident in school. Not the least of the problems with reasearch in the home are the representativeness of the small samples of behavior observed and the reactivity of the parents to being observed. For example Johnson and Lobitz (1974) showed clearly parents' ability to make their children's behavior look good or bad to home observers when instructed to do so. This kind of dissimulation is thus a potential problem in behavioral observation just as it is in relation to interviews and pencil-and-paper personality tests.

What Types of Reinforcement and Punishment Should Be Used?

In a Pollyanna world perhaps all persons would refrain from disturbing others because it is wrong or act out of consideration for others' feelings. In the same world learning no doubt would occur because of a sheer desire for mastery of difficult problems or the joy of discovery. However in the world with which we are all more familiar, behavior and learning are also influenced by more mundane extrinsic rewards and punishments. As Glynn (1970) notes, educators must not object to extrinsic reinforcers on *absolute* grounds, since grades, promotions, degrees, diplomas, and medals are in widespread use. In the family, despite the desirability of unconditional (or noncontingent) positive regard of parent for child, there will no doubt always be a role played by extrinsic rewards, such as expressions of affection, reciprocal performance of domestic chores, gifts, food, and money in the form of allowances.

On a priori grounds one might wish to place reinforcements and punishments in a hierarchy of desirability. The authors do this simply on the basis of their own values, hoping that others will find the ranking not too different from their preferences:

1. Intrinsic rewards and punishments (those that are inherent in an activity).
2. Rewards and punishments which are a natural consequence of the action.
3. Extrinsic rewards and punishments which are culturally normative for individuals in a given situation.
4. Extrinsic rewards and punishments which are culturally normative for persons in some situations, but which are unusual for the individual in those particular circumstances.
5. Unusual or needlessly coercive rewards and punishments.

Other things being equal the incentives at the top of this list are to be preferred to those lower down; rewards are in general preferable to punishments. This way of defining the desirability of incentives makes it clear that it is not simply the nature of the reward or punishment in itself that may be objectionable, but whether it is socially appropriate for that person in that situation, for example food is an acceptable reinforcer for a toddler learning correct use of the fork—it may not be suitable for behavior control of a junior high student.

Of course decisions about the clinical use of incentives depend not only upon their desirability, but also on their efficacy in controlling behavior. It is this concern which sometimes leads to escalation to more powerful if less desirable incentives when milder ones do not prove effective.

Intrinsic Reward

Many activities seem to be performed because of qualities inherent in the activity itself. Thus in Piagetian theory (Ginsburg and Opper, 1969), children's cognitive development is considered to be largely the result of intrinsically motivated activity. Similarly Gibson and Levin (1975) argue that the usual motive for reading is an intrinsic one, namely the meaning which is obtained in the process. If ways of enhancing the intrinsic reinforcement value of academic tasks could be discovered, this would be of considerable interest.

For the behavior-modifier one important reason for identifying intrinsically reinforcing activities is that they can themselves often be used as rewards to increase the frequency of other, lower probability activities. Further their identification helps one avoid the possibility of undermining intrinsic rewards by unnecessary extrinsic rewards or surveillance. The purported danger of turning play into work, so to speak, has been a much debated topic in the recent literature. Some years ago Harlow and his colleagues (Davis, Settlage, and Harlow, 1950; Harlow, 1950; Harlow, Harlow, and Meyer, 1950) demonstrated that rhesus monkeys would learn to solve mechanical puzzles and continue to engage in this activity day after day without any extrinsic reward. In fact the introduction of food rewards for this task initially disrupted performance somewhat, apparently because it led the animals to try to open the final device in the puzzle (with food beneath it) without going step by step by starting with the first of the several restraining devices making up the puzzle.

Deci (1971) stated the hypothesis that giving subjects extrinsic rewards, such as money, would decrease their intrinsic motivation on the same tasks. Deci reasoned that receiving money would lead the subjects to a cognitive reevaluation of their interest in the tasks as simply a financial one. Although the three experiments with college students Deci (1971) reported had various flaws (a ceiling effect, inappropriate use of individuals as the unit of analysis, and apparent initial differences between subjects in different conditions), his hypothesis has been influential. Deci (1972) reported another more satisfactory experiment in which college students who were given financial rewards for working Soma puzzles subsequently spent less time voluntarily working the puzzles than other subjects who were either given money before doing the puzzles (but for whom the money was not viewed as a reward) or those given no money.

Some parallel studies have now been done with pre-school children showing the apparent undermining of intrinsic motivation by extrinsic reward and by the kind of adult surveillance or monitoring which often goes with it (Lepper and Greene, 1975; Lepper, Greene, and Nisbett, 1973). Lepper, Greene, and Nisbett offered an overjustification hypothesis which states that a person's intrinsic interest in an activity may be reduced by inducing the person to engage in the activity as a means to an extrinsic goal. Lepper, Greene, and Nisbett, (1973) caution that their hypothesis may apply only to behaviors in which a person has great initial interest, and say that it would be a mistaken overgeneralization to apply their results to proscribe the use of token-economy programs which, after all, are used mainly to increase rates of initially low probability behaviors.

Social Reinforcement

Many of the behavior modification studies already reviewed made use of ordinary social rewards such as attention, praise, or good grades. The use of such rewards seems uncontroversial and would mostly fit into the category of rewards which are usual and culturally normative. Even persons who are concerned about preserving intrinsic motivation seem unconcerned about social rewards. Deci (1971, 1972) in fact argues that verbal reinforcement may even enhance intrinsic interest in a task.

Token Economies

Token rewards would probably be culturally normative for persons in some situations but would not be culturally normative for the situations in which they are used. The first research using token rewards with children was that of Staats, et al., (1962) which we already discussed. Less than 10 years later, O'Leary and Drabman (1971) reported that there were more than 100 token reinforcement programs under way with children and adults in the U. S. These authors concluded that such programs had clearly demonstrated their effectiveness in changing the academic and social behaviors of many different populations of children. Token programs seemed to have a greater effect on children's social behavior than on their academic performance. The problems O'Leary and Drabman reported with token programs were: (1) that they sometimes fail (though few reports of these failures appear in print); (2) that some particular children seem resistant to their effects, and (3) that so far there has been little evidence of long-term effects or of generalization across settings. The broader review of token economies by Kazdin and Bootzin (1972) also concluded that the programs were generally effective in the particular setting where they were employed but did not generalize. They agreed with the comment of Zimmerman, et al., (cited in Kazdin and Bootzin, 1972) that token economies tend to be prosthetic rather than therapeutic in their effects.

A number of recent attempts have been made to modify token programs in the direction of greater generalization of their effects, for example Johnson (1970) showed that teaching subjects to reinforce themselves led to initially greater resistance to extinction than did external reinforcement. Drabman, Spitalnik, and O'Leary (1973) first had disruptive children match teacher evaluations of their behavior. They worked out an elaborate four-stage process for fading out direct reinforcements for correct self-ratings, apparently establishing honesty as a peer-group norm. They then were able to demonstrate generalization of the effects of the token reward system to times of day when the program was not in effect.

Use of Tangible Rewards

O'Leary, Poulos, and Devine (1972) provide a useful discussion of the pros and cons of tangible reinforcers for children. While such rewards unquestionably are effective in changing behavior, O'Leary, Poulos and Devine note common objections to their use, for example that a child should not be reinforced for doing what was only the child's moral duty, that one should avoid undermining the child's intrinsic motivation, and that the use of such rewards can teach greed and avarice. O'Leary and coworkers advise that tangible rewards be used only after less powerful means of behavior modification have been tried and found unsuccessful.

Use of Punishment

Most behavior modification research has emphasized the use of positive reinforcement rather than punishment. Nevertheless sometimes judicious use of punitive procedures is indicated. Perhaps the mildest type of punishment and one that is culturally normative is receiving the information that one is incorrect. Paris and Cairns (1972) found that in a discrimination learning task, negative comments ("wrong") after after incorrect responses greatly facilitated learning, while positive comments ("good") after correct responses had little effect. Their subjects were children in a class for the educable mentally retarded (EMR) and an observational study of teacher behavior in several EMR classes suggested that negative teacher comments in the EMR classroom were much more likely to carry information than positive comments, which tended to be used indiscriminately.

A second type of mild punishment involves the use of response-cost procedures. These are often used in token systems in the form of point fines contingent upon undesirable behaviors. An example of how effective response cost can be was provided by the Brent and Routh (1978) study already discussed.

The only other type of punishment commonly used in behavior-modification research related to MBD is time-out (isolation). A review of the basic research on time-out from positive reinforcement by Leitenberg (1965) supported the tentative conclusion that time-out was indeed an effective aversive stimulus. Drabman and Spitalnik (1973) found that brief social isolation reduced out-of-seat and aggressive behaviors in a class for emotionally disturbed children.

It should be emphasized again that, although punishment can be an effective means of controlling behavior, its use should be reserved for situations in which less aversive procedures have been unsuccessful.

Summary

Behavior modification clearly works with children when contending with circumscribed behaviors, including behaviors of concern in MBD. It can be used to induce children to sit still, reduce their disruptive behaviors in class, and pay attention. It can be used to improve children's performance on a variety of school tasks, and since good academic performance seems to be somewhat incompatible with disruptive classroom behavior, it is often better strategy to concentrate mostly on task performance rather than directly upon the child's disruptive behavior. Behavior-modification procedures can also be taught to parents and used by them to deal with children's behavior problems at home. Reinforcers can be arranged in a hierarchy of desirability with intrinsic motivation at the top and unusual extrinsic rewards and punishments at the bottom of the list. In general it would seem advisable to use the mildest behavioral approaches that are effective, reserving token systems, tangible rewards, and the use of punishment for the most severe problems.

In concluding this section, it can be stated that behavioral procedures have proven quite effective in arranging prosthetic environments for the short-term management of children's behavior. Much additional work needs to be done before we can say we know how to reprogram the social environment to achieve generalization across settings and behavior change which is still apparent to follow-up evaluation.

We turn now to the consideration of a variety of psychological and environmental intervention procedures.

ENVIRONMENTAL INTERVENTION

The Over-Stimulation Hypothesis

The excessive stimulation of the classroom environment as a source of problems for certain children was one of the key principles emphasized by Strauss and Lehtinen (1947) in their book, *Psychopathology and Education of the Brain-Injured Child.* They viewed the brain-injured child as excessively distractible and therefore recommended that all extraneous stimulation such as brightly colored pictures or flower arrangements be removed from the classroom. They suggested that the child be given an individual study carrel. The teacher was directed to dress plainly, to use no jewelry or excessive makeup, and even to move deliberately. Cruickshank, et al., (1961) designed a complete educational program for brain-injured children based on these principles and carried out a one-year longitudinal study to test its effectiveness. The results of the study however were equivocal with no significant differences in standard achievement test scores between treatment and control children.

There is some research indicating that, under certain conditions, extraneous stimulation can increase children's activity and that decreased stimulation can be educationally beneficial. The amount of such research is however surprisingly small considering the fact that the hypothesis has been in existence for 30 years and has long been used as a justification for educational practice. Reiber (1965) placed normal five- and six- year-old children in a playroom with a number of toys which required the child to act in order to operate them, for example a train that could be operated by a mechanical crank, a spring-type rocking horse, and a series of lever-press activated lights. When music was played the children in this situation were more active (in terms of crank turns, lever presses) than with no music; the faster the music, the higher the activity and so on. In a study with more apparent educational relevance, Jenkins, Gorrafa, and Griffiths (1972) examined the effect of providing children with small, isolated study rooms. These were educable retarded children in a classroom operating under a token economy. Their work output (pages of programmed text completed) was significantly greater when they were in the isolated rooms than in the classroom.

Another reason for isolating a hyperactive or disruptive child in a carrel rather than keeping the child in the classroom might be because of the effect on'other children. Kasper and Lowenstein (1971) observed school-age boys individually in a free-play situation, and then retested low-activity children alone or together with a highly active child. The presence of a high-activity child had the effect of dramatically increasing the observed activity of the low-activity child.

The Under-Stimulation Hypothesis

Some recent writers have taken a position quite the opposite of Strauss and Lehtinen. Zentall (1975), for example theorized that hyperactive behavior may be an attempt by an under-aroused child to optimize stimulation rather than a reaction to over-stimulation. If this view is correct, an under-stimulating situation may only make the child's behavior worse, and higher levels of stimulation might act to normalize behavior.

Studies supporting the under-stimulation view are numerous. Gardner, Cromwell, and Foshee (1959) simply asked their subjects to sit in a chair and listen to recorded music. All subjects, including those considered hyperactive, were more active in the sense of moving around in the chair in the situation with reduced visual stimulation. When there was more visual stimulation (Chistmas tree lights, toys, and trinkets displayed on a black screen) the subjects were less active. Forehand and Baumeister (1970) found that both visual and auditory stimulation had the effect of reducing the activity of severely retarded, institutionalized subjects. Reardon and Bell (1970) found that severely retarded boys were less active with fast rock-and-roll music than when slower Bach chorales were played. Zentall and Zentall (1976) observed hyperactive children in two situations: one in which the child was supposed to sit and wait for the experimenter to return and another in which the child was to carry out a simple, repetitive academic task. In both situations the children engaged in significantly less activity in the high stimulation condition, which featured such attractions as flashing Christmas tree lights, mice in a transparent cage, and popular rock music. Performance on the academic task was however not affected significantly by the amount of extraneous stimulation provided.

Reconciling Opposites

The conflicting evidence concerning the over-stimulation and under-stimulation views leaves the classroom teacher and the enviromental designer at a loss. It seems conceivable to the authors that some MBD children could be both insufficiently aroused and excessively distractible at the same time. If so, it might be important both to minimize the amount of extraneous stimulation and to make the materials to which the child is to attend as interesting and varied as possible. It must be the goal of future research to tell us how to do this. A hopeful beginning in encouraging children's attention has been made by the producers of the children's television program, *Sesame Street*. In research analyzing the appeal of segments of this program to children, Anderson and Levin (1976) found that one-year-olds would watch no longer than 60 seconds at a time, whereas four-year-olds' attention could be held for up to seven minutes. A number of particular program attributes, for example animation, sound effects, motion through space, and change to an essentially familiar scene, were found partially to account for the increasing attention-holding power of the program with age. It remains to draw the implications of such findings for the classroom and other settings where sustained attention and task persistence are important.

Structure versus Openness in the Classroom

The conventional wisdom in special education seems to be that children with learning and behavior problems need much more structure than do normal children. It might be thought therefore that a self-contained classroom might be, in general, more appropriate for such children than the looser structure of the so-called open classroom. If anything, the research on this issue suggests the opposite conclusion.

Flynn and Rapoport (1976) found that teachers rated the behavior of hyperactive children as better when they were in open classrooms than when they were in self-contained classrooms. Jacob, O'Leary, and Rosenblad (1978) carried out classroom observations of hyperactive children and controls in formal and informal (open) classrooms. They found that the hyperactive children behaved in about the same way in the two types of settings. The control children in contrast were less active and less noisy in the formal classroom where their behavior differed significantly from that of the hyperactive children. Thus the *same* behaviors of the hyperactive children appeared deviant in the formal classroom, but not unusual in the informal one. It is interesting that the direction of these results did not support O'Leary's (1972) previously expressed preference for a structured classroom for children with social and academic problems. Neither of the above studies however examined the effects of the two types of classroom on children's academic achievement. This type of comparison needs to be included in future studies of traditional versus open classrooms.

Parent Counseling

By default the heaviest emphasis of this chapter has been upon behavior modification as a technique for clinical and educational management of the MBD child. This is not because there are no other types of approaches to psychological and environmental intervention but because this approach has received the most attention—and the most validation—in the published research literature.

In this final section of the chapter we wish to redress the balance by at least brief allusion to some different approaches for dealing with the entire social network of which the child is a part. Hobbs (1966) forcefully emphasized the importance of the whole social ecology of the disturbed child (which surely would include the MBD child): family; school; community and neighborhood; social agencies; and professionals, including the clergy, physicians, dentists, and so on. Hobbs argued for rejection of the traditional child psychotherapy model in favor of a systems approach focused on parent and teacher interaction with the child. Haley (1973) showed how clinicians in a child guidance center might reconceptualize their cases as family problems: the most common one being the child who is overinvolved with some adult (usually the mother), with another adult available but peripheral (usually the father), and an absence of any close relationship between the child and peers. Haley suggested that at the end of successful treatment the adults in the family should be involved with each other and the child involved with peers.

Feighner and Feighner (1974) presented the most comprehensive clinic based treatment program for the hyperkinetic child that the authors have seen to date. This program, in which the social worker appeared to play a key role, involved the use of stimulant drugs if indicated, regular parent and teacher groups, and frequent phone contacts with the teacher. So far however there has been little research on the effectiveness of such multimodality treatment approaches. We believe that research of this type is possible, and indeed that it is essential to the goal of helping the MBD child develop into a competent adult. As a recent demonstration of the possibility of this kind of research, we would cite Tavormina's (1975) recent evaluation of the relative effectiveness of two types of parent group counseling with a different clinical population, the parents of mentally retarded children. We close with the hope that the next edition of such a handbook as this might include a discussion of parent counseling approaches solidly based on research findings relevant to subpopulations now falling under the MBD conceptual umbrella.

REFERENCES

Ackerson, F. *Children's Behavior Problems.* Chicago: University of Chicago Press, 1942.

Allen, K. E., L. B. Henke, F. R. Harris, D. M. Baer, and N. J. Reynolds. "Control of hyperactivity by social reinforcement of attending behavior." *Journal of Educational Psychology*, 58, 231–237, (1967).

Anderson, D. R., and S. R. Levin. "Young children's attention to 'Sesame Street'." *Child Development*, 47, 806–811, (1976).

Ayllon, T., and M. D. Roberts. "Eliminating discipline problems by strengthening academic performance." *Journal of Applied Behavior Analysis*, 7, 71–76, (1974).

Bailey, J. S., M. M. Wolf, and E. L. Phillips. "Home-based reinforcement and the modification of pre-delinquents' classroom behavior." *Journal of Applied Behavior Analysis*, 3, 223–233, (1970).

Barnard, J. D., E. R. Christophersen, and M. M. Wolf. "Teaching children appropriate shopping behavior through parent training in the supermarket setting." *Journal of Applied Behavior Analysis*, 10, 49–59, (1977).

Barrish, H. H., M. Saunders, and M. M. Wolf. "Good behavior game: Effects of individual contingencies for group consequences on disruptive behavior in a classroom." *Journal of Applied Behavior Analysis*, 2, 119–124, (1969).

Baumrind, D., and A. E. Black. "Socialization practices associated with dimensions of competence in preschool boys and girls." *Child Development*, 38, 291–327, (1967).

Becker, W. C., and R. S. Krug. "A circumplex model for social behavior in children." *Child Development*, 35, 371–396, (1964).

Bender, L. "A visual-motor Gestalt test and its clinical use." *American Orthopsychiatric Association Research Monograph*, No. 3., (1938).

Benowitz, M. L., and T. V. Busse. "Effects of material incentives on classroom learning over a four-week period." *Journal of Educational Psychology*, 68, 57–62, (1976).

Blackwood, R. "The operant conditioning of verbally mediated self-control in the classroom." *Journal of School Psychology*, 8, 251–258, (1970).

Brent, D. E., and D. K. Routh. "Response cost and impulsive word recognition errors in reading disabled children." *Journal of Abnormal Child Psychology*, b, 211–219, (1978).

Broden, M., R. V. Hall, A. Dunlap, and R. Clark. "Effects of teacher attention and a token reinforcement system in a junior high school special education class.'" *Exceptional Children*, 36, 341–349, (1970).

Clements, S. D. *Minimal Brain Dysfunction in Children: Terminology and Identification.* Washington, D.C.: U.S. Department of HEW, 1966.

Cohn, R. "Arithmetic and learning disabilities," in H. R. Myklebust, ed., *Progress in learning disabilities*, vol. 2. New York: Grune & Stratton, 1971.

Cruickshank, W., F. Bentzen, F. Ratzburg, and M. Tannhauser. *A Teaching Method for Brain-Injured and Hyperactive Children.* Syracuse, N.Y.: Syracuse University Press, 1961.

Davis, R. T., P. H. Settlage, and H. F. Harlow. "Performance of normal and brain-operated monkeys on mechanical puzzles with and without food incentive." *Journal of Genetic Psychology*, 77, 305–311, (1950).

Deci, E. L. "Effects of extrinsically mediated rewards on intrinsic motivation." *Journal of Personality and Social Psychology*, 18, 105–115, (1971).

——"Intrinsic motivation, extrinsic reinforcement, and inequity." *Journal of Personality and Social Psychology*, 22, 113–120, (1972).

Douglas, V. I., P. Parry, P. Marton, and C. Garson. "Assessment of a cognitive training program for hyperactive children." *Journal of Abnormal Child Psychology*, 4, 389–410, (1976).

Drabman, R. S., and R. Spitalnik. "Social isolation as a punishment procedure: A controlled study." *Journal of Experimental Child Psychology*, 16, 236–249, (1973).

Drabman, R. S., R. Spitalnik, and K. D. O'Leary. "Teaching self-control to disruptive children." *Journal of Abnormal Psychology*, 82, 10–16, (1973).

Dreger, R. "A progress report on a factor analytic approach to classification in child psychiatry," in R. Jekins and J. Cole, eds., *Research report No. 18.* Washington, D.C.: American Psychiatric Association, 1964.

Eysenck, H. J. *The Structure of Human Personality.* New York: Wiley, 1953.

Feighner, A. C., and J. P. Feighner. "Multimodality treatment of the hyperkinetic child." *American Journal of Psychiatry*, 131, 459–463, (1974).

Ferritor, D. E., D. Buckholdt, R. L. Hamblin, and L. Smith. "The noneffects of contingent reinforcement for attending behavior on work accomplished." *Journal of Applied Behavior Analysis*, 5, 7–17, (1972).

Flynn, N. M., and J. L. Rapoport. "Hyperactivity in open and traditional classroom environments." *Journal of Special Education*, 10, 285–290, (1976).

Forehand, R., and A. A. Baumeister. "Effects of variations in auditory-visual stimulation on activity levels of severe mental retardates." *American Journal of Mental Deficiency*, 74, 470–474, (1970).

Gardner, W. I., R. L. Cromwell, and J. G. Foshee. "Studies in activity level: II. Effects of distal visual stimulation in organics, familials, hyperactives, and hypoactives." *American Journal of Mental Deficiency*, 63, 1028–1033, (1959).

Garvey, M., and N. Gordon. "A follow-up study of children with disorders of speech development." *British Journal of Disorders of Communication*, 8, 17–28, (1973).

Gibson, E. J., and H. Levin. *The Psychology of Reading.* Cambridge: MIT Press, 1975.

Gillespie, S. K., and E. B. Cooper. "Prevalence of speech problems in junior and senior high schools." *Journal of Speech and Hearing Research*, 16, 739–743, (1973).

Ginsburg, H., and S. Opper. *Piaget's Theory of Intellectual Development: An Introduction.* Englewood Cliffs, N.J.: Prentice-Hall, 1969.

Glynn, E. L. "Classroom applications of self-determined reinforcement." *Journal of Applied Behavior Analysis*, 3, 123–132, (1970).

Goodenough, F. L. *Measurement of Intelligence by Drawings.* Chicago: World, 1926.

Griffiths, C. P. S. "A follow-up study of children with disorders of speech." *British Journal of Disorders of Communication*, 4, 46–56, (1969).

Haley, J. "Strategic therapy when a child is presented as the problem." *Journal of the American Academy of Child Psychiatry*, 12, 641–659, (1973).

Hall, R. V., D. Lund, and D. Jackson. "Effects of teacher attention on study behavior." *Journal of Applied Behavior Analysis*, 1, 1–12, (1968).

Harlow, H. F. "Learning and satiation of response in intrinsically motivated complex puzzle performance by monkeys." *Journal of Comparative and Physiological Psychology*, 43, 289–294, (1950).

Harlow, H. F., M. K. Harlow, and D. R. Meyer. "Learning motivated by a manipulation drive." *Journal of Experimental Psychology*, 40, 228–234, (1950).

Hawkins, R. P., R. F. Peterson, E. Schweid, and S. W. Bijou. "Behavior therapy in the home: Amelioration of problem parent-child relations with the parent in a therapeutic role." *Journal of Experimental Child Psychology*, 4, 99–107, (1966).

Hay, W. M., L. R. Hay, and R. O. Nelson. "Direct and collateral changes in on-task and academic behavior resulting from on-task versus academic contingencies." *Behavior Therapy*, 8, 431–441, (1977).

Herjanic, B. M., and E. C. Penick. "Adult outcome of disabled child readers." *Journal of Special Education*, 6, 397–410, (1972).

Hewitt, L. E., and R. L. Jenkins. *Fundamental Patterns of Maladjustment: The Dynamics of Their Origin*. Chicago: State of Illinois, 1946.

Hobbs, N. "Helping disturbed children: Psychological and ecological strategies." *American Psychologist*, 21, 1105–1115, (1966).

Hopkins, B. L., R. C. Schutte, K. L. Garton. "The effects of access to a playroom on the rate and quality of printing and writing of first-and second-grade students." *Journal of Applied Behavior Analysis*, 4, 77–87, (1971).

Jacob, R. G., K. D. O'Leary, and C. Rosenblad. "Formal and informal classroom settings: Effects on hyperactivity." *Journal of Abnormal Child Psychology*, 6, 47–59, (1978).

Jacobson, J. M., D. Bushell, Jr., and T. Risley. "Switching requirements in a Head Start classroom." *Journal of Applied Behavior Analysis*, 2, 43–47, (1969).

Jenkins, J. R., S. Gorrafa, and S. Griffiths. "Another look at isolation effects." *American Journal of Mental Deficiency*, 76, 591–593, (1972).

Johnson, S. M. "Self-reinforcement versus external reinforcement in behavior modification with children." *Developmental Psychology*, 3, 147–148, (1970).

Johnson, S. M., and G. K. Lobitz. "Parental manipulation of child behavior in home observations." *Journal of Applied Behavior Analysis*, 7, 23–31, (1974).

Jung, C. G. *Psychological Types*. New York: Harcourt, Brace, 1924.

Kaspar, J. C., and R. Lowenstein. "The effect of social interaction on activity levels in six-to eight-year-old boys." *Child Development*, 42, 1294–1298, (1971).

Kassebaum, G. G., A. S. Couch, and P. E. Slater. "The factorial dimensions of the MMPI." *Journal of Consulting Psychology*, 23, 226–236, (1959).

Kazdin, A. E., and R. R. Bootzin. "The token economy: An evaluative review." *Journal of Applied Behavior Analysis*, 5, 343–372, (1972).

Kohn, M. and B. L. Rosman. "Relationship of preschool social-emotional functioning to later intellectual achievement." *Developmental Psychology*, 6, 445–452 (1972).

Leitenberg, H. "Is time-out from positive reinforcement an aversive event?" *Psychological Bulletin*, 64, 428–441, (1965).

Lepper, M. R., and D. Greene. "Turning play into work: Effects of adult surveillance and extrinsic rewards on children's intrinsic motivation." *Journal of Personality and Social Psychology*, 31, 479–486, (1975).

Lepper, M. R., D. Greene, and R. E. Nisbett. "Undermining children's intrinsic interest with extrinsic reward: A test of the 'overjustification' hypothesis." *Journal of Personality and Social Psychology*, 28, 129–137, (1973).

Meichenbaum, D., and J. Goodman. "Training impulsive children to talk to themselves: A means of developing self-control." *Journal of Abnormal Psychology*, 77, 115–126, (1971).

Mendelson, W., N. Johnson, and M. A. Stewart. "Hyperactive children as teenagers: A follow-up study." *Journal of Nervous and Mental Disease*, 153, 273–279, (1971).

Menkes, M. M., J. S. Rowe, and J. H. Menkes. "A twenty-five year follow-up on the hyperkinetic child with minimal brain dysfunction." *Pediatrics*, 39, 393–399, (1967).

Minde, K., G. Weiss, and N. Mendelson. "A 5-year follow-up study of 91 hyperactive school children." *Journal of the American Academy of Child Psychiatry*, 11, 595–610, (1972).

O'Leary, K. D. "Behavior modification in the classroom: A rejoinder to Winett and Winkler." *Journal of Applied Behavior Analysis*, 5, 505–511, (1972).

O'Leary, K. D., and R. Drabman. "Token reinforcement programs in the classroom." *Psychological Bulletin*, 75, 379–398, (1971).

O'Leary, K. D., R. W. Poulos, and V. T. Devine. "Tangible reinforcers: Bonuses or bribes?" *Journal of Consulting and Clinical Psychology*, 38, 1–8, (1972).

O'Leary, K. D., K. F. Kaufman, R. E. Kass, and R. S. Drabman. "The effects of loud and soft reprimands on the behavior of disruptive students." *Exceptional Children*, 37, 145–155, (1970).

Osborne, J. G. "Free-time as a reinforcer in the management of classroom behavior." *Journal of Applied Behavior Analysis*, 2, 113–118, (1969).

Osgood, C. E., G. J. Suci, and P. H. Tannenbaum. *The Measurement of Meaning*. Urbana: University of Illinois Press, 1957.

Packard, R. G. "The control of classroom attention: A group contingency for complex behavior." *Journal of Applied Behavior Analysis*, 3, 13–28, (1970).

Paine, R. S., J. S. Werry, and H. C. Quay. "A study of minimal cerebral dysfunction." *Developmental Medicine and Child Neurology*, 10, 505–520, (1968).

Palkes, H., M. Stewart, and J. Freedman. "Improvement in maze performance of hyperactive boys as a function of verbal-training procedures." *Journal of Special Education*, 5, 337–342, (1972).

Palkes, H., M. Stewart, and B. Kahana. "Porteus maze performance of hyperactive boys after training in self-directed verbal commands." *Child Development*, 39, 817–826, (1968).

Paris, S. G., and R. B. Cairns. "An experimental and ethological analysis of social reinforcement with retarded children." *Child Development*, 43, 717–729, (1972).

Passini, F. T., and W. T. Norman. "A universal conception of personality structure?" *Journal of Personality and Social Psychology*, 4, 44–49, (1966).

Patterson, G. R., and G. Brodsky. "A behavior modification programme for a child with multiple problem behaviours." *Journal of Child Psychology and Psychiatry*, 7, 277–295, (1966).

Peckham, C. S. "Speech defects in a national sample of children aged seven years." *British Journal of Disorders of Communication*, 8, 2–8, (1973).

Premack, D. "Toward empirical behavior laws: I. Positive reinforcement." *Psychological Review*, 66, 219–233, (1959).

Quitkin, F., and D. F. Klein. "Two behavioral syndromes in young adults related to possible minimal brain dysfunction." *Journal of Psychiatric Research*, 7, 131–142, (1969).

Rawson, M. B. *Developmental Language Disability: Adult Accomplishments of Dyslexic Boys*. Baltimore: Johns Hopkins University Press, 1968.

Reardon, D. M., and G. Bell. "Effects of sedative and stimulative music on activity levels of severely retarded boys." *American Journal of Mental Deficiency*, 75, 156–159, (1970).

Rieber, M. "The effect of music on the activity level of children." *Psychonomic Science*, 3, 325–326, (1965).

Rodin, E., A. Lucas, and C. Simson. "A study of behavior disorders in children by means of general purpose computers," in K. Enslein, ed., *Proceedings of the 1963 Rochester*

Conference on data acquisition and processing in biology and medicine, vol. 3. New York: Pergamon, 1963.

Routh, D. K., and R. D. Roberts. "Minimal brain dysfunction in children: Failure to find evidence for a behavioral syndrome." *Psychological Reports*, 31, 307–314, (1972).

Salzberg, B. H., A. J. Wheeler, L. T. Devar, and B. L. Hopkins. "The effect of intermittent feedback and intermittent contingent access to play on printing of kindergarten children." *Journal of Applied Behavior Analysis*, 4, 163–171, (1971).

Schaefer, E. S. "Converging conceptual models for maternal behavior and for child behavior," in J. C. Glidewell, ed., *Parental attitudes and child behavior*. Springfield, Ill.: Thomas, 1961.

———— "Factors that impede the process of socialization," in M. J. Begab and S. A. Richardson, eds., *The mentally retarded and society: A social science perspective*. Baltimore: University Park Press, 1975.

Schmidt, G. W., and R. E. Ulrich. "Effects of group contingent events upon classroom noise." *Journal of Applied Behavior Analysis*, 2, 171–179, (1969).

Silver, A. A., and R. A. Hagin. "Specific reading disability: Follow-up studies." *American Journal of Orthopsychiatry*, 34, 95–102, (1964).

Spivack, G., and M. Shure. *Social Adjustment of Young Children: A Cognitive Approach to Solving Real-Life Problems*. San Francisco: Jossey-Bass, 1974.

Staats, A. W., C. K. Staats, R. E. Schutz, and M. Wolf. "The conditioning of textual responses using extrinsic reinforcers." *Journal of the Experimental Analysis of Behavior*, 5, 33–40, (1962).

Strauss, A. A., and L. E. Lehtinen. *Psychopathology and Education in the Brain-Injured Child*. New York: Grune & Stratton, 1947.

Tavormina, J. B. "Relative effectiveness of behavioral and reflective group counseling with parents of mentally retarded children." *Journal of Consulting and Clinical Psychology*, 43, 22–31, (1975).

Vogt, D. K. *Literacy Among Youths 12-17 Years: United States*. Washington, D.C.: U.S. Department of HEW, 1973.

Wahler, R. G. "'Setting generality: Some specific and general effects of child behavior therapy." *Journal of Applied Behavior Analysis*, 2, 239–246, (1969).

Weiss, G., K. Minde, J. S. Werry, V. Douglas, and E. Nemeth. "Studies on the hyperactive child: VIII. Five-year follow-up." *Archives of General Psychiatry*, 24, 409–414, (1971).

Werry, J. S. "Developmental hyperactivity." *Pediatric Clinics of North America*, 15, 581–599, (1968).

Winett, R. A., and R. C. Winkler. "Current behavior modification in the classroom: Be still, be quiet, be docile." *Journal of Applied Behavior Analysis*, 5, 499–504, (1972).

Wolf, M. M., E. L. Hanley, L. A. King, J. Lachowicz, and D. K. Giles. "The timer-game: A variable interval contingency for the management of out-of-seat behavior." *Exceptional Children*, 36, 113–117, (1970).

Zentall, S. S. "Optimal stimulation as theoretical basis of hyperactivity." *American Journal of Orthopsychiatry*, 45, 549–563, (1975).

Zentall, S. S., and T. R. Zentall. "Activity and task performance of hyperactive children as a function of environmental stimulation." *Journal of Consulting and Clinical Psychology*, 44, 693–697, (1976).

CHAPTER 26

Coordinating Multiple Interventions

Thomas J. Kenny and Aden Burka

To meet effectively the needs of children is a challenging and potentially rewarding endeavor. The child with minimal neurological dysfunction has been brought to society's attention by presenting a set of problems or dysfunctions that suggest a need to provide remedial efforts. Our social values make children's needs an emotionally appealing concern and tend to produce an instant initial response. Another characteristic of our society is a reflex that says "more is better" and often culminates in a service delivery overkill. The system which values highly trained consultant specialists is in constant jeopardy of expanding itself to the point of logistic chaos.

The complex and multifaceted nature of the problem called MBD clearly requires the special skills of a variety of professionals. This fact has led to the evolution of the so-called multidiscipline approach to the MBD child. The disciplines of medicine, education, psychology, speech and hearing, social work, physical therapy, and others have all played a part in serving children with MBD. It is a diagnostic entity with multiple manifestations and etiologies which disrupt both the social and educational adjustment of the child. MBD elicits interest from multiple professionals because of its manifold problems. It pulls distant relative professionals together on whom it is then incumbent to communicate and follow through. MBD is an elusive and exasperating area in which mental health professionals, pediatricians, and educators must look to one another for help and collaboration.

The involvement of so many specialists is both a benefit and a problem. The skill and interest of these disciplines represent the benefit, but the often overlooked problem is the absence of effective coordination of complex interrelations. When coordination is effective, the focused skills of the group can be as precise and as powerful as a laser beam; when it is not, it becomes an operation that dissipates its energy by protecting the territory and position of each individual profession.

To facilitate the best outcome of efforts aimed at helping the MBD child, this chapter will critically view the problems and potentials of multiple intervention. The process will involve a review of the evolution of the multidisciplinary approach with its merits and deficiencies. Historical origins of multiple interventions and the research related to the issues will be reviewed and types of interventions in common use will be summarized. Interventions used in MBD can be performed by a number of professional disciplines, many of which can overlap in their service functions. Initial focus will be on person-oriented interventions which will be followed by a discussion of systems approaches. The number of therapeutic interventions used to manage MBD has steadily increased over the years. Many more professionals want to participate because they believe they have something to contribute. Indeed the deficits related to MBD may be so varied (neurological, motoric, cognitive, perceptual-motor, linguistic, behavioral, interpersonal or intrapsychic) that many professionals can rightly claim that the deficits fall within their bailiwick. Issues related to professional territory, interdisciplinary communication, and prioritization of interventions will be discussed subsequently.

DIAGNOSIS VERSUS INTERVENTION

The process of establishing a multidisciplinary approach to MBD seems clearly to have had its origin in two interrelated factors, First, the process of diagnosing MBD and second, in the official Task Force Report on the definition of MBD (Clements, 1966). The nature of the problem as defined by the Task Force included medical-neurological factors, educational problems, and psycho-social-behavioral difficulties. The difficulty in diagnosing MBD led to a situation in which experts sought confirmation from other experts to establish the child's diagnosis. Thus the multidisciplinary approach grew out of the process of identification and diagnosis rather than by virtue of the intervention skill of the particular professional. In its simplest form the intervention process usually evolved from the multiple recommendations of the diagnosticians and was all too often relatively uncoordinated. The physician was usually thrust into the central role in the intervention program and, thus, was perceived as the captain of the intervention team. The preeminent concern with the neurologic component of the diagnostic process led to physicians being placed in the position of directing the diagnostic evaluation and subsequently coordinating the intervention or management program. The most common symptom noted in the MBD syndrome is hyperactive behavior. The focus on this behavioral manifestation resulted in an intervention strategy that saw medication as the key management process. This served to set the physician in the central position for both diagnosis and management of the MBD child. Real progress toward effective intervention strategies has been impaired by the assumption that the diagnostician and therapist must necessarily be one and the same. In the zeal to identify the problem-child, the professional has tended to focus on the indentification process and let the management follow as if it were an inevitable prescription. This concept is rooted in the so called medical model which sees the diagnosis as the preliminary and prerequisite step to prescription, and the unwarranted assumption that a useful prescription is necessarily available for every diagnosis. This is an optimistic, but unrealistic, expectation in the case of the MBD child. The results of this approach is often a set of overlapping and sometimes conflicting recommendations. As a verification of the tendency to confuse assessment with management, the recent book by Ross and Ross (1976) on hyperactivity, an area usually subsumed under MBD, has a thirty-page chapter titled "Management." In that chapter twenty pages actually deal with aspects of the assessment process, while only ten pages have anything to do with intervention procedures. The emphasis in the area of MBD has been to gain acceptance of the existence of the problem, which is an identification or diagnostic function, and only as an afterthought does the concern shift to long-term management. There is an urgent need to acknowledge the imprecisions and imperfections in the definition of MBD. We may then accept that in the population of exceptional children there is a group that has various manifestations of the MBD syndrome. In this way we can begin to concentrate not on recognition, but on intervention. Children with MBD have been recognized for a minimum of thirty years. It is now important to assess our effectiveness in helping these children.

The growth of therapeutic interventions for MBD is correlated with the increasing number of professionals involved in the diagnostic process. As we have widened the scope of causative and contributing factors, our treatment programs have changed qualitatively and increased in number.

The experience of research in schizophrenia and mental retardation should teach us that a specific etiology is not necessary in developing a variety of effective intervention procedures for MBD children. It is possible to identify the needs of the individual and use those needs as a basis for intervention. Indentifying the etiology of these syndromes might be important to the prevention of the problem, but does not rule out effective management strategies.

Medical Management

Medical management of MBD includes both the use of pharmacological agents and counseling related to the use of medications. Approximately 2% or 300,000 to 400,000 children in the United States are currently on some form of stimulant medication to control hyperactive behavior (Safer and Allen, 1976), much of which is assumed to be associated with minimum brain dysfunction, although clear evidence for this is lacking. Considerably fewer, but a significant number of children, are receiving other forms of medication such as phenothiazines, anticonvulsants or antihistamines to control hyperactive behavior. With such large numbers of children on medication, one wonders how many of these children are being given only medication? A more basic question is whether the research investigating the effects of such pharmacological interventions supports the widespread use of these medications?

Although much research has been conducted on this topic, most experiments lack the scientific rigor needed to draw firm conclusions. Whether one argues for or against the use of medication with hyperactive MBD children, there is research to support the thesis.

Some of the highest estimates of effectiveness come from pediatric research. Haslem and Valletutti (1971) cite a 60 to 80% effectiveness rate; Safer and Allen (1976) state that 35 to 50% of children show dramatic positive responses to stimulant medication, 30 to 40% show moderate benefit, and 15 to 20% show no benefit; Kenny and Clemmens (1975) estimate the effectiveness of such medication between 33 and 66%. It must be noted that the benefits of medication usually relate only to the reported hyperactive behavior manifest by these children and not to brain function per se. As in schizophrenia the medication may alter behavior, but there is no evidence that it cures the problem.

Several notes of caution must be sounded when confronting such data. First, one cannot be sure that all the children in the above cited studies were actually MBD children. Although all were diagnosed as hyperactive, such a label does not necessarily denote MBD. Secondly, many of the measurements of improvement were gathered by using global rating scales. As Wulbert and Dries (1977) point out, such observation systems are of unknown value as reliable and valid indices of actual behavior change. Millichap, Gordon, and Boldrey (1967) reported that even when a child was rated as globally improved, activity level (measured by a stabilimeter) actually increased with medication. Thirdly, more and more investigators are beginning to understand the situational nature of behavior change. Thus a medicated child may show improvement in the classroom setting, but manifest no change at home. (Wahler, 1969; Wulbert, et al., 1974; Wulbert and Dries, 1977). A fourth issue concerning the effectiveness of medication concerns its effects on intellectual functioning. Current research strongly suggests that there is little evidence of any long-term benefit in the area of learning associated with the use of medication. (Rie, H., et al., 1976; Barkly, R., 1977). A correlate problem concerns the extent to which placebo effects play a role in the changes observed following medication. Unfortunately most data on this topic have been collected in laboratory settings, which reduces generalizing to classroom and home settings. Considerable data (Sykes, 1972; Campbell, 1969; Sprague, Barnes, and Werry, 1975) report that such medication decreases distractibility and enhances the efficiency of processing task-revelant information. Sroufe (1975) argues that the stimulant medication does not enhance abstract reasoning skills. On the other hand Connors (1972) presents data showing improved WISC scores following medication. The latter study however did not demonstrate that cognitive functioning was enhanced above and beyond what would be expected from increased capacity to attend. The safest conclusion to be drawn is that hyperactive MBD children respond to stimulant medication in a highly variable fashion and that it is hard to predict whether learning and/or behavior will be improved.

In a long-term follow-up study conducted by Weiss, et al., (1975), comparisons were made between hyperactive children treated with stimulant medication, chlorpromazine, and no treatment. The three groups were matched on age, IQ, SES, sex. The results indicated that while stimulant medication made children more manageable at home and school, it did not affect greater change in a positive or negative direction than did the other two conditions. Their impressions are summed up in the following comments,

> It was wishful thinking on our part that a useful drug alone would change the outcome of a fairly serious condition like severe, chronic, hyperactivity with multiple etiologic factors and multiple and various manifestations.

One other factor that must be considered in the use of medication with MBD children is the implicit message being given both to the children and to those around them. Medication assigns the locus of responsibility within the child, even though his behavior may be out of his control. In a sense, by medicating the child, those significant adults in his or her life may feel releived of major responsibility for managing the child's hyperactive behavior as well as other symptoms which may be related to MBD. Behaviorists however have made us quite aware of the role environment plays in perpetuating behavioral patterns. Studies such as Ayllon, Layman and Kendel (1975) or Wulbert and Dries (1977) demonstrate that control of environmental contingencies is sometimes as effective in reducing hyperactivity as stimulant medication. What is being argued here is that medication has a symbolic impact on the child and his or her surrounding environment. Related to this point, Weiss, et al., (1975) found an interaction between stimulant medication and healthy family functioning. The authors suggest that other treatment modalities, such as family counseling, behavior modification, or optimal classroom environments serve to enhance the effectiveness of medication.

Physiotherapy and Occupational Therapy

Some MBD children have perceptual motor dificulties which may interfere with their social and academic adjustment. The dysfunction may occur at the sensory in-put level, during integration, or at the motor out-put stage. A breakdown in any one of these areas can seriously disrupt the acquisition of information and concepts which normally occur in school. Children who are clumsy may also find themselves ostracized by their peers. Being unable to compete with peers or feeling self-conscious because of their lack of coordination, MBD children may shy away from participation in games. Ericcson (1968) emphasized the struggle school-age children go through trying to experience themselves as someone who can, as opposed to cannot. To the extent that his/her perceptual-motor difficulties impede his/her success, the MBD child's self-concept will suffer.

Occupational therapists, physiotherapists, and special educational personnel have begun the task of intervening in perceptual motor difficulties. Abbe (1974) reviews the five major physiotherapeutic approaches to treat perceptual-motor problems associated with MBD. The Ayres method (1966) emphasized stimulation of tactile and vestibular systems. Although Ayres does not claim that her method will improve neural organization, she does think subcortical sensory-integration exercises supplement classroom tutoring. The Doman-Delacato system (1963) is based on the theory of phylogenetic recapitulation. Children are presumably taken back to the level at which the motor development was fixated and given stimulation to progress through more advanced stages until cortical dominance has been reached. Some rather fantastic claims have been made by adherents of this method, such as in Doman's book *How to Teach Your Baby to Read*, but no empirical research has supported them.

Frostig's method (1968) focuses on identification and remediation of perceptual deficits. These two approaches however have been criticized as perhaps missing the target for effectualy remediating learning problems associated with MBD (Abbe, 1974). Similarly Kephart's (1964) approach to treatment utilized exercises to develop laterality, space and form perception, and ocular control. His intervention, which draws from Piagetian theory, also includes training in feedback and matching between sensory and motor process. Kinsbourn (Abbe, 1974) questions whether such specific training will improve reading processes that are more complex in nature.

Naville's (1970) program of psychomotor therapy makes no claim to improve MBD children's learning. However through more efficient movement, the child is thought to experience achievement, gratification, and the sense of competence which support improved self-concept and interpersonal relations. Naville envisions a program of this nature to be a part of a broader treatment intervention. The method, actually developed by Naville and deGuriaqueva in Switzerland, has not received wide attention in this country.

Psychotherapy with MBD Children

Although the etiology of MBD is thought to be somatogenic, many of its symptoms, such as emotional or behavioral dysfunctions, may be treated through a variety of interventions. Pschologists, psychiatrists, and social workers all utilize the various forms of therapy to help the MBD child. The history of mental health interventions with MBD is similar to that of other diagnostic entities. Adherents of various therapeutic approaches interpreted the problem from their own perspective and assimilated MBD into their treatment strategies. That analytically and behaviorally oriented professionals have not integrated their treatment approaches to MBD is more a function of theoretical bias than of the nature of minimal brain dysfunctions.

It seems popular to characterize MBD as refractory to psychotherapy (Stewart and Olds, 1973; Wender, 1971). Eisenberg, et al., (1961) reported that brief psychotherapy was ineffective in treating hyperkinetic children. Unfortunately their results are limited due to the idiosyncratic form of psychotherapy utilized. The particular MBD child who has difficulties with abstraction, distractibility, and reflection would not seem to be a good candidate for traditional, insight oriented psychotherapy. However Gardner (1974) provides another perspective of the usefulness of psychotherapy with MBD children. He claims that often these children have very low self-esteem, are socially isolated, and may even deny their difficulties. Gardner recognized the inappropriateness of the traditional psychotherapy model for children in general and MBD patients in particular. He developed a number of games to keep the child engaged while transmitting therapeutic messages. Through the use of a story telling technique, Gardner seems to captivate the interest of his child patients, while providing a corrective focus and sense of understanding of their problems. Gardner (1975) has also written a book on MBD children that offers objective information about MBD in addition to instilling a sense of hope. Although no empirical data have been reported on his work, it does not seem like a promising set of interventions.

An additional problem in utilizing psychotherapy with MBD children is that parents and/or teachers often seek immediate nonpsychotherapeutic help for symptoms of hyperactivity. By the time a child is brought for therapy, a crisis has usually occurred. Psychotherapeutic procedures require time to be effective and even if the child experiences emotional growth or gains a better self-concept, his hyperactivity may not have diminished. Thus the nature of psychotherapy does not fit well with the management of MBD symptoms. However, if the measure of success is not solely associated with reducing hyperactivity, therapy can be more effectively utilized in dealing with psychogenic problems which are secondary to MBD.

Behavior Therapy

To handle the demand for managing behavioral symptoms associated with MBD in a relatively brief period of time, behavioral interventions have emerged as the psychological treatment of choice. Environment plays an important role in perpetuating various behavioral problems. Applied behavioral analysis and behavioral modification are a conceptual system and set of related strategies which rearrange the environment to alter the conditions that perpetuate the problems. Behavior modification has several distinct advantages. First, it is empirically based, which allows for parents and therapists to chart the child's progress. Secondly, its concepts are easy for parents and teachers to understand. Although the language of behavior modification sometimes scares people, concepts such as Grandma's law of "eat your peas before you get your dessert" seem commonsensical. Thus parents and teachers can more easily talk to one another about various goals and progress towards those goals. Thirdly, the model has applicability to both home and school and allows for coordination between these two spheres.

A few statements of caution should be made about the use of behavioral modification. It is not unusual for parents or teachers to see rapid changes for the better when using this approach. The mistake made at this point is to assume that the child has changed. Hence the motivation to continue the treatment program, which may have involved considerable effort on the part of parents or teachers, is lost. Such a withdrawal of treatment often leads to deterioration in the behavior of the MBD child because the environmental contingencies which supported the behavioral changes are no longer operative.

Recently a number of articles (Abikoff, Gloisten, and Kates, 1976; Stableford, Butz, 1976; Ayllon, Layman, and Kandel, 1975; Shafto and Sulzbacher, 1977; Wulbert and Dries, 1977; Christensen and Sprague, 1973) have compared the relative effectiveness of stimulant medication and behavior modification. These studies report data collected not only in schools, but also in clinics and home settings. There is no way to be sure if the children are properly diagnosed as MBD, although all the hyperactive children appeared to have many MBD symptoms.

At the heart of this set of studies lies heated debate and controversy. The opposing factions appear to be medically oriented professionals who favor stimulant medication and behaviorists who believe that equally effective results can be obtained through behavior modification without the risk of medications. Although no unequivocal conclusions can be drawn from the research, a number of issues and useful treatment strategies have emerged:

1. Stableford, et al., (1976) demonstrated that stimulant medication could gradually be replaced by behavior therapy with little disrupting effect.

2. With some children, a behavioral-educational approach is more effective than stimulant medication in decreasing hyperactive behavior and increasing learning (Ayllon, Layman, and Kandel, 1975). Other data (Klein, et al., 1976) show pharmacological approaches more effective in changing behavior, although neither showed significant positive effects. This latter study pointed to the usefulness of combining methylphenidate (Ritalin) and behavior modification for some children.

3. Careful assessment which includes analyses of changes in learning and behavior in multiple settings is the exception rather than the rule (Wulbert and Dries, 1977; Wahler, 1969, Rie, et al., 1976).

Parent Counseling — Parent Training

Another set of mental health interventions is parent counseling. Parent interventions might usefully be divided into three types: education, counseling, and training. Parent education about the nature of MBD provides general principles of management as a useful first step in the intervention process. Often parents blame themselves for their child's dysfunction and experience unnecessary guilt. Knowledge about MBD can help relieve such feelings.

Intervention with parents can be extended beyond education to focus on attitudes and/or emotional reactions of parents. Such counseling is helpful when parents have unrealistic expectations for their MBD child or when the therapist wants to work with the parents as they try to make changes in their interactions with their child. This form of counseling may be either behaviorally or emotionally focused, but in either case requires an additional set of skills to educational counseling.

A third parent intervention which has become increasingly popular is parent training. This type of intervention differs from education and counseling in that the emphasis is on training parents in specific skills to manage their children. Such skills usually include observation of behavior, pinpointing, data taking, strategies of reinforcement, and punishment and extinction derived from learning theory. Behavior-modification training groups have burgeoned recently, since they so well meet the needs of parents who want to learn more effective ways of coping with hyperactive behavior. The reader is reminded however to consider the limitations pointed to earlier in using behavior modification.

Group Therapy and Recreational Therapy

Although very little has been published on the use of group therapy for MBD children, the technique may hold some promise. MBD children are deficient in perceptual-motor skills as they apply to learning situations, some are also deficient in interpersonal contexts. Gardner (1974) notes that his MBD patients manifest difficulties in social perception. They are less likely to grasp the subtleties of cooperative games, such as baseball or tag, and thus become further alienated from peers.

Remediations of such deficits may be achieved through the use of structured group therapy or recreational therapy. In this modality it would be important to integrate activities which captivate the children's interests and provide a format for learning basic skills in cooperation and social perception.

Family Therapy

Not infrequently the MBD child has become enmeshed in family turmoil. The symptoms associated with MBD often put a strain on the entire family. Brothers and sisters may shun their MBD sibling or feel jealous over the amount of attention he/she is receiving. Other children in the family may feel angry at their parents for not being able to discipline the MBD child.

At the same time the parents feel exasperated over their own ineffectiveness and their childrens' withdrawal from the problem. It is hard for siblings to understand the disadvantage at which their MBD brother or sister is placed because the handicap is not strikingly apparent.

Given these considerations, it is not difficult to see how the MBD child could be scapegoated by other family members (Vogel and Bell, 1968). The MBD child is an easy target on whom to displace family difficulties. Another role which this child might play within the family system is a negative bond which holds a wavering marriage together. From a systems perspective, the symptomology of MBD may serve a function for the family, such as scapegoating or negative bonding. If so, efforts to help the MBD child may be subtley undermined to preserve family disequilibrium.

Unlike other therapeutic interventions mentioned thus far, family therapy does not focus on the MBD child directly. As Satir (1967) has stated, the entire family, its role delineation, methods of communication, and ways of handling feelings become the primary target. No one person is blamed for the problems which exist because each person's behavior is interdependent with that of other members. For the MBD child and for the parents, a systems perspective may come as a relief with responsibility for family difficulties distributed more evenly across family members.

Educational Intervention

Educators for some time have recognized the need for special education when working with MBD children. The pendulum of educational strategies however seems to swing back and forth on the issue of whether MBD children and learning-disabled pupils should remain in special classrooms which remove them from their peers. Advantages and disadvantages on both sides seem to have forced the pendulum to the middle, so that today the concept of mainstreaming with resource help is emphasized.

The primary educational interventions used to advance the MBD child's learning usually include a mixture of small classroom size, individualized instruction, remedial help, ungraded evaluations, and some behavioral management. Approximately 200,000 children in this country are being educated in classrooms for the specific learning disabled (SLD), many of whom may be MBD children. The SLD classroom usually has 8 to 10 children with one teacher and often a half-time teacher's aide. The small size is ideal for providing individualized instruction and close attention to each child's progress. Ideally the classrooms are designed to reduce distractive stimuli, but in reality many have to cope with make-shift facilities.

The SLD classroom has clear advantages, among them easing the regular classroom teacher's burden, however several objections have been raised (Safer and Allen, 1976). Beside being very expensive, these classrooms have rarely advanced their pupils to the point where they can return to the regular classroom. Often SLD children are labelled as mental or elicit a variety of other derogatory comments by peers which contribute to a damaged self-concept. There is also the chance of increased negative modeling when all the children in a class have problems and manifest atypical behavior. These negative points and others have cast a shadow over the optimism which was expressed when SLD classes were introduced.

Remedial instruction for MBD children is aimed at improving their basic learning skills, but special educators differ in their approaches to remedial instruction. The developmental method for example is based upon identification of learning defects (such as auditory or visual perceptual discrimination) and training to strengthen those targeted areas. Some of the different developmental strategies were mentioned in the section on physiotherapies. Another remedial approach is the task analytic method (Safer and Allen, 1976). In this strategy educational goals, such as reading, writing, or arithmetic, are pursued more directly. If reading is the target skill, then the MBD child will be taught the rules of phonics or word recognition directly. At this point the burden seems to be on the developmentalists to demonstrate that their approach is worth the effort and time that it requires.

Another important intervention in the education of MBD children is the use of behavioral management. The same advantages and disadvantages outlined earlier in the section on social interventions obtain in the schools. Behavior modification can be used to either decrease the negative or hyperactive behavior of the MBD child or to increase learning skills or prosocial behavior. Too often in the past behavioral programs have been used to keep children "still, quiet and docile" (Winett and Winkler, 1974), without shaping appropriate active participation.

The Multidisciplinary Approach

The difficulty in establishing a diagnosis was the real basis for establishing multidisciplinary teams. In the usual evolution of the process a child was identified through poor school performance or adjustment. The diagnostic model set up by the Clements Task Force (1966) had elements of physical status, cognitive function, and behavior in its description. The presence of these elements and the difficulty in reaching a clear diagnosis had the result of involving a number of experts in the process. If the problem had been strictly medical, the process would have been covered by the consultant model in which the primary physician refers the patient to specialists who assist in the diagnosis and management. In this model each consultant performs his function, diagnosis, or management and, on completion, releases the patient to the primary physician. There is little coordination required in that each consultant has a relatively independent responsibility. The problems in MBD went beyond physical development and resulted in referrals to nonmedical specialists, including psychologists, speech and hearing specialists, educational specialists, and social workers to name a few. This procedure became the multidisciplinary approach as opposed to the consultant model. Unfortunately the change in names did not really produce a change in procedure. Too often each professional approached the patient as a consultant and did the diagnosis and management related to his special competence and returned the child to the primary physician. As in the consultant model this led to minimal coordination and, as a matter of convenience, put the primary physician in the position of insuring continuity of management. This was an unfortunate outcome, since there was no basis for putting the physician in this position other than the traditional assumption of the physician's willingness to assume authority and responsibility. The primary physician usually had no special training in the process of diagnosing MBD, let alone any experience in overseeing the functions of speech pathologists, special educators, or psychologists. The consultant model allowed for this lack of special expertise by reducing the role of the coordinator to that of serving as a repository for the records of the patient. The physician's concern for the child served by this model and his realization that this was not the most effective way to function was probably the central force in the development of the team approach. In an effort to improve the coordination and to provide the physician with some support, professionals involved in the evaluation process met as a group or team to share their findings and to plan for the needs of the child.

The major shortcoming of the development of this team approach is that it evolved or grew out of practical needs but without any special planning. Most especially this multidisciplined approach was practiced by professionals who were not trained in the system.

Multiple interventions represent a new system with which most professionals are unaccustomed. The model requires a frame of reference that includes shared responsibility and mutual respect, but it also calls for specific skills which are usually omitted in the training of those who work with MBD children.

There is a need to spell out the skills and responsibilities needed to coordinate multiple intervention. A number of disciplines can serve as coordinator of intervention programs and each has some particular resource to bring to the role, but all could benefit from some additional training.

Training the Intervention Coordinator

In an early section of this chapter various intervention approaches were outlined. Many of these interventions fell into the domain of several professional disciplines. The disciplines that could serve as coordination for this intervention approach were discussed, including the training available to each discipline and the additional functions needed to carry out the job responsibility more effectively. In addition it is necessary to outline the basic steps or requirements that should be involved in managing ongoing intervention approaches for the MBD child.

There are four major functions basic to managing effective intervention:

1. A willingness to accept the central role and responsibility for coordinating management.
2. An awareness of the resources needed and available for the MBD child.
3. The responsibility for taking the evaluation data and translating it into a simple, unified treatment plan.
4. A built-in system to check on progress of the treatment plan over an extended time period.

Each of these factors seems obvious and relatively simple. However a critical examination of the discipline involved in providing treatment services will point up weak points in each profession that would benefit from further training or a new emphasis for the professional involved. Let us now consider those professionals who provide treatment for the MBD child. While there are many individual disciplines that provide some of the services, for convenience these functions can be grouped so they fall into these broad groups—medical, mental health, and educational.

In the group of medical practitioners managing MBD problems one must include pediatricians, family physicians, nurses, and psychiatrists. The latter would also fall into the group of mental-health professionals, which would also include psychologists, social workers, and mental-health counselors. The educational group would include teachers as well as special educators; diagnostic and prescriptive teachers; school guidance counselors and other remedial personnel, such as speech therapists, physical therapists, occupational therapists, and so on.

Considering the four basic requirements to manage intervention previously listed, let us examine each of these groups of professionals both for the opportunity and the training needed to meet those requirements.

Medical Professionals

The pediatrician has long occupied the central role in managing intervention for the MBD child. This role evolved in relation to the early concept that the key need in the problem was a good medical dignosis that would lead to a treatment prescription. The prescription that resulted in these cases was all too often a simple management approach relying on medication as answer to the problem. Current information strongly indicates that this is a very limited approach to a complex problem. Medication as a treatment has some benefit in the short-term behavioral management of some of the behavioral aspects of the MBD problem, namely hyperkinesis. The limitation of this approach has been discussed in an earlier section, in that all MBD children are not hyperactive and, even when they are, there are other important environmental and educational aspects of MBD that are not altered by medication alone. Most MBD children eventually are referred to a facility which is medically based or oriented. Pediatricians have early and ongoing contact with children in providing health-care services and as a result can be a key identification source for the child manifesting MBD symptoms. Children, not first identified by a pediatrician, are usually referred to the pediatrician by school personnel who may raise the question of MBD. In this way the physician becomes the person who accepts the central role in managing diagnosis and subsequently intervention strategies.

The other major asset of the pediatrician is his position to coordinate intervention relates to ongoing contact with the child and the family. The pediatrician is a long term careperson for the child and serves as a convenient repository for records of diagnostic reports and follow-up reports by other disciplines. This role is more the result of the medical consultant model than a demonstration of any practical benefit in the treatment processes. The presence of the information is not a guarantee of effective utilization of the information.

There is a potential danger for a data overload in which information is routinely filed without a meaningful response. The physician has to evolve a new and more comprehensive caretaking role to utilize the information sent to him and to direct effectively the management process for an MBD child and his family. There is a need to have the physician consider the needs of the whole child and family and acquire skills in managing psychosocial and educational interventions. The pediatrician must become behaviorally oriented and learn the skills of an effective psychological interview, managing social systems, identifying community resources, and dealing in educational programming. The physician must gain training in those behaviorally related areas to be an effective member of an intervention team and certainly this is necessary if he is to fill the role as coordinator of these intervention strategies. This is an important role in terms of the pediatrician's position as a long-term caretaker and his involvement with the family.

The American Academy of Pediatrics has indicated that pediatricians must prepare themselves to fill this expanded service-delivery role and to become involved in identifying and managing the problems of the MBD child and the learning-disabled or hyperkinetic child. The W. T. Grant Foundation has funded a pediatric training program that will provide experiences in this new role. In this program pediatric residents spend two months in their first-and second-year program on a rotation totally devoted to this training. The training curriculum was designed and is taught by faculty from pediatrics, child psychiatry, and pediatric psychology and includes experiences in the school system. As a result of this venture the foundation has considered applications from other institutions who wish to begin similar training programs.

Family practice training programs are in a situation similar to pediatrics. They would have the advantage of a long-term care relationship and contact with the family, but would have a similar lack of training experience in psychosocial and educational areas.

Psychiatry has had a more limited contact with the MBD population in that psychiatry has served in a consultant role to the primary physician or to a social or educational agency. This consultant role usually results in the psychiatrist serving as an acute intervention agent. The short supply of psychiatric resources, the expense of services, and the traditional time-limited involvement of the psychiatrist are shortcomings in psychiatrists serving as the prime coordinator of intervention strategies. Psychiatrists tend to be pure-treatment people. Spending time in coordinating or doing routine follow-up is not a regular occurrence, especially for the psychiatrist in private practice. In an agency setting a psychiatrist may serve as the director of an interdisciplinary team, but in this role he usually functions as a super consultant rather than the regular patient-contact person. In the traditional mental-health, child-guidance-clinic model, the psychiatrist would use the other disciplines for the social systems management.

In summary pediatricians and family physicians have the advantage of early and ongoing contact with a child and family as an asset in managing MBD problems. They have a set of intervention skills in using medication that provides some short-term management benefits, but they need more training in psychosocial, educational, and behavioral areas. The psychiatrist has training in many of those skills, but has traditionally filled a consultant role and has not fully developed a long-term management system. In addition the limited resource of psychiatric time and the expense of psychiatric services has held back the development of the psychiatrist as the central coordinator of multiple interventions.

Psychology and Social Work

Psychiatrists, psychologists, and social workers have usually constituted the traditional mental-health intervention team.

Psychologists bring many skills into the service system for the MBD child. The diagnostic skills of the psychologist play a major role in identifying MBD children. The assessment of cognitive development has been a major part of the evaluation of MBD. The psychologist also contributes important information about academic achievement and emotional adjustment.

The training of a clinical or pediatric psychologist includes interview skills to produce important information about family function and adjustment. In the area of intervention approaches the psychologist is trained to provide a variety of therapeutic services. These have been reviewed in the section on intervention strategies and include various forms of psychotherapy, including individual, family, and group therapy; behavior management; parent training and counseling. The psychologist usually works with school personnel, social agencies, and physicians, so they have a knowledge of existing social systems and community resources. This experience can be valuable in helping to organize an intervention plan for an MBD child and having it relate effectively to the programs and skills avaliable in the community. The major shortcoming of the psychologist as an intervention coordinator is their tendency to function as acute intervention agents or diagnosticians. The independent practicing psychologist has come to function as a free-standing treatment person in the role model of the psychiatrist. In serving the MBD child and his family this does not usually provide a regular follow-up procedure that would allow the psychologist to coordinate ongoing treatment programs being provided by other professionals. The psychologist must develop a check-back or follow-up process that would routinely return the child and his family for consultation about progress and facilitate supervision of treatments that had been recommended.

This problem is similar for a psychologist working as an agent for a community resource. In that setting the psychologist would serve as a team member and responsibility for long-term follow-up would be dictated by agency practice and would vary markedly from system to system. Mental-health professionals give great importance to follow-up, but as a practical matter it is a most difficult process to accomplish. It involves many complex factors, including the time pressure of both the agency and the patient, expense for service, the desire of the patient to detach from the dependency, and the simple variable of establishing a good follow-up procedure.

In summary the psychologist has strong skills in psychodiagnostics that puts him in a central position in working with the MBD child and his family. The psychologist is able to identify the problem and describe assets and deficits that should be involved within the treatment process. The diagnostic skills of the psychologist touch on cognitive, educational, and emotional factors involved in working with the child, the family, and the support systems in the community. In the intervention process the psychologist has a variety of useful therapeutic approaches to manage the problems manifested in relation to MBD. These include a variety of psychotherapy approaches and counseling. In addition the psychologist can interact with the skills of a number of professionals to help coordinate an effective treatment plan. The major shortcoming psychologists must remedy is a questionable record as long-term care providers. Their history has been to serve as acute intervention agents. To benefit the MBD child and manage effectively a coordinated treatment program, psychologists must work to develop an effective check-back or follow-up system.

Social workers have many useful intervention tools but, unlike the physician and psychologist, they are not usually seen as identifiers or diagnosticians. The social worker can effectively develop a family history and look at the family system or the individual functioning in the family, but these functions have usually been performed as part of a team in which other members had the identification role or the diagnostic responsibility. The strength of social workers' functions in managing MBD problems lies in their experience in data gathering, concern with family units, and familiarity with community systems and resources. In addition the social worker, more than the physician or psychologist, will go into the family environment to deliver service. Social workers have had experience doing family evaluations in the home. This gives them a unique and valuable perspective on the interacting factors that can be a part of the MBD problems. To be able to effectively help MBD children, it is almost always necessary to organize the family effectively and to structure the environment to provide maximum support.

Social casework intervention can take many forms that could be useful in helping manage the problems related to MBD. Family counseling or therapy has been mentioned as an intervention approach and is an area covered by the skills of a social worker. Social workers also provide various types of individual theapeutic interventions that can facilitate a better adjustment by the MBD child. In addition to this intervention skills, social workers have an orientation to long-term follow-up that is necessary for effective management of MBD children.

The limited diagnostic skills of social workers have produced situations in which these professionals usually serve at the direction of an identifying or referral resource and so tend to be team members rather than service coordinators. The nature of the presenting problems in MBD are such that it is unusual for the child to be seen initially by a social worker. There are times when a social worker in a school setting will be asked to organize a referral for a child for evaluation. In this role the social worker usually facilitates the referral, but does not direct it. In reality there is no reason demonstrated why the social worker could not direct the process but the usual habit of the system has seldom allowed for this.

The summation of the assets of social workers in coordinating service to MBD children would include skills in interviewing, a knowledge of community systems and resources, skills in family and individual therapeutic intervention, a history of entering the environment for assessment and treatment purposes, and a willingness to engage in long-term management and follow-up.

The basic limitation of social workers lies in their limited diagnostic or identification skills, which has put them in a position of team members rather than team leaders. In addition the usual manifestations of MBD problems are such that the child is usually sent to other professionals before they would be sent to a social worker.

Educationally Related Specialists

The major disabling manifestations of MBD are behavior disorders or learning disabilities. Not all MBD children have these problems, but the large majority of those who require significant amounts or degrees of assistance will have problems in one or both of these areas. Educationally related programs constitute a major array of interventions designed to remediate the problems of MBD children. It is difficult to group the professionals that deliver services in this area. In this discussion the group will include: classroom teachers; special education teachers; reading specialists; speech, hearing and communication specialists; and physical, occupational, and recreational therapists. School psychologists, social workers, and guidance counselors should probably be included in this group because they tend to provide their services around the educational adjustment or achievement of the child as opposed to functioning in broader mental health role. These professionals practice in a child guidance clinic or community agency.

The major demand on children is to succeed in school. MBD tends to place a child at risk in this critical area and so requires special interventions that will minimize this risk for the child. The various types of interventions have been previously reviewed, so that in this section we shall consider the potential role of the educational personnel as the overall coordinators of services to the MBD child.

The basic and overwhelming value of this group of porfessionals is their ability to remediate the child's educationally related deficit. If the child is able to over-come his problem with educational subjects, speech or language, or the motor skills involved in athletics or recreation, society will usually tend to see them as acceptable members. The frustration of failure to achieve in any of the above areas is the frequent source of adjustment and behavior problems, so that educational remediation can be of two-fold benefit. The problems encountered by most MBD children tend to be long-term in nature and so require an ongoing system of remedial efforts. The school and educational personnel have a long-term relation-ship with this group of children during the critical points of the child's greatest need. This relationship has the potential to be of great value in serving the MBD population.

However in current practice it is unusual for people in the educational system to capitalize on this potential. In practice educational services tend to separate them-selves from other nonschool related services and even from the family environ-ment. When managing MBD problems, school personnel all too frequently refer the problems to the family or other professionals to have them managed. All too often parents are told that their child cannot sit still in class and they should take him to a physician for some help. This situation may be a reaction to society's questioning of the school functioning. As a result educationally related systems have created an island of resources that can interact with other services. However they seldom show the committment necessary to accept the broad responsibilities of coordinating multiple interventions involving several professional disciplines and extending into the home environment. The move toward educational main-streaming or the educational continuum may produce changes that create flexibil-ity in the system that will help meet the needs of the MBD children. The resources of educationally related professionals covers many of the areas of need of the MBD child, but the system of delivery tends to fractionate itself so that coordina-tion is not the rule. Programs tend to be mutually exclusive rather than comple-mentary. A child will have to be classified either as a learning problem or a behavior problem, either as a communication disorder or mentally retarded, and the program for the child will be set by the classification. It is difficult for children to be between classifications or to draw program resources from two classifica-tions. A child is usually "in" special education or "out" of special education, so that special resources are compartmentalized by virtue of some artificial program labels. If a real educational continuum could evolve, then children could receive the services from the variety of professionals that their problem indicates and move from more intensive to less intensive service needs as they progress through the system.

In summary educationally related professionals have much to offer the MBD child. Their skills can be helpful in remediating some of the more serious conse-quences of the MBD problem. A child who receives effective educational reme-diation is more likely to succeed in managing the manifestations of MBD and entering more fully into the general society. Educational personnel have a long-term contact with the child and can be available to intercede when the child shows signs of needing additional help.

The basic shortcomings of the educational professionals have been their unwill-ingness to extend their influences beyond the school system. They have long since established a pattern of referral to medical or social resources that results in the educational personnel separating from coordination responsibility. The educational system tends to compartmentalize itself and is often seen as a separate entity by other community resources. Other professionals dealing with MBD children do not readily go into the school system to function and the school personnel do not easily venture into community-based treatment programs. New forces in education may help resolve this problem. The previously mentioned continuum programs may encourage programmatic flexibility, Public Law 94–142, which mandates education for all the handicapped, could provide the stimulus for greater interdisciplinary functioning in the school system. This law would require the in-put of many professionals to develop an adequate program for a handicapped child.

Factors Affecting Coordination

There are many factors that impact on the process of achieving effective coordination of service intervention. Some of these factors are in the nature of problems and can range from readily apparent to unspoken and unseen. The most basic problem faced in coordinating multiple interventions is the relative lack of training to fill that role. No single discipline has prepared its students to handle the task. It seems to be an unspoken assumption that all professionals acquire this skill by virtue of learning their own special skills. Professional training today emphasizes an independent practitioner model. Each discipline trains its students to provide their services to consumers and to do it in a freestanding role model. The confidence and skill related to meeting this role model may help facilitate good treatment, but it does little to insure effective coordination of various treatments for MBD children. In fact the overlap of treatment skills among various professionals who can provide the same or similar service has impeded coordination. There is a strong need for each discipline to prove its expertise and the result is a situation where professional territory-protecting takes precedent over the need of the MBD child. To correct the problem of territoriality effectively, it is necessary for each discipline to accept fully the skills and competence of the other disciplines. There must be a willingness to accept leadership from the person who undertakes the coordination effort. Acceptance must be based on the best interests of the child and not predicated on the credentials of the person serving as coordinator. The roles of each team member should be clearly defined and functionally related to the needs of the MBD child. This can be achieved by the efforts of an effective coordination of the many of the disciplines discussed in this chapter.

An unacknowledged problem that complicates the effort to coordinate multiple interventions is the lack of a clear reward for the effort. All too often this role is merely an extra burden, a situation requiring special effort, which is not appreciated by the other disciplines involved in the delivery of service. As a result of this lack of clear reward, the job of coordinator all too often evolves by default of most of the members of the intervention team.

A practical consideration related to satisfaction in the coordination role is the question of payment for service. In the private service system there is no ready mechanism to charge for the time spent organizing the services of other professionals or the time spent in follow-up checking of the progress of the child and the need for continued services. Since much of this effort takes place away from the patient, it may be difficult for a professional to render a bill for the time expended.

The final two problems in coordinating multiple intervention are products of the routine of the present service delivery system. The first problem relates to the loss of enthusiam by the professional resulting from the time lapse between the diagnostic evaluation and the onset of treatment. Too often the multidisciplinary diagnostic team will make its recommendations and then begin to set up the intervention program. When the intervention requires the services of a professional outside the diagnostic team, it usually takes considerable time to contact the other professionals, arrange meetings, explain the need for service from the professional, and process the request through the service delivery system.

The second problem is the tendency of the system to close a case. Record keeping seems to require that intervention take place quickly, the patient be cured, and the case closed. MBD problems do not fit this model and obviously effective long-term supervision of the needs of an MBD child would suffer from this approach. To remedy this situation, intervention strategies must be considered management projects that require long-term supervision contact.

On the positive side of the situation there are basic procedures that can be used effectively to facilitate the management of MBD children. The first is the willingness of the professional to accept the central role in coordinating management. This willingness should reflect an awareness of the problems involved in training to facilitate an effective application of professional skills to meet the MBD child's needs. Second, the coordinating professional must have an awareness of the resources available and needed to meet the needs of the MBD child. This requires an effort to search the local community to find resources and to be available to meet with and evaluate the effectiveness of the services provided by the various professionals and facilities in the community. Third, the coordinator must take the responsibility for taking the evaluation and diagnostic data and see that it becomes a simple, efficient intervention program. This will necessitate weeding out overlapping referral recommendations and holding down the number of interventions to the minimum. The role of the coordinator should be to keep the management plan as simple as possible, while meeting the child's needs. Along this line it is necessary and important to see the intervention recommendations take into consideration such factors as the ability to finance the services needed, the ability of the family to reach the location of this service, the identification of a resource to provide the service recommended, and the ability of the family to organize a time schedule to comply with the recommendations. Finally, there is a need for the coordinator to have an effective check-back system.

An Overview of the Problem

In approaching the topic of coordinating multiple intervention, several main points have evolved:

1. There must be a clear realization that diagnosis and recommendations are a beginning of intervention, but do not insure coordinated intervention.
2. The results of the diagnostic evaluation should set priorities for the intervention strategy.
3. There are multiple types of interventions that are applicable to the problems manifested by MBD children.
4. The treatment approaches fall in the skills and domain of a number of disciplines and the territories often overlap.

5. The decision for leadership in coordinating the intervention program must be approached on a systematic basis. Leadership should be delegated on a functional rather than hierarchial basis.

An important factor in working towards a service system that will effectively manage interdisciplinary treatment programs lies in clearly accenting the importance of treatment. Currently there is a greater satisfaction in the more limited responsibility attached to the role of diagnosis, which makes this a convenient role for most professionals dealing with MBD children. It is always easier to tell someone else what is wrong and what to do about it. On the other hand there has been much frustration and failure attached to the role of the long-term treatment agent. The division among disciplines, the abrogation of leadership roles, and the defense of territorial prerogatives have contributed to the problem. It is time the interdisciplinary process becomes a matter of accepting each professional for his competence and the relation of that skill to the central needs of the patient. We need to abandon a notion of hierarchial leadership to focus on the most efficient way to meet the needs of the child. As often happens in working with children, adult authority needs prevail when the child should be the major concern. It is simple to believe that we must work for the child and not the system, but the system has a long history of trapping the child and it also has unconsciously trapped the helping professions. A renewed commitment to selflessness by the adult authorities would be a critical step in facilitating optimal treatment for the MBD child.

REFERENCES

Abbe, M. "Treatment of minimal brain dysfunction." *Physiotherapy*, 60, 203–207, (1974).

Abrams, J. C., and F. Kaslow. "Family systems and the learning disabled child: Intervention and treatment." *Journal of Learning Disabilities*. 10, 27–31, (1977).

Ayllon, T., D. Layman, and H. J. Kandal. "A behavioral-educational alternative to drug control of hyperactive children." *Journal of Applied Behavior Analysis*, 8, 137–146, (1975).

Ayres, A. J. "Interrelation of perception, function, and treatment." *Physical Therapy*, 16, 741, (1966).

Campbell, S., V. Douglas, and G. Morgenstern. "Cognitive Styles in hyperactive children and the effect of methylphenidate." (Paper presented at the annual meeting of the Canadian Psychological Association, Toronto, (June 1969).

Christensen, D. E., and R. L. Sprague. "Prediction of hyperactive behavior by conditioning procedures alone and combined with methylphenadate (Ritalin)." *Behavior Research and Therapy*, 11, 331–334,)1973).

Clements, S. D. *Minimal Brain Dysfunction in Children*. NINDB, Monograph No. 3. Washington, D. C.: U. S. Department of HEW, 1966.

Connors, C. K. "Symposium: Behavior modification by drugs II: Psychological effects of stimulants drugs in children with minimal brain dysfunction." *Pediatrics*, 49, 702–708, (1972).

Delacato, C. *The Diagnosis and Treatment of Speech and Reading Problems*. Springfield, Ill.: C. Thomas, 1963.

Doman, G. *How to Teach Your Baby to Read*. New York: Random House, 1964.

Eisenberg, L., A. Gilbert, L. Cytryn, and P. Molling. "The effectiveness of psychotherapy alone and in conjunction with perphenazine or placebo in treatment of neurotic and hyperactive children." *American Journal of Psychiatry*, 117, 1088–1093, (1961).

Ericson, E. *Identity, Youth and Crisis*. New York: Norton, 1968.

Frostig, M. "Sensory-motor development." *Special Education*, 57, 18, (1968).

Gardner, R. "The mutual storytelling technique in the treatment of psychogenic problems secondary to minimal brain dysfunction." *Journal of Learning Disabilities*, 7, 135–143, (1974).

Gardner, R. *Psychotherapeutic Approaches to the Resistant Child*. New York: Aronson, 1975.

Gittelman, G. et al. "Relative efficacy of methylphenadate and behavior modification in hyperactive children: An interim report." *Journal of Abnormal Psychology*, 4, 361–379, (1976).

Haslem, R. and P. J. Valletutti. *Medical Problems in the Classroom*. Baltimore: University Park Press, 1975.

Holmberg, N. J. "Serving the child with MBD and his family—In a health maintenance organization." *Nursing Clinics of North America*, 10, 381–391, (1975).

Kenney, T. J., R. L. Clemmens, B. W. Hudson, G. A. Lentz, R. Cicci, and P. Nair. "Characteristics of children referred because of hyperactivity." *Journal of Pediatrics*, 79, 618–622, (1971).

Kephart, N. C. "Perceptual-Motor Aspects of learning disabilities." *Exceptional Children*, 31, 201 (1964).

Millichap, J. Gordon, and E. E. Boldrey. "Studies in hyperactive behavior II. Laboratory and Clinical Evaluation of Drug Treatments." *Neurology*, 17, 467–472, (1967).

Naville, S. "Psychomotor therapy." *Remedial Education*, 10, 13, (1970).

Rie, H., E. Rie, S. Stewart, and J. P. Ambuel. "Effects of ritalin on underachieving children: A replication." *American Journal of Orthopsychiatry*, 46, 313–322, (1976).

Rie, H. "Hyperactivity in Children." *American Journal of Diseases of Children*, 129, 783–789, (1975).

Ross, D., and S. Ross. *Hyperactivity: Research, Theory, Action*. New York: Wiley, 1976.

Safer, D., and R. P. Allen. *Hyperactive Children: Diagnosis and Management*. Baltimore: University Park Press, 1976.

Satir, V. *Conjoint family Therapy*. Palo Alto, Cal.: Science and Behavior Books, 1967.

Shafto, F., and Sulzbacher. "Comparing treatment tactics with a hyperactive pre-school child: Stimulant medication and programmed teaching intervention." *Journal of Applied Behavior Analysis*, 10, 13–20, (1977).

Sprague, R. L., K. R. Barnes, and J. S. Werry. "Methlyphenadate and thioridazine: Learning, reaction time, activity, and classroom behavior in disturbed children." *American Journal of Orthopsychiatry*, 40, 615–628, (1975).

Sroufe, L. A. "Drug treatment of children with behavior problems," in F. Horowitz, ed., *Review of Child Development Research*, 4, 347–407, (1975).

Stewart, M., and S. Olds. *Raising a Hyperactive Child*. New York: Harper and Row, 1971.

Sulzbacher, S. I. "Behavior analysis of drug effects in the classroom," in G. Semb, ed., *Behavior Analysis and Education—1972*. Lawrence: University of Kansas Press, 1973.

Sykes, D., V. Douglas, and G. Morgenstern. "The effect of methlyphenadate (Ritalin) on sustained attention in hyperactive children." *Psychopharmacologia*, 25, 19–85, (1972).

Vogel, E., and N. Bell. *A Modern Introduction to the Family*. New York: Free Press, 1964.

Wahler, R. G. "Setting generality: Some specific and general effects of child behavior therapy." *Journal of Applied Behavior Analysis,* 2, 239–246, (1969).

Wender, P. *Minimal Brain Dysfunction in Children.* New York: Wiley, 1971.

Weiss, G., E. Kruger, U. Danielson, and M. Elmore. "Effects of long-term treatment of hyperactive children with methylphenadate." *Canadian Medical Association Journal,* 112, 159–165, (1975).

Winett, R. A. and R. C. Winkler. "Current behavior modification in the classroom: Be still, be docile, be quite." *Journal of Applied Analysis,* 5, 499–504, (1972).

Wulbert, M., "The generalization of newly acquired behaviors by parents and children across three different settings: A study of an autistic child." *Journal of Applied Behavior Analysis,* 2, 87–93, (1974).

Wulbert, M., and R. Dries. "The relative efficay of methlyphenadate (Ritalin) and behavior modification techniques in the treatment of a hyperactive child." *Journal of Applied Behavior Analysis,* 10, 21–31, (1977).

PART NINE

Research Methods and Problems

Chapter 27

Minimal Brain Dysfunctions: An Appraisal of Research Concepts and Methods

Paul Satz and Jack M. Fletcher

The original purpose in writing this chapter was to provide a critical appraisal of research in the area broadly defined as minimal brain dysfunction (MBD). After reviewing much of this research which spans nearly four decades, it became painfully clear that the task was too complex to be accomplished within a single chapter. The major problem, which continuously confronted the authors, concerned the manner in which this term was used and conceptualized in the literature. It was often impossible to determine which target children were selected from one study to another. Terms such as minimal brain dysfunction (Clements, 1966), hyperkinetic behavior syndrome (Laufer and Denhoff, 1957), hyperkinesis (Wender, 1973), developmental hyperactivity (Werry, 1968), hyperactivity (Safer and Allen, 1976), specific learning disability (USOE, 1968), specific reading disability (Money, 1962), specific dyslexia (de Hirsch, Jansky and Langford, 1966), developmental dyslexia (Waites, 1968), primary reading retardation (Rabinovitch, de Jong, Ingram and Withey, 1954), educationally handicapped (Owen, 1978), psychoneurological learning disability (Myklebust, 1968) continue to be used almost interchangeably in research and clinical practice. The terms refer to an elusive and heterogeneous group of children, primarily in the elementary and middle schools, who are having unexpected academic and/or behavioral difficulties.

In attempts to categorize this research it was felt that the studies fell into three broad, but partially overlapping, divisions. One major group of studies seemed to address behavioral problems in children in which signs of hyperactivity, distractibility, and poor attention span coexisted with various academic-learning difficulties. For descriptive convenience, this group will be referred to as hyperactive-learning disabilities. However it should be pointed out that in most of these studies, the target children are selected primarily on the basis of hyperactivity, learning disability, or both. Because of this selection bias, there is varying overlap in symptoms both within and among studies. However, if the selection is made primarily on the basis of hyperactivity, then a majority of the children will show evidence of specific learning disabilities (Safer and Allen, 1976; Fine, 1977; Douglas, 1976). Within this division terms such as hyperkinetic behavior syndrome, hyperkinesis, hyperactivity, developmental hyperactivity, specific learning disability, and psychoneurological learning disability are commonly used.

The second major group of studies can more easily be classified on the basis of their primary interest in academic underachievement. The vast majority of children in this group demonstrate significant problems in reading, spelling, and writing. A smaller number demostrate specific problems in related learning skills, such as mathematics and visuo-spatial integration. Although some of these reading-or learning-disabled children may also show signs of hyperactivity, selection is usually made only on the basis of achievement criteria. For descriptive convenience children within this broad research category will be referred to as reading and learning-disabilities. Frequently these two terms are used interchangeably. Also most of the children labeled as learning disabled reveal a primary disturbance in reading (Owen, 1978). Within this division terms such as specific reading disability, specific learning disability, educationally handicapped, primary reading retardation, specific dyslexia, and developmental dyslexia are commonly used.

The third group of studies refer more to a general concept rather than to a specifiable group of children. As a concept, it is defined as an umbrella term which subsumes virtually all of the target children designated in the preceding two categories. The term is minimal brain dysfunction and, at present, it enjoys increasingly wide acceptance in both research and clinical settings. The concept, as presently defined, is felt to present one of the most persistent hurdles to progress in this area of child mental health. In fact the concept is so loosely defined that it defies attempts to determine its prevalence, course, and prognosis. For this reason the present chapter is addressed to a critical review of the concept of minimal brain dysfunction followed by an appraisal of current research developments in the broad areas of hyperactivity/learning disabilities and reading/learning disabilities.

MBD: MYTH OR FACT?

Of all the terms used to describe children at risk, the concept of minimal brain dysfunction is the most popular and controversial. The term also exemplifies much of the confusion that results when a concept is loosely defined both in terms of behavior and inferred etiology. As Benton has pointed out:

'Minimal brain dysfunction' is a behavioral concept with neurological implications. It must be called a 'behavioral' concept because it is defined by certain behavioral features rather than, as is usually the case in adult patients, by infrabehavioral evidence of cerebral abnormality. A patient can have clearly evident disease of the brain without showing any functional (including behavioral) abnormality, at least as disclosed by present methods of investigation. But a child (or an adult) cannot have minimal brain dysfunction without showing behavioral abnormalities, since the designation in fact means behavioral deviation. [1973, p. 29]

The concept springs from the early work of Kahn and Cohen (1934) who speculated on a relationship between school behavior problems and neurological damage. The authors noted that symptoms of hyperkinesis, distractibility, short attention span, and impulsivity were commonly seen in encephalitic disorders of childhood and in some childhood behavioral disorders without evidence of brain damage. Kahn and Cohen (1934) referred to this latter group as "organic driveness" and postulated an underlying brain-stem lesion.

Strauss (1947) also noted a relationship between behavioral disturbances in motor control, particularly hyperactivity, and severely brain damaged children. This relationship was later extended to include presumably normal school children who showed a pattern of high activity, distractibility and explosivity. Strauss and Kephart (1955) speculated that despite evidence of classical neurological signs of perinatal complications in these children, the behavioral patterns suggested a minor deviation in the brain. Hence the term minimal brain damage was invoked to refer to these behavior problem children.

This relationship between childhood behavioral disturbances and suspected CNS dysfunction was expanded to include children with learning problems (Laufer and Denhoff, 1957). The authors noted a pattern of hyperactivity, distractibility, impulsivity, and poor attention span in children following severe head trauma, encephalitis, and measles encephalopathy. They also noted a similar behavioral pattern in some children who presented no clear-cut history or signs of brain disease. These children, who were referred to as hyperkinetic impulse disorder, also showed signs of academic underachievement and visual-motor difficulties.

Hence the concept was broadened to include both behavioral and academic problems with the clear implication of an underlying neurological basis.

The concept of minimal brain damage, as a presumtive diagnosis based on purely behavioral signs, soon came under critical attack. In 1962 the Oxford Study Group (Bax and MacKeith, 1963) recommended that the term should be abandoned because of its disease connotation and its reliance on behavioral signs alone. They suggested that the word minimal should also be avoided when possible. The word minimal is bad for several reasons.

> The term suggests that either the symptoms or signs are minimal and that the brain lesion is too, but this is frequently not the case. All syndromes may have minimal or maximal manifestations but a minimal manifestation of a syndrome does not create a new syndrome entity. [p. 96]

According to Koupernik, MacKeith, and Francis-Williams (1975), the word minimal was used to refer to the abnormal neurological signs (soft and classical) that occur in some of these children with severe behavioral problems (for example hyperactivity, distractibility, and so on). But the same distractibility pattern is seen in children with severe epilepsy, cerebral palsy, or mental deficiency. As Koupernik, MacKeith, and Francis-Williams state,

> their troubles are minimal neither as regards their behavior nor as regards their neurological signs. [p. 122]

Notwithstanding these criticisms, the concept gained new impetus and respectability following the task force cosponsored by the Easter Seal Research Foundation and the National Institute of Neurological Diseases and Blindness (Clements, 1966). The word dysfunction was substituted for damage, but without any explicit change in meaning. More seriously the concept of minimal brain dysfunction, like hyperkinetic impulse disorder, was expanded to include a much broader class of childhood behavioral and learning disabilities.

> The term 'minimal brain dysfunction syndrome' refers . . . to children of near average, average, or above average general intelligence with certain learning or behavioral disabilities ranging from mild to severe, which are associated with deviations of functions of the central nervous system. These deviations may manifest themselves by various combina-

tions of impairment in perception, conceptualization, language, memory, and control of attention, impulse, or motor function. [p. 9–10]

This definition can be faulted at a number of levels. First, it implies that learning or behavioral problems in children with below average intelligence who show impairment in perception, language, and so on, are due to more severe deviations of central nervous system function. Second, the definition fails to specify how discrepancies between intelligence and achievement are to be determined. Third, it fails to specify how these IQ-achievement discrepancies are to be treated in the culturally disadvantaged. One is merely told that this determination represents an equally complex but different problem (unspecified). Fourth, and most serious, the definition states that deviations of central nervous system function in these learning or behavioral disabilities (unspecified) are evidenced by impairment in behavioral-cognitive performance (also unspecified). Stated more formally, the concept is defined as follows:

1. A severe learning or behavioral disability (unspecified).
2. Average-above average intelligence (unspecified).
3. Impairment in perception; conceptualization; language; memory; and control of attention, impulse, or motor function (unspecified).

Events 1. and 2. represent necessary but not sufficient conditions. Event 3. must also be present before the diagnosis of MBD can be made. Clements (1966) defends this presumptive inference as follows:

With our limited validated knowledge concerning relationships between brain and behavior, we must accept certain categories of deviant behavior, developmental dyscrasias, learning disabilities, and visual-motor perceptual irregularities as valid indices of brain dysfunctioning. They represent neurologic signs of a most meaningful kind, and reflect disorganized central nervous system functioning at the highest level. [P. 6–7]

Despite the vagueness and circularity in this definition, the concept of MBD was given uncritical acceptance by the National Advisory Committee on Handicapped Children some two years later (USOE, 1968). Essentially the MBD concept was translated into educational terms as specific learning disability (SLD):

Children with specific learning disabilities exhibit a *disorder* in one or more of the basic psychological processes involved in understanding or in using spoken or written language. These may be manifested in disorders of listening, thinking, talking, reading, writing, spelling, or arithmetic. They include conditions which have been referred to as perceptual handicaps, brain injury, minimal brain dysfunction, dyslexia, developmental aphasia, etc. They do not include learning problems which are due primarily to visual, hearing, or motor handicaps, to mental retardation, emotional disturbance, or to environmental disadvantage. [P. 34]

Despite the attempts to derive an equivalent educational definition for MBD, the USOE definition, by emphasis on academic achievement, excluded those behavioral symptoms of hyperactivity, distractibility, impulsivity, motor clumsiness, and short attention span that were traditionally part of the minimal brain damage or dysfunction syndrome (Strauss and Lehtinen, 1947; Laufer and Denhoff, 1957).

In an attempt to resolve the discrepanices between the SLD and MBD definitions, the concept of MBD was uncritically elevated to the status of a hypothetical class of cerebral dysfunctions which subsumed smaller discrete and overlapping

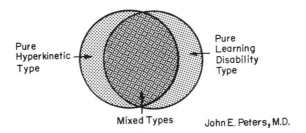

Figure 27-1.

subsets of academic and/or behavioral disabilities (Peters, Davis, Goolsby, Clements, 1973; Connors, 1976; Wender, 1976).

The formulations of Peters, et al., (1973) are instructive here. Figure 27-1 illustrates two partially overlapping circles which subsume three subsets of the MBD syndrome: a pure hyperkinetic type, a pure learning disability type, and a much larger mixed type with features of the two pure types.
According to Peters, et al., (1973):

> When these two circles overlap, the part of the circle on the left which extends out as 'unmixed' shows that there is a small percentage of these children who have only hyperactivity, impulsiveness, and short attention span, sometimes referred to as the hyperkinetic syndrome. The other part of the circle on the right, where it is 'unmixed,' indicates that there is a small percentage of children who do not have hyperactivity and impulsiveness; they have a pure form of learning disability (such as developmental dyslexia) with few other signs. In fact, they may be hypoactive. The area of overlap corresponds with the MBD children who have both hyperactivity *and* a specific learning disability—the 'mixed' group as indicated in the figure. This is the largest segment of MBD. [P. 5-6]

Virtually the same formulation was advanced by Wender (1976). He stated that the syndrome of minimal brain dysfunction (MBD) bears a close relationship to and may perhaps include the syndrome of learning disabilities. According to Wender (1976):

> MBD is one of a number of designations for a common behavioral syndrome of childhood for which a variety of other terms and phrases have previously been employed, including the hyperactive child syndrome, hyperactivity, hyperkinesis, minimal brain damage, minimal cerebral function. . . . The signs fall into two major realms: (1) behavioral and (2) perceptual and cognitive (learning disabilities). These signs occur in MBD children in all three logical combinations. [P. 111]

The purpose in presenting this brief historical account is to show that despite obvious terminological looseness in the concept and its definition, the use of the term has continued to enjoy increasing acceptance in both research and clinical practice. The concept has also become an umbrella term that subsumes the vast majority of academic and/or behavioral disabilities in children within a neurological net. Although opponents have referred to minimal brain dysfunction as an empty term, "used to save us the trouble of thinking clearly about what we are talking about" (Koupernik, MacKeith, and Francis-Williams, 1975, p. 125), or "merely a sophisticated statement of ignorance" (Grinspoon and Singer, 1973) or as "maximal neurological confusion" (Gomez, 1967), the concept has remained impervious to critical scrutiny. Why? Wolff and Hurwitz (1973) pointed out that

> . . . if experience can teach us anything, it is more than likely that a concept as vague and

global as minimal brain dysfunction will sooner or later be hypostasized, just as similar diagnoses were in the past. The concept MBD will then begin to demand respect in its own right, without ever having been subjected to the tedious work of classification that is necessary to determine the concept's actual significance. [P. 107]

The word hypostasis derives from a deeply theological term implying the essence as opposed to what is attributed.

As stated earlier in this chapter, the term MBD is a behavioral concept with neurological implications. Benton (1973) argued that it must be called a behavioral concept because it is defined by behavioral features, not by infrabehavioral evidence of cerebral dysfunction. Yet the inference from these behavioral signs to the brain is unwarranted at the present time, and is potentially reckless if the diagnosis leads to specific modes of drug treatment. These concerns were originally expressed by the International Study Group on Child Neurology in 1963 (Bax and MacKeith):

It became clear that this term (MBD) has, for most people, the anatomical and aetiological implications that there has been an episode of injury and that this has produced an anatomical change. Yet, closer examination makes it clear that evidence of anatomical change is usually absent, that evidence or history of an injury process is often absent and that disorder of functions is the evidence for applying the diagnostic label of minimal brain dysfunction.

Unfortunately disorder of function, whether expressed in terms of academic achievement, behavioral motility, or cognitive performance, provides no valid basis for inferring a deviation in central nervous system functioning (Birch, 1964). There are multiple factors that have long been recognized to account for academic underachievement as well as for behavioral and cognitive difficulties. These factors are too numerous to repeat here, but include constitutional as well as environmental variables (Thomas and Chess, 1977). Deviations in cerebral functioning represent only one subset of underlying causes.

As presently defined the term MBD represents an inference concerning an unknown deviation in the brain based on unexpected academic failure and/or signs of behavioral disturbance (primarily hyperactivity). This inference is reckless and unwarranted and leads to circularity in reasoning. Moreover the concept is defined to exclude children with evidence of gross neurological damage. Yet the vast majority of children who are labelled MBD have no consistent evidence of soft neurological signs, perinatal complications or electroencephalographic abnormalities (Koupernik, MacKeith, and Francis-Williams, 1975; Stevens, Sachdev, and Milstein, 1968; Satterfield, 1973; Fine, 1977; Safer and Allen, 1976). Finally there are many severely brain-injured children who show no evidence of academic difficulty nor behavioral impulse problems (Fine, 1977; Birch, 1964).

These comments inevitably lead to the conclusion that the concept of MBD is indeed an empty and superfluous term. As such it represents a myth that should be discarded as illusory. In fact the concept is not even necessary. What is urgently needed is a more descriptive and operational class of definitions for these target children without any presumption as to etiology. Inferences should only be entertained on selected subgroups of the target children based on systematic behavioral, electrophysiological, and/or pharmacological measures. Only then will it be possible to move beyond a descriptive nomenclature. As Douglas (1976) has pointed out, "good neurologizing cannot precede accurate operational definition of symptoms" (p. 414).

HYPERACTIVITY/LEARNING DISABILITIES

Definition Problems

In recent years attempts have been made to redefine the concept of MBD in terms of one of its major characteristics—namely, the hyperkinetic behavior syndrome first proposed by Laufer and Denhoff (1957). This has in part been accomplished by stripping the concept of its surplus neurological meaning and by using more descriptive terminology. Through these efforts the concept of developmental hyperactivity was advanced and defined as follows:

. . . a level of daily motor activity which is clearly greater (ideally by more than two standard deviations from the mean) than that occurring in children of similar sex, mental age, socioeconomic and cultural background and which is not accompanied by clear evidence of major central nervous system disorder or childhood psychosis and-which has been present consistently since the earliest years of life. [Werry, 1968, p. 583]

Similar defining criteria have been proposed by Douglas (1976):

1. The hyperactive behavior must be present since early childhood, sustained throughout the day, and the major complaint of both parents.

2. The child must be of normal intelligence, attending regular school classes, and living at home with at least one parent.

3. No evidence of gross psychiatric or neurological disability must be present.

Other definitions have been equally descriptive:

Hyperactivity (HA) is simply defined as a long term childhood pattern characterized by excessive restlessness and inattentiveness. It is a developmental disorder which begins in early to midchildhood (ages 2–6), and begins to fade during adolescence. During childhood, the pattern is consistent year after year. [Safer and Allen, 1976, p. 5]

Most of these definitions, which stress hyperactivity as the necessary feature, do recognize an associated pattern of primary and secondary symptoms. These symptoms generally include inattentiveness, learning problems, impulsivity, excitability, antisocial behavior, low self-concept, and immaturity (Safer and Allen, 1976; Cantwell, 1975). There is however considerable variability in how these symptoms are ranked. Some authors report that the primary disturbance in hyperactive children is a severe learning disability involving reading, mathematics, and/or visual-motor skills (Douglas, 1976; Safer and Allen, 1976; Connors, 1969; Ambrosimo and Del Fonte, 1973; Laufer, 1971). Other authors rank the learning difficulties as secondary symptoms (Cantwell, 1975; Denckla, 1978). If evidence of a learning disability is part of the selection criteria (Connors, Taylor, Meo, Kurtz and Fournier, 1972), then by definition it should rank as a primary symptom. Unfortunately most definitions are vague with respect to the selection criteria used. This latter problem inevitably leads to variability in the type of children selected.

Thus children labeled hyperactive by one set of criteria would be excluded by another. The study of Kenny, et al., (1971) illustrates this point. One hundred children who were labeled as severely hyperactive were referred to a multidisciplinary setting for separate clinical examinations. Although there was close agreement among examiners, over half of the children were not considered hyperactive by any examiner. Only a third of the children in fact were deemed hyperactive by the majority of examiners. Of the 78 children who were also given electroence-phalograms, 38 were normal. Nor was any significant relationship found among the neurological examination, EEG findings, and final diagnosis.

More disturbing findings concern the low incidence of this behavioral disturbance (hyperactivity) in other cultural groups. For example, epidemiological surveys in Great Britain (Rutter, Graham, and Yule, 1970) revealed only 2 cases of hyperkinesis in a population of 2189 school children between the ages of 9–11. Bax (1972) on the other hand found not a single case of the hyperkinetic syndrome in a study of 1200 five-year olds living in the Isle of Wight. Similar findings have also been reported for Chinese-American children in New York and among mainland Chinese children (Sollenberger, 1968). Yet these prevalence estimates contrast with estimates derived from school and clinic samples in North America. For example, when teachers are asked to identify those children who have a primary degree of hyperactivity and inattentiveness, and have had it since the beginning of elementary school, the estimates range between 3 to 10% of the school population (Fine, 1977; Safer and Allen, 1976). The vast majority of these children are boys and, in contrast to specific reading disabilities, the ratios range from 4:1–9:1 (Stevens, Sachder, and Milstein, 1968; Gross and Wilson, 1974; Safer and Allen, 1976). Stewart, et al., (1966), using a different questionnaire approach, reported a similar incidence ranging between 4 to 10%. These estimates however are markedly increased when computed on atypical samples of emotionally disturbed, mentally retarded, learning-disabled and brain-damaged children (Fine, 1977; Safer and Allen, 1976). Here the estimates range from 10 to 30%.

Differences in the preceding estimates reflect a number of problems that continue to exist in this area. Differences exist in how the term is defined (descriptive or otherwise); the type of cultural group selected; whether a measure of academic achievement is included in the definition; whether children showing the target behavior are selected on the basis of IQ, age, and SES status; and whether estimates are based on school samples, clinic samples, or population surveys.

Clinically the concept of hyperactivity is applied to children of average intelligence who are characterized by restlessness, hyperactivity, distractibility, poor attention span, low frustration tolerance, emotional lability, immaturity, and aggressive behavior. Although descriptive in nature, the concept utilizes terms that refer to a broad and heterogeneous class of behaviors. As such the concept shares some of the inherent weaknesses of the MBD concept. According to Shrag and Divorky (1975),

Teachers have traditionally assumed that between a fourth and a third of their students would be academic losers, and mothers have always complained that their children can't sit still. [P. 47].

In an epidemiologic study of behavior characteristics (Lapouse and Monk, 1958), the authors found that half of the mothers regarded their own children as overactive. Similarly in a later survey questionnaire concerning childhood behavior problems, teachers reported that 53% of the boys and 30% of the girls in an entire school system were having problems associated with overactivity.

Symptoms of restlessness, hyperactivity, emotional lability, and so on, could reflect the effects of environmental and cultural problems as well as the effects of organic, maturational, and constitutional problems. In fact Marwitt and Stenner (1972) have proposed two patterns of hyperactivity: (1) a psychological pattern called hyper-reactive and (2) an organic-constitutional pattern called hyperactive. Because of differences in the way the concept of developmental hyperactivity is defined, children with hyper-reactive patterns of behavior may well be mislabeled as hyperactive. Support for this possibility is seen in the frequent reports of environmental deprivation and conflict in the families of hyperactive children. For example Kenny, et al., (1971) found that

Sixty-four percent of the families had evidence of major environmental pathology. Nearly one third of the children lived in one-parent families or did not live with either parent. Thirty-eight of the families were considered to be overly unstable, including history of parental institutionalization for emotional disturbance, alcoholism, drug addiction, or criminal acts. Environmental deprivation was noted in fourteen homes. [P. 620]

Similar findings of parental conflict and rejection have been reported by Stewart (1970), Chess (1960), Fine (1977), and Battle and Lacey (1972). Stevens, et al. (1968) also found that disturbed family relations represented the most prominent feature in their electroencephalogic study of hyperactive/learning disabled children. In fact the presence of abnormal EEG patterns was more related to these adverse familial disturbances than to predisposing prenatal and perinatal complications in the probands. These findings, while not discrepant with the concept of an organic or constitutional subgroup of hyperactive children, clearly illustrate the importance of environmental factors in both the etiology and management of hyperactive children. Sollenberger (1968) has already discussed how stable child-rearing practices may account for the low incidence of hyperactivity in Chinese-Americans and in mainland Chinese.

The preceding findings again illustrate how problems with definition and selection criteria can obscure attempts to evaluate research findings in this area. Although the concept of developmental hyperactivity, in contrast to MBD, is defined in more descriptive terms, the terms vary considerably with respect to the selection criteria employed. The concept also refers to too broad a class of behavioral characteristics in children. As Koupernik, MacKeith, and Francis-Williams (1975) have stated:

Certainly not all high activity is associated with distractibility, impulsivity, learning difficulties. Some of the situations in which high activity are seen are: (1) most normal two- or three- year old children (2) other children with mental age of two or three years (3) highly intelligent children with a strong exploratory drive (4) children reacting to environmental influences such as nagging by a parent or teacher (5) anxious children (6) some depressed children (7) many deprived children, especially those who are also mentally handicapped. [P. 121]

Kornetsky (1975) advanced a similar point when he stated that

. . . the terms used to define the characteristics are terms used to describe, to a lesser or greater degree, the behavior of all children at some time. [P. 453]

It is little wonder, in view of these definitional problems, that studies continue to report discrepant findings with respect to etiology, behavioral and electrophysiological correlates, and prognosis. Many of these target children are most probably misdiagnosed as hyperactive, which would tend to obscure group differences on diagnostic and treatment variables. It would also tend to obscure attempts to derive meaningful subtypes within the concept of hyperactivity if a significant number of the children were not hyperactive. This point will be addressed later.

Maturation Problems

The concept of maturation as it relates to developmental hyperactivity has yet to be fully understood. Yet this concept continues to be suggested as a possible clue in the etiology of this disorder and more remotely, to reading and learning disabilities. The concept of maturation also raises the question as to whether the performance or performance or behavioral decrements in hyperactive children are best explained in terms of an individual difference, delay, or deficit model (Kinsbourne, 1975).

Developmental hyperactivity is characterized by the following maturational phenomena.

Developmental Course

Most investigators have reported that the hyperactivity commences in early to midchildhood (ages 2 to 6) and begins to fade during adolescence at which time signs of learning, emotional, or antisocial problems become more prominent in many of the children (Fine, 1977; Safer and Allen, 1976; Minde, Weiss, and Mendelson, 1972; Weiss, et al., 1971; Dykman, Peters, and Ackerman, 1973; Mendelson, Johnson, and Stewart, 1971; Laufer, 1972). Variables that have an adverse influence on these later outcome results are low IQ, grade repeats, poor reading skill, and poor emotional adjustment during childhood (Safer and Allen, 1976; Minde, Weiss, and Mendelson, 1972).

Resemblance to Younger Developmental Behavior Patterns

Investigators have long reported that symptoms of hyperactivity, distractibility, and impulsivity represent normal developmental patterns in younger children (Koupernik, MacKeith, and Francis-Williams, 1975; Kornetsky, 1975; Kagan, 1965; Fine, 1977; Kinsbournce, 1973). It is only when these behavioral patterns persist into late childhood that they are considered developmental deviations. During infancy behavior is less organized and differentiated, particularly in the control and modulation of motor and attentional systems (Werner, 1957; Caldwell, 1968; Piaget, 1952). This is also the period in which the immature brain is undergoing enormous structural, electro-physiological, and biochemical changes (Lenneberg, 1967; Geschwind, 1974).

Developmental psychologists such as Werner (1957) have stated that,

> wherever development occurs it proceeds from a state of relative globality and lack of differentiation to a state of increasing differentiation, articulation, and hierarchic integration. [P. 126]

As the individual progresses through the sensorimotor, perceptual, and conceptual phases of development, each earlier phase is presumed to become reorganized in a way that permits it to become hierarchically integrated within the subsequent, higher phase. This position is compatible with the views of Bruner (1968) and Piaget (1952) which postulate that the transition to symbolic representation marks the final and most important stage in cognitive development. This later ontogenic stage frees the child from dependence upon the concrete and immediate aspects of perceptual representation and, through language internalization, facilitates a so-called second-signal system (Luria, 1973) in which experience can

be both represented and transformed. Witkin's (1962) concept of field dependence-independence is also compatible with this developmental position. Witkin
(1962) has suggested that the constuct of field-dependence represents the primary
cognitive style of younger normal children characterized by a more global and less
differentiated perceptual mode. This particular approach to problem-solving situations is often associated with

. . . impulse control problems, a poorly developed sense of responsibility and a lack of
resources and initiative. [Witkin, 1962, p. 212-213]

Kagan's (1965) work on impulsivity-reflectivity also sheds additional light on the
importance of maturational factors and cognitive styles in developmental hyperactivity. Kagan has shown that the normal impulsive child differs from the reflective child by his greater physical activity, higher distractibility, and poorer control
of attentive and motor processes in problem situations with high response uncertainty. Kagan also states that

. . . the results are persuasive insuggesting that a tendency for reflection increases with
age, is stable over periods as long as 20 months, manifests pervasive generality across
varied task situations, and is linked to some fundamental aspects of the child's personality
organization. [P. 134]

The preceding findings, in summary, show that many of the physical symptoms
of developmental hyperactivity recede during early adolescence when the brain is
known to reach more mature levels of maturation and cerebral lateralization
(Lenneberg, 1967; Luria, 1973). The findings also suggest that many of the behavioral characteristics of hyperactivity, distractibility, impulsivity, and inattention
seen in older hyperactive children are also observed in younger normal children.
Consequently when these less mature and differentiated behavioral patterns are
shown to persist into late childhood (and are associated with learning disabilities),
a lag in brain maturation and/or cognitive development has been postulated to
underlie the disorder (Bender, 1958).

Neurological Studies

Four recent studies have reported evidence of a lag in neurological development
in children labeled as learning disabled and/or hyperactive. Dykman, et al., (1971)
conducted an extensive neurological examination of 82 learning disabled boys and
34 normal controls (boys) between the ages of 8 and 12. Children with IQs less
than 90 and with evidence of gross physical defects were excluded from the study.
Approximately one-third of the learning disabled group were labeled as hyperactive. The examination consisted of classical responses (choreiform jerks, athetoid
movements, diadochokinesis, visual and cranial nerve integrity, and so on) and
paraclassical (soft) responses (mixed laterality, directionality, two-point tactile
discrimination, finger agnosia, and so on). Results showed that responses to both
the classical and paraclassical times differentiated groups. The most intriguing
finding, according to the authors, was the age factor. When learning-disability
children were divided into two age groups of below 10 years and over 10, it was
found that the older group differed significantly from the controls on only 11 of the
45 items that discriminated all learning-disability children and controls. The fact
that the older learning-disability group (> 10 years) had fewer signs than the

younger learning-disability group (<10 years) was interpreted as evidence of a neurodevelopmental lag.

Similar age effects were reported recently by Peters, Romine, and Dykman (1975). An extensive neurological examination was administered to 82 learning-disabled boys and 45 normal controls (boys) between the ages of 8 and 11. Children with IQs less than 90 and with evidence of gross physical defects were excluded from the study. Approximately one-third of the learning-disabled group were labelled as hyperactive. In contrast approximately 75% of the index cases revealed a significant reading disability. The results showed that over half of the items in the special neurological examination discriminated groups with the learning-disability group showing the positive findings. When the results were computed by age it was again shown that with increasing age the incidence of special neurological signs decreased in children with learning disabilities. In other words, more of the neurological items discriminated groups at the younger ages (< 10 years) than at the older ages (> 10 years). The younger index children showed four times the number of discriminatory signs compared with the older learning disabled and control Ss. According to the authors,

These findings indicate that children with learning difficulties tend to have a delay in motor development and that improvement occurs first in gross motor functioning and body orientation. This developmental delay is assumed to be due to a delay in neurological maturation. [P. 74]

Additional support for the concept of an underlying physiological imaturity in learning-disabled children was demonstrated through estimates of bone-age development (Oettinger, et al., 1974). Single anterior-posterior X-rays of the left wrist and hand were evaluated on ''. . . 53 children diagnosed as having minimal brain dysfunction by the criteria of Clements (1966).'' X-ray films were read independently by three physicians (two radiologists and an endrocrinologist) familiar with interpretation of bone-age radiographs. These radiographs were then compared to a standard chart. Unfortunately no separate control was used nor were subjects divided into different age categories within groups. The results revealed an overall discrepancy between mean chronological age (8.5 years) and mean bone age (8.0 years). In approximately two-thirds of the MBD children, bone age was lower than chronological age. Ten of these children had bone ages which were more than two standard deviations below the norm, while one had a significant increase in bone age. This study, while subject to a number of methodological flaws, suggests that the technique of bone-age radiographs could provide more direct test of physiological maturation in hyperactive/learning-disabled children.

Denckla and Rudel (1977) reported similar developmental anomolies of motor function in a group of hyperactive children without evidence of learning disability. A brief motor examination was administered to 82 hyperactive boys between the ages of 5 and 12. Performance was then compared to normative data collected by the authors on normal children in the same age range. The motor tasks included toe-tapping, heel-toe alteration, hand patting, hand pronation-supination, finger-to-thumb repetitive, and successive finger-to-thumb oppositions. Results showed that performance on these motor tasks discriminated hyperactive and control groups only at the younger ages (ages 7 to 9), not at the older ages (ages 10 to 12). The authors found that a floor effect occurred at the youngest ages (5 to 6) in both groups, rendering these measures insensitive as discriminators. However the measures revealed robust differences in the middle-age range (ages 7 to 9) when motor coordination in children is normally taking a developmental spurt. At these ages the younger hyperactive boys were significantly delayed relative to their younger controls.

Electrophysiological Studies

A number of EEG studies have reported an increased incidence of abnormal findings in hyperactive/learning-disabled children (Stamm, 1977). Despite numerous methodological and conceptual problems in this research (Hughes, 1978; Denckla, 1978), studies have often reported patterns of occipital or diffuse slow wave activity in some of these children (Gross and Wilson, 1974; Capute, Niedermeyer, and Richardson, 1968; Hughes, 1971; Hughes and Park, 1968; Ingram, Mason and Blackburn, 1970; Satterfield, 1973; Stevens, et al., 1968; Wikler, Dixon, and Parker, 1970). This wave from pattern is of particular interest because it has been shown to decline with age (Gibbs and Gibbs, 1951). In fact excessive slow wave activity, when present, is more commonly seen in younger normal and older hyperactive children (Satterfield, 1973).

Studies using auditory-or visual-evoked potentials have also reported more immature responses in hyperactive/learning-disabled children. For example Satterfield (1973) found a significant increase in latency of the auditory-evoked response (AER) in a small group of MBD (that is hyperactive/learning-disabled) children who were matched for age and sex with a group of normal children. Although WISC Full Scale IQs were in the average range in both groups, the MBD children had significantly lower IQs (118 versus 104). The fact that AER latencies have been shown to decrease with age in normal children (Schenkenberg, 1970; Dustman and Beck, 1969) led Satterfield to postulate a delay in central nervous system maturation in some MBD children. This delay hypothesis was further strengthened by the greater response to amphetamine treatment in those children who showed evidence of both excessive EEG slow wave activity and soft signs on the neurological examination.

More direct support for this hypothesis was reported by Buchsbaum and Wender (1973). Visual and auditory-average-evoked responses (AERs) were studied in 24 children vaguely defined as MBD and 24 age- and sex-matched normal controls. The MBD children showed AERs characteristic of relatively younger normal children. For example the MBD children revealed larger amplitude-evoked responses than the normal children in the visual intensity experiment. In addition the normal children had a slower rate of increase of amplitude with increasing stimulus intensity than the MBD children. Also when analyses were made on latencies of the AER, the normal group showed evoked responses (P200) which decreased in latency with increasing intensity, whereas the MBD group showed evoked responses which increased in latency with increased stimulus intensity. Of particular significance was the relationship between AER and response-to-amphetamine treatment. Those MBD children who showed a positive drug response also showed the more immature AER patterns at pretreatment.

Buchsbaum and Wender (1973) suggested that the results provided indirect support for the concept of delayed CNS maturation in some hyperactive/learning-disabled children. They did however note certain interpretive problems regarding the amplitude differences. According to the authors:

Amplitude may be a function of a-frequency, slower frequencies being associated with greater AER amplitudes. Previous studies have shown that MBD children as a group have slower a-frequencies than age-matched controls. Since a-frequency increases with age and since AER amplitude decreases with age, the finding of greater AER amplitude in MBD children may be another reflection of age-related increases in a-frequency. Again, MBD appears associated with having electroencephalographic and AER characteristics typical of younger children. [1973, p. 770]

Critique of Neurological and Electrophysiological Studies

Despite the appeal which these results give to the concept of a neuromaturational lag, a number of methodological and theoretical problems still remain. First, selection criteria for the target children continue to be poorly defined. To label a child MBD, as in the Buchsbaum and Wender (1973), Oettinger, et al., (1974), and Satterfield (1973) studies tells us absolutely nothing about what types of children were selected. For example were behavioral (hyperactivity) and/or academic (reading/learning) problems included and—if so—in what proportions? Also, loosely defined selection criteria will most probably increase variability within the index group and wash out between group effects. More seriously it could subject certain children, incorrectly labeled as MBD or hyperactive, to unnecessary risk in the measurement or treatment condition. This risk was most probably present in both the bone-age (Oettinger, et al., 1974) and amphetamine studies (Buchsbaum and Wender, 1973; Satterfield, 1973). Approximately one-third to one-half of the subjects in these studies failed to show the measurement or treatment effect.

Second, in virtually all of these studies the children were not matched or equated on IQ level. Selection of children (index and controls) with IQs greater than 85 provides no control for between-group differences on this variable. In such studies the index group, while of average intelligence, is still 10 to 20 IQ points lower than the control group (Satz, Friel, and Rudegeair, 1976). Nor have attempts been made to partial out the effects of these IQ differences on the dependent measures when they occur. Third, studies on developmental age effects may easily be confounded by floor and/or ceiling effects in the tasks. This is particularly true of the neurological studies which reported differences between younger and older learning disabled and/or hyperactive children (Dykman, Ackerman, Clements, and Peters, 1971; Peters, Romine, and Dykman, 1975; Denckla and Rudel, 1977. Floor effects, as in the youngest age group in the Denckla and Rudel study (1977), means that the tasks were inappropriate or insensitive as discriminators at these ages (5 to 6). In contrast ceiling effects may have occurred in the older age groups of the Dykman, Peters, and Ackerman, (1971) and Peters, Romine, and Dykman (1975) studies which may have accounted for the ease with which the older index and control cases performed on these measures. In fact, if the items were too easy for the older children, then one would be unable to separate out delay from deficit effects. This problem speaks to the broader issue of appropriate age norms for any task variable, behavioral or electrophysiological —particularly when comparisons to younger normal children are invoked.

Fourth, in none of the studies have repeated measurements been made on the same children over time. Virtually all of the studies have employed cross-sectional designs, on small groups of children, which increases the chance of sampling bias in the between-age comparisons. Longitudinal studies, based preferably on representative normal samples, would provide more valid information of developmental changes in the characteristic with age, which would then allow one to address the more difficult question of delay versus deficit hypotheses in hyperactive/learning-disability children (Rourke, 1976; Fletcher and Satz, 1978). This latter issue leads to the fifth problem which is basically theoretical. In what context and how is a difference, when it occurs, to be interpeted? The preceding studies were selected not because of their methodological merits, but because of their results. If correct, they provided compelling alternatives to the deficit explanations that have dominated the research literature in this area. To assume that an observed difference, when it occurs between index and control cases, is due to an underlying defect in the CNS is both reckless and unwarranted, regardless of whether the difference is based on behavioral and/or electrophysiological evidence. At the present time we lack substantial understanding of the normal developmental acquisition rates in most of our tests. This is particularly true for the electrophysiological measures (Dustman and Beck, 1969). Lacking this information should caution any attempts, premature or otherwise, to invoke explanations based on unobserved and inferred CNS etiologies. Such explanations, while probably true for some hyperactive/learning-disability children, should not be entertained until alternative delay hypotheses have also been evaluated. Even then interpretations can be obscured by failure to designate what is meant by a difference when the associated event or performance is construed neither as a deficit nor a delay. Kinsbourne (1975) defines the difference model as follows:

Individual differences are no less to be expected in cognitive than in physical development. Differences in not only the child's overall intelligence but also the degree of excellence he achieves with respect to the various components of that intelligence can exist. Just like adults, some children will show more aptitude for verbal tasks, others for spatial tasks. Some will be more systematic, others more creative. . . . The difference model, then, deals in variability of brain development (genetic component) but emphasizes the interaction between early experience and learning skills. [P. 1066]

The preceding reference to difference and delay models in learning disability is made to illustrate equally viable alternative approaches to the deficit model. As Divorky (1974) has said:

To see every variation from the norm as a 'disability' is to remorselessly limit the boundaries of what passes for normalcy. And to treat what are in fact social problems— nonreaders, nonconformists, nonstudents—as medical problems is to admit the bankruptcy of both the schools and the society in finding real solutions. [P. 25]

In a recent review of this literature, Hallahan (1975) came to a similar view:

. . . because of the generally pervasive problems related to methodology and because of the relatively recent movement toward using experimental laboratory tasks instead of standardized tests, we find ourselves in an extremely primitive stage of knowledge concerning the psychological characteristics (i.e., differences) of learning disabled compared to normal children. [P. 53]

Hallahan (1975) argued that the developing field of learning disabilities might be able to profit from some of the concepts advanced from the field of mental retardation:

For many years, the comparative studies within mental retardation were confined to comparisons between retardates and normals equated on on CA. Lower task scores by retardates in these situations resulted in the inference that they were different or defective in comparison to normals. Zigler (1969), however, has popularized another research paradigm and has claimed that when educable retardates are equated with normals on MA, no differences obtain. Zigler thus has proposed a developmental theory of educable mental retardation which in his estimation directly opposes those theories which hold that retardates are defective or different from normals. [P. 54]

Zigler's (1969) position is as follows:

Employing a stage or levels approach to cognitive development, the normal variation viewpoint generated in my thinking the rather parsimonious view that the cognitive development of the familially retarded is characterized by a slower progression through the same sequence of cognitive stages (a rate phenomenon) and a more limited upper stage of cognition (a levels phenomenon) than is characteristic of the individual of average intellect. [P. 537]

Zigler's developmental model of cognitive growth (1969) can be seen in Figure 27–2. The single vertical arrow represents the passage of time. The horizontal arrows represent environmental events impinging on the individual who is represented as a pair of vertical lines. The individual's cognitive development appears as an internal ascending spiral, in which the numbered loops represent successive stages of cognitive growth.

Although Zigler recognized some of the simplicity and ambiguity in the model, it does represent a formal and testable alternative to the deficit model discussed in this chapter. Of most importance, the model incorporates both a rate factor (delayed acquisition of cognitive stages) and a levels factor (a more limited upper stage of cognition) which, in essence, correspond to the delay and difference models discussed by Kinsbourne (1976).

The model as stated makes specific predictions regarding the performance of educable retardates and normals. When matched on MA, the developmental model predicts no difference in psychological performance between older retardates and younger controls. The value of this model is that it could be directly applied to the field of learning disabilities by simply matching index and control cases on achievement measures and, perhaps, IQ level. Consequently a defect model would predict group differences dispite this matching procedure, whereas a developmental delay model would predict similar performance between groups. One should note that this matching procedure would generate a comparison test between older learning disabled and younger normal control children. Similar performance between groups would suggest that although learning-disabled children progress slower in those psychological abilities important for achievement, they do pass through the same stages of development. A more likely outcome might be that the predictions vary as a function of the type of cognitive task sampled. For example skills which have an earlier and faster rate of acquisition ontogenetically (such as sensori-motor perceptual) might yield negligible group differences in line with Zigler's developmental model. However skills which have a slower and later rate of acquisition ontogenetically (such as syntactic and semantic language) may continue to reveal differences after this matching strategy. Unfortunately these concepts have yet to be applied to hyperactive/learning-disabled children. Preliminary applications of these concepts will be discussed and evaluated in the following section.

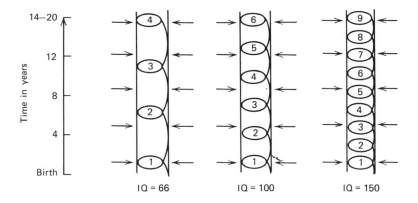

Figure 27–2. Developmental model of cognitive growth. The single vertical arrow represents the passage of time. The horizontal arrows represent environmental events impinging on the individual who is represented as a pair of vertical lines. The individual's cognitive development appears as an internal ascending spiral, in which the numbered loops represent successive stages of cognitive growth.

READING AND LEARNING DISABILITIES

Definition and Epidemiology

It would appear that the problem of defining reading/learning disabilities would prove a relatively simple task. The major identifying characteristic of these children is academic underachievement, so that operationalizing the meaning of academic underachievement should be straightforward. However the difficulty of providing an adequate definition of these disabilities has led to many of the problems discribed for MBD and hyperactivity/learning disabilities. Once again it is evident that a very heterogeneous group of children falls under the rubric of reading/learning disabilities. As a consequence considerable controversy exists concerning the definition of these disabilities.

One simple approach to the definition merely specifies the degree of academic underachievement necessary to label a child disabled. For example reading disabilities are often defined as a two-year lag in reading achievement relative to the child's age. This definition has at least made epidemological studies possible and it is known that the prevalence of severe reading disabilities in the United States and northern Europe is about 15% (Kline, 1972; Satz, et al., 1978). The empirical basis for these estimates however has come under serious criticism.

> Definitions differ and classifications differ, depending upon whether they are based upon a medical or educational model; or whether they are based primarily on cause, symptoms or treatment. [CELDIC Report, 1970, p. 51]

Many of these prevalence studies are based on highly selected samples that fail to differentiate backward readers from children who have specific reading handicaps (Rutter, 1978). Despite these definitional problems, the consistency of these estimates in recent years is more prominent than their variability (CELDIC Report, 1970).

A more serious problem with this definition is that merely specifying a discrepancy in age and achievement obscures the meaning of reading/learning disabilities. These disabilities are also notable because they are somehow unexpected or specific. In other words these disabilities arise in children who are apparently capable of age-appropriate achievement. In addition these disabilities are presumably specific, that is involve no additional disabilities. The attempt to embody these characteristics is a prominent feature of almost every definition of reading/learning disabilities. This worthy attempt is exemplified by the World Federation of Neurology definition of specific developmental dyslexia:

A disorder manifested by difficulties in learning to read despite conventional instruction, adequate intelligence, and socio-economic opportunity. It is dependent upon fundamental cognitive disabilities which are frequently of constitutional origin. [Critchley, 1970, p. 11]

The problems with this definition are multiple and apply to most definitions of reading/learning disabilities. Almost all definitions define by exclusion, that is merely specify what the disabilities are not (Benton, 1975; Doehring, 1978; Ross, 1976; Rutter, 1978). Ross (1976) attributed the following problems to exclusionary definitions:

Stripped of clauses which specify what a learning disability is not, this definition is circular, for it states, in essence, that a learning disability is an inability to learn. It is a reflection of the rudimentary state of knowledge in this field that every definition in current use has its focus on what the condition is not, leaving what it is unspecified and thus ambiguous. [P. 11]

Rutter (1978) described additional problems with exclusionary definitions in a broadly based critique of the World Federation of Neurology definition of specific developmental dyslexia. He subdivided this definition into three components: (1) the exclusionary criteria; (2) concept of cognitive deficits; and (3) concept of constitutional origin. The first part of this definition, Rutter argued, merely begs the question on several issues. It fails to specify the meaning of conventional instruction, average intelligence, and sociocultural opportunity. As Rutter observed, the exclusionary criteria

suggest that if all the known causes of reading disability can be ruled out, the unknown (in the form of dyslexia) should be invoked. [P. 9]

Rutter noted that the second part of the definition is more helpful since it makes a statement about cognitive characteristics present in the disability. However he also noted that

without further elaboration, this is too vague to be at all helpful in the individual child. [P. 10]

In other words a wide variety of cognitive deficits are correlated with reading disabilities, all of which are not present in each child. These correlated deficits may change with age and the reading problem may persist even when these developmental deficits are no longer apparent (Fletcher and Satz, 1978, 1979).

The third part of this definition, concerning constitutional origins, was criticized by Rutter because of the vagueness of this clause. As Rutter observed, constitutional factors may be prominent for many reading problems, dyslexic or not. For example studies concerning a genetic component are helpful for evaluating constitutional factors. They generally show that reading disorders "run in the family" and affect more boys than girls (4:1 ratio). However definition and sampling methods vary greatly from study to study. Moreover these studies are not overly helpful in partitioning biological and social factors. Other constitutional factors, especially neurological theories, are often vague speculations and as Benton (1975) observed, nothing more than slogans.

Rutter concluded

that the World Federation of Neurology attempt to provide an operational definition for dyslexia is unsatisfactory and unworkable. It is not that the basic notions are unsound but rather that not only does the definition fall short on logic . . . but also it fails to provide effective guidance for today's clinical practice. [P. 11]

The problems Rutter described are similar to those illustrated for the MBD concept. The consequences of these problems are also similar. Different target children will be used from study to study. Unproven etiological theories will become hypostasized and will inappropriately guide clinical practice. Most important the basic work in classification will not be completed because of the pervasiveness of this definition. The target children under the reading/learning disabilities rubric are heterogeneous and may represent several distinctive subtypes of disability. In this respect Rutter described three basic distinctions that must guide attempts to classify reading/learning disabilities. First, initial failure to learn these academic skills must be distinguished from later loss because of a failure to make sufficient scholastic progress. Second, the range of academic strengths and weaknesses must be described more fully. Children with reading problems may or may not suffer deficiencies in mathemates and spelling. It might be added that children with reading problems may or may not present additional behavioral or neurological problems (for example hyperactivity or soft neurological signs). The third distinction represents Rutter's starting point for classification. It concerns a

basic distinction between *general backwardness* (i.e., low achievement in relation to the average for that age, but withoug taking IQ into account) and *specific retardation* (i.e., achievement which is low after taking both age and IQ into account. [Rutter, 1978, p. 12]

The value of this distinction is twofold. Reading problems may be further classified according to: (1) patterns of cognitive functioning and (2) presumed etiology (for example presence or absence of brain damage, SES, and so on).

A review of research concerning the classification problem is beyond the scope of this chapter. The point has been to illustrate definitional problems and their impact on reading/learning disabilities.

Major Research Thrusts

In concluding the section on hyperactivity/learning disabilities it was suggested that the behavioral characteristics of these disabilities may vary with the age (and cognitive level) of the child. For this section the possibility of age-dependent relationships in the behavioral correlates of reading/learning disabilities will be explored. Age-dependency is another way of referring to developmental change, an important aspect of research and theory on cognitive development. In general developmental changes represent shifts in the rate of acquisition and the importance of different cognitive abilities underlying the acquisition of information-processing skills. These changes can be described for the acquisition of language

(Palermo and Molfese, 1972), memory (Hagen, Jongeward, and Kail, 1975), and reading (Doehring, 1976; Gibson and Levin, 1975).

The importance of developmental changes for reading/learning disabilities research accrues from the need to consider developmental factors for interpreting the multiple correlates of these disabilities. Several recent reviews of research on reading/learning disabilities (Benton, 1975; Hallahan, 1975; Torgesen, 1975; Vellutino, 1978) attest to the number and variety of behavioral factors associated with these disabilities. However interpreting these differences may depend on the age and cognitive level of the child. Torgesen (1975) clearly implicated the importance of these developmental factors by suggesting that

> studies using subjects at one age may identify deficits associated with reading disability which are different from those found at other ages. [P. 421]

From a methodological standpoint failure to recognize, control, and appropriately manipulate the age variable may distort research outcomes. Moreover investigating possible age-dependent relationships may help to interpret the multiple behavioral correlates of these disabilities (Satz, et al., 1978).

A substantive review of literature on reading/learning disabilities is beyond the scope of this chapter. Rather the current status of research in two areas will be reviewed. These areas concern: (1) the perceptual-deficit hypothesis and (2) the linguistic-deficit hypothesis. In some respects different versions of these hypotheses jointly dominate reading/learning disabilities research and are sometimes viewed as competing (Vellutino, 1978). The purpose of reviewing these two areas of research is to illustrate the importance of developmental factors for interpreting the performance correlates of these disabilities. In addition an attempt will be made to illustrate some additional methodological problems that may potentially retard research in reading/learning disabilities.

Perceptual-Deficit Hypothesis

The hypothesis that reading/learning disabilities result from a basic deficiency in visual-perceptual function was advanced as early as 1917 (Bronner). Orton (1937) expanded the perceptual-deficit hypothesis by relating it to the reading errors of disabled readers and to hypotheses concerning incomplete cerebral dominance (Satz, 1976). The perceptual-deficit hypothesis is still prominent and the subject of considerable controversy, as witnessed by at least four major reviews since 1975 (Benton, 1975; Hallahan, 1975; Torgesen, 1975; Vellutino, 1978). Of these reviews, Hallahan (1975) accepts the traditional viewpoint and concludes that deficits in visual-perceptual function play a major role in reading/learning disabilities. Torgesen (1975) concludes that although disabled readers seem to perform more poorly on measures of perceptual function, this relationship is complex and does not provide useful information for remediation. Benton (1975) reiterates the conclusion of an earlier review (Benton, 1962), concluding that the relationship between visual-perceptual skills and reading disorders is weak. If there is a relationship, Benton (1962, 1975) concludes that it exists primarily for younger reading groups, which does not explain the persistence of reading disabilities into adolescence. Vellutino (1978) actually accepts the null hypothesis and concludes that visuo-spatial skills are unrelated to reading failure. He concludes that reading disabilities are due to a primary defect in verbal mediation.

The different conclusions reached by these reviews show that there is considerable controversy concerning the perceptual-deficit hypothesis. The data are conflicting and the studies concerning this problem present a number of methodological and conceptual problems. In this section several major studies supporting the alternative interpretations of the perceptual-deficit hypothesis will be reviewed to show how methodological and conceptual problems may have inflamed the controversy.

THERE IS NO PERCEPTUAL DEFICIT.   Vellutino (1978) has argued most convincingly against the perceptual-deficit hypothesis. His point of view is consistent with several other studies which apparently found no evidence for a perceptual deficit in disabled readers (Denckla and Rudel, 1976; Liberman and Shankweiler, 1976; Symes and Rapoport, 1972). Although Vellutino (1978) reviewed many studies concerning the perceptual-deficit hypotheses, the strongest support for his position derived from three studies which attempted critical tests of the perceptual deficit hypothesis (Allington, Gormley, and Truex, 1976; Vellutino, Smith, Steger and Kaman, 1975; Vellutino, Steger, and Kandel, 1972). Although these studies are interpreted as evidence against the perceptual-deficit hypothesis, a closer examination reveals that certain empirical and theoretical factors limit the degree to which these studies refute the hypothesis.

The basic procedure for each of these three studies comprised a comparison of good and poor readers on recognition tasks defined as visual-visual, visual-verbal, and verbal-verbal. Visual-visual tasks required reading groups to copy visually presented geometric designs, while visual-verbal tasks required copying and naming of visually presented scrambled letters and words. The verbal-verbal task required pronunciation of visually presented words. Because good and poor readers apparently performed equally well on the visual-visual and visual-verbal tasks, it was concluded that "poor readers do not necessarily sustain a visual-spatial deficit" (Allington, et al., 1976, p. 295). In contrast to these null (not negative) results, good and poor readers differed significantly on the verbal-verbal task, which led the authors to argue for a verbal-mediational deficit.

This research, which has been widely accepted as disproving the visual-spatial-deficit hypothesis, may be criticized at the level of constuct validation (cf. Fletcher and Satz, 1979). For example visual-visual and visual-verbal tasks required recognition and memory processing by the children. Consequently differences on these tasks would be confounded by this memory component. In addition the visual-verbal task was a simply letter-copying task. This type of test has seldom been employed as a measure of visual-perceptual processing and sensitivity of such a task to the perceptual and discrimination skills involved in learning to read (cf. Gibson and Levin, 1975) is certainly questionable. These skills involve more than the simple optical confusions and letter reversals often interpreted as visual-spatial processing errors (Denckla and Rudel, 1976; Shankweiler and Liberman, 1972; Vellutino, Steger, and Kandel, 1972; Vellutino, et al., 1975).

Problems with construct validity are also apparent for the verbal-verbal (pronunciation) task. Since pronunciation of words could involve several phonological and semantic strategies, the nature of verbal-mediation required by the verbal-verbal task is difficult to specify. Moreover the reading measures used to form the comparison groups were based in part on word recognition. As such performance on the verbal-verbal task (pronunciation) was probably highly correlated with the reading criterion, in effect stacking the cards in favor of accepting the null hypothesis. Although pronouncing letters and words is integral to certain aspects of reading, differences between groups defined on the basis of word recognition sheds little light on the underlying nature of the disability.

Additional problems with test ceilings affect the interpretation of these three studies. In reviewing these studies Benton (1975) noted that copying and naming letters are rather easy tasks, even for 8- and 12-year old children. As such ceiling effects on the visual-verbal tasks may have occurred because of the reduced stimulus demands. In the Vellutino, Steger, and Kandel (1972) and Vellutino, et al. (1975) studies, reading groups at all ages were generally correct in 90 to 100% of their responses in most conditions. Such high levels of performance could easily mask potential group differences on the visual-verbal tasks. The only condition in which a ceiling effect was not evident was for the second-grade poor readers used by Vellutino, et al. (1975). In this study increased task complexity (number of letters) for naming and copying letters produced statistically significant differences between good and poor readers. The results, which were compatible with a visual-copying deficit in the younger disabled reader groups (if the construct dimensions of the task are accepted) were dismissed by Vellutino, et al., (1975).

These methodological problems, involving construct validity and ceiling/floor effects limit the degree to which these three studies refute the perceptual deficit hypothesis. It is notable that few of the studies reviewed by Vellutino (1978) considered chronological age as a variable for interpreting their findings. For example Shankweiler and Liberman (1972) observed that reversal errors accounted for a very small proportion of the oral reading of good and poor second-grade readers. Since reversal errors are often interpreted as indicants of perceptual processing, the authors concluded that visual-perceptual skills are not an important component of reading disabilities. However reversal errors are more prominent in normal children learning to read in kindergarten and the first grade. Futhermore this period (ages 5 to 7) accounts for much of the basic development of those perceptual skills involved in learning to read. Therefore it is unlikely that second-grade children would show a high proportion of reversal errors, since they are beyond this stage of learning to read. Similar problems, especially concerning the age factor, are apparent for other studies which accept the null hypothesis (Denckla and Rudel, 1976; Symes and Rapoport, 1972).

THERE IS A PERCEPTUAL DEFICIT.   Hallahan (1975) and Hallahan and Cruickshank (1973) concluded that deficits in visual-perceptual functioning play a major role in reading and learning disabilities. On the basis of their conclusion, they also justified training programs to remediate these deficits and presumably, the reading disability. There are a number of problems with this conclusion. First, many of the problems with construct validity described for the Vellutino, Steger, and Kandel (1972) and Vellutino, et al., (1975) studies also affect studies which find evidence for a perceptual deficit. This problem is particularly apparent for studies which use a psychometric measure as the measure of visual-perceptual function. For example the measurement characteristics of the Bender Gestalt are poorly defined. Although it does seem related to reading disabilities, the basis for this relationship is obscure (cf. Torgesen, 1975). Excution of the Bender designs requires perceptual synthesis and integration of motor and conceptual operations. It is difficult to simply accept the Bender Gestalt as a measure of visual perceptual functioning. Second, there are many studies which find no evidence for deficits on these skills (cf. Benton, 1975; Vellutino, 1978). The absence of differences on the visual-visual (design-copying) task employed by Vellutino, Steger, and Kandel, (1972) and Vellutino, et al., (1975) is a case in point. Finally, as Vellutino, et al., (1977) conclude, evidence that perceptual-motor training remediates the disorder is limited and certainly does not justify the extent to which these programs are employed.

CRITIQUE: A DEVELOPMENTAL INTERPRETATION   In reviewing the literature concerning the perceptual deficit hypothesis, it is evident that only limited progress has been made since Orton (1937) regarding its evaluation. The paradigm for much of this research assumes that a single psychological deficit can explain both the reading/learning problems and a wide variety of correlative deficits. If the perceptual deficit is viewed as one of many skills which are correlated with reading/learning disabilities, the studies tend to fall into place. The most obvious fact is that some studies find evidence for perceptual problems in disabled readers, while others do not. Benton (1962) first noted that perceptual problems were more often found by studies employing younger reading groups (age 7 to 8) than in studies employing older reading groups (ages 9 to 11). As such it may be that perceptual problems are more characteristic of younger children with reading/learning disabilities.

More recent studies support this notion, showing that measures of visual-perceptual discrimination skills are predictive of reading/learning disabilities in younger children. These studies also suggest that the relationship of these skills to reading/learning disabilities diminishes with age. Rourke and Orr (1977) addressed the relative accuracy of a number of reading and spelling tests, two measures of psychometric intelligence (WISC and PPVT) and a speeded visual-discrimination task (Underlining Test) in predicting reading achievement (4 years) from grades 1 to 2 (ages 7 to 8) to grades 4 to 5 (ages 11 to 12). Results of the stepwise regression analysis showed that performance on the Underlining Test was

. . . a far more potent means of identifying retarded readers who are 'at risk' (at ages 7-8) with respect to eventual reading and spelling achievement (at ages 11-12) than are the measures of psychometric intelligence, reading, or spelling which were used. [P. 18]

Sabatino and Hayden (1970) conducted a principle component analysis of several psycholinguistic and perceptual measures which were given to a younger (ages 7 to 9) and older (ages 11 to 14) group of disabled learners (N=472). They identified a primary loading on perceptual deficits in the younger children and a psycholinguistic deficit in the older children. Consistent with the developmental hypotheses already discussed, the authors concluded

. . . that six years to nine years is the maximum growth period for perceptual functional performance. After age 10, integrated language skills become of prime importance. [P. 411]

Gruen (1972) compared the predictive accuracy of a battery of perceptual-motor and cognitive-intellectual tasks administered to a large group of first-grade (N=204) and third-grade Ss (N=202) in a one-year follow-up. Multiple regression analyses showed that the perceptual-motor tests accounted for more of the explained variation in reading achievement scores (vocabulary and comprehension) for first-grade boys and girls. In contrast the cognitive-intellectual tests accounted for more of the explained variation in reading achievement scores (vocabulary and comprehension) for third-grade boys and girls.

Sobotka, Black, Hill and Porter, (1977) conducted a cross-sectional study comparing reading disabled and nondisabled children at ages 7, 9, 11, and 13 years on a variety of perceptual and linguistic measures. This study is remarkable in terms of the care taken to define cases of pure reading disability. Over 400 disabled readers were screened to exclude children with reading problems attributable to cultural deprivation, intellectual and neurological impairment, and emotional disorders. Results indicated that group differences on the perceptual measures (WISC Performance Scale, Bender Gestalt) were more apparent at ages 7 and 9, diminishing by age 11. These results replicate earlier cross-sectional studies (Satz, Rardin, and Ross, 1971; Satz and Van Nostrand, 1973) which employed less rigorous selection criteria for reading level.

A recent six-year longitudinal study (Fletcher and Satz, 1978) provided strong support for developmental changes in the relationship of perceptual (and linguistic) skills to reading achievement. For this study the entire kindergarten population of white males (N=497) entering school in Alachua County, Florida, was administered a battery of tests assessing a variety of perceptual and linguistic skills. Repeat administrations of these tests (with adjustments for floor and ceiling effects) and representative reading achievement measures were obtained on a large proportion of these children (at least 85%) at the end of grades 2 and 5 (3- and 6-year follow-up). Both the 3- and 6-year follow-ups (age 5 to ages 8 and 11) revealed that the greater proportion of the predictive validity of the test battery was explained by measures of sensorimotor-perceptual ability. However with advances in age, the relationship (concurrent validity) between these measures receded, with other (largely linguistic) measures accounting for more of the variability in reading achievement.

In summarizing this evidence developmental changes in the relationship of perceptual skills to reading achievement are apparent. These skills have a higher correlational (and predictive) relationship with reading achievement prior to age seven. After this age the magnitude of this relationship diminishes. The reasons for this relationship are not clear. At least two factors seem important. Visual-perceptual motor skills develop primarily between ages three to nine (cf. Satz and Van Nostrand, 1973). In other words they have an earlier ontogenetic development than other types of skills. In addition visual-perceptual discrimination skills are more important for the initial stages of learning to read (Gibson and Levin, 1975). Their importance diminishes as the child moves on to higher level stages of reading acquisition. It is apparent that these explanatory hypotheses require additional cross-sectional and longitudinally based research. Their evaluation is heavily dependent on advances in research and theory on cognitive development and learning to read. In the next section these hypotheses will be reconsidered for their value in explaining developmental changes in the relationship between linguistic skills and reading achievement.

Linguistic-Deficit Hypothesis

The hypothesis that reading/learning disabilities result from a basic language deficiency actually represents a variety of hypotheses concerning different linguistic skills. Some of these skills are clearly involved in the reading process, while others arise from mere observations of the language performance of disabled readers. In the present section research on some of the linguistic correlates of reading disability will be reviewed with an eye towards developmental change. This literature represents a more recent research emphasis and is expanding rapidly. It has not to our knowledge received a thorough review and evaluation. In addition to highlighting some of the major research thrusts of this literature, an attempt will be made to illustrate some of its shortcomings.

PHONETIC-SEGMENTATION SKILLS. Gibson and Levin (1975) have summarized considerable research which shows that the ability to decompose words into their representative phonemic units (phonetic segmentation) is one underlying component of the initial stages of learning to read. These decoding skills are particularly important for bridging the gap between written and spoken language. Much of the current research on phonetic segmentation stems from work by Liberman and Shankweiler and has been summarized in several recent publications (Liberman and Shankweiler, 1976; Liberman, Shankweiler, Liberman, Fowler and Fischer, 1977; Shankweiler and Liberman, 1976). Although these authors have explored phonetic-segmentation skills in several contexts, only research concerning the child's developing awareness of phonetic segments in language will be reviewed in this chapter.

The child's awareness of the number of phonetic segments in a word develops primarily between the ages of four and eight (Gibson and Levin, 1975). Liberman, et al., (1974) explored the ability of four-, five-, and six-year-olds (prekindergarten to grade 1) to identify the number of phonetic and syllabic segments in spoken utterances. The task used required the child to tap a wooden dowel for each of the segments in a list of verbal utterances. At age four no children could identify phonemic segments, while half could identify syllabic segments. At age six however 70% of the children could identify phonemic segments and 90% could identify syllabic segments. Liberman, et al., (1977) continued this study with a comparison of the segmentation skills of good and poor readers in the six-year-old children about four months after initial testing (beginning of grade 2). Half of the children in the lowest third of the reading achievement distribution failed the phonetic-segmentation task, while all of the top third of the distribution passed the task.

More rigorous investigations have strengthened the relationship of phonetic-segmentation skills and early reading achievement. Helfgott (1976) measured segmentation and blending skills in kindergarten children in an attempt to predict first-grade reading achievement. Segmentation of spoken CVC words in kindergarten correlated at .72 with the first-grade word recognition subtest of the *Wide Range Achievement Test.* Zifcak (1976) found a significant correlational relationship between phonetic segmentation on a dowel tapping task and reading achievement in first-grade children. Treiman (cf. Liberman, et al., 1977), in a study of first- and second-grade inner city children (largely blacks), also found a high correlation between phonetic segmentation (measured by a variation of the tapping task) and reading ability.

These results, on diverse samples with different criterion reading measures, provide preliminary evidence that the child's ability to decompose linguistic units into phonetic segments has a strong relationship to early reading achievement. This relationship, while impressive, can only be described as preliminary for several reasons. First, the Liberman, et al., (1974; 1977) studies, while employing a four-month longitudinal follow-up, report only a frequency relationship. Such a relationship does not necessarily indicate that these skills are predictive of reading achievement. Second, the correlational relationships reported by other studies may be based on rather small samples. For example the correlation reported by Helfgott (1976) was based on just 31 subjects. Although significant, the magnitude of the correlation is undoubtedly inflated because of the sample size. Third, although adequate reading measures were employed in all these studies, the criteria by which good and poor readers were defined is unclear. In the Liberman, et al., (1977) study children were merely divided according to classroom rankings on an achievement test. Finally, the method of investigation presumes a unitary deficit hypothesis which implies that the underlying cause of reading disability is a deficiency in phonetic segmentation. It is noteworthy that Shankweiler and Liberman (1976) devote considerable energy to refuting the perceptual-deficit hypothesis on the basis of research with children no younger than eight years of age. It would be interesting to compare performance of disabled readers prior to age eight on phonetic-segmentation and perceptual-discrimination tasks; both develop earlier and are important for early stages of learning to read. Research of this sort would shed light on the developmental precursors of reading/learning disabilities, which are probably multiple.

RAPID AUTOMATIZED NAMING.   Another prominent linguistic area of research in reading disabilities concerns speed of digit and object naming in good and poor readers. Spring (1975) attempted to predict first-grade reading achievement ($N=44$) with a simple measure of digit naming speed. After a five-month follow-up, a correlation of .53 between digit-naming speed and reading achievement was found. In the large scale longitudinal-predictive study of Jansky and de Hirsch (1972), a picture-naming test was among the best kindergarten predictors of grade 2 reading ability, correlating at .53.

With relatively older readers, Spring (1976) examined speed of digit, color, and picture-naming in small samples of poor readers ($N=24$) and good readers ($N=24$ from 7 to 13 years of age. Overall results indicated that disabled readers named more slowly than good readers across the age range. Denckla and Rudel (1976) measured performance on several naming tasks in a large sample of reading-disabled children (with and without neurological problems) and normal children at four levels: 7.5, 8.5, 9.5, and 11.5. Age related group differences were found on all tasks, with a strong trend towards an Age by Group interaction.

Denckla and Rudel (1976) attempted to relate these error patterns to the naming errors of adult aphasics. A more parsimonious interpretation of these findings attributes reduced naming-speed to slower phonological coding in disabled readers (Spring and Farmer, 1975). In this respect both the phonetic-segmentation studies and the oral-naming studies suggest the importance of phonological skills for early reading achievement. In contrast to phonetic-segmentation skills, the relationship of these naming skills to phonological development has not been systematically investigated. Similarly, while these skills seem related to reading achievement, it is not clear to what aspect of reading and learning to read these tasks relate. It is also unfortunate that these naming skills have not been more systematically related to reading-group differences across age since important evidence regarding developmental change could be forthcoming. Although the Denckla and Rudel (1976) study employed an excellent cross-sectional design, the statistical analysis may have been inappropriate. Four naming tasks were employed and treated as repeated measures in an analysis of variance design. Such a design however carries the assumption of equal covariance among the four measures. This assumption is difficult to meet in developmental research and is especially pertinent for this study because of the age differences emerging for the four tasks. A multivariate design which treated the four tasks as dependent variables would have obviated the need for this assumption and would have provided a more powerful test of the Age by Group interaction. Despite the use of a less powerful univariate design, the interaction approached significance (p .07). This trend suggests that developmental change may be an important consideration for research on rapid automatized naming in reading/learning disabilities.

SYNTACTIC SKILLS.   With recent advances in developmental psycholinguistics, the relationship between syntactic development and reading achievement has become a popular area of research. For reading acquisition, syntactic skills are an important part of learning to use higher-level sources of redundancy for reading. As such these skills involve the extraction of meaning in units larger than the single word and are important for more advanced stages of learning to read (Doehring, 1976; Gibson and Levin, 1975). In the present section three types of studies will be reviewed, concerning (1) morphological knowledge; (2) oral reading errors; and (3) syntactic comprehension.

MORPHOLOGICAL KNOWLEDGE.   Morphemes are the smallest meaningful grammatical units. In essence they are phonemes which have meaning (for example -ed, -s). Just as syntactic rules can refer to the set of formation rules used to generate meaningful sentences, morphemes can be considered a set of word formation rules for creating meaningful words (Dale, 1976).

Numerous studies have used the Grammatic Closure subtest of the Illinois Test of Psycholinguistic Abilities (Kirk, McCarthy, and Kirk, 1968) to explore potential differences in morphology between good and poor readers. Grammatic Closure is a test of morphological knowledge using real words as response-eliciting stimuli. Studies employing this test with reading/learning disabilities are generally poorly designed. Few studies control for chronological age and few employ children younger than grade 2. Nonetheless a simple generalization can be made for good and poor readers at and above the second grade. In summarizing the many studies of the ITPA and academic achievement, Hammill, Parker, and Newcomer (1975) concluded that,

Only Grammatic Closure, the most linguistic of the ITPA subtests, consistently predicted academic achievement in that it evidenced significant predictive and diagnostic relationships in this study. [P. 351]

Summarily, Grammatic Closure almost always separates second grade and older good and poor readers.

A similar approach to the study of morphology in good and poor readers is based on an important early study in developmental psycholinguistics (Berko, 1958). Berko measured first and second-graders' knowledge of a variety of morphemes using nonsense word stimuli. Berko found that the second-graders in her study had acquired most of the morphological forms measured, though other studies have suggested some caution regarding this conclusion (Palermo and Molfese, 1972).

In looking at reading group differences, Brittain (1970–1971) correlated performance on the stimuli employed by Berko (1958) with reading achievement in grades 1 and 2. A partial correlation (correcting for IQ) of only .36 was obtained with first-grade achievement, while the correlation with second-grade achievement was .70. Wiig, Semel, and Crouse (1973) gave Berko's stimuli to groups of high-risk children (age 4.4) and learning-disabled children and controls (age 9.5). The high-risk Ss were defined in terms of a history of neonatal trauma with subsequent neurological disability. Differences were found between experimental and control groups at their respective age levels. Vogel (1975) gave a variant of the Berko's testing procedure, the Berry-Talbot Test of English Morphology (Berry, 1969), and the Grammatic Closure subtest to groups of second-grade good and poor readers. Robust differences were found on both measures between these well-defined groups. Fletcher, Satz, and Scholes (1978) administered the Berry-Talbot and Grammatic Closure tests to groups of good and poor readers at three age levels: 5.5, 8.5, and 11 years of age. The 5.5-year-old groups were comprised of children (N=40) who received the morphological measures in kindergarten and criterion reading measures in the second grade (three-year follow-up). Robust differences between groups across all ages were found.

It is evident that poor readers perform more poorly on measures of morphological knowledge across several age levels. The basis for this difference is not clear because the construct characteristics of these different morphological tests have not been clarified. For example Grammatic Closure generally loads on the Verbal-Comprehension factor usually found in factor analyses of the WISC (Newcomer, et al., 1975). Correlations with vocabulary tests are uniformly high (cf. Fletcher, et al., 1978). The net effect of these findings is to question the suggestion of some authors (Vogel, 1975; Wiig and Semel, 1976) that morphological knowledge is a specific underlying factor in reading disability. The tests used to assess these skills may also tap additional linguistic and intellectual skills. Therefore caution must be exercized in interpreting findings concerning morphological knowledge in disabled readers.

ORAL READING ERRORS.   Two oral reading studies, concerned with the use of grammatical sources of redundancy, investigated linguistic error patterns of good and poor first-grade readers (Biemuller, 1970–1971; Weber, 1970). In both studies 90% of the oral reading errors of good and poor readers made sense given the preceding grammatical context. Somewhat different results were reported by Little (1975), who analyzed oral reading errors of third-grade average and disabled readers. These errors were also compared with performance on the Developmental Sentence Scoring Test (Lee and Canter, 1971). Although no relationship between oral reading errors and syntactic development was evident, the errors of average readers did conform more to grammatical constraints within stimulus sentences than the errors of poor readers. Isakson and Miller (1976) defined groups of fourth-grade children equivalent on word recognition skills, but differing in comprehension ability. Results, based on oral reading errors at the verb position, revealed that poor comprehenders were less disturbed by syntactic (and semantic) violations of sentence structure than good comprehenders, in whom error rates increased. This study replicated similar findings by Clay and Imlach (1971) and Weinstein and Rabinovitch (1971) showing that (relatively older) poor readers seemed less sensitive to grammatical constraints in language, processing words one at a time. Less use was made of syntactic (and semantic) contextual cues necessary for processing larger groups of words.

The latter studies provide a clear contrast to the Biemuller (1970–1971) and Weber (1970) studies. This contrast provides preliminary evidence suggesting that older (but not younger) poor readers make less use of the organizational constraints provided by grammatical sources of redundancy in written text. This evidence can only be considered preliminary for several reasons. First, assessment of errors was different in each of these studies. Second, studies were restricted to a single age level. Cross-sectional and longitudinal designs are necessary for the evaluation of this developmental interpretation. Finally, oral reading errors are limited as indices of linguistic function because of the influence of instructional methods on learning to read and the fact that there are many ways of reading successfully (Gibson and Levin, 1975).

SYNTACTIC COMPREHENSION.   Almost all the studies described so far for syntactic skills are based on measures requiring language production. The present section will examine studies based on sentence comprehension to see if poor readers may be deficient in grammatical comprehension.

For younger reading groups, two studies are pertinent. Falk (1977) compared the ability of good and poor first and second-grade readers to answer questions about 23 spoken sentences varying in syntactic complexity. A significant age effect was observed, but reading group differences were apparent only for second-grade (not first-grade) readers. Taylor (1977) dichotomized first- and second-grade readers on the basis of Metropolitan Achievement Test Scores. He then asked these children to judge the grammatical acceptability of disrupted sentences. Correct judgements increased with age, with semantic disruptions more easily identified and correlated with achievement at both grade levels. Syntactic disruptions however were significantly correlated with reading achievement only at the second-grade level (not first-grade).

With older reading groups Vogel (1975) failed to find differences between second-grade reading groups on the Northwestern Syntax Screening Test (Lee, 1971), a task requiring picture selection on the basis of different sentence types. In contrast Semel and Wiig (1975) found differences on this measure between reading groups sampled across a broader age range (7 to 11.5 years) which was slightly older (about one year). Berger (1975) and Wiig and Semel (1976) examined comprehension of different sentence types in older reading groups (age 11 years) using sentence-repetition tasks. Differences in sentence comprehension were found in both studies. Guthrie (1973) examined the relationship between sentence comprehension and the use of syntactic cues during silent reading. Disabled readers, about 10 years of age, were selected across a broad age range, while younger (7.5 years) and older (10 years) control groups were employed. The task required children to read silently and select different words from contrasting syntactic classes that would make the sentence passages acceptable. Results indicated that while comprehension was lower in disabled readers, the pattern of errors was quite similar. Rabinovitch and Strassberg (1968) also showed that syntactic cues did not facilitate comprehension in fourth-grade poor readers using sentence repetition and sentence learning tasks.

The study by Fletcher, Satz and Scholes (1978) also employed a measure of syntactic comprehension. This measure had a solid foundation in formal linguistics, required no reading of the children, and was used in a number of earlier developmental studies with normal children (cf. Scholes, 1977). Several different linguistic forms with different developmental rates were employed, all of which required picture selection based on the child's comprehension of syntactic structure. Analysis of performance on these linguistic forms revealed an Age by Group interaction showing larger differences between older reading groups. Moreover the degree to which the different linguistic forms contributed to this interaction corresponded almost exactly with the developmental sequence of acquisition defined by the studies on normal development. In other words reading groups did not differ on linguistic forms which developed earlier. Rather, group differences were apparent only between older reading groups (age 11) on linguistic forms with a later development. Such a finding can be related to Gibson and Levin's (1975) observation that the use of higher-order linguistic skills becomes important for reading after the fourth grade.

CRITIQUE: LINGUISTIC-DEFICIT HYPOTHESIS.   The syntactic comprehension studies reveal a number of methodological and conceptual problems that complicate an interpretation of the results. For example many studies confound the age variable either by using disabled readers from a broad age range (for example Semel and Wiig, 1975) or by failing to sample groups across the entire age range (5 to 14 years). These studies, especially in the comprehension area, uniformly fail to manipulate variables clearly described as syntactic. Identifying target words (Guthrie, 1973), repeating sentences of different syntactic complexity (Wiig and Semel, 1976; Weinstein and Rabinovitch, 1971), or selecting pictures on the basis of two sentences differing in single word meanings (for example Northwestern Syntax Screening Test), manipulate a number of lexical, semantic, conceptual, and syntactic variables. These variables, all important for reading comprehension, may develop at different rates and may have different relationships with other cognitive abilities (for example intelligence). Furthermore, because a variety of linguistic and nonlinguistic factors are related to reading competency, it is not clear that tasks requiring reading of the child (for example Guthrie, 1973) yield conclusions specific to linguistic skills in disabled readers. Finally few of the studies relate substantively to current knowledge concerning language development and the acquisition of reading. Good and poor readers differ on a wide variety of linguistic and nonlinguistic skills. The meaning of these differences is difficult to specify when the relationship to the reading process is not specified.

Some evidence did emerge for developmental changes. In these studies reading group differences were more apparent between older children (ages 10 to 14) than younger children (ages 5 to 7). Such findings suggest that at older ages the reading process has changed from the initial decoding stages in which visual-perceptual and phonological factors are important components of the reading process. For more advanced levels of reading acquisition children learn to read in units larger than the single word. Comprehension of meaning in larger chunks, facilitated by grammatical sources of redundancy, becomes more important for these advanced reading stages (Smith, 1971; Doehring, 1978; Gibson and Levin, 1975). Therefore the conclusion that higher-order linguistic skills are more related to reading/learning disabilities at older ages is consistent with data on the acquisition of reading in nondisabled children.

The Fletcher, Satz, and Scholes, (1978) study also suggested that the relationship between linguistic skills and reading achievement varied because of ontogenetic sequence of development. In other words group differences were more apparent for later-developing linguistic forms. Additional evidence for this interpretation is provided by several studies previously reviewed (Fletcher and Satz, 1978a; Gruen, 1972; Sabatino and Hayden, 1970; Satz, Rardin, and Ross, 1971; Satz and Van Nostrand, 1973). In addition to the perceptual measures, each of these studies employed measures of language skill which emphasized semantic and conceptual processing. These components of language appear to proceed more slowly through childhood (Hagen, Jongeward, and Kail, 1975; Palermo and Molfese, 1972; Thurstone, 1955). Differences on these measures were more apparent between older reading groups (age 10 to 14) than younger reading groups (age 5 to 8).

These findings are consistent with a recent cross-sectional study (Tarver, et al., 1976) concerning semantic factors in memory. This study revealed age-dependent performance differences between learning-disabled and nondisabled children at 8.5 and 10 years of age, and an additional 13.5-year-old learning-disabled group on the Hagen Central Incidental learning task (a serial-learning recall task). Results revealed the presence of a primacy effect in the older rather than younger disabled readers. Furthermore the primacy effect exhibited by 10-year-old disabled readers resembled that of 8-year-old normals, with performance by the 13.5-year-old disabled group resembling normal 11-year-old performance. Tarver, et al., (1976) summarized their results by noting that "the evidence suggests that a developmental lag of about 2 years is characteristic of the learning disabled" (p. 383).

For the other linguistic skills reviewed, different methodological problems precluded strong conclusions regarding developmental change. The major problem was that the age variable had not been systematically manipulated in this research. This shortcoming is particularly apparent for research on phonetic segmentation skills. These skills develop earlier and are important components of the initial stages of learning to read (Gibson and Levin, 1975). It would be interesting to know whether the relationship between these skills and reading diminishes with time.

Three studies provide some preliminary information concerning this possibility. The first study (Calfee, Lindamood, and lindamood, 1973) measured the performance of children from kindergarten through the twelfth grade on the Lindamood Auditory Discrimination Test, a type of phonetic segmentation task. The subjects were also administered an age-appropriate reading (or reading-readiness) test. Groups of good and poor readers were selected by dividing children according to their classroom rank on the group-administered reading test. On the subtest with the easier stimuli, larger differences were apparent between kindergarten achievement groups, with differences diminishing by the fourth grade. The two more difficult subtests may have been too difficult for children prior to the second grade (that is, floor effect). After this grade large differences between achievement groups were obtained, which persisted through the tenth grade. Interpretation of this study is difficult because children were merely split into good and poor reading groups. It is not evident that severely disabled readers were used. In addition a cross-sectional study does not permit statements about poor readers prior to the second grade.

The Calfee, Lindamood, and Lindamood, (1973) study certainly suggests that it would be fruitful to study the relationship of phonetic segmentation and reading achievement across time. Two other studies which concern an earlier developing source of intraword redundancy (letter-sound correspondence) support this suggestion. Calfee, Venezky, and Chapman (1969) explored the relationship between the child's knowledge of letter-sound correspondences and reading. Synthetic words, incorporating regular and irregular letter-sound patterns, were presented for pronounciation to good and poor readers in third grade, fifth grade, high school, and college. Correlations between pronounciation and reading achievement were highest in third-graders, decreasing substantially after that age as variables, such as IQ, accounted for much more of the variability in reading achievement. Differences between good and poor readers were larger at the third-grade level, decreasing with age except on more complex patterns. A subsequent study (Venezky and Johnson, 1973) gave similar synthetic words to first-, second-, and third-grade reading groups. Correlations with reading comprehension were at 77 for first-grade readers, dropping to .63 for third-grade readers, a significant decrease. Both studies provide some evidence for developmental changes on the relationship between earlier developing linguistic skills and reading. Of course the relationship is merely correlational; it is not clear that severely disabled readers were employed.

Conclusions: Developmental Change

It was suggested at the close of the preceding section (hyperactivity/learning disabilities) that group differences on cognitive and behavioral tasks may be age-dependent. It was also suggested that these differences might be predicted on the basis of the nature of the skill (for example perceptual versus linguistic). In evaluating this possibility in the present section (reading/learning disabilities), developmental changes were demonstrated for earlier developing perceptual skills and later developing linguistic skills. In addition some preliminary evidence was cited for developmental changes in the relationship of earlier developing linguistic skills and reading level. In general age-dependent relationships were more apparent during the period when these different perceptual and linguistic skills are important for learning to read.

The research reviewed in these two sections shows that developmental factors are important for the interpretation of research on reading/learning disabilities. The meaning of these developmental factors is difficult to specify. Age-dependent relationships seem to emerge regardless of the nature of the skill (for example perceptual versus linguistic). These relationships are also apparent at different stages in cognition and reading. If there is a common denominator underlying these age-dependent relationships, it may concern the child's developmental readiness for meeting the task demands of reading at different ages (cf. Fletcher and Satz, 1979). Developmental readiness is a difficult concept to describe and evaluate. In general it is intended as a statement concerning the child's degree of cognitive/behavioral development. The cognitive/behavioral performance of children will reflect in part their level of developmental maturity. A child who is developmentally immature will display a variety of apparent cognitive/behavioral problems depending on the sensitivity of the assessment instrument to his developmental level. These problems will appear as deficits only if the child is compared with children at the same age who are developmentally more advanced. In this respect a study by Waber (1976) concerning possible sex differences in the development of spatial abilities is instructive. Waber found that sex differences which are sometimes found for the development of spatial skills may reflect earlier and more rapid physical maturation in girls than boys. Children of both sexes who demonstrated more advanced physical maturation had better spatial skills than their same-aged counterparts who were less advanced in physical maturation.

Waber's (1976) study suggests that differences on cognitive/behavioral tasks are related to the child's general level of development. Waber (1977) reviewed additional literature concerning sex differences in field dependence which also supported this developmental relationship. However a more complete test of this hypothesis requires matching children on variables which are felt to reflect developmental level. For example matching children on variables measuring physical maturation should eliminate differences on tasks measuring spatial development. Confirming this prediction would provide strong support for Waber's contention that biological-maturational factors are important underlying components of performance on cognitive/behavioral tasks.

Developmental factors apparent for reading/learning disabilities may also be related to the developmental factors cited for hyperactivity/learning disabilities. The age-dependent relationships which emerge for cognitive/behavioral skills and reading achievement may reflect a greater degree of developmental immaturity in reading/learning-disabled children. Testing this hypothesis, which is a variant of the familiar maturational lag hypothesis, requires a test similar to that outlined by Zigler (1969) and Hallahan (1975) in the preceding section. Matching children on reading achievement should eliminate differences on cognitive/behavioral tasks. To date only a few studies have even indirectly addressed this possibility. The most recent research (Guthrie and Seifert, 1977) comprised a longitudinal study of the acquisition of letter-sound correspondence rules in good and poor readers in the first, second, and third grades. Children were matched only on reading level, so that the disabled reader group (age=9.35 years) was substantially older than the control group (age=6.3 years). During the course of the year children were evaluated three times with different word-identification tasks. Results revealed a definite sequence in the acquisition of letter-sound correspondence rules based on the complexity of the rules. For our purposes the important finding was that, "Good and poor readers manifested similar developmental phases" (Guthrie and Seifert p. 695). In other words the developmental sequence governing the acquisition of these rules was similar. Both groups acquired simpler rules before they learned more complex rules.

It should be noted that this study only indirectly addressed the developmental hypotheses outlined in this section. Extrapolation of these results may be premature and the conclusions can be considered tentative at best. Direct tests using the Zigler (1969) model are likely to be influenced by a number of factors, including (1) type of reading measure employed; (2) prior reading experience; (3) instructional methods; and (4) academic expectations. These factors may limit the confirmation of hypotheses based on the Zigler strategy. In addition Rourke (1975, 1976) has eloquently demonstrated that the age-dependent relationships described in this chapter may be subject to a variety of interpretations. These differing interpretations concern whether age-dependent relationships truly refute a deficit interpretation. As Rourke (1976) demonstrated, a variety of developmental findings are apparent, some of which may be more plausibly approached from a deficit model. At present it is difficult to evaluate whether findings in this broad area of research are best explained within a difference, delay, or deficit model. It was suggested that a developmental model might provide an heuristic approach for unravelling at least some of this controversy. The issue is not whether a model is right or wrong, but whether it yields useful, testable hypotheses. The final section of this chapter will attempt to show the utility of a developmental approach in future research.

FUTURE DIRECTIONS FOR RESEARCH: A SUMMARY

The present chapter was written with three purposes in mind: (1) to highlight promising areas of research in hyperactivity/learning disabilities and reading/learning disabilities, (2) to illustrate the value of approaching this research from a developmental model, and (3) to highlight some of the methodological problems that continue to retard progress in these areas. In large part these problems reflect the continued use of a research paradigm which assumes that impairment of a single behavioral-construct (for example perception) forms the "underlying" cause of the disorder.

Single Syndrome Paradigm

Most unitary deficit hypotheses are based on a research paradigm termed by Doehring (1978) as the "single syndrome paradigm." This paradigm makes extensive use of a contrasting groups approach in which disabled and nondisabled children are separated according to criteria for the different disorders (for example reading and intelligence scores for developmental dyslexia). The tests which are presumed to measure some psychological construct (such as perception) are given to the two groups. If a difference emerges, then the single deficit can be used as the basis of a theory of the disorder. For example, if a measure of perception separates dyslexic and control groups, then evidence for a perceptual deficit is invoked to explain the disability. If no difference emerges, then the researcher is faced with the necessity of accepting the null hypothesis, an event which occurs all too frequently with this paradigm.

Although this approach may seem reasonable, there are several problems which make this paradigm inadequate for research in hyperactivity/learning disabilities and reading/learning disabilities. These problems are discussed below.

Definition: The Problem of Classification

Major problems with defining the target group continue to plague the area. This problem was particularly acute for research subsumed under the MBD rubric where it was shown that the term was empty and misleading, particularly with respect to its presumptive neurological basis. The wide acceptance of the MBD rubric in applied settings illustrates the potential harm of a diagnostic term whose existence merely obscures many of the basic problems which led to its creation.

Definitional problems provide serious shortcomings for the single syndrome paradigm because of the need to contrast groups composed of disabled and non-disabled children. Throughout this chapter it was shown that these disabled children are heterogeneous in terms of neurological, behavioral, and academic criteria. Some children may have abnormal neurological signs, no hyperactivity, and academic problems. Others may be hyperactive without neurological or academic problems. Few studies actually report this information. Even disabled readers may represent a very heterogeneous group. Doehring (1978) cautioned that reading is not a homogeneous phenomenon and even in impaired groups many different types of reading skills may be represented. As such there are probably multiple types of impairment. This possibility highlights the importance of reporting basic variables, such as age, IQ, reading level, and type of reading test.

The problem of subtypes constitutes an issue to which substantial research should be devoted. When children globally diagnosed as MBD or SLD are placed into an experimental group, differences on the dependent variable may be influenced by surplus sources of variance stemming from the heterogeneity of the group formation variable. This variability in the independent variable may distort the interpretation of the results, especially within the single syndrome paradigm. More importantly information regarding these sources of variability are discarded in the search for unitary deficits. Future research progress clearly awaits some resolution of the classification problems currently plaguing the area.

Construct Validation

The problem of defining what different tests actually measure is crucial for unitary deficit hypotheses. Unfortunately most studies simply assume the measurement characteristics of their instuments These assumptions are questionable because of the absence of construct validation studies of the instuments. Such studies would be difficult, due in part to the lack of acceptance in the scientific community regarding the nature of these constructs and how they should be measured (Doehring, 1978). However the fact that disabled children differ on so many tasks must reflect in part some impurity in the experimental measures, resulting in extraneous sources of variance which influence performance. In other words the tasks used to measure a single construct are probably sensitive to several other contructs, so that the assessment of a single skill is contaminated by the instrument's lack of specificity.

Problems with construct validity were apparent in every major research heading reviewed in this chapter. This problem was specifically highlighted in the Vellutino, Steger, and Kandel, (1972) and Vellutino, et al., (1975) studies, the results of which may have fueled the controversy concerning the perceptual deficit hypothesis. This type of controversy, with its basis in task definition, is inherent in the single syndrome paradigm because of the need for purely defined constructs.

Chronological Age

Throughout this chapter developmental factors were emphasized. It was shown that the performance patterns of disabled readers vary considerably with chronological age (for example Benton, 1962; Fletcher and Satz, 1978). In the hyperactivity/learning disabilities section the problem of maturational problems was described in some detail. It was shown that some of the behavioral and neurological correlates of these disabilities diminish with age. Similarly it was shown that some of these so-called behavioral and neurological deficits are observed in normal younger children.

The possibility of developmental factors in reading/learning disabilities has been noted for some time (Benton, 1962). A review of the research revealed some support for the concept of developmental changes in the correlative performance patterns of these children. Failure to consider these factors could lead to misleading conclusions. Deficits associated with disabled children at one age may not characterize these children at a different age (Fletcher and Satz, 1979; Torgesen, 1975). An additional problem concerns test ceilings and floors and was described for several studies (for example Vellutino, Steger and Kandel, 1972; Vellutino, et al., 1975). Other studies reported results that were contaminated by inadequate control for chronological age, studies including children from different ages in the same group (for example Symes and Rapoport, 1972).

Appropriate manipulation of the age variable is crucial in order to examine possible changes in the developmental performance correlates over time. The fact that most studies which rejected the perceptual deficit hypothesis were based on older retarded readers highlights the importance of developmental considerations. Such considerations however seem incompatible and unnecessary in the search for unitary deficit explanations.

Making Inferences and Building Theories

Additional difficulties arise for the single syndrome paradigm when problems of inferences and theories are considered. These difficulties result from at least two sources: (1) confusion of correlation and causation and (2) confusion of intervening variables and hypothetical constructs.

Correlation and causation are often confused in behavioral research. The problem is particularly acute for research on hyperactivity/learning disabilities and reading/learning disabilities because of the pervasiveness of unitary deficit hypotheses. Doehring (1978) described the problem as follows:

> The single syndrome implies a single cause leading to a single effect. Such reasoning makes it easier to impose order on events, but differences between groups or correlations between variables do not prove cause-and-effect relationships. Although a child's home life, socio-economic status, and educational opportunity can be considered antecendents rather than consequences of his reading problems, there is no more reason to classify his intelligence, personality, perceptual, memory, and language abilities as consequences than as antecedents of reading disabilities. [P. 9–10]

In short psychological investigations are inevitably and necessarily directed to the correlates of the disability. Separating these correlates into antecedents and consequences is virtually impossible on the basis of the single syndrome paradigm. As Doehring noted, reading/learning disabilities are correlated with a variety of nonreading skills. Attributing the reading problem to deficits in the correlated skills has no better an inferential basis than attributing deficits in the correlated skills to the reading problem.

When correlation is confused with causation another problem results which concerns the confusion of intervening variables with hypothetical constructs. MacCorquodale and Meehl (1948) defined intervening variables as concepts which: (1) contain no meaning beyond the sum of the empirical statements supporting them and (2) depend solely for their validity on the validity of these empirical statements. In contrast, hypothetical constructs: (1) contain surplus meaning beyond the empirical statements supporting them and (2) are not necessarily dependent on these particular empirical statements for their validity. A hypothetical construct need not be observable, but its factual reference should be compatible with existing knowledge.

For example consider the relationship between perceptual tasks and reading/learning disabilities. When an investigator concludes that a deficit in perception is related to reading failure, the perceptual deficit represents an intervening variable comprising what is known about the task and groups employed. If it is concluded that reading/learning disabilities result from (are caused by) a perceptual deficit, the statement attains the status of a hypothetical construct. This status accrues from the attribution of causality to the perceptual deficit, which is a source of meaning beyond the statements relating performance on the perceptual task to reading/learning desabilities.

The single syndrome paradigm leads inevitably to this confusion because of the assumption of a singular cause-effect relationship. To give a perceptual deficit the status of a hypothetical construct requires appeal to other empirical statements which relate the disability to all the other skills correlated with reading/learning disabilities. The difficulty of adequately producing these statements tends to make any unitary deficit hypothesis incongruent with current knowledge, which is why these statements should represent intervening variables. In reality, since the psychological construct of perception is merely correlated with the disability, conclusions regarding a perceptual deficit can only be considered an intervening variable. Disabilities subsumed under the hyperactivity/learning disabilities and reading/learning disabilities rubric are associated with a wide variety of performance differences. Focusing on one deficiency and using it to form the basis of a theory is inherently reductionistic and unlikely to explain the wide variety of correlated differences.

Multiple Syndrome Paradigm

In concluding his methodological critique of behavioral research on reading disabilities, Doehring (1978) called for "multiple syndrome paradigms" which can accomodate the considerable heterogeneity of reading disabilities and their correlative behavioral patterns. Doehring (1978) also suggested that some of the problems with cause-and-effect relationships, construct validation, and subtypes be dealt with by studying the covariance of variables associated with reading disabilities. Such an approach recognizes that the psychological variables of interest are multiple and probably correlated in different ways and to different degrees with the various disabilities. The basic research problem is that of untangling the complex behavioral relationships manifested by these disabilities and their multiple sources of variability. These suggestions should be applied to the entire spectrum of research on hyperactivity/learning disabilities and reading/learning disabilities and reflect the need for multivariate models. Multivariate models enable the researcher to represent these disabilities along multiple dimensions of variability. Instead of attempting to control for certain dimensions (such as age) as in the single syndrome paradigm, multivariate methods permit the building of more complex models which incorporate these dimensions. Most importantly, as opposed to looking for group differences, the focus is on the variety of correlational relationships which make up these disabilities. Of course caution should be exercised regarding the basic methodological requirements of multivariate techniques.

Concommitant with the need for covariance based multivariate models is the need for developmental models of these disabilities. If the performance correlates vary with age, then the covariance relationships underlying the multiple syndrome approach should also vary with age. In this respect there is an increasing need for longitudinal and cross-sectional studies of these disabilities. It is unfortunate that so much emphasis has been placed on the problems with longitudinal designs. These problems can be dealt with and do not outweigh the clear advantage of the longitudinal design (cf. McCall, 1977). Longitudinal/cross-sectional studies would provide important information regarding the general issue of developmental change. In addition, information pertaining to long-term outcomes and prognosis may be vital for understanding the heterogeneity characteristic of these disabilities. A developmental model and its emphasis on change has important implications for the way we think about disabled children. If we assume that these children, despite their handicaps, continue to develop (albeit differently) and are capable of learning, the prospects for continued study and eventual remediation are much brighter. Relating these disabilities to a static unitary deficit hypothesis or to a model of adult function introduces a negative and potentially iatrogenic bias in the way these children are treated on an everyday basis.

In closing this chapter it must be noted that the major value of any approach to research concerns not only its validity, but also whether it is useful. The multivariate developmental model suggested in this chapter provides an empirical and theoretical rationale for research with these children which is more heuristic than that provided by the single syndrome paradigm. Research is more difficult within the multiple syndrome paradigm and it may still be useful to test very specific hypotheses from the single syndrome paradigm. However there is a strong need to upgrade research standards in these areas. Pursuing a developmental model, even if the early theoretical formulations it generates do not prove to be valid, should improve research quality and bring us closer to understanding and remediating these childhood disabilities.

REFERENCES

Allington, R. L., K. Gormley, and S. Truex. "Poor and normal readers achievement on visual tasks involving high frequency-low discriminability words." *Journal of Learning Disabilities,* 9, 292–296, (1976).

Ambrosimo, S. V., and T. Del Fonte. "A psychoeducational study of the hyperkinetic syndrome." *Psychosomatics*, 14, 207–213, (1973).

Battle, E. S., and B. Lacey. "A context for hyperactivity in children, over time." *Child Development*, 43, 757–773, (1972).

Bax, M. "The active and the over-active school child." *Developmental Medicine and Child Neurology*, 14, 83–86, (1972).

Bax, M., and R. MacKeith, eds., *Minimal Cerebral Dysfunction*. London: Heinemann, 1963.

Bender, L. "Problems in conceptualization and communication in children with developmental alexia," in P. H. Hoch and J. Zubin, eds., *Psychopathology of Communication*. New York: Grune & Stratton, 1958.

Benton, A. L. "Dyslexia in relationship to form perception and directional sense," in J. Money, ed., *Reading Disability: Progress and Research Needs in Dyslexia*, 81–102. Baltimore: John Hopkins University Press, 1962.

———"Minimal brain dysfunction from a neuropsychological point of view," in F. F. de la Cruz, B. Fox, and R. H. Roberts, eds., *Minimal brain dysfunction*. Annals of the New York Academy of Sciences, 205, 29–37, (1973).

———"Developmental dyslexia: Neurological aspects," in W. J. Friedlander, ed., *Advances in Neurology*, vol. 7, 1–46. New York: Raven, 1975.

Berger, N. "An investigation of the literal comprehension and organizational processes of good and poor readers." *Dissertation Abstracts International*, 36B 1899–1900, (1975).

Berko, J. "The child's learning of English morphology." *Word*, 14, 150–177, (1958).

Berry, M. F. *Language Disorders of Children: The Basis and Diagnoses*. New York: Appleton-Century-Crafts, 1969.

Biemuller, A. "The development of the use of graphic and contextual information in children learning to read." *Reading Research Quarterly*, 6, 75–96, (1970–1971).

Birch, H. G., ed., *Brain-Damage in Children: The Biological and Social Aspects*. Baltimore: Williams & Wilkins, 1964.

Brittain, M. "Inflectional performance and early reading." *Reading Research Quarterly*, 6, 34–48, (1970–1971).

Bronner, A. F. *The Psychology of Special Abilities and Disabilities*. Boston: Little, Brown, 1917.

Bruner, J. S. "The course of cognitive growth," in N. S. Endler, L. K. Boulter, and H. Osser, eds., *Contemporary Issues in Developmental Psychology*. New York: Holt, Rinehart & Winston, 1968.

Buchsbaum, M., and P. H. Wender. "Average evoked responses in normal and minimally brain dysfunctioned children treated with amphetamine." *Archives of General Psychiatry*, 29, 764–770, (1973).

Caldwell, B. M. "The usefulness of the critical period hypothesis in the study of filiative behavior," in N. S. Endler, L. R. Boulter, and H. Osser, eds., *Contemporary Issues in Developmental Psychology*, pp. 213–223. New York: Holt, Rinehart & Winston, 1968.

Calfee, R., P. Lindamood, and C. Lindamood. "Acoustic-phonetic skills and reading—Kindergarten through twelfth grade." *Journal of Educational Psychology*, 64, 293, (1973).

Calfee, R., R. Venezky, and R. Chapman. "Pronunciation of synthetic words with predictable and unpredictable letter-sound correspondences." Technical Report No. 71. Wisconsin Research and Development Center for Cognitive Learning, 1969.

Cantwell, D. P. "Genetic studies of hyperactive children: Psychiatric illness in biologic and adopting parents," in R. R. Fieve, D. Rosenthal, and H. Bull, eds., *Genetic Research in Psychiatry*, 273–280, Baltimore: Johns Hopkins University Press, 1975.

Capute, A. J., E. F. L. Niedermeyer, and F. Richardson. "The electroencephalogram in children with minimal cerebral dysfunction." *Pediatrics*, 41, 1104–1114, (1968).

CELDIC Report. *One Million Children.* A national study of Canadian Children with emotional and learning disorders. L. Crainford, 1970.

Clay, M. M., and R. H. Imlach. "Juncture, pitch, and stress as reading behavior variables." *Journal of Verbal Learning and Verbal Behavior*, 10, 133–139, (1971).

———— *Minimal Brain Dysfunction in Children.* NINDB Monograph No. 3. Washington, D. C.: U. S. Department of HEW, 1966.

Connors, C. K. "A teacher rating scale for use in drug studies with children." *American Journal of Psychiatry*, 126, 884–888, (1969).

————"Learning disabilities and stimulant drugs in children: Theoretical implications," in R. Knights and D. J. Bakker, eds., *The Neuropsychology of Learning Disorders*, 389–404. Baltimore: University Park Press, 1976.

Connors, C. K., E. Taylor, G. Meo, M. Kurtz, and M. Fournier. "Magnesium pemoline and dextroamphetamine: A controlled study in children with minimal brain dysfunction." *Psychopharmacologia*, 26, 321–336, (1972).

Critchley, M. *The Dyslexic Child.* Springfield, Ill.: Thomas, 1970.

Dale, P. S. *Language Development: Structure and Function.* New York: Holt, Rinehart, & Winston, 1976.

de Hirsch, K., J. J. Jansky, and W. S. Langford. *Predicting Reading Failure.* New York: Harper & Row, 1966.

Denckla, M., and R. Rudel. "Anomalies of motor development in hyperactive boys without traditional neurological signs." 1977 [Preprint]

Denckla, M. B. "Critical review of electroencephalographic (EEG) and neurophysiological studies in dyslexia by John R. Hughes," in A. L. Benton and D. Pearl, eds., *Dyslexia: An Appraisal of Current Knowledge*, New York: Oxford U. Press, 241–250, 1978.

————"Rapid 'automatized' naming (R.A.N.): Dyslexia differentiated from other learning disabilities." *Neuropsychologia*, 14, 471–479, (1976).

Divorky, D. "Education's latest victim: The I.D. kid." *Learning*, 3, 20–25, (1974).

Doehring, D. G. "Acquisition of rapid reading responses." *Monographs of the Society for Research in Child Development*, 41, 1–54, (1976).

Doehring, D. G. "The tangled web of behavioral research on developmental dyslexia," in A. L. Benton and D. Pearl, eds., *Dyslexia: An Appraisal of Current Knowledge*, New York: Oxford U. Press, 123–138, 1978.

Douglas, V. I. "Effects of medication on learning efficiency. Research findings review and synthesis," in P. Anderson and C. G. Halcomb, eds., *Learning Disability/Minimal Brain Dysfunction Syndrome: Research Perspectives and Applications.* Springfield, Ill.: Thomas, 1976.

Dustman, R. E., and E. C. Beck. "The effects of maturation and aging on the wave form of visually evoked potentials." *Electroencephalography and Clinical Neurophysiology*, 26, 2–11, (1969).

Dykman, R. A., J. E. Peters, and P. T. Ackerman. "Experimental approaches to the study of minimal brain dysfunction: A follow-up study," in F. F. de la Cruz, B. Fox, and R. H. Roberts, eds., *Minimal Brain Dysfunction.* Annals of the New York Academy of Science, 205, 93–108, 1973.

Dykman, R.A., P. T. Ackerman, S. D. Clements, and J. E. Peters. "Specific learning disabilities: An attentional deficit syndrome," in H. R. Myklebust, ed., *Progress in Learning Disabilities*, Vol. II. New York: Grune & Stratton, 56–93, 1971.

Falk, J. W. "A comparison of the comprehension of syntax in spoken language by poor and average pre-readers in first grade and poor and average readers in second grade." *Dissertation Abstracts International*, 37A, 4921–4922, (1977).

Fine, M. J. "Hyperactivity: Where are we?" in M. J. Fine, ed., *Principles and Techniques of Intervention with Hyperactive Children*. Springfield, Ill.: Thomas, 3–46, 1977.

Fletcher, J. M., and P. Satz. "Developmental changes associated with reading disability: A multivariate test of a theory." [1978] in preparation.

————"Unitary deficit hypotheses of reading disabilities. Has Vellutino led us astray?" *Journal of Learning Disabilities*, 1979, 12(3), in press.

Fletcher, J. M., P. Satz, and R. J. Scholes. "Developmental changes in the linguistic performance correlates of reading disabilities." [1978] in preparation.

Geshwind, N. *Selected Papers on Language and the Brain*. Boston: D. Reidel, 1975.

Gibbs, F. A., and E. L. Gibbs. *Atlas of Electroencephalogy*, vol. I. Reading, Mass.: Addison-Wesley, 1951.

Gibson, E. J., and H. Levin. *The Psychology of Reading*. Cambridge: MIT Press, 1975.

Gomez, M. R. "Minimal cerebral dysfunction (maximal neurologic confusion)." *Clinical Pediatrics*, 6, 589, (1967).

Grinspoon, L., and S. B. Singer. "Amphetamines in the treatment of hyperkinetic children." *Harvard Educational Review*, 43(4), 515–555, (1973).

Gross, M. B., and W. C. Wilson, *Minimal Brain Dysfunction*. New York: Brunner/Mazel, 1974.

Gruen, R. S. "Prediction of end-of-year reading achievement for first and third grade pupils." *Proceedings of the American Psychological Association*, 7, 563–564, (1972).

Guthrie, J. T. "Reading comprehension and syntactic responses in good and poor readers." *Journal of Educational Psychology*, 65, 294–299, (1973).

Guthrie, J. T., and M. Seifert. "Letter-sound complexity in learning to identify words." *Journal of Educational Psychology*, 69, 686–696, (1977).

Hagen, J. W., R. H. Jongeward, and R. V. Kail. "Cognitive perspectives on the development of memory," in H. W. Reese, ed., *Advances in Child Development and Behavior*, vol. 10, 57–101, 1975.

Hammill, D., R. Parker, and P. Newcomer. "Psycholinguistic correlates of academic achievement." *Journal of School Psychology*, 13, 248–254, (1975).

Hallahan, D. P. "Comparative research studies on the psychological characteristics of learning disabled children," in W. M. Cruickshank and D. P. Hallahan, eds., *Perceptual and Learning Disabilities. Vol. I; Psychoeducational Practices*. Syracuse, N.Y.: Syracuse University Press, 1975.

Hallahan, D. P., and W. M. Cruickshank. *Psychoeducational Foundations of Learning Disabilities*. Englewood Cliffs, N. J.: Prentice-Hall, 1973.

Helfgott, J. "Phonemic segmentation and blending skills of kindergarten children: Implications for beginning reading acquisition." *Contemporary Educational Psychology*, 1, 157–169, (1976).

Hughes, J. R. "Electroencephalography and learning disabilities," in H. R. Myklebust, ed., *Progress in Learning Disabilities*, vol. 2. New York: Grune & Stratton, 1971.

Hughes, J. R. "Electroencephalographic (EEG) and neurophysiological studies in dyslexia." in D. Pearl and A. Benton, eds., *Dyslexia: An Appraisal of Current Knowledge*, New York: Oxford U. Press, 205–240, 1978.

Hughes, J. R., and G. E. Park. "The EEG in dyslexia," in P. Kellaway and I. Peterson, eds., *Clinical Electroencephalography of Children*. Stockholm: Almquist and Wiksell, 307–327, 1968.

Ingram, T. T. S., A. W. Mason, and K. Blackburn. "A retrospective study of 82 children with reading disability." *Developmental Medicine and Child Neurology*, 12, 271–281, (1970).

Isakson, R. L., and J. W. Miller. "Sensitivity to syntactic and semantic cues in good and poor comprehenders." *Journal of Educational Psychology*, 68, 787–792, (1976).

Jansky, J., K. de Hirsch. *Preventing Reading Failure*. New York: Harper & Row, 1972.

Kagan, J. "Impulsive and reflective children: Significance of conceptual tempo." in J. D. Krumboltz, ed., *Learning and the Educational Process*. Chicago: Rand McNally, 1965a.

Kahn, E., and L. H. Cohen. "Organic driveness: A brain stem syndrome and an experience—With case reports." *New England Journal of Medicine*, 210, 748–756, (1934).

Kenney, T. J., R. L. Clemmens, B. W. Hudson, G. A. Lentz, R. Cicci, and P. Mair. "Characteristics of children referred because of hyperactivity," in S. Chess and S. Thomas, eds., *Annual Progress in Child Psychiatry and Child Development*. New York: Brunner/Mazel, 1971.

Kinsbourne, M. "Minimal brain dysfunction as a neurodevelopmental lag," in F. F. de la Cruz, B. Fox, and R. H. Roberts, eds., *Minimal Brain Dysfunction*. Annals of the New York Academy of Sciences, 205, 268–273, (1973).

"Models of learning disability: Their relevance to remediation." *Journal of Psychological Association*, 113, 1066–1068, (1976).

Kirk, S., J. McCarthy, and W. Kirk. *The Illinois Test of Psycholinguistic Abilities*, rev. ed. Urbana: University of Illinois Press, 1968.

Kline, C. L. "The adolescents with learning problems: How long must they wait?" *Journal of Learning Disabilities*, 5, 127–144, (1972).

Kornetsky, C. "Minimal brain dysfunction and drugs," in W. M. Cruickshank and D. P. Hallahan, eds., *Perceptual and Learning Disabilities in Children. Vol. 2, Research and Theory*, 446–481, 1975.

Koupernik, C., R. MacKeith, and L. Francis-Williams. "Neurological correlates of motor and perceptual development," in W. M. Cruickshank and D. P. Hallahan, eds., *Perceptual and Learning Disabilities in Children, Vol. 2: Research and Theory*, 104–135. Syracuse, N.Y.: Syracuse University Press, 1975.

Lapouse, R., and M. A. Monk. "An epidemiologic study of behavior characteristics in children." *American Journal of Public Health*, 48, 1134–1144, (1958).

Laufer, M. W. "Long-term management and some follow-up findings on the use of drugs with minimal cerebral syndromes." *Journal of Learning Disabilities*, 4, 55–58, (1971).

———"Brain disorders," in A. M. Freedman and H. I. Kaplan, eds., *The Child: His Psychological and Cultural Development*, vol. 2. New York: Atheneum, 1972.

Laufer, M. W., and E. Denhoff. "Hyperkinetic behavior syndrome in children." *Journal of Pediatrics*, 50, 463–474, (1957).

Lee, L. *Northwestern Syntax Screening Test*. Evanston, Ill.: Northwestern University Press, 1971.

Lee, L., and S. Canter. "Developmental sentence scoring: A clinical procedure for estimating syntactic development in children's spontaneous speech." *Journal of Speech and Hearing Disorders*, 36, 315–317, (1971).

Lenneberg, E. H. *Biological Foundations of Language*. N.Y.: Wiley, 1967.

Liberman, I. Y., and D. Shankweiler. "Speech, the alphabet, and teaching to read," in L. Resnick and P. Weaver, eds., *Theory and Practice of Early Reading*. Hillsdale, N. J.: Lawrence Erlbaum, 1976.

Liberman, I. Y., D. Shankweiler, F. W. Fischer, and B. Carter. "Explicit syllable recognition and phonemic segmentation in the young child. *Journal of Experimental Child Psychology*, 18, 201–212, (1974).

Liberman, I. Y., D. Shankweiler, A. M. Liberman, C. Fowler, and F. W. Fischer. "Phonetic segmentation and recoding in the beginning reader," in A. S. Reber and D. Scarborough, eds., *Reading: Theory and Practice*. Hillsdale, N. J.: Lawrence Erlbaum, 1977.

Little, L. J. "A study of the relationship between syntactic development and oral reading substitution measures of average and disabled readers." *Dissertation Abstracts International*, 35A, 5971, (1975).

Luria, A. R. *The Working Brain: An Introduction to Neuropsychology*. London: Penguin, 1973.

Marwitt, S. J., and A. J. Stenner. "Hyperkinesis: Delineation of two patterns." *Exceptional Child*, 38, 401–406, (1972).

McCall, R. B. "Challenges to a science of developmental psychology." *Child Development*, 48, 333–344, (1977).

MacCorquodole, and K., and P. E. Meehl. "On a distinction between hypothetical constructs and intervening variables." *Psychological Review*, 55, 95–107, (1948).

Mendelson, W., and N. Johnson, M. A. Stewart. Hyperactive children as teenagers: A follow-up study." *Journal of Nervous and Mental Diseases*, 153, 273–279, (1971).

Minde, K., G. Weiss, and N. Mendelson. "A 5-year follow-up study of 91 hyperactive school children." *Journal of the American Acadamy of Child Psychiatry*, 11, 595–610, (1972).

Money, J., ed., *Reading disability: Progress and Research Needs in Dyslexia*. Baltimore: Johns Hopkins University Press, 1962.

Myklebust, H. R., ed., *Progress in Learning Disabilities*, Vol. I. New York and London: Grune & Stratton, 1968.

Newcomer, P., B. Hare, D. Hammill, and J. McGettigan. "Construct validity of the Illinois Test of Psycholinguistic Abilities." *Journal of Learning Disabilities*, 8, 220–231, (1975).

Oettinger, L., L. V. Majorski, G. A. Limbeck, and R. Gauch. "Bone age in children with minimal brain dysfunction." *Perceptual and Motor Skills*, 39, 1127–1131, (1974).

Orton, S. T. *Reading, Writing, and Speech Problems in Children*. New York: Norton, 1937.

Owen, F. "Dyslexia: Genetic aspects," in A. L. Benton and D. Pearl, eds., *Dyslexia: An Appraisal of Current Knowledge*. New York: Oxford U. Press, 265–284, 1978.

Palermo, D. S., and D. L. Molfese, "Language acquisition from age five onward." *Psychological Bulletin*, 78, 409–428, (1972).

Peters, J. E., J. S. Davis, C. M. Goolsby, and S. P. Clements, *Physicians Handbook: Screening for MBD CIBA Medical Horizons*, 1973.

Peters, J. E., J. S. Romine, and R. A. Dykman. "A special neurological examination of children with learning disabilities." *Developmental Medicine and Child Neurology*, 17, 63–78, (1975).

Piaget, J. *The Origins of Intelligence in Children*. New York: International Universities Press, 1952.

Rabinovitch, M. S., and R. Strassberg. "Syntax and retention in good and poor readers." *The Canadian Psychologist*, 9, 142–153, (1968).

Rabinovitch, R. D., A. L. Drew, R. de Jong, W. Ingram, and L. A. Withey. "A research approach to reading retardation." *Association for Research in Nervous and Mental Disease*, 34, 363–396, (1954).

Ross, A. D. *Psychological Aspects of Learning Disabilities and Reading Disorders.* New York: McGraw Hill, 1976.

Rourke, B. P. "Brain-behavior relationships in children with learning disabilities." *The American Psychologist*, 30, 911–920, (1975).

———"Reading retardation in children: Developmental lag or deficit," in R. Knights and D. J. Baker, eds., *The Neuropsychology of Learning Disorders: Theoretical Approaches.* Baltimore: University Park Press, 1976.

Rourke, B. P., and R. R. Orr. "Prediction of the reading and spelling performances of normal and retarded readers: A four year follow-up." *Journal of Abnormal Child Psychology*, 5, 9–19, (1977).

Rutter, M. "Prevalence and types of dyslexia," in A. L. Benton and D. Pearl, eds., *Dyslexia: An Appraisal of Current Knowledge.* New York: Oxford U. Press, 3–28, 1978.

Rutter, M. and W. Yule. "The concept of specific reading retardation." *Journal of Child Psychology and Psychiatry*, 16, 181–197, 1975.

Rutter, M., P. Graham, and W. Yule. "A neuropsychiatric study of childhood." *Clinics in Developmental Medicine*, 35–36. London: SIMP/Heinemann, 1970.

Sabatino, D. H., and D. L. Hayden. "Variation on information processing behaviors." *Journal of Learning Disabilities*, 3, 404–412, (1970).

———*Hyperactive Children.* Baltimore: University Park Press, 1976.

Satterfield, J. H. "EEG issues in children with minimal brain dysfunction." *Seminars in Psychiatry*, 5, 35, (1973).

Satz, P. "Cerebral dominance and reading disability: An old problem revisited," in R. Knights and D. J. Bakker, eds., *The Neuropsychology of Learning Disorders: Theoretical Approaches.* Baltimore: University Park Press, 1976.

Satz, P. and G. K. Van Nostrand. "Developmental dyslexia: An evaluation of a theory," in P. Satz and J. Ross, eds., *The Disabled Learner: Early Detection and Intervention*, 121–148. Rotterdam, The Netherlands: The Rotterdam University Press, 1973.

Satz, P., J. Friel, and F. Rudegeair. "Some predictive antecedents of specific reading disability: A two-, three- and four-year follow-up," in J. T. Guthrie, ed., *Aspects of Reading Acquisition.* Baltimore: Johns Hopkins University Press, 1976.

Satz, P., D. Rardin, and J. Ross. "An evaluation of a theory of specific developmental dyslexia." *Child Development*, 42, 2009–2021, (1971).

Satz, P., H. G. Taylor, J. Friel, and J. M. Fletcher. "Some developmental and predictive precursors of reading disabilities: A six year follow-up." in A. L. Benton and D. Pearl, eds., *Dyslexia: An Appraisal of Current Knowledge:* New York: Oxford U. Press, 313–348, 1978.

Schenkenberg, T. "Visual, auditory, and somatosensory evoked responses of normal subjects from childhood to senescence" (Ph. D. diss., University of Michigan, 1970). [Microfilmed]

Scholes, R. J. "Syntactic and lexical aspects of sentence comprehension," in A. Caramazza and E. Zuril, eds., *The acquisition and breakdown of language.* Baltimore: John Hopkins University Press, 1977.

Semel, E. S., and E. H. Wiig,. "Comprehension of syntactic structures and critical verbal elements by children with learning disabilities." *Journal of Learning Disabilities*, 8, 46–58, (1975).

Shankweiler, D., and I. Y. Liberman. Misreading: A search for causes," in J. F. Kavanagh and I. G. Mattingly, eds., *Language by Ear and by Eye.* Cambridge: MIT Press, 1972.

———"Exploring the relations between reading and speech," in R. M. Knights and D. J.

Bakker, eds., *Neuropsychology of Learning Disorder: Theoretical Approaches.* Baltimore: University Park Press, 1976.

Shrag, P., and D. Divorky. *The Myth of the Hyperactive Child.* New York: Dell, 1975.

Smith F. *Understanding Reading: A Psycholinguistic Analysis of Reading and Learning to Read.* New York: Holt, Rinehart & Winston, 1971.

Sobotka, K. R., W. Black, S. D. Hill, and R. J. Porter. "Some psychological correlates of developmental dyslexia." *Journal of Learning Disabilities,* 10, 363–369 (1977).

Sollenberger, R. T. "Chinese-American child rearing practices and juvenile delinquency." *Journal of Social Psychology,* 74, 13–23, (1968).

Spring, C. "Norming speed as a correlate of reading ability." *Perceptual and Motor Skills,* 41, 134, (1975).

———"Encoding speed and memory span in dyslexic children." *Journal of Special Education,* 10, 35–40, (1976).

Spring, C., and R. Farmer. "Perceptual span of poor readers." *Journal of Reading Behavior,* 12, 90–97, (1975).

Stamm, J., and Kreder, S. "Minimal brain dysfunction," in M. S. Gazzaniga, ed., *Handbook of Behavioral Neurobiology.* New York: Plenum Press, 119–150, (1979).

Stevens, J. R., K. Sachdev, and V. Milsteen. "Behavior disorders of childhood and the electroencephalogram." *Archives of Neurology,* 18, 160–177, (1968).

Stewart, M. A. "Hyperactive children." *Scientific American,* 222, 94–98, (1970).

Stewart, M. A., F. N. Pitts, A. G. Craig, and N. Dieraf. "The hyperactive child syndrome." *American Journal of Orthopsychiatry,* 36, 861–867, (1966).

Strauss, A. A., and N. C. Kephart. *Psychopathology and Education of the Brain-Injured Child. Vol. II: Progress in Theory and Clinic.* New York: Grune & Stratton, 1955.

Strauss, A. A., and L. Lehtinen. *Psychopathology and Education of the Brain-Injured Child.* New York: Grune & Stratton, 1947.

Symes, J. S., and J. L. Rapoport. "Unexpected reading failure." *American Journal of Orthopsychiatry,* 42, 82–91, (1972).

Tarver, S. G., D. P. Hallahan, J. M. Kaufman, and D. W. Ball. "Verbal rehearsal and selective attention in children with learning disabilities: A developmental lag." *Journal of Experimental Child Psychology,* 22, 375–385, (1976).

Taylor, N. S. "An investigation of children's awareness of the acceptability of selected grammatical and semantic structures and their relationship to reading achievement." *Dissertation Abstracts International,* 37A, 4190, (1977).

Thomas, A., and S. Chess. *Temperament and Development.* New York: Brunner Mazel, 1977.

Thurstone, L. L. *The Differential Growth of Mental Abilities.* Chapel Hill: University of North Carolina Psychometric Laboratory, No. 14, 1955.

Torgesen, J. K. "Problems and prospects in the study of learning disabilities," in M. G. Hetherington, ed., *Review of Child Development Research,* Chicago: University of Chicago Press, 1975.

United States Office of Education. First Annual Report of the National Advisory Committee on Handicapped Children. Washington, D. C.: U. S. Department of HEW, 1968.

Vellutino, F. R. "Toward an understanding of dyslexia: Psychological factors in specific reading disability," in D. Pearl and A. Benton, eds., *Dyslexia: An Appraisal of Current Knowledge.* New York: Oxford U. Press, 61–112, 1978.

Vellutino, F. R., J. A. Steger, and G. Kandel. "Reading disability: An investigation of the perceptual deficit hypothesis." *Cortex,* 8, 106–118, (1972).

Vellutino, F. R., H. Smith, J. A. Steger, and M. Kaman. "Reading disability: Age differences and the perceptual-deficit hypothesis." *Child Development*, 46, 487–493, (1975).

Vellutino, F. R., B. M. Steger, S. C. Moyer, C. J. Harding, and J. A. Niles. "Has the perceptual deficit hypothesis led us astray?" *Journal of Learning Disabilities*, 10, 375–385, (1977).

Venezky, R., and D. Johnson. "Development of two letter-sound correspondences in grades one through three." *Journal of Educational Psychology*, 64, 109–113, (1973).

Vogel, S. A. *Syntactic Abilities in Normal and Dyslexic Children.* Baltimore: University Park Press, 1975.

Waber, D. P. "Sex differences in mental abilities: A function of maturation rate." *Science*, 192, 572–574, (1976).

——"Biological substrates of field dependence. Implications of the sex difference." *Psychological Bulletin*, 6, 1076–1087, (1977).

Waites, L. "World Federation of Neurology: Research group on developmental dyslexia and world illiteracy." *Report of Proceedings*, 22, (1968).

Weber, R. M. "First graders' use of grammatical context in reading," in H. Levin and J. P. Williams, eds., *Basic Studies on Reading.* New York: Basic Books, 1970.

Weinstein, R., and M. S. Rabinovitch. "Sentence structure and retention in good and poor readers." *Journal of Educational Psychology*, 62, 25–30, (1971).

Weiss, G., K. Minde, J. S. Werry, V. Douglas, and E. Nemeth. "Studies on the hyperactive child: VIII. Five year follow-up." *Archives of General Psychiatry*, 24, 409–414, (1971).

Wender, P. H. "Some speculations concerning a possible biochemical basis of minimal brain dysfunction." *Annals of the New York Academy of Sciences*, 205, 18–27, (1973).

——"Hypothesis for a possible biochemical basis of minimal brain dysfunction," in R. M. Knights and D. J. Bakker, eds., *The Neuropsychology of Learning Disorders. Theoretical Approaches.* Baltimore: University Park Press, 1976.

Werner, H. A. "The concept of development and organismic point of view," in D. B. Harris, ed., *The Concept of Development: An Issue in the Study of Human Behavior.* Minneapolis: University of Minnesota Press, 1957.

Werry, J. S. "Developmental hyperactivity." *Pediatric Clinics of North America*, 15, 581–599, (1968a).

Wiig, E. S., and E. H. Semel. *Language Disabilities of School Age Children and Adolescents.* Columbus, Ohio: Merrill, 1976.

Wiig, E. S., E. H. Semel, and M. B. Crouse. "The use of English morphology by highrisk and learning disabled children." *Journal of Learning Disabilities*, 6, 457–465, (1973).

Wikler, A., J. F. Dixon, and J. B. Parker. "Brain function in problem children and controls: Psychometric, neurological, and electroencephalographic comparisons." *American Journal of Psychiatry*, 127, 634–645, (1970).

Witkin, H. A. *Psychological Differentiation.* New York: Wiley, 1962.

Wolff, P. H., and I. Hurwitz. "Functional implications of the minimal brain damage syndrome." in S. Walzer and P. H. Wolff, eds., *Minimal Cerebral Dysfunction in Children.* New York: Grune & Stratton, 1973.

Zifcak, M. "Phonological awareness and reading acquisition in first grade children" (Ph.D. diss., University of Connecticut, 1976).

Zigler, E. "Developmental versus difference theories of mental retardation and the problem of motivation." *American Journal of Mental Deficiency*, 73, 536–556, (1969).

NAME INDEX

SUBJECT INDEX